Control of Breathing during Sleep

Control of Breathing during Sleep

From Bench to Bedside

Edited by

Susmita Chowdhuri, MD, MS
Professor of Internal Medicine
Wayne State University School of Medicine
Staff Physician and Section Chief of Sleep Medicine
John D Dingell VA Medical Center
Detroit, Michigan, USA

M Safwan Badr, MD, MBA
Professor and Chair of Internal Medicine
Wayne State University School of Medicine
Staff Physician, John D Dingell VA Medical Center
Detroit, Michigan, USA

James A Rowley, MD
Professor of Medicine and Division Chief of Pulmonary/
Critical Care and Sleep Medicine
Wayne State University School of Medicine
Medical Director, Detroit Receiving Hospital Sleep Disorders Center
Program Director, Pulmonary/Critical Care Fellowship
Detroit Medical Center
Detroit, Michigan, USA

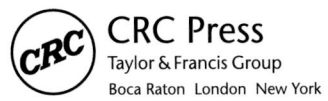

CRC Press
Taylor & Francis Group
Boca Raton London New York

CRC Press is an imprint of the
Taylor & Francis Group, an **informa** business

First edition published 2023
by CRC Press
6000 Broken Sound Parkway NW, Suite 300, Boca Raton, FL 33487-2742

and by CRC Press
4 Park Square, Milton Park, Abingdon, Oxon, OX14 4RN

CRC Press is an imprint of Taylor & Francis Group, LLC
© 2023 Taylor & Francis Group, LLC

Library of Congress Cataloging-in-Publication Data

Names: Chowdhuri, Susmita, editor. | Badr, M. Safwan, editor. | Rowley, James A., editor.
Title: Control of breathing during sleep : from bench to bedside / edited by Susmita Chowdhuri, M. Safwan Badr, James A. Rowley.
Description: First edition. | Boca Raton, FL : CRC Press, 2022. | Includes bibliographical references and index. | Summary: "This book describes control of ventilation during sleep in both health and disease states. The topics are presented in a fashion that can be easily comprehended with many figures to illustrate complex concepts. Thus, a wide range of topics, starting from the site of normal respiratory rhythm generation to chemoreceptor control of sleep apnea, description of the apneic threshold, pathophysiology of upper airway closure, novel techniques to measure control of breathing, effect of cerebral blood flow on breathing, effect of opioids on ventilation, effect of heart failure on ventilation, genetic aspects of breathing disorders, age and gender differences, and various therapies are discussed"-- Provided by publisher.
Identifiers: LCCN 2022000122 (print) | LCCN 2022000123 (ebook) | ISBN 9780367430115 (paperback) | ISBN 9780367556259 (hardback) | ISBN 9781003000631 (ebook)
Subjects: MESH: Sleep Apnea Syndromes--physiopathology | Sleep Apnea Syndromes--therapy | Sleep--physiology | Respiration | Respiratory Physiological Phenomena
Classification: LCC RC737.5 (print) | LCC RC737.5 (ebook) | NLM WF 143 | DDC 616.2/09--dc23/eng/20220323
LC record available at https://lccn.loc.gov/2022000122
LC ebook record available at https://lccn.loc.gov/2022000123

ISBN: 978-0-367-55625-9 (hbk)
ISBN: 978-0-367-43011-5 (pbk)
ISBN: 978-1-003-00063-1 (ebk)

DOI: 10.1201/9781003000631

Typeset in Palatino
by KnowledgeWorks Global Ltd.

Table of Contents

Foreword ix

Preface x

About the Editors xi

List of Contributors xii

Section I. Anatomy, Development, Aging, and Mechanisms of Control of Ventilation 1

1. Anatomy of the Respiratory Neural Network 2
   Christopher A Del Negro and Christopher G Wilson

2. Chemoreception: Pathways, Plasticity, and Pathophysiology 24
   Barbara J Morgan and Jerome A Dempsey

3. Developmental Changes in the Respiratory System of the Neonate-Child 42
   Ahuva Brown, Liran Tamir Hostovsky, and Estelle B Gauda

4. Control of Breathing in Older Adults 58
   Susmita Chowdhuri

5. Breathing Control in Exercise 70
   Philippe Haouzi

6. Control of the Upper Airway during Sleep 80
   Leszek Kubin

Section II. Pathophysiology of Sleep-Disordered Breathing 97

7. Pathophysiology of Sleep-Disordered Breathing in Children and Neonates 98
   Sofia Konstantinopoulou and Ignacio E Tapia

8. Pathogenesis of Sleep-Disordered Breathing in Adults: Overview 108
   Thomas M Tolbert, Indu Ayappa, and David M Rapoport

9. Risk and Causality by Genetics, Gender, and Age 118
   Moshe Y Prero, Nardine Zakhary, Sally Ibrahim, and Kingman P Strohl

10. The Influence of Cerebral Blood Flow and Cerebrovascular Responsiveness on
    Ventilatory Control 133
    Jay MJR Carr, Gustavo Vizcardo-Galindo, and Philip N Ainslie

11. Central Apnea: Propensity and Plasticity 146
    M Safwan Badr

Section III. Sleep-Disordered Breathing in Different Conditions and Disease States 153

12. Sleep-Disordered Breathing due to Heart Failure 154
    Shahrokh Javaheri and Robin Germany

13. Breathing at Altitude 168
    David Patz

14. Sleep-Disordered Breathing Associated with Chronic Lung Diseases 182
    Bernie Y Sunwoo, Ana Sanchez-Azofra, and Atul Malhotra

15. Obesity Hypoventilation Syndrome 193
    Amanda Piper

Section IV. Pathophysiology-Directed Therapies for Sleep-Disordered Breathing 201

16. Effect of Positive Airway Pressure on Ventilatory Control and Sleep-Disordered Breathing 202
    James A Rowley

17. Mild Intermittent Hypoxia and Supplemental Oxygen: Potential Therapeutic Interventions to Treat Breathing Instability 209
    Sreenavya Gandikota and Jason H Mateika

18. Pharmacological Management of Sleep-Disordered Breathing 221
    Thomas J Altree, Peter G Catcheside, Sutapa Mukherjee, and Danny J Eckert

19. Neural Mechanisms Regulating Opioid-Induced Respiratory Depression and Therapeutic Strategies to Alleviate the Respiratory Side-Effects of Opioid Drugs 233
    Jean-Philippe Rousseau and Gaspard Montandon

20. Pharmacologic Intervention Studies to Mitigate Breathing Instability – Animal Studies . . . 246
    Carla Freire, Lenise J Kim, and Vsevolod Y Polotsky

Index 258

Foreword

The regulation of breathing has intrigued scientists since the time of Whelan, who believed ventilation served to control body temperature and that the brain was the site of ventilatory control. European physiologists, in the late 19th through mid-20th centuries, introduced us to chemoreception and the importance of investigating the adaptability of the respiratory system to various acute and chronic stressors. It is the past three decades that have provided dramatic advances in our understanding of this essential biological rhythm and its clinical relevance. I refer to three categories of advances which also provide the core of this book. Firstly, we have witnessed the unmasking of the respiratory neuronal network, its locations, neural connections, and even some of its vast, complex integrative capabilities in deciphering sensory inputs. Secondly, we became intimately familiar with the mechanisms, the plasticity, and adaptability of chemoreceptors and most recently with their potentially pivotal role in the pathogenesis and treatment of cardiorespiratory disease. Finally, these mostly neuroscience-based advances have laid the foundations for clinical investigation into sleep-disordered breathing— its prevalence, pathogenesis, and treatment. In turn, this massive clinical problem has been responsible for promoting novel basic research into such problems as state effects, coordination of respiratory pump/upper airway caliber control, aging and developmental influences, chemoreceptor plasticity, and control of respiratory motor output stability. These basic science/clinical applications form the core of this book, which also includes bold attempts to introduce novel new personalized treatments for sleep apnea based on the underlying mechanisms.

To paraphrase my longtime friend Dr Thomas Hornbein, this text is filled with science, some philosophy, and an anticipation that the best is yet to come. This book, edited by Drs Susmita Chowdhuri, Safwan Badr, and James Rowley, will not disappoint in meeting these expectations.

Editors Chowdhuri, Badr, and Rowley are experienced investigators who have contributed for many years to our understanding of sleep-disordered breathing. They are to be congratulated for assembling an authorship of distinction and for their considerable efforts in producing this comprehensive treatment of respiratory control and its clinical applications.

Jerome A Dempsey, PhD
Madison, Wisconsin

Preface

Human fascination with breathing control probably dates back to the ancient yogic practices of *Pranayam*, described by Patanjali's aphorisms about 2,500 years ago, where the practitioner focuses on learning regulated breathing maneuvers to control the mind and enhance well-being. *Pranayam* may even be the earliest treatise alluding to the interplay between the brain and the respiratory and autonomic systems.

Over the years, many outstanding books have provided in-depth reviews of the physiologic mechanisms of control of breathing while also examining the various experimental models and techniques used to examine the regulation of respiration during wakefulness and sleep. However, these detailed complex research deliberations are not easily incorporated into the everyday life of sleep clinicians or trainees in clinical fellowships. Hence, knowledge about the remarkable intricacies linking the regulation of breathing and sleep is sometimes *"lost in translation"* and, inadvertently, may remain within the purview of research scholars.

Therefore, the focus of this book was to distill and bring to the clinical sleep practitioner and trainees, a collection of chapters examining ventilatory control of breathing in simple "everyday fashion." These chapters, in combination, explore the anatomy and development of the respiratory system, the fundamental physiologic mechanisms controlling breathing, links between chemoreceptors and cerebral blood flow, hypoxia/hyperoxia, hypercapnia/hypocapnia, genetics, sex, aging, and obesity, while portraying how these factors, separately or in unison, may conspire to either exacerbate breathing instability or to stabilize breathing during sleep, in both health and disease states.

Thus, the book is divided into four sections. The first examines the anatomy, development, and mechanisms of ventilatory control, the second and third sections discuss the pathophysiology of sleep-disordered breathing (SDB) in different scenarios, whereas the fourth section examines pathophysiology-driven targeted therapies for SDB. Nevertheless, many unknowns limit our understanding of the key pathophysiologic mechanisms that contribute to breathing instability and apnea during sleep, and, hence, the chapters also briefly allude to questions that have eluded answers thus far. We envision that these unanswered questions will kindle future hypotheses and research. And the relentless quest for *Truth* resumes in the realm of respiratory control.

We are completely indebted to all the contributors of the chapters for bringing their expertise to the readers while keeping a clinical slant on the topics and for affording their valuable time to this book in the midst of a ravaging pandemic. We are especially grateful to Jerry Dempsey, a giant in the field of "regulation of breathing", for conveying the essence of this book in his foreword. We also deeply thank the reviewers for their careful corrections and comments and the publishers of other journals and books, who granted us permission to reproduce illustrations. We are beholden to the publisher, Taylor & Francis Group, along with their managing staff, Shivangi Pramanik and Himani Dwivedi, for their unstinted support to the authors and editors and for collaborating ceaselessly to bring this book to fruition.

Susmita Chowdhuri
M Safwan Badr
James A Rowley

About the Editors

Susmita Chowdhuri, MD, MS

Dr Chowdhuri is a Professor of Internal Medicine at Wayne State University School of Medicine and a Staff Physician and the Section Chief of Sleep Medicine at the John D Dingell VA Medical Center in Detroit, Michigan. She is also the Medical Director of the Sleep Wake Disorders Center at the John D Dingell VA Medical Center.

Dr Chowdhuri received her medical degree from Maulana Azad Medical College in New Delhi, India, and went on to complete a residency in Internal Medicine at Albert Einstein College of Medicine-Jacobi Medical Center in New York, followed by fellowships in Pulmonary and Critical Care at Syracuse, New York, and in Sleep Medicine at Stanford University Sleep Disorders Center, California. In addition, she completed a Master's in Science degree at the University of Michigan, Ann Arbor, Michigan.

Dr Chowdhuri's research focuses on deciphering the pathophysiologic mechanisms sleep-disordered breathing in high-risk populations, including older adults and opioid users, with a translational goal of developing therapies that target control of breathing during sleep. Dr Chowdhuri has served on several national and local professional committees. She has contributed to the development of many clinical practice guidelines for sleep disorders. She is also passionate about mentoring a new generation of clinical scholars and has received many awards from sleep fellowship trainees for her dedication to teaching.

M Safwan Badr, MD, MBA

Dr Badr is a Professor and Chair of Internal Medicine at Wayne State University School of Medicine and a Staff Physician at the John D Dingell VA Medical Center.

Dr Badr completed a residency in Internal Medicine at Cook County Hospital in Chicago, followed by clinical and research fellowships in Pulmonary, Critical Care and Sleep Medicine at the University of Wisconsin, Madison. In addition, he completed a Master of Business Administration degree at the University of Tennessee.

Dr Badr has served on multiple national and international medical societies. He has served on the Board of Directors of the American Thoracic Society (ATS) and the American Academy of Sleep Medicine (AASM). He was the President of the AASM from 2013 to 2014. Dr Badr currently serves on the Board of Directors for the American Board of Internal Medicine (ABIM).

Dr Badr is an internationally known sleep disorders researcher and research mentor with an extensive record of funding, publication, and mentoring. He has mentored numerous trainees and junior faculty members who have launched successful academic careers.

Dr Badr is invested in outstanding medical education. He was the founding director of the Wayne State University School of Medicine Sleep Medicine Fellowship program and he teaches and mentors students in multiple departments across the medical school. He has mentored many trainees and junior faculty who went on to develop successful clinical and academic careers.

James A Rowley, MD

Dr James A Rowley is a professor of medicine and division chief of pulmonary/critical care and sleep medicine at Wayne State University School of Medicine in Detroit, Michigan. He is also the medical director of the Detroit Receiving Hospital Sleep Disorders Center and program director of the pulmonary/critical care fellowship at Detroit Medical Center, where he is chair of the DMC Pharmacy & Therapeutics Committee. After receiving his medical degree from the New York University School of Medicine, he completed a residency in internal medicine at the University of Chicago Hospital and a fellowship in pulmonary/critical care medicine at the Johns Hopkins Medical Institutions, where he developed his interest in sleep medicine. Dr Rowley's research has focused on clinical aspects of obstructive sleep apnea, upper airway physiology, and control of breathing during sleep. Dr Rowley has served on the board of directors of the American Thoracic Society and the American Academy of Sleep Medicine. He has served as President of the American Academy of Sleep Medicine Foundation and is presently the Secretary-Treasurer of the AASM.

Contributors

Philip N Ainslie, PhD
Centre for Heart, Lung and Vascular Health
University of British Columbia—Okanagan
    Campus
School of Health and Exercise Sciences
Kelowna, BC, Canada

Thomas J Altree, MD
Flinders Health and Medical Research
    Institute/Adelaide Institute for Sleep Health
Flinders University
Bedford Park, South Australia

Indu Ayappa, PhD
Division of Pulmonary, Critical Care, and Sleep
    Medicine
Mount Sinai Hospital
New York, NY

M Safwan Badr, MD, MBA
Professor and Chair of Internal Medicine
Wayne State University School of Medicine
Staff Physician
John D Dingell VA Medical Center
Detroit, MI

Ahuva Brown, MD
The Hospital for Sick Children
Toronto, ON, Canada

Jay MJR Carr, PhD Candidate
Centre for Heart, Lung and Vascular Health
University of British Columbia—Okanagan
    Campus
School of Health and Exercise Sciences
Kelowna, BC, Canada

Peter G Catcheside, PhD
Flinders Health and Medical Research
    Institute/Adelaide Institute for Sleep Health
Flinders University
Bedford Park, South Australia

Susmita Chowdhuri, MD, MS
Professor of Internal Medicine
Wayne State University School of Medicine
Staff Physician and the Section Chief of Sleep
    Medicine
John D Dingell VA Medical Center
Detroit, MI

Christopher A Del Negro, PhD
Professor of Applied Science and Neuroscience
Integrated Science Center III
William & Mary
Williamsburg, VA

Jerome A Dempsey, PhD
John Rankin Laboratory of Pulmonary
    Medicine and Department of Population
    Health Sciences
School of Medicine and Public Health
University of Wisconsin-Madison
Madison, WI

Danny J Eckert, PhD
Flinders Health and Medical Research
    Institute/Adelaide Institute for Sleep Health
Flinders University
Bedford Park, South Australia

Carla Freire, MD, PhD
Division of Pulmonary and Critical Care
    Medicine
Department of Medicine
Johns Hopkins University
School of Medicine
Baltimore, MD

Sreenavya Gandikota, MS
John D Dingell Veterans Affairs Medical
    Center
Department of Physiology
Wayne State University School of Medicine
Detroit, MI

Estelle B Gauda, MD
The Hospital for Sick Children
Toronto, ON, Canada

Robin Germany, MD, FACC
Clinical Assistant Professor of Medicine
Division of Cardiovascular Disease
University of Oklahoma
Oklahoma City, OK

Philippe Haouzi, MD, PhD
Professor of Medicine
Division of Pulmonary and Critical Medicine
Penn State University, College of Medicine
Hershey, PA

Liran Tamir Hostovsky, MD
Sheba Medical Center
Ramat Gan, Israel

Sally Ibrahim, MD
Associate Professor of Pediatrics
Case Western Reserve University
Rainbow Babies and Children's Hospital
Cleveland, OH

Shahrokh Javaheri, MD
Sleep Physician
Division of Pulmonary and Sleep Medicine,
  Bethesda North Hospital
Adjunct Professor of Medicine
Division of Cardiology, The Ohio State
  University, Columbus
Emeritus Professor of Medicine
Division of Pulmonary and Sleep Medicine,
  University of Cincinnati
Cincinnati, OH

Lenise J Kim, PhD
Division of Pulmonary and Critical Care
  Medicine
Department of Medicine
Johns Hopkins University
School of Medicine
Baltimore, MD

Sofia Konstantinopoulou, MD
Pediatric Pulmonology
Sheikh Khalifa Medical City
Abu Dhabi, United Arab Emirates

Leszek Kubin, PhD
Department of Biomedical Sciences
School of Veterinary Medicine
University of Pennsylvania
Philadelphia, PA

Atul Malhotra, MD
Research Chief of Pulmonary, Critical Care,
  Sleep and Physiology
Peter C Farrell Presidential Chair
Tenured Professor of Respiratory Medicine
University of California San Diego
San Diego, CA

Jason H Mateika, PhD
John D Dingell Veterans Affairs Medical
  Center
Departments of Physiology and Internal
  Medicine
Wayne State University School of Medicine
Detroit, MI

Gaspard Montandon, PhD
Keenan Research Centre for Biomedical Science
St Michael's Hospital
Unity Health Toronto
Department of Medicine
University of Toronto
Toronto, ON, Canada

Barbara J Morgan, PhD
John Rankin Laboratory of Pulmonary
  Medicine and Department of Orthopedics
  and Rehabilitation
School of Medicine and Public Health
University of Wisconsin-Madison
Madison, WI

Sutapa Mukherjee, MD, PhD
Flinders Health and Medical Research
  Institute/Adelaide Institute for Sleep Health
Flinders University
Bedford Park, South Australia
Respiratory and Sleep Services
Southern Adelaide Local Health Network, SA
  Health
Adelaide, South Australia

David Patz, MD
Sleep Medicine Clinic
Division of Pulmonary Medicine
University of Colorado School of Medicine,
  Anschutz Campus
Aurora, CO

Amanda Piper, PhD
Department of Respiratory and Sleep Medicine
Royal Prince Alfred Hospital
Camperdown, NSW, Australia

Vsevolod Y Polotsky, MD, PhD
Division of Pulmonary and Critical Care
  Medicine
Department of Medicine
Johns Hopkins University
School of Medicine
Baltimore, MD

Moshe Y Prero, MD
Assistant Professor of Pediatrics
Case Western Reserve University
Rainbow Babies and Children's Hospital
Cleveland, OH

David M Rapoport, MD
Division of Pulmonary, Critical Care, and Sleep
  Medicine
Mount Sinai Hospital
New York, NY

Jean-Philippe Rousseau, PhD
Keenan Research Centre for Biomedical Science
St Michael's Hospital, Unity Health Toronto
Toronto, ON, Canada

James A Rowley, MD
Professor of Internal Medicine
Chief, Division of Pulmonary, Critical Care and
  Sleep Medicine
Wayne State University School of Medicine
Detroit, MI

Ana Sanchez-Azofra, MD
Postdoctoral Research Fellow
University of California San Diego
Department of Medicine
Division of Pulmonary, Critical Care and Sleep
  Medicine
San Diego, CA
Hospital Universitario de la Princesa
Universidad Autónoma de Madrid
Madrid, Spain

Kingman P Strohl, MD
Professor of Medicine
Case Western Reserve University
University Hospitals Cleveland Medical Center
Cleveland, OH

Bernie Y Sunwoo, MBBS
Associate Professor of Medicine
Department of Medicine
Division of Pulmonary, Critical Care and Sleep
  Medicine
University of California San Diego
San Diego, CA

Ignacio E Tapia, MD
Division of Pulmonary and Sleep Medicine
Children's Hospital of Philadelphia
Associate Professor of Pediatrics
Perelman School of Medicine
University of Pennsylvania
Philadelphia, PA

Thomas M Tolbert, MD
Division of Pulmonary, Critical Care, and Sleep
  Medicine
Mount Sinai Hospital
New York, NY

Gustavo Vizcardo-Galindo, BSc
Centre for Heart, Lung and Vascular Health
University of British Columbia—Okanagan
  Campus
School of Health and Exercise Sciences
Kelowna, BC, Canada

Christopher G Wilson, PhD
Professor of Physiology and Pediatrics
Lawrence D Longo, MD Center for Perinatal
  Biology
Loma Linda University, School of Medicine
Loma Linda, CA

Nardine Zakhary, DO
Assistant Professor of Medicine
Case Western Reserve University
University Hospitals Cleveland Medical Center
Cleveland, OH

SECTION I

ANATOMY, DEVELOPMENT, AGING, AND MECHANISMS OF CONTROL OF VENTILATION

1 Anatomy of the Respiratory Neural Network

Christopher A Del Negro* and Christopher G Wilson*

INTRODUCTION

Historical Background and Discovery of the Respiratory Network

Breathing is so fundamental to our lives, we hardly think about it—but it is simultaneously automatic and necessary for survival. Breathing-related pathophysiology can be morbid or fatal and can be traced to dysfunctions in the brain and central nervous system (CNS). The regions of the CNS that drive and control breathing are typically the last regions to stop functioning before death. Because of its automatic nature and physiological importance, the control of ventilation is one of the most important of all brain functions. Our brains *must* generate and control respiration to meet physiological needs. In this chapter, we provide an overview of respiratory system anatomy with a focus on the CNS regions that generate breathing rhythms and shape them into appropriate spatiotemporal patterns of muscle activation. We incorporate cellular and molecular level details for those CNS sites. Our goal is to provide the clinician with a state-of-the-art understanding of respiratory anatomy—neuroanatomy in particular—at the gross systemic, neural circuit (i.e., microcircuit), developmental, and molecular levels of analysis.

Historical Overview and Discovery of the Respiratory Center

During the Roman Republic, Galen served as a physician to gladiators in Pergamon and noted that upper cervical injuries would stop breathing (1). Those observations from ancient times presage the contemporary discovery that the seat for breathing rhythm lies in the lower brainstem, with critical motor relays in the cervical spinal cord. Later, in the 18th century, French physiologist Antoine Charles de Lorry performed experiments on dogs showing that the cerebrum and cerebellum were not necessary for normal pulse and respiration. He suggested that the medulla must be the locus of vital functions (2, 3). The French physiologist Julien-Jean-César Legallois (1770–1840) investigated autoresuscitation and his experiments (4) showed that

circumscribed regions of the brainstem were obligatory for breathing. Legallois sectioned the midbrain and medulla and found that cutting the medulla at the level of the vestibulocochlear cranial nerve (CN VIII) resulted in the complete cessation of breathing. These observations were consistent with Galen's experimental observations (1, 5) that localized a critical respiratory-related, possibly rhythmogenic, substrate to the medulla oblongata. Legallois' work inspired Marie-Jean-Pierre Flourens (1794–1867) to localize the breathing center with even greater precision within the medulla. Flourens originally called the entire medulla the *nœud vital* (vital node), but, by 1851, he used this term to refer to a very small region of the ventral brainstem (6). Figure 1.1A shows an illustration from his 1858 manuscript detailing his experiments on breathing in rabbits, where 3 marks the approximate location of the *nœud vital*.

In the 20th century, English scientist Lumsden (7–9) performed serial transections along the neuraxis from the midbrain to spinal cord in cats and found that breathing stopped when he transected at the spinomedullary junction (marked number 6 in Figure 1.1B). He concluded that the respiratory rhythm generator was localized within the caudal medulla—a region we now know contains the preBötzinger complex, which is inspiratory rhythmogenic and inexorable for breathing, as we elaborate later.

Later work on the anatomical structure and functional connectivity of respiratory centers in the CNS emerged from experiments on sensory feedback to central breathing circuits. Chemosensors were detected on the ventral surface of the brainstem (10–14) in an area now recognized as the parafacial respiratory group or retrotrapezoid nucleus. The parafacial respiratory group houses an expiratory-related oscillator circuit, and, as we relate later, this is now an active area of interest in breathing control. Parallel *top-down* (whole, in vivo animal behavior and physiology) and *bottom-up* approaches (single cells in slices to multiple neuron network recordings) have yielded a greater body of knowledge encompassing gross and microanatomy than any other physiological control system in mammals. In spite of this knowledge base, there has been–until now–no consolidation in one convenient

---

* Both authors contributed equally.

DOI: 10.1201/9781003000631-2

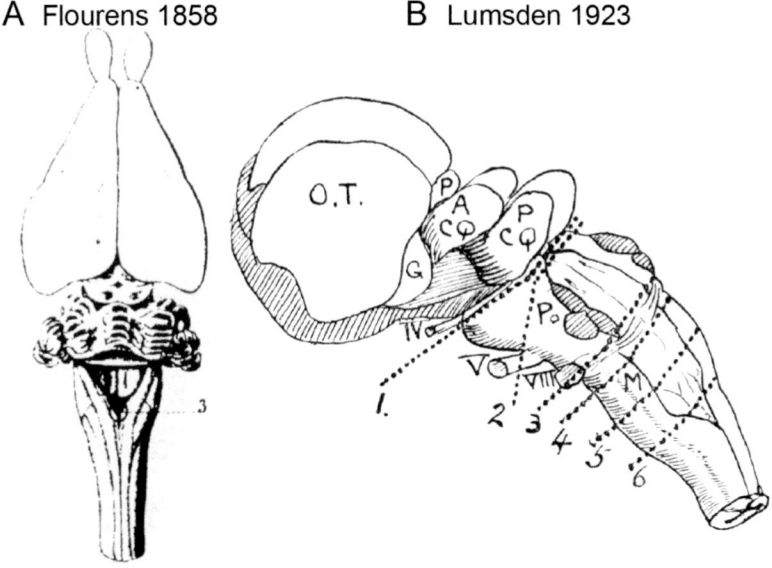

Figure 1.1 A. Illustration from Marie-Jean-Pierre Flourens' seminal work of 1858 on the respiratory center in rabbits. Transactions of the neuraxis at the level of the obex stopped breathing, consistent with a specialized rhythm-generating region located in the lowest portion of the medulla oblongata. B. Diagram from Lumsden's work localizing the respiratory center to the ventral medulla (1923). Numerals 1–6 represent transections in adult cat brains that corresponded to changes in respiration. Cut 6 stopped breathing, suggesting the location of a specialized rhythm-generating region in the lower medulla oblongata. Acronyms: ACQ (anterior colliculus, contemporary nomenclature: superior colliculus); IV (trochlear cranial nerve); M (medulla oblongata); OT (optic tectum), P (peduncle, i.e., cerebellar peduncle), PCQ (posterior colliculus, contemporary nomenclature: inferior colliculus); Po (pons); V (trigeminal cranial nerve); VIII (vestibulocochlear cranial nerve). (From Lumsden, 1923.)

corpus, which inspired (pun intended) this chapter.

MOTOR NEURON POOLS THAT SERVE BREATHING MUSCLES

We begin our discussion of respiratory neural control circuits assuming that the reader is already well familiar with the physical plant for breathing and its musculature: pump, airway resistance, and accessory muscles.

Starting from the pump muscles, our path to the CNS follows the phrenic nerve, C3–C5. Starting from the airway resistance muscles there are four paths along cranial nerves (CNs) IX, X, XI, and XII. The phrenic motor neurons are located within a column spanning ventral horns at a minimum of three cervical segments: C3–C5 in humans. Phrenic motor neurons receive recurrent inhibition via Renshaw cells like most motor neurons innervating skeletal muscles but not Ia inhibitory feedback from stretch receptors of intrafusal muscle fibers (muscle spindles), which are sparse in the diaphragm. Most diaphragmatic motor units

supply type 1 slow oxidative fibers, which aligns with the need to avoid fatigue in regular (eupneic) breathing (15, 16). The diaphragm contains non-oxidative fatigable, high force-generating motor units, but their respiratory roles are limited to episodic behaviors like expectoration, cough, or sneeze, but not eupnea (17). Phrenic motor neurons are recruited by Henneman's size principle, which allows for uniform recruitment from smallest soma size (highest input resistance) to largest soma size (lowest input resistance), a property in which somatic size maps to motor unit size and force production capability (18, 19).

The glossopharyngeal (IX) and vagus (X) nerves are key components of the respiratory motor control system in terms of regulating airway resistance. Motor neurons whose axons depart via CN X comprise the dorsal motor nucleus of the vagus (DMNX) and the *nucleus ambiguus* (NA) (Figures 1.2 and 1.3). The DMNX is located in the lower brainstem immediately dorsal to the XII motor nucleus, lateral to the 4th ventricle. Its constituents are preganglionic

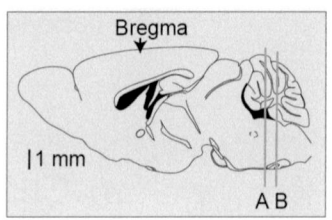

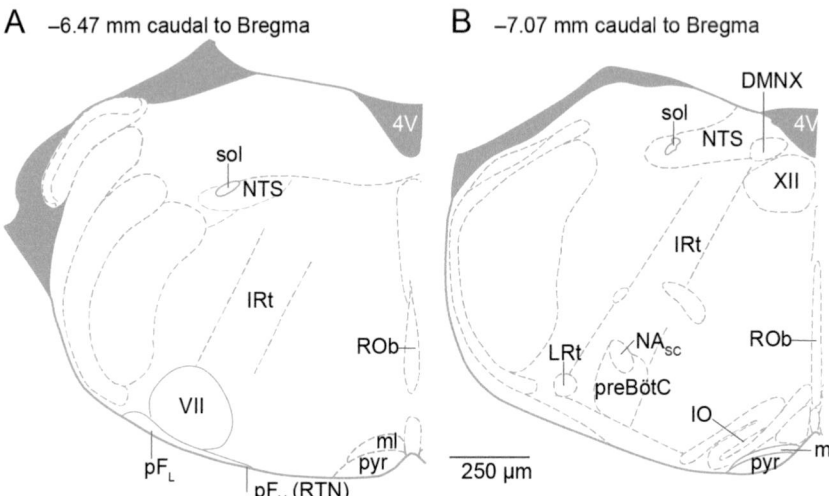

Figure 1.2 Anatomy of respiratory nuclei in transverse sections. The parasagittal section (gray inset box) indicates the location of transverse sections below labeled A and B. (Adapted from Figures 90 and 85 from Paxinos and Franklin. *The Mouse Brain in Stereotaxic Coordinates*, 5th edition. Boston: Elsevier Academic Press, 2020.) Calibration bars are shown for parasagittal and transverse sections. Position of Bregma at top and caudal distance of sections from Bregma listed for transverse sections A and B. Labeled structures include: fourth ventricle (4V), dorsal motor nucleus of vagus (DMNX), facial cranial motor nucleus (VII), hypoglossal cranial motor nucleus (XII), inferior olivary complex (IO), intermediate reticular formation (IRt), lateral parafacial nucleus (pFL), medial lemniscus (ml), nucleus of the solitary tract (NTS), semi-compact division of the *nucleus ambiguus* (NA$_{SC}$), ventral parafacial nucleus (pFV), pre-Bötzinger complex (preBötC), pyramidal tract (pyr), raphe obscurus (ROb), retrotrapezoid nucleus (RTN), solitary tract (sol), ventral parafacial nucleus (pFL). (These transverse sections were traced from outlines in G Paxinos & KBJ Franklin, editors, Paxinos and Franklin's *The Mouse Brain in Stereotaxic Coordinates*, 5th edition. Amsterdam, Boston: Elsevier Academic Press, 2020, and then modified substantially to reflect respiratory sites and nuclei and labeled according to field-specific nomenclature, which is not the same as the published atlas.)

neurons of the parasympathetic nervous system controlling gastrointestinal organs and serve no known respiratory function. The NA is ventrally situated in a column that spans from the caudal pole of the facial nucleus (VII) posteriorly to past the obex (20). Somatic motor neurons of the NA have widespread control of pharyngeal and laryngeal motor units whose functions pertain to respiration and swallowing. Esophagomotor neurons are concentrated at the dorsal end of NA, in the division referred to as the compact NA (NAc) (20). A significant fraction of NA, particularly the rostrally sited NAc motor neurons, depart via CN IX instead of CN X and its branches. The NAc is so compact that it literally appears like a bullseye in transverse sections. Caudally adjacent divisions of the NA are referred to as semi-compact (NAsc) and loose (NAl); those divisions contain middle and lower pharyngeal constrictor motor neurons and laryngeal motor neurons. Another ventral division called external NA (NAe) contains cardiovagal preganglionic motor neurons. The NAe extends the entire anterior–posterior length of the NA. The size and appearance of the NA, particularly the NAc and NAsc is a reliable diagnostic used by pathologists and neuroscientists in

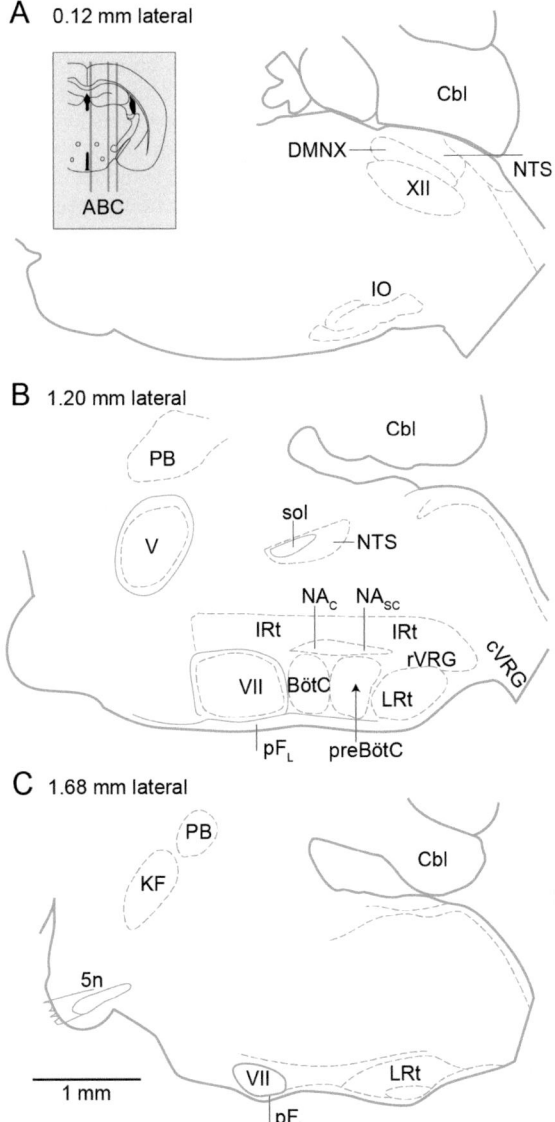

Figure 1.3 Anatomy of respiratory nuclei in parasagittal sections. The coronal section (gray inset box) indicates the location of parasagittal sections labeled A–C. (Sections are adapted from Figures 102, 111, and 115 from Paxinos and Franklin. *The Mouse Brain in Stereotaxic Coordinates*, 5th edition. Boston: Elsevier Academic Press, 2020.) The lateral distance of the parasagittal sections from the midline is listed with each section. Calibration bar applies to all sections. Labeled structures include trigeminal cranial nerve (5n), Bötzinger complex (BötC), caudal ventral respiratory group (cVRG), cerebellum (Cbl), compact division of the *nucleus ambiguus* (NA_C), dorsal motor nucleus of vagus (DMNX), inferior olivary complex (IO), intermediate reticular formation (IRt), Kölliker-Fuse nucleus (KF), semi-compact division of the *nucleus ambiguus* (NA_SC), lateral parafacial nucleus (pFL), lateral reticular nucleus (LRt), pre-Bötzinger complex (preBötC), parabrachial nucleus (PB), rostral ventral respiratory group (rVRG), nucleus of the solitary tract (NTS), solitary tract (sol), trigeminal cranial motor nucleus (V), facial cranial motor nucleus (VII). (These parasagittal sections were traced from outlines in G Paxinos & KBJ Franklin, editors, *Paxinos and Franklin's The Mouse Brain in Stereotaxic Coordinates*, 5th edition. Amsterdam, Boston: Elsevier Academic Press, 2020, and then modified substantially to reflect respiratory sites and nuclei and labeled according to field-specific nomenclature, which is not the same as the published atlas.)

preparing transverse sections for histology or physiological laboratory studies. The NAc is located, in parallel, with the Bötzinger complex in the anterior–posterior axis (Figure 1.3). The transition from NAc to NAsc reliably maps to the anterior border of the preBötzinger complex (21–23). In both examples, the respiratory nuclei lie ventral to NAc and NAsc (Figure 1.2).

Accessory muscles such as the sternocleidomastoid and trapezius have their motor neurons within pools of the ventral horn located at C1–C2. Scalene motor neurons are dispersed within cervical segments 3–6, at least in mice. Interestingly, their motor axons ascend to exit the neuraxis via the Accessory CN XI, which is above the cervical spinal cord. The quadratus lumborum is the lowest of abdominal accessory respiratory muscles. It is innervated by motor axons from T12–L4, whose motor neurons are located in the corresponding ventral horns.

Airway resistance is also regulated via the position of the tongue in the oropharynx. Motor neurons for the genioglossus, geniohyoid, and styloglossus muscles reside in the hypoglossal motor nucleus in the dorsomedial region of the lower medulla (Figures 1.2 and 1.3). A portion of the XII nucleus is located posterior to the obex, thus formally a part of the cervical spinal cord. Motor axons serving motor units of all three muscles depart via CN XII (24–28).

PREMOTOR NEURONS (FIRST ORDER) OF THE MEDULLA AND CERVICAL SPINAL CORD

Three sets of respiratory premotor neurons are well understood: phrenic premotor neurons of the upper cervical spinal cord and hypoglossal premotor neurons of the lower (dorsal) medulla, which are inspiratory, as well as abdominal premotor neurons of the lower cervical spinal cord, which are expiratory (29–32). The sites and nuclei described below can be located in Figures 1.2 and 1.3.

Phrenic Premotor Neurons

A network of phrenic premotor neurons reaches from the ventral brainstem to the upper cervical spinal cord (33–39). This network is generally called the rostral ventral respiratory group (rVRG). Phrenic premotor neurons are glutamatergic (excitatory) and a significant subset, particularly located at the rostral-most portion of the rVRG, express neurokinin-1 peptide receptors (40–42); the cognate ligand is substance P, a neuropeptide closely linked to generation and modulation of inspiratory rhythm and motor pattern (43).

The diaphragm contracts as a unit and this functionality is reflected in the organization of premotor neurons and motor units. Phrenic premotor neuron axons often bifurcate to project bilaterally to phrenic motor neurons of the left and right motor pools. Conversely, a modified rabies virus tracer injected into diaphragm muscle fibers unilaterally, with the ability to leap just one synapse upstream from its motor neuron, retrogradely labels efferent phrenic premotor neurons on both left and right sides of the cervical spinal cord (29).

Excitatory inspiratory drive to phrenic motor neurons, as described above, comes from the rVRG. However, we also recognize inhibitory drive to phrenic motor neurons, which comes from long-range axon projections from the Bötzinger complex. Generally, Bötzinger neurons discharge during expiration. They inhibit phrenic motor neurons as well as rVRG phrenic premotor neurons (44–47).

Hypoglossal Premotor Neurons

Because XII-innervated tongue muscles serve a wide array of orofacial behaviors, their premotor neurons are found throughout the lower brainstem, within nuclei that surround the trigeminal motor nucleus of the pons and in the midbrain reticular formation (48). Confining our presentation to respiratory function, in which XII motor neurons protrude the tongue during inspiration, those XII premotor neurons are found in the intermediate reticular formation (IRt), extending anterior-posteriorly in register with the XII motor neurons that they innervate (30, 31, 49–52).

Abdominal Premotor Neurons

The ventral respiratory column continues posteriorly following the population of rVRG phrenic premotor neurons. The transition from inspiratory premotor neurons to expiratory premotor neurons is marked by a name change from rVRG to caudal ventral respiratory group (cVRG). The cVRG contains premotor neurons for abdominal motor neurons of the lumbar spinal cord (L1–L3), which serve expiratory pump functionality (53–58). Abdominal premotor neurons with expiratory function are also found in the rVRG, just caudal to obex (32).

RHYTHM-GENERATING NUCLEI AND HIGHER ORDER INTERNEURONS IN THE BRAINSTEM AND PONS

There are at least two distinct rhythmogenic microcircuits, the pre-Bötzinger complex (preBötC) for inspiratory rhythm and the lateral parafacial (pFL) for expiratory rhythm. The sites and nuclei described in the following sections are illustrated in Figures 1.4–1.6 with an overview diagram in Figure 1.7.

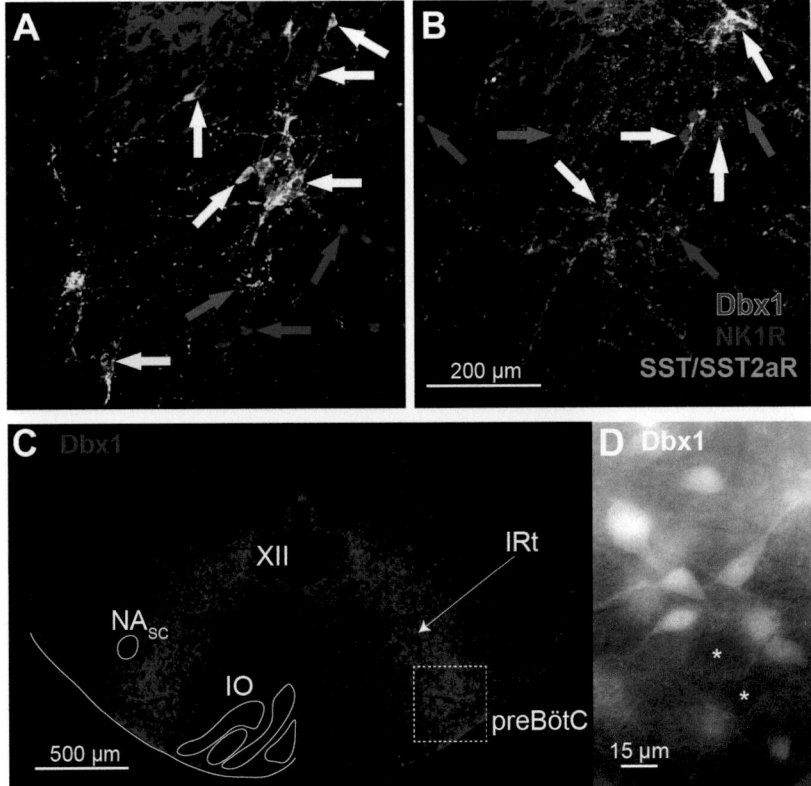

Figure 1.4 Cellular composition of the preBötC. A and B show preBötC neurons in a Dbx1[nlsLacZ] reporter mouse, which expresses the bacterial *LacZ* reporter gene only in Dbx1-derived cells. Those nuclei were stained blue by antibodies directed at ß-galactosidase (ß-gal, the *LacZ* gene product). NK1Rs stained red by immunohistochemistry. Note the heavy labeling of neurons in the NA_{SC} at the top of each field of view. SST (A) and SST2a receptors (SST2aRs, B) stained green by immunohistochemistry. White arrows indicate triple labeled neurons: Dbx1 (ß-gal), NK1R, and SST/SST2aR. Yellow arrows indicate NK1R and SST labeling on a non-Dbx1 neuron. Blue arrows indicate Dbx1-derived cells (possibly glia). Purple arrows indicate Dbx1 (ß-gal) and SST/SST2aR labeled neurons. (Data in A and B were adapted from Gray et al. J Neurosci 30:14883, 2010.) C and D show Dbx1-derived cells (neurons and glia) in an intersectional mouse genetic model, Dbx1[CreERT2]; Rosa26[tdTomato], in which Cre recombinase expression in Dbx1-derived cells facilitates fluorophore tdTomato expression. C shows a transverse section from the medulla at the level of the preBötC (near to section shown in Figure 1.5B). Labels are the same as Figures 1.5 and 1.6. D shows a high magnification view from panel C, where Dbx1-derived neurons are pseudo-colored white for maximum contrast. Asterisks show non-Dbx1 neurons. Panel D reflects typical imaging during patch-clamp experiments targeting preBötC neurons in vitro. (Data in C and D were adapted from Ruangkittisakul et al. Sci Rep 2:e12111, 2014.)

pre-Bötzinger Complex

The inexorable rhythm for breathing is inspiratory. That rhythm emanates from the preBötC (59), located in the lower ventral medulla. It spans 250–500 μm in the anterior–posterior axis (depending on species and age), approximately in parallel with the XII motor nucleus. The caudal border of the preBötC is slightly caudal to the obex, where preBötC merges with the rVRG. The preBötC-rVRG border is ill-defined because rhythmogenic propriobulbar interneurons (whose axons project within the medulla) and phrenic premotor bulbospinal interneurons (whose axons project to cervical spinal cord) intermingle in this anatomic gray area (29, 40–42, 59).

Functional and Anatomic Definition of the preBötC

At first, the definition of the preBötC was functional; it represented the portion of the ventral respiratory column that was necessary and sufficient to generate inspiratory-related

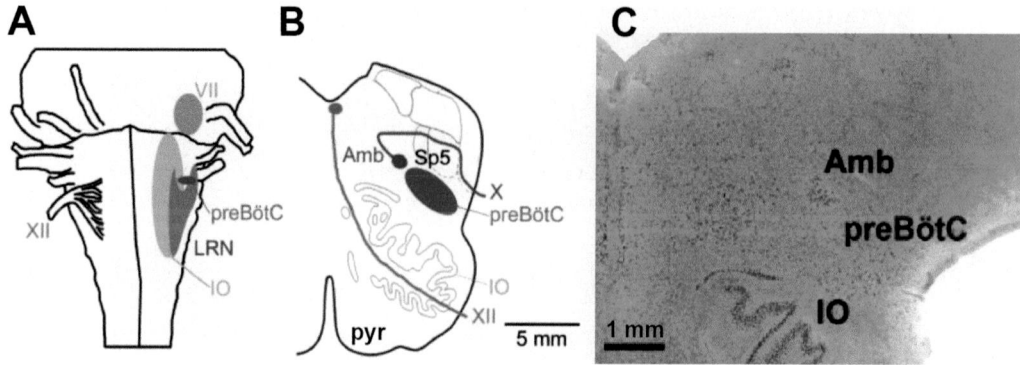

Figure 1.5 Human preBötC. A and B show the location of the preBötC in humans via schematics from the ventral brainstem (A) and in transverse sections 9 mm from the obex (B). C shows a Nissl-stained transverse section at the level of the preBötC in B. (Data and diagrams adapted from Schwarzacher et al. Brain 134:24, 2011.) Note, the authors used "Amb" for the *nucleus ambiguus*, which is called "NA" in the present manuscript. Sp5 refers to the spinal trigeminal nucleus. All other abbreviations are consistent with the present manuscript.

rhythm and motor output *in vitro*. Perturbations that elevated excitability in preBötC sped up respiratory rhythm, whereas perturbations that depressed its excitability slowed the rhythm down. Those results established that preBötC contained a rhythmogenic microcircuit linked paucisynaptically to motor outputs of the phrenic and XII motor nerves (59), but it did not specify its cellular constituents or definitively establish its borders.

The following anatomical discoveries advanced understanding of the preBötC by augmenting its functional definition. Neuropeptide and peptide receptor expression patterns define the borders of preBötC (40–43, 60). preBötC neurons selectively express neurokinin-1 receptors (NK1Rs), μ-opioid receptors (μORs), as well as somatostatin (SST) and SST receptors (61–63). NK1R, as well as SST and SST2a receptors, are illustrated in Figures 1.4A and B.

Fortuitously, those peptide markers could be used to probe preBötC function too. Substance P sped up inspiratory rhythms *in vitro* (43, 64–67) acting directly to depolarize putatively rhythmogenic preBötC interneurons as well as motor output-related neurons therein (68, 69). Furthermore, substance P, conjugated to the ribosomal toxin saporin, injected into the preBötC of adult rats caused progressive breathing deficits over several days culminating in severe respiratory pathology and death (70, 71). Unilateral ablation of NK1R-expressing neurons in the preBötC caused compatible, albeit less severe, breathing deficits (72).

Those experiments bolstered confidence that the preBötC was not just necessary for inspiratory rhythm and motor output *in vitro*

but was necessary for real breathing in living animals. That last point was not universally accepted in the 1990s because *in vitro* preparations from neonates were not yet widely accepted as experimental models of the respiratory neural control system in adults. Some even argued that *in vitro* rhythms reflected fictive gasping (73), despite the fact that *in vitro* preparations, measured via oxygen- and pH-sensitive electrodes (74, 75), are normoxic to depths of several hundred micrometers. The disparity of motor patterns *in vitro* compared to motor patterns in adults *in vivo* can be explained by three factors: developmental stage, temperature, and sensorimotor integration. In adults, the phrenic motor nerve discharges with an incremental pattern, whereas in neonates, the pattern is often decrementing, as observed *in vitro* at physiological temperature. Decreasing temperature to ~27°C, which increases the duration of time *in vitro* preparations are viable in the laboratory, enhances that decremental pattern of phrenic nerve discharge. Finally, the inspiratory rhythm is considerably slower *in vitro*, and each decremental cycle more long lasting, because of the lack of vagal sensory feedback (76, 77).

The other peptide markers (μORs and SST) provide functional insights that also help define the preBötC and characterize its role(s) in rhythmogenesis and motor pattern formation. Regarding μORs, the recreational use of opioid drugs slows and stops breathing (78, 79). Opioids diminish the rhythmogenic functionality of preBötC neurons (43, 80–83) by modulating G-protein-coupled inwardly rectifying K[+] (GIRK) channels (84) as well as depressing presynaptic drive (85–87).

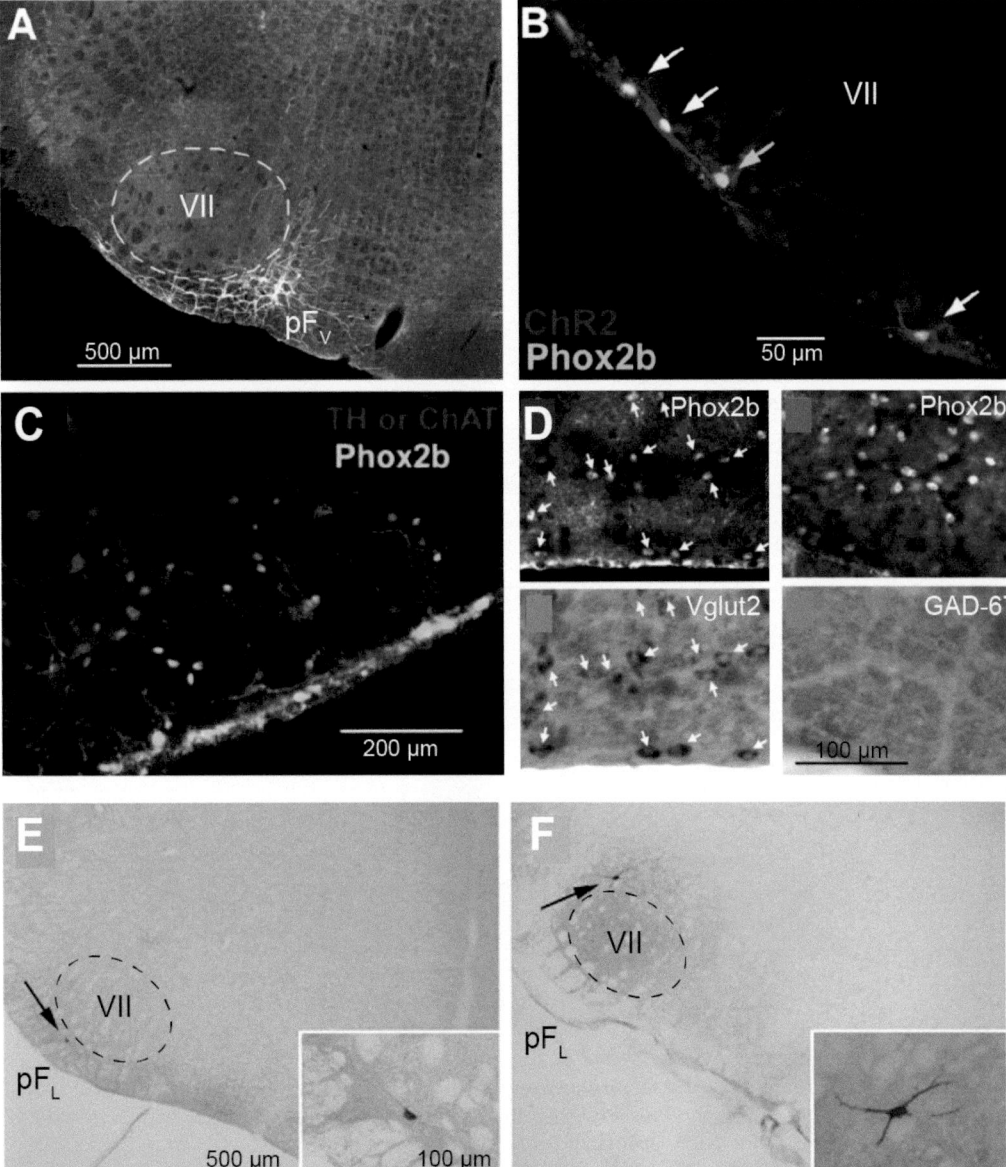

Figure 1.6 The parafacial (pF), a.k.a., retrotrapezoid (RTN) nuclei. A and B, transverse sections showing fluorescent reporter protein in Phox2b-expressing pFV/RTN neurons transduced to also express channelrhodopsin2 (ChR2). Subsequent photostimulation of those Phox2b- and ChR2-expressing pFV neurons sped up breathing and induced active expiration. (Data adapted from Abbott et al. J Neurosci 29:5806, 2009.) Phox2b reporter pseudo-colored white in A and green in B. C shows that Phox2b-expressing pFV neurons are neither catecholaminergic C1 nor cholinergic VII motor neurons, which are located in the vicinity of the pFV. TH refers to tyrosine hydroxylase; ChAT refers to choline acetyl cholinesterase. D shows that Phox2b-expressing pFV neurons are glutamatergic and not GABAergic. Vglut2 refers to vesicular glutamate transporter 2 (Slc17a6); GAD-67 refers to glutamic acid decarboxylase (GAD1). Arrows indicate double Phox2b and Vglut2 labeling. (Data adapted from Stornetta et al. J Neurosci 26:10305, 2006.) E and F, transverse sections that mark a single pF$_L$ neuron (E) and a VII motor neuron (F). Insets in E and F show recorded neurons at higher magnification. Scale bars in E apply to E and F. (Data adapted from Pagliardini et al. J Neurosci 31:2895, 2011.)

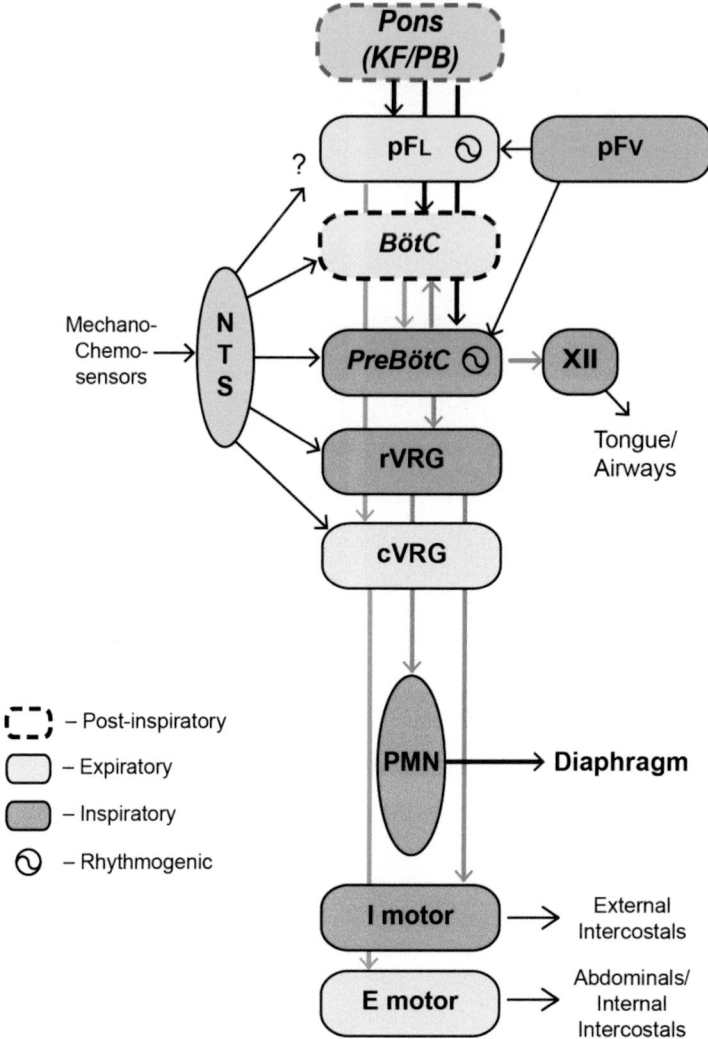

Figure 1.7   Block diagram of the respiratory regions of the CNS. Regions marked with gold are inspiratory related and regions in blue are expiratory related. During inspiration, bursts initiate in the preBötC and project to the inspiratory premotor neurons in the rVRG, which in turn excite phrenic and external intercostal motor neurons to contract the diaphragm and inspiratory-related intercostal muscles. The BötC is active in early expiration (E1), also known as post-inspiration. Given sufficient respiratory drive, the lateral parafacial (pF$_L$) becomes active in late expiration (E2) to drive cVRG neurons and thus expiratory motor pools in the spinal cord. Abbreviations: Bötzinger complex (BötC); caudal ventral respiratory group (cVRG); hypoglossal motor nucleus (XII); Kölliker Fuse (KF); lateral parafacial (pFL); nucleus tractus solitarius (NTS); parabrachial nucleus (PB); preBötzinger complex (preBötC);ventral parafacial (pFV).

The direct effects of opioids on preBötC neurons emphasize the preeminence of the preBötC for inspiratory rhythm generation. Nevertheless, we recognize a caveat, because opioids are administered orally or intravenously, their respiratory depressant effects can be attributed to sites in the pons too (88), although the effects in the preBötC appear to be the most significant for respiratory depression (82, 83, 89) (see Haouzi et al. in this volume). Given the social and medical implications of opioid abuse (90, 91) and the need to employ opioids for pain management (92) while minimizing addictions (93), it is imperative that we advance the current state of understanding regarding how μOR activation impacts the preBötC and other respiratory sites.

SST-expressing neurons also occupy the preBötC core. They do not populate the rVRG like NK1R-expressing neurons do, and thus SST-expressing neurons appeared to be better markers for the preBötC core (42). A molecularly engineered receptor that activates K^+ channels was installed in the preBötC of adult rats. Whether the animals were awake or anesthetized, the activation of those receptors diminished the frequency and amplitude of breathing movements until total apnea resulted—the rats needed mechanical ventilation until they recovered from the experiment (94). Follow-up studies examined the underlying cellular mechanisms and found that SST-expressing preBötC neurons serve predominantly output functions. They are intermingled in the preBötC with rhythm-generating neurons, and their function is to coactivate and pass on inspiratory rhythm to dedicated populations of inspiratory premotor and motor neurons residing outside of the preBötC (95, 96).

To recap: the preBötC is the preeminent respiratory oscillator. We know that because its constituent interneurons can be distinguished by NIK1Rs, μORs, and SST, each having functional significance. NK1Rs mapped the preBötC borders, SP modulated inspiratory rhythms *in vitro*, and killing NK1R-expressing preBötC neurons caused pathologic ataxic breathing. μORs map the preBötC too. Opioid effects on breathing also suggest the preeminence of the preBötC. SST further maps the preBötC core, and SST-expressing neurons are breathing essential, but their role is output-related rather than rhythmogenic.

Genetic Definition of the preBötC

What is the cellular rhythmogenic core of preBötC? We are certain that core rhythm generators are glutamatergic interneurons that express NK1Rs and probably not SST. We are confident that they interconnect with one another and that they generate collective activity via recurrent excitation, a network-based rhythmogenic mechanism (95–101). The feature, at present, that uniquely distinguishes core preBötC neurons is their genetic origin: those interneurons are unambiguously derived from progenitors that express transcription factor *Dbx1* (developing brain homeobox 1) during embryonic development (Figure 1.4). *Dbx1*-derived preBötC neurons are glutamatergic; they are rhythmically active *in vitro* in sync with the inspiratory rhythm and motor output. *Dbx1*-derived preBötC neurons express NK1Rs as well as SST and SST receptors (102, 103). Selective laser

ablation of *Dbx1*-derived preBötC neurons in rhythmic slice preparations diminishes and then irreversibly stops inspiratory rhythm and motor output (104). In living animals, optogenetic stimulation or silencing of *Dbx1*-derived preBötC neurons accelerates or decelerates (then stops) inspiratory breathing movements in both anesthetized and awake intact mice (95, 105–107).

Dbx1 is an advantageous marker for core preBötC interneurons, but there are important caveats. First, *Dbx1* is only expressed during embryonic development (102, 108, 109), which makes it more challenging to use as a marker or a tool to manipulate neuronal function (23, 110) compared to a transcription factor like *Phox2b* that is expressed into adulthood in parafacial respiratory neurons (see Ventral Parafacial [pF$_V$ or Retrotrapezoid Nucleus [RTN], below). Second, *Dbx1*-expressing progenitors also give rise to output-related preBötC neurons and inspiratory hypoglossal premotor neurons in the intermediate reticular formation (31, 111) as well as phrenic premotor neurons in the rVRG (29).

Inhibitory preBötC Neurons

Approximately half of preBötC interneurons are inhibitory: glycinergic or GABAergic (112–116). Inhibitory preBötC neurons modulate the amplitude as well as the frequency of the rhythmic inspiratory bursts (117, 118). These inhibitory populations receive sensorimotor information from the nucleus of the solitary tract (NTS), located in the dorsomedial medulla near the XII motor nucleus and DMNX. Inhibitory neurons project to core rhythmogenic preBötC neurons (61, 63, 119). During normal breathing, inhibitory neurons in the preBötC are recruited periodically during each breath to hasten inspiratory termination. That role profoundly influences phase transition from inspiration to post-inspiration, then expiration, and that speeds up breathing cycles (107, 120). Without preBötC inhibitory microcircuits, the breathing rhythm is slower overall and "stiff" in the sense that its frequency plateaus even when faced with normally effective respiratory drive like CO_2 or SP (107, 120). Inhibitory preBötC neurons also inhibit parafacial expiratory rhythmogenic neurons (see Lateral Parafacial [pF$_L$] below).

preBötC in Perspective

This chapter is dedicated to anatomical properties of the respiratory neural networks. Here, in the section on preBötC, we have delved deeper than in previous (and following) sections into cellular constituents, their functions, and their molecular genetic origins. Why such detail? It is foremost because the preBötC is so important: it gives rise to the only inexorable and indispensable respiratory rhythm, i.e., inspiration. Another reason is because so much is known about constituent preBötC interneurons therefore it is possible to provide those levels of detail. Given its preeminent respiratory role and depth of knowledge, we hope these hard-won details can be leveraged by clinicians to develop prophylaxis or treatments for respiratory disorders, including treatments for opioid-induced respiratory depression (78, 92), congenital central hypoventilation syndrome (CCHS), Apnea of Prematurity in newborns, and sudden infant death syndrome (SIDS). For these kinds of disorders, agents that reduce tonic inhibition of the preBötC (such as caffeine) or low-level enhancement of excitatory inputs to the preBötC—including new drugs such as ampakines (121–124)—may prove effective and sufficiently selective to treat patients who are not responsive to caffeine. This objective is eminently feasible because the preBötC has been well characterized in humans (125) (Figure 1.5).

Parafacial Nucleus (pF)

The next two sections describe the parafacial respiratory group (pF). That nomenclature refers to a mixed group of interneurons that are located at the ventral (Figures 1.6A–D) and lateral (Figure 1.6E) margins of the facial (VII) cranial motor nucleus (Figure 1.6F shows a VII motor neuron). Parafacial respiratory interneurons serve two functions: central chemosensitivity and generation of expiratory rhythm, which is conditional (not inexorable). We present expiratory function first, then proceed to central chemosensitivity.

Lateral Parafacial (pF$_L$)

Expiratory parafacial interneurons are concentrated at the lateral margin of VII thus we apply the shorthand pF$_L$ (parafacial lateral) (Figure 1.6E). VII motor neurons are not located at the ventral margins like pF$_L$ neurons (e.g., compared Figures 1.6E–F). In neonatal rodent preparations *in vitro*, pF$_L$ interneurons exhibit peri-inspiratory discharge patterns. That is, they activate prior to inspiration for ~0.5–1 s and then are actively silenced during inspiration, but then recover and spike vigorously again in post-inspiration.

These parafacial neurons were first considered inspiratory rhythmogenic because of their activation during the preinspiratory phase, and indeed they were first dubbed "preinspiratory neurons" (126–130) between 1989 and 1993. Parafacial interneurons were studied in parallel with the preBötC during the 1990s. At that time, the preBötC was a relatively new discovery and its status as the inspiratory rhythmogenic site was still being corroborated. Constituent preBötC neurons also activated prior to inspiration (~300–600 ms latency), and were equivalently dubbed "preinspiratory" and hypothesized to be rhythmogenic (77, 131, 132).

The competing ideas positing two populations of rhythmogenic preinspiratory neurons were in conflict: parafacial and preBötC interneurons were separated by hundreds of microns in the anterior–posterior axis; both could not be inspiratory rhythmogenic. However, by the mid-2000s, the solution was apparent. The rhythm observed in parafacial neurons matched active expiration, in that context, late-stage expiratory activity coincided with the period immediately prior to inspiration. Parafacial neurons generated another bout of activity that occurred during post-inspiration (133, 134). The parafacial neurons were able to generate expiratory rhythmic activity, which was periodically interrupted during inspiration by synaptic inhibition relayed from preBötC. The rhythm of expiration is state-dependent and conditional. Autonomous expiratory rhythmicity from the pF$_L$ can be evoked by disinhibition via application of GABA$_A$ and glycine receptor antagonists, hypercapnia, muscarinic neuromodulation, or exogenous recruitment via optogenetic stimulation of pF$_L$ neurons. In all cases, the pF$_L$ is recruited by elevated neural excitability to become rhythmically active (135–140).

Interestingly, the pF$_L$ does not express µORs so its rhythmicity is opioid insensitive. When activity in the preBötC is shut down via opioid agonists, the expiratory rhythm persists independently (80, 133, 134).

Under normal physiological conditions, the preBötC operates as the master oscillator governing inspiratory rhythm. If active expiration is evoked, then pF$_L$ microcircuits, which have excitatory inputs to the preBötC, hasten inspiration. In turn, the preBötC sends inhibitory projections to pF$_L$, which transiently silence it during inspiration. pF$_L$ active resumes during post-inspiration (137, 138, 141).

Ventral Parafacial (pF$_V$) or Retrotrapezoid Nucleus (RTN)

Central chemosensor neurons are situated at ventral and medial margins of the VII nucleus. Those pF$_V$ chemosensors are derived from *Atoh1* (a.k.a., *Math1*) and *Egr2* (a.k.a., *Krox20*) expressing progenitor cells (142, 143), and they express the transcription factor *Phox2b* throughout development into adulthood (144–146). *Phox2b* expression has proved to be a convenient marker to identify pF$_V$ neurons anatomically and a tool to manipulate them experimentally and thus probe their functions. pF_V neurons are excitatory (glutamatergic) rather than inhibitory (Figures 1.6A–D).

Phox2b-expressing pF_V neurons become rhythmically active earlier in embryonic development than the preBötC (144). At this stage, the site is called e-pF (embryonic parafacial). In the absence of an active preBötC, the embryonic parafacial neurons are intrinsically rhythmic and synchronized. Once the preBötC comes online, like their pF_L neighbors, pF_V neuronal discharge becomes biphasic: they discharge during late expiration and post-inspiration in rhythmically active neonatal rodent preparations (144, 147, 148). pF_V neurons are opioid-insensitive during neonatal stages of development and in juvenile and adult rodents (85).

Respiratory rhythmic activity in pF_V neurons goes away with age such that in adult rodents, the pF_V neurons spike tonically without evidence of respiratory rhythmicity. Instead, their firing rate is modulated by pH and CO_2 (145, 149). Nevertheless, even while embryonic *Phox2b*-expressing pF_V neurons are respiratory rhythmic, their status as a central chemoreceptor is already well established (150). The mechanism of chemosensation depends on GPR4 receptors that bind protons and then regulate TASK2-type K^+ channels (151, 152). KCNQ (i.e., K_V7) type K^+ channels also play a role in the chemosensory function of pF_V neurons (153, 154).

Central chemoreception also involves astrocytes in the parafacial region, whose mechanism depends on pH-mediated inhibition of inwardly rectifying K^+ channels and purinergic signaling (155–158).

pF_V neurons are glutamatergic and their activity, as modulated by CO_2 and pH, boosts excitability throughout the respiratory networks to both evoke active expiration and speed-up breathing frequency overall (159–161). Their activity widely supports respiratory rhythmogenesis from embryonic stages onward. This seems to be directly related to central chemosensitivity modulating the excitability of the entire respiratory neural control system. CO_2 is the strongest stimulus to breathe; elevation of the partial pressure of CO_2 in the blood and tissues lowers pH, which is sensed by pF_V neurons and then translated into widespread excitation of respiratory microcircuits from midbrain to spinal cord.

Regarding nomenclature, the parafacial region was identified by retrograde tract tracing experiments before its physiological roles were characterized. At that time, the site was dubbed *retrotrapezoid nucleus* (RTN) (36) and that nomenclature has persisted. Gradually, the name RTN has become attached to pF_V and chemosensation rather than active expiration and pF_L. The name RTN is still in widespread usage and always associated with chemosensation (152).

Postinspiratory Sites: Kölliker-Fuse and Parabrachial Nucleus

Post-inspiration immediately follows inspiration. It is generally present—and beneficial—during eupnea but not obligatory. Post-inspiration is generally lost *in vitro* because brainstem-spinal cord preparations retain inspiratory rhythmogenic (preBötC) and expiratory rhythmogenic (pF_L) sites. Slice preparations retain only the preBötC. Nevertheless, preparations that include the pons can generate postinspiratory activity measurable via CN IX and CN X (162, 163).

Given those constraints, postinspiratory activity has been attributed to pontine sites like the Kölliker-Fuse nucleus (KF) and the lateral parabrachial nucleus (164, 165). In living animals with intact mechanical sensory feedback from the lungs, via CN X, the KF acts in concert with vagal feedback to enforce inspiratory–expiratory phase transition and postinspiratory activity generally. Mechanistically, the KF may modulate the threshold value of lung inflation that triggers the end of inspiration (166, 167).

The KF projects to laryngeal motoneurons of the *nucleus ambiguus*, particularly those controlling glottal constriction. Therefore, the KF controls the valve for air being exhaled during post-inspiration (164). Its projections to glottal constrictors are important for airway defensive behaviors like sneeze, cough, swallow, and emesis. Glottal constriction allows for the buildup of high intraabdominal pressures whose release generates expulsive expiratory efforts for sneezing and coughing. For swallowing and emesis, KF-mediated glottal closure prevents foodstuffs from entering the trachea.

Parabrachial and Kölliker-Fuse neurons are derived from *Atoh-1* expressing progenitors. Their relationship to *Atoh-1* expression is noteworthy because this transcription factor is critical for the development of other important respiratory nuclei like the pF_V (and perhaps pF_L). And it is consistent with a general role for *Atoh-1* in patterning key respiratory sites and nuclei (143, 168).

KF neurons can be distinguished from parabrachial neurons by *FoxP2* expression. *FoxP2* is associated with speech and vocalization. It is logical that an area with control of laryngeal muscles that regulates inspiration-expiratory phase transition, as well as post-inspiration, could be important for speech and vocalization. Further, in support of a KF role in speech and vocalization, the KF projects directly to the NTS, wherein a key subpopulation is essential for vocalization in mice (169). However, the relevance to human vocal control has not been established.

The well-established role of the KF in post-inspiration notwithstanding, one lab proposed that post-inspiration is generated by an independent (third) respiratory oscillator in the medulla. A set of glutamatergic and cholinergic neurons, characterized by oscillatory post-inspiratory activity, were identified in the region immediately medial and caudal to the VII nucleus in mice. This region was dubbed the *postinspiratory complex* (PiCo) (170). Although silent under baseline conditions *in vitro*, it becomes rhythmically active in the presence of norepinephrine. The PiCo appears to have a reciprocally inhibitory interaction with the preBötC, which makes sense given that inspiratory and postinspiratory motor patterns must occur in sequence and never simultaneously for effective ventilation.

However, enthusiasm for PiCo must be tempered for the time being. Its discovery in 2016 has not been corroborated by any follow-up studies. Further, one group that did attempt to verify the PiCo instead found the same glutamatergic and cholinergic neurons located medial and caudal to VII, but they were autonomic relays for respiratory and swallowing-related sympathetic output (171). Another group surveyed the entire ventral respiratory medulla and pons using arrays of microelectrodes and observed no post-inspiratory activity in the putative PiCo region, yet post-inspiration was expressed within the KF (172). So, post-inspiratory rhythmicity of this putative PiCo region may be an artifact attributable to *in vitro* conditions that modify its constituent neuron behaviors in the absence of an autonomic control system.

Apart from their roles in post-inspiration, the Kölliker-Fuse and parabrachial nuclei broadly elevate excitability throughout the ventral respiratory column to help maintain rhythmicity. The PB nuclei are involved in arousal from sleep apnea (173). However, the KF and PB are opioid-sensitive and may play a role in opioid-induced respiratory depression (82, 88).

Bötzinger Complex (BötC)

This region is associated with expiratory activity. Its constituent inhibitory interneurons send their axons throughout the respiratory medulla and to phrenic motor neurons (174–177). Some BötC neurons project to the pF_V (i.e., RTN) (177, 178). BötC neurons in rodent animal models are predominantly glycinergic (177, 179, 180), but also some are GABAergic (181, 182).

BötC neurons show either augmenting expiratory activity, i.e., their discharge rate increases during expiration (dubbed E-Aug), or decrementing activity that peaks during post-inspiration and then slows down during the remaining expiratory phase (dubbed E-Dec). Lung inflation excites E-Dec BötC neurons, yet it inhibits E-Aug BötC neurons (174, 183). E-Dec neurons clearly contribute to the Breuer-Hering inflation reflex. In the context of sensorimotor integration, the role of E-Aug neurons is less clear. In general, as inhibitory and expiratory interneurons, BötC neurons influence both rhythm and motor pattern. BötC neurons inhibit inspiratory activity during postinspiratory and late expiratory phases (184, 185). BötC neurons contribute to generating post-inspiration via their projections to KF (186). Stimulating BötC neurons slows breathing by shortening inspiration as well as (i) lengthening late expiration (187), (ii) prolonging post-inspiration (65), or (iii) prolonging both post-inspiration and late expiration (188).

BötC neurons constrain the expiratory rhythmogenic pF_L neurons under normoxic and normocapnic conditions (189).

Some posit that BötC inhibitory neurons form an integral part of a tripartite rhythmogenic circuit that also includes inhibitory neurons of the preBötC (190, 191). We do not advocate that mechanism, however, because multiple experimental interventions that block synaptic inhibition in the preBötC and BötC do not stop breathing *in vivo*, and in reduced preparations *in vitro* or *in situ* (117, 118, 192). Our view, consistent with all existing data sets, is that synaptic inhibition is an important modulator of breathing motor pattern. Bottom line: BötC neurons restrain active expiration under normal breathing conditions, and also influence via inhibition inspiratory activity in rhythmogenic and motor-related sites; BötC neurons promote phase transitions.

Nucleus of the Solitary Tract

NTS neurons are concentrated in the dorsal region of the lower medulla adjacent to the obex and area postrema (Figures 1.2 and 1.3). They are a collection of second-order sensory neurons often called the dorsal respiratory group (DRG). NTS neurons comprise a collection of subnuclei (commissural, medial, ventrolateral, etc.), which receive sensory inputs via CNs X and IX.

Slowly adapting pulmonary stretch receptor afferents of CN X communicate the distension of mechanoreceptors in the terminal bronchioles of the lung. *Rapidly adapting receptor* afferents detect lung inflation, too, as well as irritants like noxious gases, smoke, dusts, and cold air. Two classes of Aδ and C-fibers detect chemical substances in pulmonary and bronchial circulation. Afferents of CN IX pertain to oxygen levels in arterial blood and blood pressure.

Vagal Inputs and NTS Neurons

Slowly adapting pulmonary stretch receptor afferents are myelinated fibers that excite a class of NTS cells called *pump* neurons. The discharge frequency of afferents and pump neurons maps to lung inflation (193–195). NTS pump neurons mediate the Breuer-Hering reflex. During lung inflation, pump neurons inhibit inspiration via GABAergic projections to the preBötC and to the pF_V or RTN (196–200).

NTS neurons that respond to lung inflation like pump cells but also show rhythmic discharge in phase with inspiration are called I-ß (beta) neurons. Unlike pump neurons, they are excitatory and project to phrenic motor neurons (201). Given their inspiratory rhythmic firing pattern and excitatory projection to phrenic, they might be phrenic premotor neurons whose activity is modulated by stretch receptor feedback.

Rapidly adapting receptors are myelinated fibers, although less sensitive to lung inflation than their slowly adapting counterparts. Rapidly adapting irritant receptor afferents are excitatory and project throughout the medulla and pons (202, 203). The subset of those irritant relay neurons that also show inspiratory rhythmic activity are called I-γ (gamma) (204). In general, NTS neurons that receive irritant receptor afferents may not project directly to conventional rhythm and pattern generating parts of the central respiratory networks but rather to less well-known microcircuits that mediate airway-defense reflexes.

Unmyelinated C-fibers that project to the NTS are found throughout the lungs and airways. Bronchopulmonary C-fibers line the airways and blood vessels of bronchial and pulmonary circulation. Juxtacapillary (J-receptors) are found in the mesh of capillaries at the gas exchange site. Collectively these afferents detect acids, tissue damage, edema, as well as other irritating stimuli and can then trigger autonomic responses, cough, and apnea followed by tachypnea (195, 205, 206).

Glossopharyngeal Inputs and NTS Neurons

Specialized sensory organs that detect oxygen in the arterial blood and blood pressure are located in the carotid bodies and ascending aorta. Cells therein have properties like neurons and glia but also epithelial cells. We recommend contemporary reviews (207, 208). Their afferents ascend via the carotid sinus nerve of CN IX and synapse on NTS neurons in the commissural and medial subnuclei. Those neurons project to the central chemoreceptor site in the pF (RTN) (209), which makes sense physiologically since each set of neurons is tasked with modulating respiration based on key physiological factors (CO_2, pH, O_2, and blood pressure).

NTS Vocalization Neurons

A group of excitatory NTS neurons is essential for innate vocalization in mice (169), as mentioned above. While it is clear that lung and peripheral chemoreceptor afferents in the NTS are present in humans, whether a homologous vocalization-related subpopulation of NTS neurons exists in humans remains unknown.

CONCLUSIONS AND PERSPECTIVE

We show the known anatomy and connectivity of central sites that generate and control breathing. In addition, we recap the transcription factors and genetic substrates (when known) that influence the development and function of the respiratory neural network and provide an overview of diseases and syndromes that are attributable to dysfunction or abnormal development of respiratory regions and their interconnections. Our goal has been to provide the most up-to-date distillation of the corpus of knowledge gathered over the past 30 years into a useful overview of the respiratory system for the medical student, clinician, and researcher.

The neuroanatomy we have reviewed comes from studies predominantly in rodent models. So far, every mammalian species studied (rats, mice, cats, dogs, goats, bats, hamsters, sheep, and humans) has a preBötC. The phrenic nuclei and the *nucleus tractus solitarii* have also been found in numerous mammals. However, many other sites have only been described in rodent models and are not yet entered in the neuroanatomical atlases for humans. Nevertheless, we remain confident that the sites characterized in rodents will have analogs in the human respiratory neural control system.

By no means do we have a complete understanding of how respiratory rhythm is generated nor how chemo- and mechanoafferents modulate breathing—much less a comprehensive armamentarium to treat respiratory disease—but one should appreciate how well described the respiratory neural control system is and how that provides unique insight into this key physiological behavior.

Figure 1.7 shows an overview of the interrelationships between the respiratory regions we have discussed and their activity during inspiration and expiration, thus providing a simple overview of functional connections that are known based on the work we have cited in this chapter. We are confident that the advent of modern bioinformatics and genomic data science will further unravel the molecular and developmental mechanisms that form respiratory neural control networks. Thus, we anticipate an even deeper understanding of respiratory physiology and pathophysiology in the coming years. Breathing may be the first mammalian behavior whose neural bases are *truly* understood at multiple levels of analysis.

REFERENCES

1. The Writings of Hippocrates and Galen—Online Library of Liberty [Internet]. [cited 2020 May 20]. Available from: https://oll.libertyfund.org/titles/hippocrates-the-writings-of-hippocrates-and-galen

2. Finger S. Origins of Neuroscience: A History of Explorations into Brain Function. Oxford University Press; 2001. 462 p.

3. Finger S. Brain damage, development, and behavior: early findings. Dev Neuropsychol. 1991 Jan 1;7(3):261–74.

4. Cheung T. Limits of life and death: Legallois's decapitation experiments. J Hist Biol. 2013 Summer;46(2):283–313.

5. Furley DJ, Wilkie JS. Galen: On Respiration and the Arteries. Princeton University Press; 1984. 298 p.

6. Flourens M. Nouveaux eclaircissementss sur le noeud vital. Compte Rendu des Seacnes de L' Academie de Sciences. 1859;48:1136–8.

7. Lumsden T. The regulation of respiration: Part I. J Physiol. 1923 Oct 22;58(1):81–91.

8. Lumsden T. The regulation of respiration: Part II. Normal Type. J Physiol. 1923 Dec 28;58(2–3):111–26.

9. Lumsden T. Observations on the respiratory centres in the cat. J Physiol. 1923 Mar 21;57(3–4):153–60.

10. Mitchell RA, Loeschcke HH, Massion WH, Severinghaus JW. Respiratory responses mediated through superficial chemosensitive areas on the medulla. J Appl Physiol. 1963 May 1;18(3):523–33.

11. Schlaefke ME, See WR, Loeschcke HH. Ventilatory response to alterations of H+ ion concentration in small areas of the ventral medullary surface. Respir Physiol. 1970 Sep;10(2):198–212.

12. Schlaefke ME, Kille JF, Loeschcke HH. Elimination of central chemosensitivity by coagulation of a bilateral area on the ventral medullary surface in awake cats. Pflugers Arch. 1979 Jan 31;378(3):231–41.

13. Schlaefke ME, See WR, Herker-See A, Loeschcke HH. Respiratory response to hypoxia and hypercapnia after elimination of central chemosensitivity. Pflugers Arch. 1979 Sep;381(3):241–8.

14. Schläfke ME, Pokorski M, See WR, Prill RK, Loeschcke HH. Chemosensitive neurons on the ventral medullary surface. Bull Physiopathol Respir. 1975 Mar;11(2):277–84.

15. Miller AD, Bianchi AL, Bishop BP. Neural Control of the Respiratory Muscles. CRC Press; 2019. 320 p.

16. Fogarty MJ, Mantilla CB, Sieck GC. Breathing: motor control of diaphragm muscle. Physiology. 2018 Mar 1;33(2):113–26.

17. Mantilla CB, Sieck GC. Phrenic motor unit recruitment during ventilatory and non-ventilatory behaviors. Respir Physiol Neurobiol. 2011 Oct 15;179(1):57–63.

18. Seven YB, Mantilla CB, Sieck GC. Recruitment of rat diaphragm motor units across motor behaviors with different levels of diaphragm activation. J Appl Physiol. 2014 Dec 1;117(11):1308–16.

19. Sieck GC. Recruitment and Frequency Coding of Diaphragm Motor Units During Ventilatory and Non-Ventilatory Behaviors. In: Swanson GD, Grodins FS, Hughson RL, editors. Respiratory Control: A Modeling Perspective. Boston, MA: Springer US; 1989. p. 441–50.

20. Bieger D, Hopkins DA. Viscerotopic representation of the upper alimentary tract in the medulla oblongata in the rat: the nucleus ambiguus. J Comp Neurol. 1987 Aug 22;262(4):546–62.

21. Ruangkittisakul A, Schwarzacher SW, Secchia L, Poon BY, Ma Y, Funk GD, et al. High sensitivity to neuromodulator-activated signaling pathways at physiological [K+] of confocally imaged respiratory center neurons in on-line-calibrated newborn rat brainstem slices. J Neurosci. 2006 Nov 15;26(46):11870–80.

22. Ruangkittisakul A, Panaitescu B, Ballanyi K. K(+) and Ca^2(+) dependence of inspiratory-related rhythm in novel "calibrated" mouse brainstem slices. Respir Physiol Neurobiol. 2011 Jan 31;175(1):37–48.

23. Ruangkittisakul A, Kottick A, Picardo MCD, Ballanyi K, Del Negro CA. Identification of the pre-Bötzinger complex inspiratory center in calibrated "sandwich" slices from newborn mice with fluorescent Dbx1 interneurons. Physiol Rep [Internet]. 2014 Aug 1;2(8). Available from: http://dx.doi.org/10.14814/phy2.12111

24. Sakamoto Y. Morphological features of the branching pattern of the hypoglossal nerve. Anat Rec. 2019 Apr;302(4):558–67.

25. Wealing JC, Cholanian M, Flanigan EG, Levine RB, Fregosi RF. Diverse physiological properties of hypoglossal motoneurons innervating intrinsic and extrinsic tongue muscles. J Neurophysiol. 2019 Nov 1;122(5):2054–60.

26. Brozanski BS, Guthrie RD, Volk EA, Cameron WE. Postnatal growth of genioglossal motoneurons. Pediatr Pulmonol. 1989;7(3):133–9.

27. Núñez-Abades PA, He F, Barrionuevo G, Cameron WE. Morphology of developing rat genioglossal motoneurons studied in vitro: changes in length, branching pattern, and spatial distribution of dendrites. J Comp Neurol. 1994 Jan 15;339(3):401–20.

28. Mazza E, Núñez-Abades PA, Spielmann JM, Cameron WE. Anatomical and electrotonic coupling in developing genioglossal motoneurons of the rat. Brain Res. 1992 Dec 11;598(1–2):127–37.

29. Wu J, Capelli P, Bouvier J, Goulding M, Arber S, Fortin G. A V0 core neuronal circuit for inspiration. Nat Commun. 2017 Sep 15;8(1):544.

30. Koizumi H, Wilson CG, Wong S, Yamanishi T, Koshiya N, Smith JC. Functional imaging, spatial reconstruction, and biophysical analysis of a respiratory motor circuit isolated in vitro. J Neurosci. 2008 Mar 5;28(10):2353–65.

31. Revill AL, Vann NC, Akins VT, Kottick A, Gray PA, Del Negro CA, et al. Dbx1 precursor cells are a source of inspiratory XII premotoneurons. Elife [Internet]. 2015 Dec 19;4. Available from: http://dx.doi.org/10.7554/eLife.12301

32. Janczewski WA, Onimaru H, Homma I, Feldman JL. Opioid-resistant respiratory pathway from the preinspiratory neurones to abdominal muscles: in vivo and in vitro study in the newborn rat. J Physiol. 2002 Dec 15;545(3):1017–26.

33. Feldman JL, Loewy AD, Speck DF. Projections from the ventral respiratory group to phrenic and intercostal motoneurons in cat: an autoradiographic study. J Neurosci. 1985 Aug;5(8):1993–2000.

34. Onai T, Saji M, Miura M. Projections of supraspinal structures to the phrenic motor nucleus in rats studied by a horseradish peroxidase microinjection method. J Auton Nerv Syst. 1987 Dec;21(2–3):233–9.

35. Ellenberger HH, Feldman JL. Monosynaptic transmission of respiratory drive to phrenic motoneurons from brainstem bulbospinal neurons in rats. J Comp Neurol. 1988 Mar 1;269(1):47–57.

36. Smith JC, Morrison DE, Ellenberger HH, Otto MR, Feldman JL. Brainstem projections to the major respiratory neuron populations in the medulla of the cat. J Comp Neurol. 1989 Mar 1;281(1):69–96.

37. Zhan WZ, Ellenberger HH, Feldman JL. Monoaminergic and GABAergic terminations in phrenic nucleus of rat identified by immunohistochemical labeling. Neuroscience. 1989;31(1):105–13.

38. Ellenberger HH, Feldman JL. Subnuclear organization of the lateral tegmental field of the rat. I: nucleus ambiguus and ventral respiratory group. J Comp Neurol. 1990 Apr 8;294(2):202–11.

39. Ellenberger HH, Feldman JL, Zhan WZ. Subnuclear organization of the lateral tegmental field of the rat. II: catecholamine neurons and ventral respiratory group. J Comp Neurol. 1990 Apr 8;294(2):212–22.

40. Wang H, Stornetta RL, Rosin DL, Guyenet PG. Neurokinin-1 receptor-immunoreactive neurons of the ventral respiratory group in the rat. J Comp Neurol. 2001 May 28;434(2):128–46.

41. Guyenet PG, Sevigny CP, Weston MC, Stornetta RL. Neurokinin-1 receptor-expressing cells of the ventral respiratory group are functionally heterogeneous and predominantly glutamatergic. J Neurosci. 2002 May 1;22(9):3806–16.

42. Stornetta RL, Rosin DL, Wang H, Sevigny CP, Weston MC, Guyenet PG. A group of glutamatergic interneurons expressing high levels of both neurokinin-1 receptors and somatostatin identifies the region of the pre-Bötzinger complex. J Comp Neurol. 2003 Jan 20;455(4):499–512.

43. Gray PA, Rekling JC, Bocchiaro CM, Feldman JL. Modulation of respiratory frequency by peptidergic input to rhythmogenic neurons in the preBötzinger complex. Science. 1999 Nov;286:1566–8.

44. Merrill EG, Fedorko L. Monosynaptic inhibition of phrenic motoneurons: a long descending projection from Bötzinger neurons. J Neurosci. 1984 Sep;4(9):2350–3.

45. Duffin J, Tian GF, Peever JH. Functional synaptic connections among respiratory neurons. Respir Physiol. 2000 Sep;122(2–3):237–46.

46. Lindsey BG, Segers LS, Shannon R. Discharge patterns of rostrolateral medullary expiratory neurons in the cat: regulation by concurrent network processes. J Neurophysiol. 1989 Jun;61(6):1185–96.

47. Segers LS, Nuding SC, Dick TE, Shannon R, Baekey DM, Solomon IC, et al. Functional connectivity in the pontomedullary respiratory network. J Neurophysiol. 2008 Oct;100(4):1749–69.

48. Stanek E 4th, Cheng S, Takatoh J, Han B-X, Wang F. Monosynaptic premotor circuit tracing reveals neural substrates for oro-motor coordination. Elife. 2014 Apr 30;3:e02511.

49. Funk GD, Smith JC, Feldman JC. Modulation of neural network activity in vitro by cyclothiazide, a drug that blocks desensitization of AMPA receptors. J Neurosci. 1995;15:4046–56.

50. Ono T, Ishiwata Y, Inaba N, Kuroda T, Nakamura Y. Hypoglossal premotor neurons with rhythmical inspiratory-related activity in the cat: localization and projection to the phrenic nucleus. Exp Brain Res. 1994;98:1–12.

51. Dobbins EG, Feldman JL. Differential innervation of protruder and retractor muscles of the tongue in rat. J Comp Neurol. 1995 Jul 3;357(3):376–94.

52. Shen L, Peever JH, Duffin J. Bilateral coordination of inspiratory neurones in the rat. Pflugers Arch. 2002 Mar;443(5–6):829–35.

53. Miller AD, Ezure K, Suzuki I. Control of abdominal muscles by brain stem respiratory neurons in the cat. J Neurophysiol. 1985 Jul;54(1):155–67.

54. Arita H, Kogo N, Koshiya N. Morphological and physiological properties of caudal medullary expiratory neurons of the cat. Brain Res. 1987 Jan 20;401(2):258–66.

55. Billig I, Foris JM, Enquist LW, Card JP, Yates BJ. Definition of neuronal circuitry controlling the activity of phrenic and abdominal motoneurons in the ferret using recombinant strains of pseudorabies virus. J Neurosci. 2000 Oct 1;20(19):7446–54.

56. Vanderhorst VG, Terasawa E, Ralston HJ 3rd, Holstege G. Monosynaptic projections from the nucleus retroambiguus to motoneurons supplying the abdominal wall, axial, hindlimb, and pelvic floor muscles in the female rhesus monkey. J Comp Neurol. 2000 Aug 21;424(2):233–50.

57. Sasaki SI, Uchino H, Uchino Y. Axon branching of medullary expiratory neurons in the lumbar and the sacral spinal cord of the cat. Brain Res. 1994 Jun 20;648(2):229–38.

58. Iscoe S. Control of abdominal muscles. Prog Neurobiol. 1998 Nov;56(4):433–506.

59. Smith JC, Ellenberger HH, Ballanyi K, Richter DW, Feldman JL. Pre-Bötzinger complex: a brainstem region that may generate respiratory rhythm in mammals. Science. 1991 Nov 1;254(5032):726–9.

60. Guyenet PG, Wang H. Pre-Bötzinger neurons with preinspiratory discharges "in vivo" express NK1 receptors in the rat. J Neurophysiol. 2001 Jul;86(1):438–46.

61. Liu Y-Y, Ju G, Wong–Riley MTT. Distribution and colocalization of neurotransmitters and receptors in the pre-Bötzinger complex of rats. J Appl Physiol. 2001 Sep;91(3):1387–95.

62. Liu Y-Y, Wong-Riley MTT, Liu J-P, Wei X-Y, Jia Y, Liu H-L, et al. Substance P and enkephalinergic synapses onto neurokinin-1 receptor-immunoreactive neurons in the pre-Bötzinger complex of rats. Eur J Neurosci. 2004 Jan;19(1):65–75.

63. Wei X-Y, Zhao Y, Wong-Riley MTT, Ju G, Liu Y-Y. Synaptic relationship between somatostatin- and neurokinin-1 receptor-immunoreactive neurons in the pre-Bötzinger complex of rats. J Neurochem. 2012 Sep;122(5):923–33.

64. Pagliardini S, Adachi T, Ren J, Funk GD, Greer JJ. Fluorescent tagging of rhythmically active respiratory neurons within the pre-Bötzinger complex of rat medullary slice preparations. J Neurosci. 2005 Mar 9;25(10):2591–6.

65. Fong AY, Potts JT. Neurokinin-1 receptor activation in Botzinger complex evokes bradypnoea. J Physiol. 2006 Sep 15;575(Pt 3):869–85.

66. Ptak K, Yamanishi T, Aungst J, Milescu LS, Zhang R, Richerson GB, et al. Raphé neurons stimulate respiratory circuit activity by multiple mechanisms via endogenously released serotonin and substance P. J Neurosci. 2009 Mar 25;29(12):3720–37.

67. Baertsch NA, Ramirez J-M. Insights into the dynamic control of breathing revealed through cell-type-specific responses to substance P. Elife [Internet]. 2019 Dec 5;8. Available from: http://dx.doi.org/10.7554/eLife.51350

68. Hayes JA, Del Negro CA. Neurokinin receptor-expressing pre-botzinger complex neurons in neonatal mice studied in vitro. J Neurophysiol. 2007 Jun;97(6):4215–24.

69. Yeh S-Y, Huang W-H, Wang W, Ward CS, Chao ES, Wu Z, et al. Respiratory network stability and modulatory response to substance P require Nalcn. Neuron. 2017 Apr 19;94(2):294–303.e4.

70. Gray PA, Janczewski WA, Mellen N, McCrimmon DR, Feldman JL. Normal breathing requires preBötzinger complex neurokinin-1 receptor-expressing neurons. Nat Neurosci. 2001 Sep;4(9):927–30.

71. McKay LC, Janczewski WA, Feldman JL. Sleep-disordered breathing after targeted ablation of preBötzinger complex neurons. Nat Neurosci. 2005 Sep;8(9):1142–4.

72. Wang H, Germanson TP, Guyenet PG. Depressor and tachypneic responses to chemical stimulation of the ventral respiratory group are reduced by ablation of neurokinin-1 receptor-expressing neurons. J Neurosci. 2002 May 1;22(9):3755–64.

73. St John WM. Medullary regions for neurogenesis of gasping: noeud vital or noeuds vitals? J Appl Physiol. 1996 Nov;81(5):1865–77.

74. Brockhaus J, Ballanyi K, Smith JC, Richter DW. Microenvironment of respiratory neurons in the in vitro brainstem-spinal cord of neonatal rats. J Physiol. 1993;462:421–45.

75. Hill AA, Garcia AJ 3rd, Zanella S, Upadhyaya R, Ramirez JM. Graded reductions in oxygenation evoke graded reconfiguration of the isolated respiratory network. J Neurophysiol. 2011 Feb;105(2):625–39.

76. Suzue T. Respiratory rhythm generation in the in vitro brain stem-spinal cord preparation of the neonatal rat. J Physiol. 1984 Sep;354:173–83.

77. Smith JC, Greer JJ Liu GS, Feldman JL. Neural mechanisms generating respiratory pattern in mammalian brain stem-spinal cord in vitro. I. Spatiotemporal patterns of motor and medullary neuron activity. J Neurophysiol. 1990 Oct;64(4):1149–69.

78. Pattinson KTS. Opioids and the control of respiration. Br J Anaesth. 2008 Jun;100(6):747–58.

79. Hall AJ, Logan JE, Toblin RL, Kaplan JA, Kraner JC, Bixler D, et al. Patterns of abuse among unintentional pharmaceutical overdose fatalities. JAMA. 2008 Dec 10;300(22):2613–20.

80. Takeda S, Eriksson LI, Yamamoto Y, Joensen H, Onimaru H, Lindahl SG. Opioid action on respiratory neuron activity of the isolated respiratory network in newborn rats. Anesthesiology. 2001 Sep;95(3):740–9.

81. Montandon G, Qin W, Liu H, Ren J, Greer JJ, Horner RL. PreBötzinger complex neurokinin-1 receptor-expressing neurons mediate opioid-induced respiratory depression. J Neurosci. 2011 Jan 26;31(4):1292–301.

82. Bachmutsky I, Wei XP, Kish E, Yackle K. Opioids depress breathing through two small brainstem sites. Elife [Internet]. 2020 Feb 19;9. Available from: http://dx.doi.org/10.7554/eLife.52694

83. Sun X, Thörn Pérez C, Halemani D N, Shao XM, Greenwood M, Heath S, et al. Opioids modulate an emergent rhythmogenic process to depress breathing. Elife [Internet]. 2019 Dec 16;8. Available from: http://dx.doi.org/10.7554/eLife.50613

84. Montandon G, Ren J, Victoria NC, Liu H, Wickman K, Greer JJ, et al. G-protein-gated inwardly rectifying potassium channels modulate respiratory depression by opioids. Anesthesiology. 2016 Mar;124(3):641–50.

85. Ballanyi K, Ruangkittisakul A, Onimaru H. Opioids prolong and anoxia shortens delay between onset of preinspiratory (pFRG) and inspiratory (preBötC) network bursting in newborn rat brainstems. Pflugers Arch. 2009 Jul;458(3):571–87.

86. Ballanyi K, Panaitescu B, Ruangkittisakul A. Indirect opioid actions on inspiratory pre-Bötzinger complex neurons in newborn rat brainstem slices. Adv Exp Med Biol. 2010;669:75–9.

87. Wei AD, Ramirez J-M. Presynaptic mechanisms and KCNQ potassium channels modulate opioid depression of respiratory drive. Front Physiol. 2019 Nov 22;10:1407.

88. Varga AG, Reid BT, Kieffer BL, Levitt ES. Differential impact of two critical respiratory centres in opioid-induced respiratory depression in awake mice. J Physiol. 2020 Jan;598(1):189–205.

89. Haouzi P, Guck D, McCann M, Sternick M, Sonobe T, Tubbs N. Severe hypoxemia prevents spontaneous and naloxone-induced breathing recovery after fentanyl overdose in awake and sedated rats. Anesthesiology. 2020 May;132(5):1138–50.

90. Rudd RA, Aleshire N, Zibbell JE, Gladden RM. Increases in drug and opioid overdose deaths–United States, 2000–2014. MMWR Morb Mortal Wkly Rep. 2016 Jan 1;64(50–51):1378–82.

91. Scholl L, Seth P, Kariisa M, Wilson N, Baldwin G. Drug and opioid-involved overdose deaths—United States, 2013–2017. MMWR Morb Mortal Wkly Rep. 2018 Jan 4;67(5152):1419–27.

92. Boyer EW. Management of opioid analgesic overdose. N Engl J Med. 2012 Jul 12;367(2):146–55.

93. Volkow ND, Jones EB, Einstein EB, Wargo EM. Prevention and treatment of opioid misuse and addiction: a review. JAMA Psychiatry. 2019 Feb 1;76(2):208–16.

94. Tan W, Janczewski WA, Yang P, Shao XM, Callaway EM, Feldman JL. Silencing preBötzinger complex somatostatin-expressing neurons induces persistent apnea in awake rat. Nat Neurosci. 2008 May;11(5):538–40.

95. Cui Y, Kam K, Sherman D, Janczewski WA, Zheng Y, Feldman JL. Defining preBötzinger complex rhythm- and pattern-generating neural microcircuits in vivo. Neuron. 2016 Aug 3;91(3):602–14.

96. Ashhad S, Feldman JL. Emergent elements of inspiratory rhythmogenesis: network synchronization and synchrony propagation. Neuron. 2020 May 6;106(3):482–97.e4.

97. Funk GD, Smith JC, Feldman JL. Generation and transmission of respiratory oscillations in medullary slices: role of excitatory amino acids. J Neurophysiol. 1993;70:1491–515.

98. Rekling JC, Shao XM, Feldman JL. Electrical coupling and excitatory synaptic transmission between rhythmogenic respiratory neurons in the preBötzinger complex. J Neurosci. 2000 Dec 1;20(23):RC113.

99. Kam K, Worrell JW, Janczewski WA, Cui Y, Feldman JL. Distinct inspiratory rhythm and pattern generating mechanisms in the preBötzinger complex. J Neurosci. 2013 May 29;33(22):9235–45.

100. Kam K, Worrell JW, Ventalon C, Emiliani V, Feldman JL. Emergence of population bursts from simultaneous activation of small subsets of preBötzinger complex inspiratory neurons. J Neurosci. 2013 Feb 20;33(8):3332–8.

101. Kallurkar PS, Grover C, Picardo MCD, Del Negro CA. Evaluating the burstlet theory of inspiratory rhythm and pattern generation. eNeuro [Internet]. 2020 Jan 15;7(1). Available from: http://dx.doi.org/10.1523/ENEURO.0314-19.2019

102. Gray PA, Hayes JA, Ling GY, Llona I, Tupal S, Picardo MCD, et al. Developmental origin of preBötzinger complex respiratory neurons. J Neurosci. 2010 Nov 3;30(44):14883–95.

103. Picardo MCD, Weragalaarachchi KTH, Akins VT, Del Negro CA. Physiological and morphological properties of Dbx1-derived respiratory neurons in the pre-Botzinger complex of neonatal mice. J Physiol. 2013 May 15;591(10):2687–703.

104. Wang X, Hayes JA, Revill AL, Song H, Kottick A, Vann NC, et al. Laser ablation of Dbx1 neurons in the pre-Bötzinger complex stops inspiratory rhythm and impairs output in neonatal mice. Elife. 2014 Jul 15;3:e03427.

105. Vann NC, Pham FD, Hayes JA, Kottick A, Del Negro CA. Transient suppression of Dbx1 preBötzinger interneurons disrupts breathing in adult mice. PLoS One. 2016 Sep 9;11(9):e0162418.

106. Vann NC, Pham FD, Dorst KE, Del Negro CA. Dbx1 pre-Bötzinger complex interneurons comprise the core inspiratory oscillator for breathing in unanesthetized adult mice. eNeuro [Internet]. 2018 May;5(3). Available from: http://dx.doi.org/10.1523/ENEURO.0130-18.2018

107. Baertsch NA, Baertsch HC, Ramirez JM. The interdependence of excitation and inhibition for the control of dynamic breathing rhythms. Nat Commun. 2018 Feb 26;9(1):843.

108. Pierani A, Moran-Rivard L, Sunshine MJ, Littman DR, Goulding M, Jessell TM. Control of interneuron fate in the developing spinal cord by the progenitor homeodomain protein Dbx1. Neuron. 2001 Feb;29(2):367–84.

109. Bouvier J, Thoby-Brisson M, Renier N, Dubreuil V, Ericson J, Champagnat J, et al. Hindbrain interneurons and axon guidance signaling critical for breathing. Nat Neurosci. 2010 Sep;13(9):1066–74.

110. Kottick A, Martin CA, Del Negro CA. Fate mapping neurons and glia derived from Dbx1-expressing progenitors in mouse preBötzinger complex. Physiol Rep [Internet]. 2017 Jun;5(11). Available from: http://dx.doi.org/10.14814/phy2.13300

111. Song H, Hayes JA, Vann NC, Wang X, LaMar MD, Del Negro CA. Functional interactions between mammalian respiratory rhythmogenic and premotor circuitry. J Neurosci. 2016 Jul 6;36(27):7223–33.

112. Shao XM, Feldman JL. Respiratory rhythm generation and synaptic inhibition of expiratory neurons in pre-Bötzinger complex: differential roles of glycinergic and GABAergic neural transmission. J Neurophysiol. 1997 Apr;77(4):1853–60.

113. Kuwana S-I, Tsunekawa N, Yanagawa Y, Okada Y, Kuribayashi J, Obata K. Electrophysiological and morphological characteristics of GABAergic respiratory neurons in the mouse pre-Bötzinger complex. Eur J Neurosci. 2006 Feb;23(3):667–74.

114. Winter SM, Fresemann J, Schnell C, Oku Y, Hirrlinger J, Hülsmann S. Glycinergic interneurons are functionally integrated into the inspiratory network of mouse medullary slices. Pflugers Arch. 2009 Jul;458(3):459–69.

115. Morgado-Valle C, Baca SM, Feldman JL. Glycinergic pacemaker neurons in preBötzinger complex of neonatal mouse. J Neurosci. 2010 Mar 10;30(10):3634–9.

116. Yang CF, Feldman JL. Efferent projections of excitatory and inhibitory preBötzinger complex neurons. J Comp Neurol. 2018 Jun 1;526(8):1389–402.

117. Janczewski WA, Tashima A, Hsu P, Cui Y, Feldman JL. Role of inhibition in respiratory pattern generation. J Neurosci. 2013 Mar 27;33(13):5454–65.

118. Sherman D, Worrell JW, Cui Y, Feldman JL. Optogenetic perturbation of preBötzinger complex inhibitory neurons modulates respiratory pattern. Nat Neurosci. 2015 Mar;18(3):408–14.

119. Koizumi H, Koshiya N, Chia JX, Cao F, Nugent J, Zhang R, et al. Structural-functional properties of identified excitatory and inhibitory interneurons within pre-Botzinger complex respiratory microcircuits. J Neurosci. 2013 Feb 13;33(7):2994–3009.

120. Cregg JM, Chu KA, Dick TE, Landmesser LT, Silver J. Phasic inhibition as a mechanism for generation of rapid respiratory rhythms. Proc Natl Acad Sci U S A. 2017 Nov 28;114(48):12815–20.

121. Ren J, Poon BY, Tang Y, Funk GD, Greer JJ. Ampakines alleviate respiratory depression in rats. Am J Respir Crit Care Med. 2006 Dec 15;174(12):1384–91.

122. Ren J, Lenal F, Yang M, Ding X, Greer JJ. Coadministration of the AMPAKINE CX717 with propofol reduces respiratory depression and fatal apneas. Anesthesiology. 2013 Jun;118(6):1437–45.

123. Ren J, Ding X, Greer JJ. Ampakines enhance weak endogenous respiratory drive and alleviate apnea in perinatal rats. Am J Respir Crit Care Med. 2015 Mar 15;191(6):704–10.

124. Ren J, Ding X, Funk GD, Greer JJ. Ampakine CX717 protects against fentanyl-induced respiratory depression and lethal apnea in rats. Anesthesiology. 2009 Jun;110(6):1364–70.

125. Schwarzacher SW, Rüb U, Deller T. Neuroanatomical characteristics of the human pre-Bötzinger complex and its involvement in neurodegenerative brainstem diseases. Brain. 2011 Jan;134(Pt 1):24–35.

126. Onimaru H, Homma I. Respiratory rhythm generator neurons in medulla of brainstem-spinal cord preparation from newborn rat. Brain Res. 1987 Feb 17;403(2):380–4.

127. Onimaru H, Arata A, Homma I. Primary respiratory rhythm generator in the medulla of brainstem-spinal cord preparation from newborn rat. Brain Res. 1988 Apr 5;445(2):314–24.

128. Onimaru H, Arata A, Homma I. Firing properties of respiratory rhythm generating neurons in the absence of synaptic transmission in rat medulla in vitro. Exp Brain Res. 1989;76(3):530–6.

129. Arata A, Onimaru H, Homma I. Respiration-related neurons in the ventral medulla of newborn rats in vitro. Brain Res Bull. 1990 Apr;24(4):599–604.

130. Onimaru H, Homma I. Whole cell recordings from respiratory neurons in the medulla of brainstem-spinal cord preparations isolated from newborn rats. Pflugers Arch. 1992 Mar;420(3–4):399–406.

131. Johnson SM, Smith JC, Funk GD, Feldman JL. Pacemaker behavior of respiratory neurons in medullary slices from neonatal rat. J Neurophysiol. 1994 Dec;72(6):2598–608.

132. Rekling JC, Champagnat J, Denavit-Saubié M. Electroresponsive properties and membrane potential trajectories of three types of inspiratory neurons in the newborn mouse brain stem in vitro. J Neurophysiol. 1996 Feb;75(2):795–810.

133. Mellen NM, Janczewski WA, Bocchiaro CM, Feldman JL. Opioid-induced quantal slowing reveals dual networks for respiratory rhythm generation. Neuron. 2003 Mar;37(5):821–6.

134. Janczewski WA, Feldman JL. Distinct rhythm generators for inspiration and expiration in the juvenile rat. J Physiol. 2006 Jan 15;570(Pt 2):407–20.

135. Pagliardini S, Janczewski WA, Tan W, Dickson CT, Deisseroth K, Feldman JL. Active expiration induced by excitation of ventral medulla in adult anesthetized rats. J Neurosci. 2011 Feb 23;31(8):2895–905.

136. Pagliardini S, Greer JJ, Funk GD, Dickson CT. State-dependent modulation of breathing in urethane-anesthetized rats. J Neurosci. 2012 Aug 15;32(33):11259–70.

137. Huckstepp RTR, Cardoza KP, Henderson LE, Feldman JL. Role of parafacial nuclei in control of breathing in adult rats. J Neurosci. 2015 Jan 21;35(3):1052–67.

138. Huckstepp RT, Henderson LE, Cardoza KP, Feldman JL. Interactions between respiratory oscillators in adult rats. Elife [Internet]. 2016 Jun 14;5. Available from: http://dx.doi.org/10.7554/eLife.14203

139. Boutin RCT, Alsahafi Z, Pagliardini S. Cholinergic modulation of the parafacial respiratory group. J Physiol. 2017 Feb 15;595(4):1377–92.

140. Saini JK, Pagliardini S. Breathing during sleep in the postnatal period of rats: the contribution of active expiration. Sleep [Internet]. 2017 Dec 1;40(12). Available from: http://dx.doi.org/10.1093/sleep/zsx172

141. Feldman JL, Del Negro CA. Looking for inspiration: new perspectives on respiratory rhythm. Nat Rev Neurosci. 2006 Mar;7(3):232–42.

142. Jacquin TD, Borday V, Schneider-Maunoury S, Topilko P, Ghilini G, Kato F, et al. Reorganization of pontine rhythmogenic neuronal networks in Krox-20 knockout mice. Neuron. 1996 Oct;17(4):747–58.

143. Rose MF, Ren J, Ahmad KA, Chao H-T, Klisch TJ, Flora A, et al. Math1 is essential for the development of hindbrain neurons critical for perinatal breathing. Neuron. 2009 Nov 12;64(3):341–54.

144. Thoby-Brisson M, Karlén M, Wu N, Charnay P, Champagnat J, Fortin G. Genetic identification of an embryonic parafacial oscillator coupling to the preBötzinger complex. Nat Neurosci. 2009 Aug;12(8):1028–35.

145. Stornetta RL, Moreira TS, Takakura AC, Kang BJ, Chang DA, West GH, et al. Expression of Phox2b by brainstem neurons involved in chemosensory integration in the adult rat. J Neurosci. 2006 Oct 4;26(40):10305–14.

146. Kang BJ, Chang DA, Mackay DD, West GH, Moreira TS, Takakura AC, et al. Central nervous system distribution of the transcription factor Phox2b in the adult rat. J Comp Neurol. 2007 Aug 10;503(5):627–41.

147. Ikeda K, Takahashi M, Sato S, Igarashi H, Ishizuka T, Yawo H, et al. A Phox2b BAC transgenic rat line useful for understanding respiratory rhythm generator neural circuitry. PLoS One. 2015 Jul 6;10(7):e0132475.

148. Onimaru H, Ikeda K, Kawakami K. CO_2-sensitive preinspiratory neurons of the parafacial respiratory group express Phox2b in the neonatal rat. J Neurosci. 2008 Nov 26;28(48):12845–50.

149. Mulkey DK, Stornetta RL, Weston MC, Simmons JR, Parker A, Bayliss DA, et al. Respiratory control by ventral surface chemoreceptor neurons in rats. Nat Neurosci. 2004 Dec;7(12):1360–9.

150. Ruffault P-L, D'Autréaux F, Hayes JA, Nomaksteinsky M, Autran S, Fujiyama T, et al. The retrotrapezoid nucleus neurons expressing Atoh1 and Phox2b are essential for the respiratory response to CO_2. Elife [Internet]. 2015 Apr 13;4. Available from: http://dx.doi.org/10.7554/eLife.07051

151. Kumar NN, Velic A, Soliz J, Shi Y, Li K, Wang S, et al. PHYSIOLOGY. Regulation of breathing by CO_2 requires the proton-activated receptor GPR4 in retrotrapezoid nucleus neurons. Science. 2015 Jun 12;348(6240):1255–60.

152. Guyenet PG, Bayliss DA. Neural control of breathing and CO_2 homeostasis. Neuron. 2015 Sep 2;87(5):946–61.

153. Hawryluk JM, Moreira TS, Takakura AC, Wenker IC, Tzingounis AV, Mulkey DK. KCNQ channels determine serotonergic modulation of ventral surface chemoreceptors and respiratory drive. J Neurosci. 2012 Nov 21;32(47):16943–52.

154. Mulkey DK, Hawkins VE, Hawryluk JM, Takakura AC, Moreira TS, Tzingounis AV. Molecular underpinnings of ventral surface chemoreceptor function: focus on KCNQ channels. J Physiol (Lond) [Internet]. 2015 Jan 21. Available from: http://dx.doi.org/10.1113/jphysiol.2014.286500

155. Funk GD, Rajani V, Alvares TS, Revill AL, Zhang Y, Chu NY, et al. Neuroglia and their roles in central respiratory control; an overview. Comp Biochem Physiol A Mol Integr Physiol. 2015 Aug;186:83–95.

156. Gourine AV, Kasymov V, Marina N, Tang F, Figueiredo MF, Lane S, et al. Astrocytes control breathing through pH-dependent release of ATP. Science. 2010 Jul 30;329(5991):571–5.

157. Wenker IC, Kréneisz O, Nishiyama A, Mulkey DK. Astrocytes in the retrotrapezoid nucleus sense H^+ by inhibition of a Kir4.1-Kir5.1-like current and may contribute to chemoreception by a purinergic mechanism. J Neurophysiol. 2010 Dec;104(6):3042–52.

158. Turovsky E, Theparambil SM, Kasymov V, Deitmer JW, Del Arroyo AG, Ackland GL, et al. Mechanisms of CO_2/H^+ sensitivity of astrocytes. J Neurosci. 2016 Oct 19;36(42):10750–8.

159. Abbott SBG, Stornetta RL, Fortuna MG, Depuy SD, West GH, Harris TE, et al. Photostimulation of retrotrapezoid nucleus Phox2b-expressing neurons in vivo produces long-lasting activation of breathing in rats. J Neurosci. 2009 May 6;29(18):5806–19.

160. Marina N, Abdala AP, Trapp S, Li A, Nattie EE, Hewinson J, et al. Essential role of Phox2b-expressing ventrolateral brainstem neurons in the chemosensory control of inspiration and expiration. J Neurosci. 2010 Sep 15;30(37):12466–73.

161. Abbott SBG, Stornetta RL, Coates MB, Guyenet PG. Phox2b-expressing neurons of the parafacial region regulate breathing rate, inspiration, and expiration in conscious rats. J Neurosci. 2011 Nov 9;31(45):16410–22.

162. Smith FG, Klinkefus JM, Kopp UC, Robillard JE. Novel recordings of renal sympathetic nerve activity

in conscious fetal sheep and newborn lambs. Am J Physiol. 1990 Jan;258(1 Pt 2):F218–21.

163. Paton JF. The ventral medullary respiratory network of the mature mouse studied in a working heart-brainstem preparation. J Physiol. 1996 Jun 15;493 (Pt 3):819–31.

164. Dutschmann M, Herbert H. The Kölliker-Fuse nucleus gates the postinspiratory phase of the respiratory cycle to control inspiratory off-switch and upper airway resistance in rat. Eur J Neurosci. 2006 Aug;24(4):1071–84.

165. Dutschmann M, Dick TE. Pontine mechanisms of respiratory control. Compr Physiol. 2012 Oct;2(4):2443–69.

166. Jenkin SEM, Milsom WK, Zoccal DB. The Kölliker-Fuse nucleus acts as a timekeeper for late-expiratory abdominal activity. Neuroscience. 2017 Apr 21;348:63–72.

167. Barnett WH, Jenkin SEM, Milsom WK, Paton JFR, Abdala AP, Molkov YI, et al. The Kölliker-Fuse nucleus orchestrates the timing of expiratory abdominal nerve bursting. J Neurophysiol. 2018 Feb 1;119(2):401–12.

168. Tupal S, Huang W-H, Picardo MCD, Ling G-Y, Del Negro CA, Zoghbi HY, et al. Atoh1-dependent rhombic lip neurons are required for temporal delay between independent respiratory oscillators in embryonic mice. Elife. 2014 May 14;3:e02265.

169. Hernandez-Miranda LR, Ruffault P-L, Bouvier JC, Murray AJ, Morin-Surun M-P, Zampieri N, et al. Genetic identification of a hindbrain nucleus essential for innate vocalization. Proc Natl Acad Sci U S A. 2017 Jul 25;114(30):8095–100.

170. Anderson TM, Garcia AJ 3rd, Baertsch NA, Pollak J, Bloom JC, Wei AD, et al. A novel excitatory network for the control of breathing. Nature. 2016 Aug 4;536(7614):76–80.

171. Toor RUAS, Sun Q-J, Kumar NN, Le S, Hildreth CM, Phillips JK, et al. Neurons in the intermediate reticular nucleus coordinate postinspiratory activity, swallowing, and respiratory-sympathetic coupling in the rat. J Neurosci. 2019 Dec 4;39(49):9757–66.

172. Dhingra RR, Dick TE, Furuya WI, Galán RF, Dutschmann M. Volumetric mapping of the functional neuroanatomy of the respiratory network in the perfused brainstem preparation of rats. J Physiol. 2020 Jun;598(11):2061–79.

173. Caille D, Vibert J-F, Hugelin A. Apneusis and apnea after parabrachial or Kölliker-Fuse N. lesion; influence of wakefulness. Respir Physiol. 1981 Jul;45(1):79–95.

174. Ezure K, Manabe M. Decrementing expiratory neurons of the Bötzinger complex. II. Direct inhibitory synaptic linkage with ventral respiratory group neurons. Exp Brain Res. 1988;72(1):159–66.

175. Jiang C, Lipski J. Extensive monosynaptic inhibition of ventral respiratory group neurons by augmenting neurons in the Bötzinger complex in the cat. Exp Brain Res. 1990;81(3):639–48.

176. Tian GF, Peever JH, Duffin J. Bötzinger-complex expiratory neurons monosynaptically inhibit phrenic motoneurons in the decerebrate rat. Exp Brain Res. 1998 Sep;122(2):149–56.

177. Ezure K, Tanaka I, Kondo M. Glycine is used as a transmitter by decrementing expiratory neurons of the ventrolateral medulla in the rat. J Neurosci. 2003 Oct 1;23(26):8941–8.

178. Rosin DL, Chang DA, Guyenet PG. Afferent and efferent connections of the rat retrotrapezoid nucleus. J Comp Neurol. 2006 Nov 1;499(1):64–89.

179. Schreihofer AM, Stornetta RL, Guyenet PG. Evidence for glycinergic respiratory neurons: Bötzinger neurons express mRNA for glycinergic transporter 2. J Comp Neurol. 1999 May 17;407(4):583–97.

180. Tanaka I, Ezure K, Kondo M. Distribution of glycine transporter 2 mRNA-containing neurons in relation to glutamic acid decarboxylase mRNA-containing neurons in rat medulla. Neurosci Res. 2003 Oct;47(2):139–51.

181. Livingston CA, Berger AJ. Immunocytochemical localization of GABA in neurons projecting to the ventrolateral nucleus of the solitary tract. Brain Res. 1989 Aug 7;494(1):143–50.

182. Krolo M, Stuth EA, Tonkovic-Capin M, Hopp FA, McCrimmon DR, Zuperku EJ. Relative magnitude of tonic and phasic synaptic excitation of medullary inspiratory neurons in dogs. Am J Physiol Regul Integr Comp Physiol. 2000 Aug;279(2):R639–49.

183. Hayashi F, Coles SK, McCrimmon DR. Respiratory neurons mediating the Breuer-Hering reflex prolongation of expiration in rat. J Neurosci. 1996 Oct 15;16(20):6526–36.

184. Ezure K. Synaptic connections between medullary respiratory neurons and considerations on the genesis of respiratory rhythm. Prog Neurobiol. 1990;35(6):429–50.

185. Ezure K, Tanaka I, Saito Y. Activity of brainstem respiratory neurones just before the expiration-inspiration transition in the rat. J Physiol. 2003 Mar 1;547(Pt 2):629–40.

186. Ezure K, Tanaka I, Saito Y. Brainstem and spinal projections of augmenting expiratory neurons in the rat. Neurosci Res. 2003 Jan;45(1):41–51.

187. Monnier A, Alheid GF, McCrimmon DR. Defining ventral medullary respiratory compartments with a glutamate receptor agonist in the rat. J Physiol. 2003 May 1;548(Pt 3):859–74.

188. Fortuna MG, Kügler S, Hülsmann S. Probing the function of glycinergic neurons in the mouse respiratory network using optogenetics. Respir Physiol Neurobiol. 2019 Jul;265:141–52.

189. Flor KC, Barnett WH, Karlen-Amarante M, Molkov YI, Zoccal DB. Inhibitory control of active expiration by the Bötzinger complex in rats. J Physiol. 2020 Nov;598(21):4969–94.

190. Smith JC, Abdala APL, Koizumi H, Rybak IA, Paton JFR. Spatial and functional architecture of the mammalian brain stem respiratory network: a hierarchy of three oscillatory mechanisms. J Neurophysiol. 2007 Dec;98(6):3370–87.

191. Ausborn J, Koizumi H, Barnett WH, John TT, Zhang R, Molkov YI, et al. Organization of the core respiratory network: insights from optogenetic and modeling studies. PLoS Comput Biol. 2018 Apr;14(4):e1006148.

192. Marchenko V, Koizumi H, Mosher B, Koshiya N, Tariq MF, Bezdudnaya TG, et al. Perturbations of respiratory rhythm and pattern by disrupting synaptic inhibition within pre-Bötzinger and Bötzinger complexes. eNeuro [Internet]. 2016 Mar;3(2). Available from: http://dx.doi.org/10.1523/ENEURO.0011-16.2016

193. Bonham AC, McCrimmon DR. Neurones in a discrete region of the nucleus tractus solitarius are required for the Breuer-Hering reflex in rat. J Physiol. 1990 Aug;427:261–80.

194. Bonham AC, Coles SK, McCrimmon DR. Pulmonary stretch receptor afferents activate excitatory amino acid receptors in the nucleus tractus solitarii in rats. J Physiol. 1993 May;464:725–45.

195. Wilson CG, Bonham AC. Effect of cardiopulmonary C fibre activation on the firing activity of ventral respiratory group neurones in the rat. J Physiol. 1997 Oct;504 (Pt 2):453–66.

196. Ezure K, Tanaka I. Pump neurons of the nucleus of the solitary tract project widely to the medulla. Neurosci Lett. 1996 Sep 6;215(2):123–6.

197. Ezure K, Tanaka I. GABA, in some cases together with glycine, is used as the inhibitory transmitter by pump cells in the Hering-Breuer reflex pathway of the rat. Neuroscience. 2004;127(2):409–17.

198. Takakura AC, Moreira TS, West GH, Gwilt JM, Colombari E, Stornetta RL, et al. GABAergic pump cells of solitary tract nucleus innervate retrotrapezoid nucleus chemoreceptors. J Neurophysiol. 2007 Jul;98(1):374–81.

199. Widdicombe J. Airway receptors. Respir Physiol. 2001 Mar;125(1–2):3–15.

200. Widdicombe JG. Pulmonary and respiratory tract receptors. J Exp Biol. 1982 Oct;100:41–57.

201. Averill DB, Cameron WE, Berger AJ. Neural elements subserving pulmonary stretch receptor-mediated facilitation of phrenic motoneurons. Brain Res. 1985 Nov 4;346(2):378–82.

202. Lipski J, Ezure K, Wong She RB. Identification of neurons receiving input from pulmonary rapidly adapting receptors in the cat. J Physiol. 1991 Nov;443:55–77.

203. Ezure K, Tanaka I. Lung inflation inhibits rapidly adapting receptor relay neurons in the rat. Neuroreport. 2000 Jun 5;11(8):1709–12.

204. Otake K, Nakamura Y, Tanaka I, Ezure K. Morphology of pulmonary rapidly adapting receptor relay neurons in the rat. J Comp Neurol. 2001 Feb 19;430(4):458–70.

205. Undem BJ, Kollarik M. The role of vagal afferent nerves in chronic obstructive pulmonary disease. Proc Am Thorac Soc. 2005;2(4):355–60; discussion 371–2.

206. Wilson CG, Zhang Z, Bonham AC. Non-NMDA receptors transmit cardiopulmonary C fibre input in nucleus tractus solitarii in rats. J Physiol. 1996 Nov 1;496 (Pt 3):773–85.

207. Lahiri S, Roy A, Baby SM, Hoshi T, Semenza GL, Prabhakar NR. Oxygen sensing in the body. Prog Biophys Mol Biol. 2006 Jul;91(3):249–86.

208. Kumar P, Prabhakar NR. Peripheral chemoreceptors: function and plasticity of the carotid body. Compr Physiol. 2012 Jan;2(1):141–219.

209. Takakura ACT, Moreira TS, Colombari E, West GH, Stornetta RL, Guyenet PG. Peripheral chemoreceptor inputs to retrotrapezoid nucleus (RTN) CO_2-sensitive neurons in rats. J Physiol. 2006 Apr 15;572(Pt 2):503–23.

2 Chemoreception: Pathways, Plasticity, and Pathophysiology

Barbara J Morgan and Jerome A Dempsey

This chapter reviews select recent advances in chemoreception, including neural pathways and their interdependence and specificity, as well as their contributions to ventilatory stability, sympathetic nerve activity, and chronic disease pathophysiology. We also provide a critique of methods for quantifying cardiorespiratory chemosensitivity in humans and animal models—their limitations and capabilities.

CAROTID BODY SENSING, SIGNAL TRANSDUCTION, AND NEURAL PATHWAYS

The carotid body (CB) peripheral chemoreceptors are polymodal receptors serving as the primary oxygen sensors but also sensing K^+, temperature, osmolality, glucose, and insulin (1). The primary sensing unit of the CB is the glomus cell, where transduction of the low O_2 signal is initiated by reciprocal changes in two gaseous transmitters. Hypoxia-induced decreases in carbon monoxide and increases in hydrogen sulfide inhibit glomus cell K^+ channels, thereby allowing increases in $[Ca^{2+}]_i$, neurotransmitter release and stimulation of afferent nerve activity (2). In glomus cells that are largely distinct from those responsive to hypoxia, acidosis is sensed when K^+ channels are inhibited by decreases in intra- and/or extracellular pH (3–5).

Anatomically distinct glomus cells and clusters of cells, each with different transmitter systems, afferent innervations, and central nervous system (CNS) targets, confer on the CB its ability to initiate responses to a wide array of stimuli in multiple organ systems. The following evidence supports the notion that such diversity results in differential control of the sympathetic and respiratory components of the carotid chemoreflex (6).

Carotid bodies contain two types of chemosensitive glomus cells with different neurotransmitters and sensitivities to mediators (6). Dopamine beta-hydroxylase (DBH)-containing cells release norepinephrine in response to hypoxia, express nicotinic receptors, are inhibited by dopamine, and project to the petrosal ganglion via A fibers. In contrast, tyrosine hydroxylase (TH)-positive cells release ATP in hypoxia, express purinergic (P2X3) receptors, are excited by angiotensin II (Ang II), and project to the petrosal ganglion via C fibers. Based on their differential sensitivities to inhibition by dopamine, it

has been proposed that DBH+ glomus cells initiate chemoreflex-mediated increases in ventilation, whereas TH+ cells initiate reflex sympathoexcitation (6).

This specificity in respiratory and sympathetic responses is carried through to central elements of the chemoreflex arc. CB afferents project to multiple sites in the nucleus of the solitary tract (NTS), again allowing the possibility of multiple, separate reflex functions (7–9). Some NTS neurons impinge on the medullary respiratory pattern generator (RPG) neurons that determine phrenic motor output, whereas others project to rostral ventrolateral medulla (RVLM) neurons that determine sympathetic outflow (10). In addition, some NTS neurons project to the paraventricular nucleus (PVN) of the hypothalamus (11). A recently described descending pathway from PVN to NTS neurons modulates cardiorespiratory responses to hypoxia by enhancing respiratory responses and reducing sympathoexcitation (12).

Findings in experimental animals and humans provide support for differential regulation of respiratory vs. sympathetic responses. Dopamine, a potent inhibitor of the hypoxic ventilatory response, had only a weak effect on the sympathoexcitatory response (13). P2X3 receptor antagonism decreased sympathetic outflow under baseline conditions and during chemoreflex stimulation without affecting ventilation (14). This mounting evidence for differential regulation has implications for cardiorespiratory chemosensitivity testing in humans (see Quantifying Cardiorespiratory Chemosensitivity).

PERIPHERAL/CENTRAL CHEMORECEPTORS AND THEIR INTERDEPENDENCE

The location and function of two distinct sets of chemoreceptors, which play key roles in regulating both ventilation and sympathetic nerve activity, have been identified. The carotid or peripheral chemoreceptors are the body's primary sensor of oxygen. In addition, hypoxic:hypercapnic combinations (*i.e.* asphyxia) interact exclusively at the level of the CB, exerting strong synergistic effects on sympathetic and ventilatory activity (15). The medullary retrotrapezoid nucleus (RTN) serves as the most sensitive site for central CO_2 reception, highly responsive to even very small CO_2/H^+ changes in its brain extracellular fluid

DOI: 10.1201/9781003000631-3

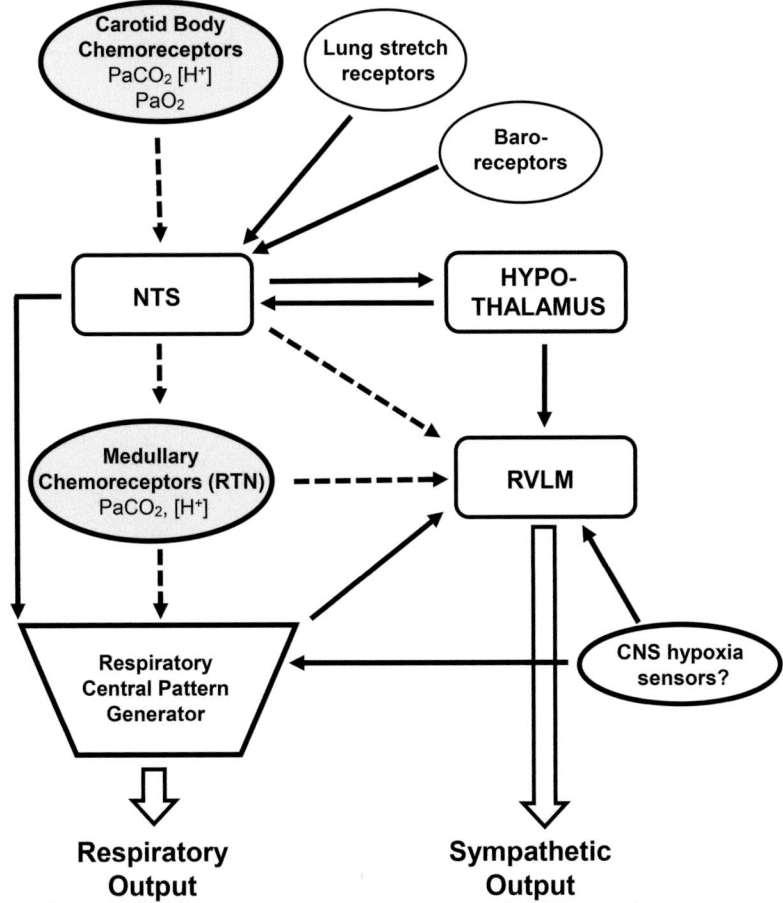

Figure 2.1 Simplified schema of central and peripheral chemoreceptors and their interconnections (dashed lines indicate neural pathways connecting carotid chemoreceptors to the RTN and regions involved in respiratory and sympathetic outputs). CB stimulates the respiratory CPG and RVLM both through and independent of the RTN. The following evidence demonstrates the interdependence of CB with RTN: (a) the gene product Phox2b is strongly expressed in neurons that are part of an uninterrupted chain that includes CB, NTS, and RTN (149); (b) hypoxic exposure activates RTN CO_2-sensitive neurons via CB stimulation (150); and (c) stimulation/inhibition of the isolated CB significantly influences central CO_2 chemosensitivity (also see Figure 2.2). The RTN also serves as an integrative site for inputs from the hypothalamus and lung stretch receptors influencing the respiratory and sympathetic output (10). Hypothalamic regions involved in respiratory and sympathetic control include the PVN and dorsomedial areas. Respiratory-sympathetic coupling is shown via connections between the respiratory CPG and RVLM. The effects of CNS hypoxia, *per se*, on both respiratory and sympathetic outputs are also included here (also see Figure 2.3). Not shown here are structures involved in parasympathetic outflow or pontine regions involved in control of breathing patterns. CB, carotid body chemoreceptor; CNS, central nervous system; CPG, central respiratory pattern generator; NTS, nucleus of the solitary tract; PVN, paraventricular nucleus of the hypothalamus; RTN, retrotrapezoid nucleus; RVLM, rostral ventrolateral medulla.

environment (16). The RTN also serves as a site of convergence of several inputs from lung stretch receptors, hypothalamus, and carotid chemoreceptors to influence cardiorespiratory control (see schema in Figure 2.1).

Experiments conducted in unanesthetized animals with isolation of the extracorporeally-

perfused CB and in humans with CB denervation (Figure 2.2) demonstrate the considerable hyperadditive influence of peripheral chemoreceptor input on central CO_2 and hypoxic ventilatory chemosensitivity. The following examples from Figures 2.2 and 2.3 point to the importance of this interdependence

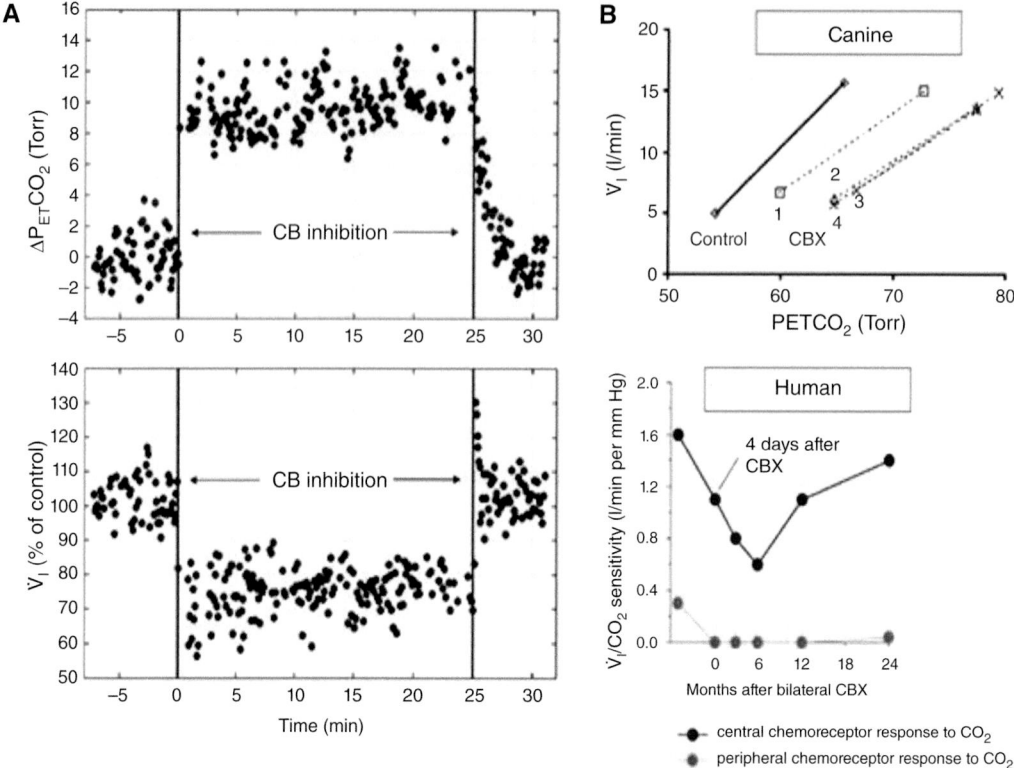

Figure 2.2 The hyperadditive effect of CB sensory input on central CO_2 sensitivity is illustrated by two types of findings. **A**: First, in awake (or sleeping) canines, one CB was denervated and the remaining CB vascularly isolated from the CNS and perfused extracorporeally. When the isolated CB was inhibited by hyperoxia combined with hypocapnia, marked alveolar hypoventilation and CO_2 retention occurred, which persisted despite substantial, sustained CNS acidosis. Also, note the immediate 60% increase in V̇E at min 25 when the tonic CB inhibition was removed, thereby further revealing the critical dependence of central CO_2 chemosensitivity on CB sensory input. Further experiments showed that the (extra-CB) central CO_2 ventilatory response slope was markedly depressed with CB inhibition and enhanced via CB stimulation using variations in CB PO_2, PCO_2, or their combination (*not shown*) (17, 37). **B**: Second, in awake humans (*bottom*) and canines (*top*), bilateral CB denervation resulted in significantly reduced ventilatory response slopes to hyperoxic hypercapnia (129, 130). In contrast to these several lines of evidence in support of hyperadditive interdependence of peripheral and central chemoreceptors, others have reported either hypoaddition in the decorticate rodent or simple addition in the intact human (151, 152). Thus, to date, evidence for hyperaddition is limited to experimental preparations with physiologic levels of CO_2 chemosensitivity and in which the peripheral and central chemoreceptors are anatomically isolated (see explanation in (37)). (Adapted from Dempsey and Smith (103).)

on ventilatory control in normally responsive physiologic mammalian preparations.

- The CBs provide a highly significant tonic contribution to the central chemoreceptor's CO_2 sensitivity and to the normal eupneic drive to breathe (17).

- Apnea elicited by transient overventilation with reductions in arterial PCO_2 during sleep is critically dependent on CB inhibition

reducing central CO_2 chemosensitivity (18) (see Pathogenesis of Sleep-Disordered Breathing).

- CNS hypoxia—by itself—provides a drive to breathe, which appears to contribute significantly to the total increase in ventilation upon coincident hypoxic exposure of both CB and CNS. CNS hyperoxia also appears to provide a stimulus to ventilation (see Figure 2.3).

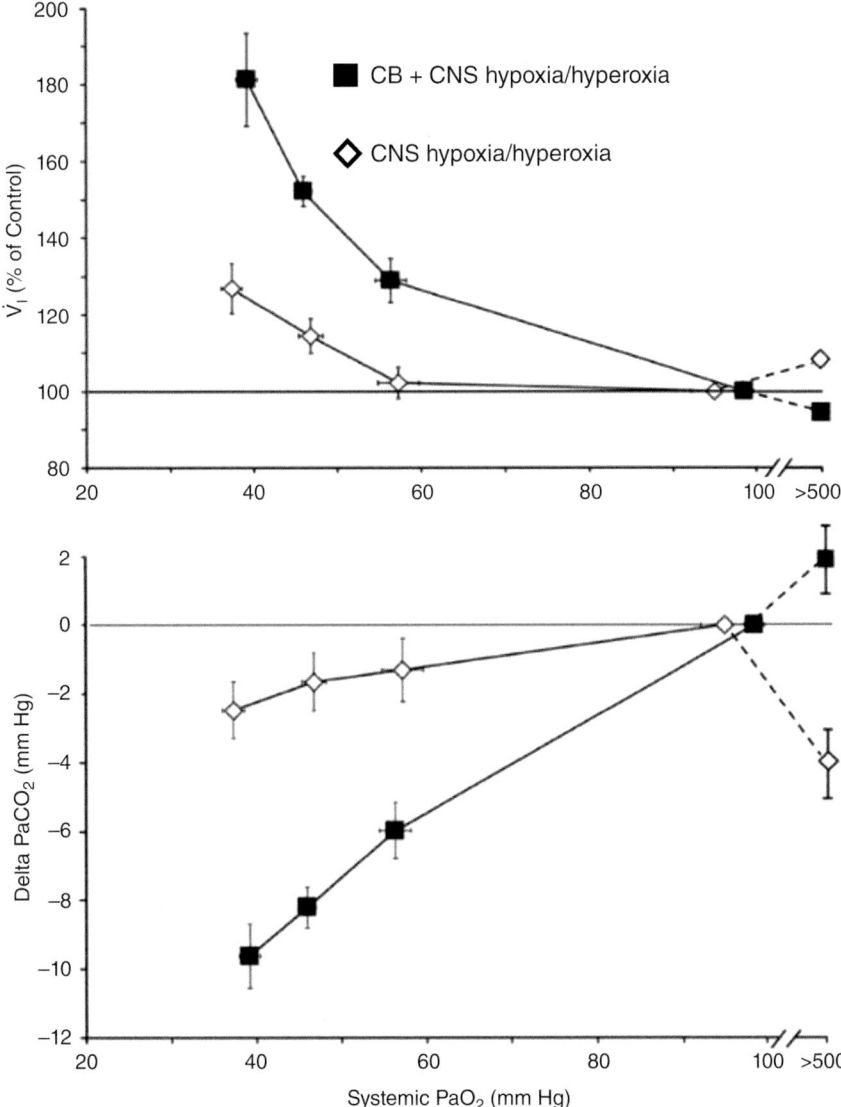

Figure 2.3 Hypoxia administered to awake CB-denervated animals has little to no effect on ventilation; however, if the isolated CB is maintained normoxic and normocapnic (*i.e.* normal tonic sensory input is preserved), then systemic hypoxia elicits a dose-dependent hyperventilation. Shown here are the steady-state ventilatory responses to CNS hypoxia/hyperoxia alone (open diamonds) vs. CNS plus CB hypoxia/hyperoxia (filled squares) in awake canines. The CNS hypoxic data were obtained using an extracorporeally-perfused carotid body canine preparation to isolate the CNS from the CB with the CB held at normoxic and normocapnic levels during inhalation of hypoxic gases (n = 11). The CNS hyperoxia data were obtained in bilaterally CB denervated dogs (n = 5). Note that when the CNS was exposed to hypoxia with CB held normoxic, dose-dependent hyperventilatory responses were initiated within 30 sec of CNS hypoxia and in the steady-state were approximately one-third of the response obtained in the intact animal when both CB and CNS were hypoxic. With CNS hyperoxia, a moderate hyperventilation occurred. The hyperventilation with CNS hypoxia was due entirely to a progressive increase in breathing frequency, whereas the hyperventilation in CNS hyperoxia was due primarily to an increase in VT (130, 153). Recent insights into potential mechanisms of CNS hypoxic/hyperoxic ventilatory stimulation are outlined in (154). (Adapted from Dempsey and Smith (103).)

RTN excitation of RVLM presympathetic neurons occurs via RPG-dependent and RPG-independent pathways (19). Central modulation of sympathetic outflow that occurs via respiratory-sympathetic coupling (*i.e.* phasic breathing-related inhibition of presympathetic neurons by input from the caudal ventrolateral medullary "depressor" area) has been demonstrated in reduced preparations (10); however, the importance of this coupling process in respiratory modulation of sympathetic outflow in intact, conscious humans has not been established (20–23).

PATHOGENESIS OF SLEEP-DISORDERED BREATHING

Sleep-induced suppression of the wakefulness drive to breathe and ventilatory stability: the loss of vigilance. Regulation of chemoresponsiveness, upper airway patency, and ventilatory stability is critically dependent on the "wakefulness drives" to breathe (24, 25). The origins of these tonic facilitatory drives have been localized to several highly state-dependent areas of the CNS. These include (a) orexinergic neurons in the hypothalamus (26) (see (27)); (b) premotor cortex and supplementary motor area neurons (28); and (c) parallel neuronal systems that link H^+ chemosensitivity to both breathing and arousal (29, 30).

Physiologically, the loss of tonic wakefulness neurogenic drives is manifest throughout sleep in the (a) increased collapsibility of the upper extrathoracic airway secondary to dilator muscle atonicity; (b) varying degrees of alveolar hypoventilation secondary to both increased airway resistance and a resetting of the CO_2 set point (31); and (c) critical dependence on CO_2 chemosensitivity above and below eupnea for the regulation of breathing stability. In turn, the breathing instability that occurs during sleep is characterized by repeated, excessive ventilatory undershoots and overshoots as if the respiratory control system had lost its "vigilance" for protecting stability and homeostasis—characteristics it displays so precisely during wakefulness.

Ventilatory undershoots via reduced $PaCO_2$/ augmented tidal volume/increased resistive loads. During wakefulness, transient hyperventilation rarely culminates in apnea or hypopnea—but does so consistently and in a dose-response manner in NREM sleep (32, 33). Dubois et al. (33) have associated maintained ventilation *i.e.* absence of apnea, following active or passive overventilation, with respiratory-related EEG activity, cortical activity that was absent when apnea accompanied hypocapnia. This association suggested a

"cortical subcortical cooperation" to preserve human ventilation during wake that would be lost during NREM sleep. Similarly, during wakefulness when inspiratory resistive or elastic loads are imposed on the airway, the inspiratory drive is augmented immediately and inspiratory time prolonged to preserve tidal volume and alveolar ventilation ($\dot{V}A$). In contrast, during NREM sleep, this immediate load compensation is absent, precipitating a reduced tidal volume until such time as CO_2 accumulates to increase inspiratory and expiratory muscle EMG activity, thereby restoring $\dot{V}E$ toward control levels (34). Studies in the sleeping canine with vascular isolation of the carotid chemoreceptor have shown that the apneas following transient hyperventilation require: (a) intact carotid chemoreceptors (35) and intact vagally mediated lung stretch receptors (36); (b) transient hypocapnia acting at *both* peripheral and central chemoreceptor sites (18); and (c) a hyperadditive interdependence of central CO_2 sensitivity on peripheral chemoreceptor sensory input (37). In subjects with inherently collapsible upper airways, airway narrowing or closure often occurs at the nadir of the ventilatory undershoot, *i.e.* central instability precipitates airway obstruction (38).

Transient ventilatory overshoots commonly occur at the termination of an apnea or hypopnea during sleep due to the synergistic action of hypercapnia plus hypoxemia at the CB on augmenting ventilatory drive. These effects of chemostimulation via asphyxia at apnea termination are further augmented because (a) the drive to resume inspiration following cessation of respiratory rhythm is delayed until arterial PCO_2 rises to a value that exceeds the pre-apneic eupneic arterial PCO_2 (39), and (b) by the common occurrence of transient cortical arousals at end-apnea which both restores upper airway patency (thereby reducing the resistive load on ventilation) and substantially augments the prevailing chemosensitive drive to breathe.

In summary, loss of wakefulness drives in NREM sleep unmasks an apneic threshold sensitive to transient hypocapnia plus lung stretch. At the same time, a sufficiently brisk synergistic responsiveness to asphyxia is retained, which, along with frequent transient arousals, mediates transient ventilatory overshoots at apnea termination. These combined effects above and below eupnea promote cyclical ventilatory instability. In phasic REM sleep, sporadic increases in medullary inspiratory neuronal activity augment breathing frequency (25) and oppose the occurrence of both hypocapnia-induced apneas and chemoreceptor-driven ventilatory overshoots (40).

Chemoresponsiveness and ventilatory instability in sleep. Excessive chemosensitivity to transient increases and decreases in CO_2 contributes importantly to central, obstructive, and mixed repeated apneas and hypopneas in health and in chronic diseases by enhancing the controller, plant, and "loop" gains of the respiratory control system, *i.e.* a dynamic measure of how close the control system is to instability (41) (see details in Figure 2.4 and figure legend).

Figure 2.4 also shows how lowering chemosensitivity/controller gain will reduce sleep-disordered breathing instability as shown via the use of nocturnal hyperoxia in patients with chronic heart failure (CHF) (42), CB denervation, or gaseous excitatory neurotransmitter blockade in rodent models of CHF (43, 44) or a single dose of morphine in obstructive sleep apnea (OSA) patients (45). Further, lowering of plant gain via acetazolamide-induced steady-state hypocapnic hyperventilation or rebreathing to raise $FICO_2$ and $PaCO_2$ reduces instability and central apneas in CHF patients and in sojourners to high altitude and even obstructive apneas in selected OSA patients (46–49).

Patients with OSA and those with ventricular dysfunction and central sleep apnea experience an increase in the frequency and duration of apneic episodes in the late vs. early hours of NREM sleep (50, 51). Can this be explained by circadian variations in chemosensitivity and, therefore, loop gain? Findings to date are conflicting. On the one hand, the CO_2 response below eupnea, as assessed via mechanical ventilator-induced transient reductions in $PaCO_2$ during NREM sleep, is increased in slope (*i.e.* the difference in $PaCO_2$ between eupnea and the apneic threshold is narrowed) in the morning vs. evening (52). Thus, this increased CO_2 response below eupnea, *per se*, would cause ventilatory instability during the night. On the other hand, the response to CO_2 above eupnea appears to be smaller, not greater, in the morning vs. evening (53, 54); however, this observation was made in healthy subjects during wakefulness, and therefore its relevance to nocturnal effects on sleep disordered breathing is unknown. Thus, alterations in chemoreceptor sensitivity below eupnea during NREM sleep over the course of the night could account for the increasing prevalence of apneas in the later sleep period. At the same time, other factors such as a change in arousal threshold (55) and accumulation of fluid in the upper airway due to prolonged recumbency (56, 57) likely also play a role.

PLASTICITY IN CAROTID CHEMOREFLEX FUNCTION

CB plasticity leading to chemoreflex hypersensitivity occurs in common diseases such as sleep apnea, hypertension, CHF, chronic obstructive pulmonary disease (COPD), and renal failure (58–63), where it often produces ventilatory instability and heightened tonic levels of sympathetic vasoconstrictor outflow. There is also some suggestion that CBs are hypersensitive in animal models and humans with obesity and insulin resistance, resulting in sympathetically mediated alterations in lipid and glucose metabolism (64).

Exposure of rats to chronic intermittent hypoxia (IH), a model of human sleep apnea, increases sympathetic outflow, elevates blood pressure, and enhances ventilatory and sympathetic responses to acute hypoxemia, all of which are dependent on intact carotid chemoreceptors, intact renal nerves, and activation of the renin-angiotensin system (65–71). Reactive oxygen species generated mainly during the reoxygenation phase of the IH cycle create an imbalance in pro- and antioxidant isoforms of hypoxia-inducible factor-α. The resultant oxidative stress increases $[Ca^{2+}]_i$, which depolarizes glomus cells and triggers sensory neuronal activity (72–78). Thus, in the CB, oxidative stress begets more oxidative stress in a feedforward manner, leading to enhanced sensory input and oxidative stress in other components of the extended chemoreflex pathway (*i.e.* NTS, RVLM, PVN), which results in increased sympathetic vasoconstrictor outflow and ventilation under baseline conditions and during hypoxia (72, 78, 79).

In human hypertension, augmented neurocirculatory and ventilatory responses to acute hyperoxia provide evidence for tonically elevated chemoreflex drive (62, 80). Blood pressure elevation in the spontaneously hypertensive rat, an animal model of neurogenic hypertension, is critically dependent on input from the CB (81). An important role for CB P2X3 receptors in causing chemoreflex hypersensitivity, heightened tonic sympathetic activity and hypertension in this model has recently been demonstrated (14). An interesting postulate is that the CB, via its own autonomic innervation, is a target of the widespread increase in sympathetic outflow observed in hypertensive states (82). This local increase in sympathetic outflow could have an excitatory effect on the CB caused, at least in part, by reductions in blood flow (83, 84). Also

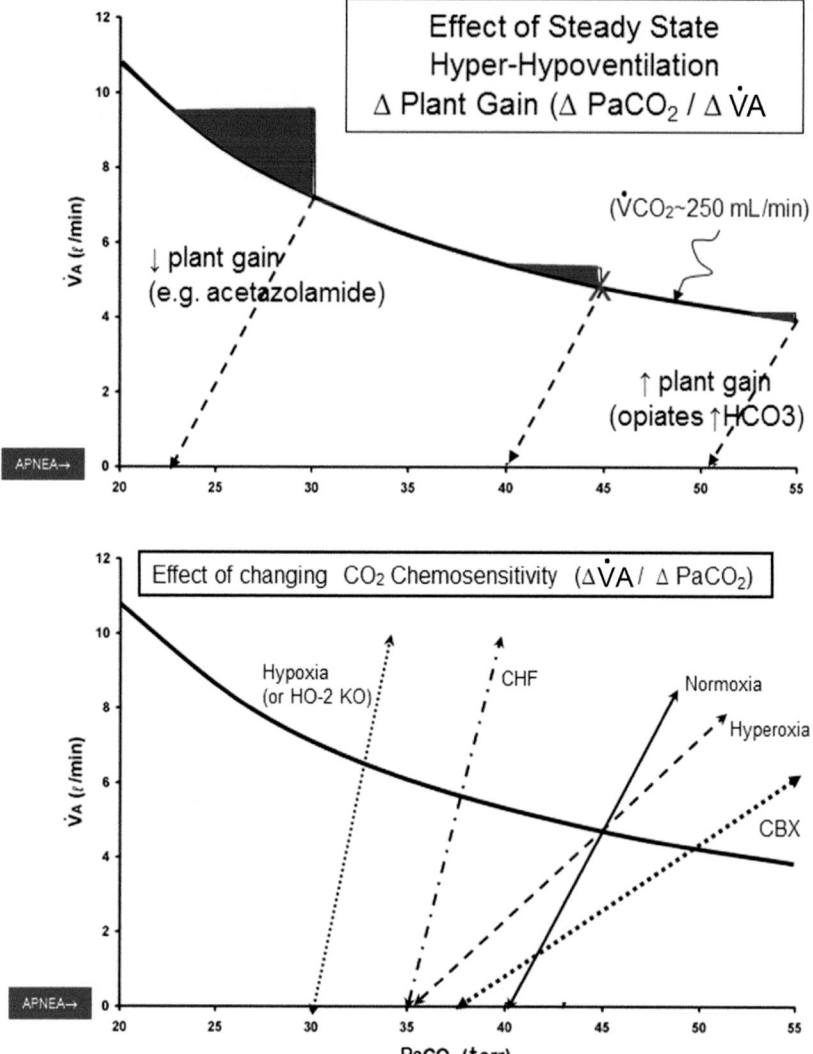

Figure 2.4 Diagram of the alveolar gas equation to illustrate the effects of loop gain components on the propensity for apnea and ventilatory instability. The equation is $PaCO_2 = \dot{V}CO_2/VA \cdot K$, where $\dot{V}CO_2 = 250$ mL/min. Each example shown is from an experimental study in sleeping humans or canines in which the apneic threshold and the slope of the CO_2 response below eupnea were measured during NREM sleep by using a mechanical ventilator in the assist-control mode to gradually raise the tidal volume and lower partial pressure of end-tidal CO_2 (PETCO$_2$) until apnea occurred. The **top panel** shows the effects of changing "plant" gain ($\Delta PaCO_2/\Delta\dot{V}A$) by itself with steady-state hyper- or hypoventilation along the iso-metabolic hyperbola. The red filled-in areas indicate the magnitude of increase in alveolar ventilation needed to reduce $PaCO_2$ sufficiently to reach the apneic threshold. For example, under control conditions in NREM sleep (eupneic $PaCO_2$ ~ 45 mm Hg, denoted by X), a transient ventilatory overshoot of about 1 l/min is required to reduce $PaCO_2$ ~ 5 mm Hg to the apneic threshold of 40 mm Hg. With steady-state hyperventilation (for example, oral acetazolamide; $PaCO_2$, 30 mm Hg), the required ventilatory overshoot to achieve apnea ($PaCO_2$, 23 mm Hg) is about twice that of control; conversely, with steady-state hypoventilation (for example, metabolic alkalosis, opiate use; $PaCO_2$ ~ 55 mm Hg), the required ventilatory overshoot to achieve apnea ($PaCO_2$ ~ 51 mm Hg) is about one-third that of control. These marked changes in the increase in $\dot{V}A$ required to reach the apneic threshold coincident with changes in steady-state $PaCO_2$ are due entirely to the hyperbolic nature of the $\dot{V}A/\Delta PaCO_2$ relationship at constant $\dot{V}CO_2$. Not illustrated here are: (a) the effects of transient arousal from sleep, which will increase the magnitude of the transient ventilatory overshoot; (b) reductions in cerebral vasculature CO_2 responsivity as often occurs in CHF will increase the ventilatory sensitivity to changes in arterial PCO_2 by widening the arterial to brain PCO_2 difference (155), and (c) the dynamic effects of lung volume on plant gain. For example, at low lung volumes, plant gain is raised; thus, the CO_2 washout from the alveoli will occur more quickly and will require smaller transient increments in ventilation to reach the apneic threshold (156). The **lower panel** shows effects of changing "controller" gain or chemoreceptor sensitivity to PCO_2 ($\Delta\dot{V}A/\Delta PaCO_2$) above eupnea (which affects the magnitude of the transient ventilatory overshoot) and below eupnea (which affects the CO_2 "reserve" or difference in $PaCO_2$ between eupneic breathing and the apneic threshold). Note the increased CO_2 response slopes above and below eupnea in chronic heart failure (CHF) and hypoxic environments and the reduced CO_2 sensitivity in hyperoxia which is further reduced with carotid chemoreceptor denervation. CBX, carotid body denervation; K, constant 0.863; $PaCO_2$, mm Hg arterial PCO_2; PCO_2, partial pressure CO_2; VA, alveolar ventilation; $\dot{V}CO_2$, CO_2 production; $\dot{V}E$, ventilation. Adapted from Dempsey (157).

intriguing is the notion that hypertension-induced remodeling of feed arteries in brainstem cardiorespiratory control regions leads to hypoperfusion that, in turn, elicits widespread sympathetic excitation via the Cushing response (85).

In humans with CHF, heightened chemoreflex sensitivity is manifest as augmented sympathetic outflow, ventilatory instability, and augmented ventilatory responses to exercise (86). Experimental heart failure in rats, canines, and rabbits produces carotid chemoreflex hypersensitivity leading to increased tonic levels of sympathetic outflow under normoxic conditions, enhanced sympathetic and ventilatory responses to acute hypoxia, and vasoconstriction of locomotor muscle vasculature during excise (87, 88). This form of CB plasticity is critically dependent on increases in locally produced Ang II, upregulation of Ang II type 1 receptors, increased expression of NADPH oxidase subunits and enhanced superoxide production (89). Thus, the CHF-induced increase in CB sensitivity is caused by a shift in redox balance toward oxidative stress. CHF-induced declines in CB blood flow, reduced shear stress, and resultant endothelial dysfunction are likely contributors to CB plasticity in this setting (90, 91).

In patients with COPD, several findings provide evidence for CB hypersensitivity: (a) heightened basal sympathetic outflow, even in the absence of overt hypoxemia (60, 92, 93); (b) larger decreases in ventilation and sympathetic nerve activity during transient hyperoxia and during low-dose dopamine infusion; and (c) augmented increases in ventilation during exposure to acute hypoxia, relative to control subjects (61). The origins of COPD-associated CB plasticity are unknown; however, this disease may impose an insult analogous to high altitude exposure—*i.e.* continuous hypoxia-induced chemoreflex hypersensitivity leading to high tonic levels of sympathetic outflow and ventilatory instability, especially during sleep (47, 94).

Several sequelae of end-stage kidney disease, for example, metabolic acidosis and chronic anemia (95, 96), are potent chemoreflex stimuli. Patients with renal failure exhibit excessive basal sympathetic outflow (97, 98) and augmented carotid chemoreflex-induced sympathoexcitation (58, 99); however, the mechanisms leading to CB plasticity remain obscure. One potential instigator is increased sympathetic outflow to the CB, which is triggered reflexly by activation of renal afferent nerves in response to hemodynamic and/or chemical derangements in the failing kidney (100–102).

Increases in sympathetic outflow produced by the plasticity-induced chemoreflex hypersensitivity described above contribute to disease progression by (a) enhancing breathing instability and raising blood pressure in sleep apnea (103); (b) causing deterioration of ventricular function in CHF (104, 105); (c) contributing to end-organ damage in hypertension (106); (d) exacerbating kidney dysfunction via vascular remodeling, increased sodium reabsorption and activation of the renin-angiotensin-aldosterone system (107); and (e) adversely affecting prognosis and cardiovascular morbidity in COPD (92, 108). Plasticity-induced increases in sympathetic outflow affect many tissues and vascular beds, and because they also target the CB, may serve to exacerbate chemoreflex hypersensitivity via effects on CB blood flow, transmitter release, or through inflammation and/or vascular remodeling, and therefore may be a cause, not only a consequence, of chemoreflex hypersensitivity (82).

Is CB plasticity reversible? Studies in experimental animals point to potential benefits of strategies aimed at reducing chemoreflex hyperexcitability (for example, CB resection, exercise training, statins, purinergic receptor blockade) (14, 43, 109–113). In human CHF, surgical resection of the CB (both bilateral and unilateral) reduced muscle sympathetic nerve activity (MSNA) and produced a modest improvement in quality of life (114). In patients with drug-resistant hypertension, unilateral CB resection reduced MSNA and blood pressure only in ~50% of individuals treated; moreover, these improvements were not maintained at 1-year follow-up (115).

These observations in animals and humans demonstrate the capacity to eliminate or at least suppress excessive chemoreceptor drive–but are these interventions safe? Extensive experience in Japan (116) with bilateral CB resection to relieve dyspnea in patients with asthma suggests that the procedure is relatively benign; however, near-total suppression of the hypoxic ventilatory response persisted in some of these patients 30 years after resection (117). Therefore, of concern is the possibility that bilateral CB resection could lead to unsafe levels of arterial oxygen saturation with air travel, sojourns at high altitude, and via apnea prolongation during sleep-disordered breathing. A more ideal treatment would reduce tonic sympathetic hyperactivity while leaving intact a normal ventilatory and sympathetic response to acute hypoxia/asphyxia. In this regard, one such treatment that holds promise is the selective pharmacologic blockade of ATP-gated ion channels (P2X3 receptors) in CB (14). The safety and efficacy of this treatment in humans with chronic disease have not yet been established.

In experimental animals, exercise training improves blood flow in CB feed arteries by ameliorating CHF-induced endothelial dysfunction (112). For decades, exercise training has been applied safely in patients with CHF, producing increases in exercise capacity and quality of life (118). Exercise-induced reversal of endothelial dysfunction in extra-CB vascular beds has been demonstrated numerous times (119).

Thus, treatments to ameliorate the causes and consequences of CB plasticity show early promise; however, complete suppression of CB sensitivity is not without potential adverse effects. For example, complete bilateral CB ablation could lead to prolonged apneas and oxygen desaturation during sleep, compromised respiratory compensation for metabolic acidosis and impaired glucose regulation. The safety, effectiveness, and ability of these interventions to reduce disease severity and/or progression must be established.

QUANTIFYING CARDIORESPIRATORY CHEMOSENSITIVITY IN THE INTACT HUMAN AND RODENT: A COMPLEX, IMPERFECT UNDERTAKING

As discussed above, recent evidence implicates excessive CB sensitivity as a cause of high levels of tonic sympathetic nerve activity in chronic diseases such as CHF, drug-resistant hypertension, COPD, and sleep apnea and of high loop gain and sleep-disordered breathing. Given the proposed attempts to suppress these high levels of chemosensitivity via, for example, CB resection, selective blockade of CB ion channels or excitatory neurotransmitters or the use of nocturnal supplemental oxygen, it is important that methods are also available to accurately and specifically quantify carotid chemoreceptor sensitivity/tonicity so that treatments can be assigned and assessed on a patient-by-patient basis.

Chemosensitivity testing. A variety of chemosensitivity tests using eucapnic hypoxia or progressive levels of hypercapnia achieved during rebreathing combined with iso-oxic levels of hypoxia and hyperoxia have been widely utilized for several decades—unfortunately, with little to no consensus as to their suitability (120–122). In some descriptive studies, chemosensitivity testing has been at least moderately successful in predicting: (a) which OSA patients would respond positively to nocturnal O_2 therapy (49, 123) or to pharmacotherapy (45) or to CO_2 supplementation (49); or (b) which patients with drug-resistant hypertension would lower their sympathetic outflow and blood pressure with unilateral CB resection (115) or for predicting survival rates in CHF patients (114). At the same time, based on findings cited above (see sections on Neural Pathways and Chemoreceptor Interdependence), we suggest that there are serious limitations that preclude attempts to equate whole-body chemosensitive ventilatory response tests in awake humans or animals to specific chemoreceptor sensitivities.

- When eupneic arterial PCO_2 differs between or within subjects, this difference will have marked synergistic effects—by itself—on the CB's eucapnic hypoxic responses (124, 125). The use of progressive increments in end-tidal PCO_2 achieved via rebreathing would be of some help for purposes of comparison of chemosensitivities by at least bracketing the different levels of prevailing arterial PCO_2 (122). The end-tidal PCO_2 at which ventilation begins to increase during hypoxic or hyperoxic rebreathing following a period of voluntary hyperventilation and apnea is also used as a "personalized" level of isocapnia with which to quantify the hypoxic response (121). It is not clear to us how closely this" threshold" truly approximates that of the carotid chemoreceptors or why this level of isocapnia is more suitable than others to use in hypoxia response assessment.

- All response tests using progressive hypercapnia combined with hypoxia or hyperoxia measure *both* central and peripheral chemoreceptor responses and their interdependence Attempts to separate out just the central chemoreceptor CO_2 response utilizing a hyperoxic background fail to consider: (a) that the CB remains responsive to hypercapnia even in the hyperoxic range (126–128); and (b) that reducing/eliminating CB sensory input markedly reduces the slope of the ventilatory response to CO_2 as assessed via open-circuit steady-state or rebreathe response tests. These findings reflect a peripheral:central chemoreceptor interdependence (37, 129–131) (see Figure 2.2).

- Use of the slope of the ventilatory response to increasing CO_2 at different iso-oxic levels to define chemosensitivity must consider that CO_2/H^+ and hypoxia are transduced at the CB through quite different underlying mechanisms (3, 4).

- The ventilatory response to hypoxia is driven primarily by the peripheral chemoreceptors but is also influenced by extra-carotid chemoreceptor CNS effects (see Figure 2.3). Further, even moderate levels of steady-state CNS hyperoxia are also stimulatory to breathing (see Figure 2.3).

In summary, we propose that the common use of tests combining variations in O_2 and CO_2 defines a "collective" ventilatory chemosensitivity of both sets of chemoreceptors and their interdependence as well as extra-chemoreceptor effects of CNS hypoxia and hyperoxia. Nevertheless, given the multiple sites of chemosensitivity and

their interdependence, such tests may still be of value in phenotyping patients to determine the suitability of certain types of treatments designed to reduce excessive chemosensitivity. Transient hyperoxic tests, using the nadir of the ventilatory or MSNA response may also be of value in assessing the magnitude of tonic levels of excessive carotid chemoreceptor activity, *per se* (132, 133) (see Figure 2.5A).

Congruence of ventilatory vs. neurocirculatory chemosensitivity. Noninvasive tests of ventilatory responses to chemoreceptor stimuli are traditionally used to make inferences about cardiovascular or sympathetic nervous system chemoresponsivity. The rationale for this dual usage comes from the generalization

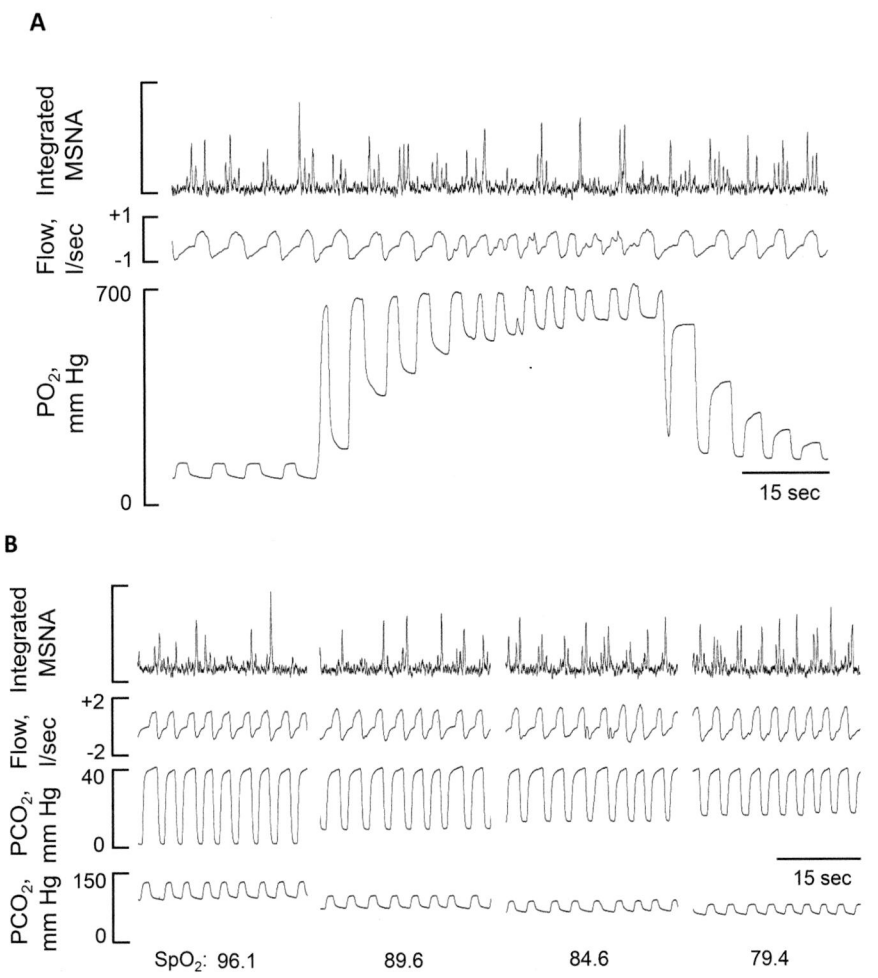

Figure 2.5 Original records showing ventilatory and muscle sympathetic nerve activity (MSNA) responses to transient (<1 min) hyperoxia (A) and to graded, eucapnic hypoxia (B). Hyperoxic responses were defined as the nadir single-breath value for ventilation (derived from respiratory airflow) and the nadir 15-sec average of MSNA. Hypoxic ventilatory and MSNA responses were defined as the slopes of the linear relationships of these variables with arterial oxygen saturation (SpO$_2$). From Prasad et al. (133).

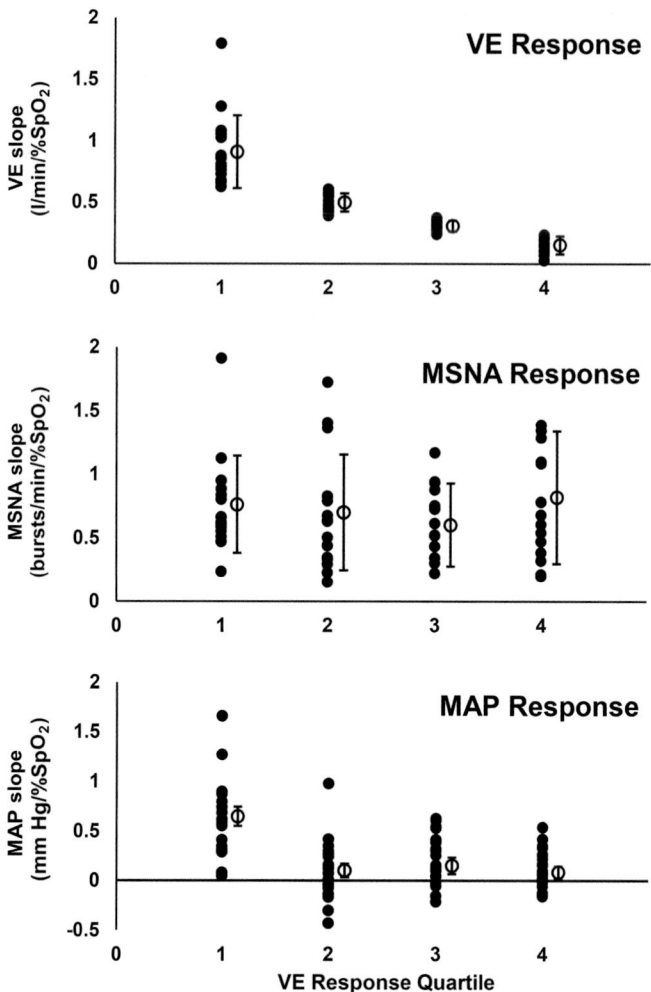

Figure 2.6 Individual and mean values of response slopes for ventilation (V̇E), muscle sympathetic nerve activity burst frequency (MSNA), and mean arterial pressure (MAP) in the four quartiles of ventilatory response to hypoxia among 82 hypertensive patients with sleep apnea. Values shown are the slopes of the linear relationships between each variable and arterial oxygen saturation. Apart from this quartile analysis, we observed a poor rank correlation coefficient (r = 0.08) between V̇E and MSNA response slopes to eucapnic hypoxia and a statistically significant but only moderate correlation among individuals between V̇E and MAP responses (r = 0.50). Note that the hypoxic response slopes, which are negative, have been converted to positive slopes for illustration purposes. Adapted from Prasad et al. (133).

that hypersensitization of CB chemoreceptors causes parallel augmentation of both ventilatory and sympathetic responsiveness. While sympathoexcitatory and ventilatory responses to acute hypoxia are *both* elevated in some patient groups (134, 135), there are also reports of non-congruence in sympathetic and ventilatory responsiveness (58, 59, 136–138). More specific tests of congruence that were used in two recent studies in normal subjects using iso-oxic hypercapnic response tests (139) and in a large group of hypertensive OSA patients using the

eucapnic hypoxia tests (133) showed a clear lack of congruence between the chemosensitivities of MSNA vs. ventilation (see Figure 2.6). Perhaps this lack of strong congruence is not surprising given the evidence that these responses are mediated by distinct pathways with different CB receptors, neurotransmitters, and central pathways (6) (see section on CB sensing, signal transduction, and neural pathways, above). The lesson here is that we need more thorough understanding of the functional specificities of components of the chemoreflex arc and how they influence the coupling or decoupling of respiratory and neurocirculatory responses to chemoreceptor stimuli.

Quantifying chemoreceptor sensitivity in small mammals. Rodents are the currently preferred animal model for investigating cardiorespiratory control mechanisms, and like other mammals, they are dependent upon intact carotid bodies for ventilatory and sympathetic responses to hypoxia (140). However, in these smaller animals, CB sensitivity influences the ventilatory response through its effects on *both* the RPG as well as (indirectly) through hypoxic-induced reductions in body temperature and metabolic rate (141, 142). The marked, dose-dependent reductions in $\dot{V}CO_2$ observed with hypoxic-induced CB stimulation coincide with reductions in sympathetic outflow to brown adipose tissue, which in turn inhibits non-shivering thermogenesis (143–145). It is well established that changing $\dot{V}CO_2$—by itself—has marked dose-dependent effects on ventilation (146, 147). Accordingly, the common use of a $\dot{V}E$ vs. FIO_2 slope to assess hypoxic responsiveness in the rodent fails to account for: (a) the large and variable (20%–40%) effects on $\dot{V}CO_2$; and (b) the variability in SpO_2 (*i.e.* the "stimulus" magnitude) generated by variations in $\dot{V}E/\dot{V}O_2$ at any given FIO_2 (142). Thus, $\dot{V}CO_2$ must be measured coincident with ventilation and the "response" slope expressed as $\dot{V}E/\dot{V}CO_2$ vs. SpO_2 (142). An inability to monitor and control $PaCO_2$ during hypoxic challenge in these small animals also greatly confounds attempts to quantify a purely hypoxic carotid chemosensitivity (142). Finally, interpretation of the chemoreflex-induced increase in sympathetic outflow will be confounded by the baroreflex-induced sympathoexcitation elicited by systemic hypotension, which occurs during acute hypoxic exposure in these animals (148). Thus, in animal models as well as humans, the complexities associated with the hypoxic (or asphyxic) exposure greatly compromise our ability to specifically quantify carotid chemoreceptor sensitivity.

ACKNOWLEDGMENTS/GRANTS

We are indebted to our Rankin Laboratory and Skatrud Laboratory colleagues for several decades of collaborative chemoreceptor research.

Funding from NHLBI (R-21 HL 137874) to J.A.D.

REFERENCES

1. Kumar P, Bin-Jaliah I. Adequate stimuli of the carotid body: more than an oxygen sensor? Respir Physiol Neurobiol. 2007;157(1):12–21.

2. Prabhakar NR, Peng YJ, Nanduri J. Recent advances in understanding the physiology of hypoxic sensing by the carotid body. F1000Res. 2018;7.

3. Lu Y, Whiteis CA, Sluka KA, Chapleau MW, Abboud FM. Responses of glomus cells to hypoxia and acidosis are uncoupled, reciprocal and linked to ASIC3 expression: selectivity of chemosensory transduction. J Physiol. 2013;591(4):919–32.

4. Lahiri S, Forster RE. CO₂/H(+) sensing: peripheral and central chemoreception. Int J Biochem Cell Biol. 2003;35(10):1413–35.

5. Tan ZY, Lu Y, Whiteis CA, Benson CJ, Chapleau MW, Abboud FM. Acid-sensing ion channels contribute to transduction of extracellular acidosis in rat carotid body glomus cells. Circ Res. 2007;101(10):1009–19.

6. Zera T, Moraes DJA, da Silva MP, Fisher JP, Paton JFR. The logic of carotid body connectivity to the brain. Physiology (Bethesda). 2019;34(4):264–82.

7. Finley JC, Katz DM. The central organization of carotid body afferent projections to the brainstem of the rat. Brain Res. 1992;572(1–2):108–16.

8. Erickson JT, Millhorn DE. Hypoxia and electrical stimulation of the carotid sinus nerve induce Fos-like immunoreactivity within catecholaminergic and serotoninergic neurons of the rat brainstem. J Comp Neurol. 1994;348(2):161–82.

9. Paton JF, Deuchars J, Li YW, Kasparov S. Properties of solitary tract neurones responding to peripheral arterial chemoreceptors. Neuroscience. 2001;105(1):231–48.

10. Guyenet PG. Regulation of breathing and autonomic outflows by chemoreceptors. Compr Physiol. 2014;4(4):1511–62.

11. King TL, Heesch CM, Clark CG, Kline DD, Hasser EM. Hypoxia activates nucleus tractus solitarii neurons projecting to the paraventricular nucleus of the hypothalamus. Am J Physiol Regul Integr Comp Physiol. 2012;302(10):R1219–32.

12. Ruyle BC, Martinez D, Heesch CM, Kline DD, Hasser EM. The PVN enhances cardiorespiratory responses to acute hypoxia via input to the nTS. Am J Physiol Regul Integr Comp Physiol. 2019;317(6): R818–R33.

13. Fisher JP, Flück D, Hilty MP, Lundby C. Carotid chemoreceptor control of muscle sympathetic nerve activity in hypobaric hypoxia. Exp Physiol. 2018;103(1):77–89.

14. Pijacka W, Moraes DJ, Ratcliffe LE, Nightingale AK, Hart EC, da Silva MP, et al. Purinergic receptors in the carotid body as a new drug target for controlling hypertension. Nat Med. 2016;22(10):1151–9.

15. Daristotle L, Engwall MJ, Niu WZ, Bisgard GE. Ventilatory effects and interactions with change in PaO₂ in awake goats. J Appl Physiol (1985). 1991;71(4):1254–60.

16. Guyenet PG, Bayliss DA, Stornetta RL, Ludwig MG, Kumar NN, Shi Y, et al. Proton detection and breathing regulation by the retrotrapezoid nucleus. J Physiol. 2016;594(6):1529–51.

17. Blain GM, Smith CA, Henderson KS, Dempsey JA. Contribution of the carotid body chemoreceptors to eupneic ventilation in the intact, unanesthetized dog. J Appl Physiol (1985). 2009;106(5):1564–73.

18. Smith CA, Chenuel BJ, Henderson KS, Dempsey JA. The apneic threshold during non-REM sleep in dogs: sensitivity of carotid body vs. central chemoreceptors. J Appl Physiol (1985). 2007;103(2):578–86.

19. Moreira TS, Takakura AC, Colombari E, Guyenet PG. Central chemoreceptors and sympathetic vasomotor outflow. J Physiol. 2006;577(Pt 1):369–86.

20. St Croix CM, Satoh M, Morgan BJ, Skatrud JB, Dempsey JA. Role of respiratory motor output in within-breath modulation of muscle sympathetic nerve activity in humans. Circ Res. 1999;85(5):457–69.

21. Fatouleh R, Macefield VG. Respiratory modulation of muscle sympathetic nerve activity is not increased in essential hypertension or chronic obstructive pulmonary disease. J Physiol. 2011;589(Pt 20):4997–5006.

22. Limberg JK, Morgan BJ, Schrage WG, Dempsey JA. Respiratory influences on muscle sympathetic nerve activity and vascular conductance in the steady state. Am J Physiol Heart Circ Physiol. 2013;304(12):H1615–23.

23. Seals DR, Suwarno NO, Joyner MJ, Iber C, Copeland JG, Dempsey JA. Respiratory modulation of muscle sympathetic nerve activity in intact and lung denervated humans. Circ Res. 1993;72(2):440–54.

24. Horner RL. Emerging principles and neural substrates underlying tonic sleep-state-dependent influences on respiratory motor activity. Philos Trans R Soc Lond B Biol Sci. 2009;364(1529):2553–64.

25. Orem J, Lovering AT, Dunin-Barkowski W, Vidruk EH. Tonic activity in the respiratory system in wakefulness, NREM and REM sleep. Sleep. 2002;25(5):488–96.

26. Nakamura A, Zhang W, Yanagisawa M, Fukuda Y, Kuwaki T. Vigilance state-dependent attenuation of hypercapnic chemoreflex and exaggerated sleep apnea in orexin knockout mice. J Appl Physiol (1985). 2007;102(1):241–8.

27. Gestreau C, Bévengut M, Dutschmann M. The dual role of the orexin/hypocretin system in modulating wakefulness and respiratory drive. Curr Opin Pulm Med. 2008;14(6):512–8.

28. Laviolette L, Niérat MC, Hudson AL, Raux M, Allard E, Similowski T. The supplementary motor area exerts a tonic excitatory influence on corticospinal projections to phrenic motoneurons in awake humans. PLoS One. 2013;8(4):e62258.

29. Williams RH, Jensen LT, Verkhratsky A, Fugger L, Burdakov D. Control of hypothalamic orexin neurons by acid and CO_2. Proc Natl Acad Sci U S A. 2007;104(25):10685–90.

30. Benarroch EE. Control of the cardiovascular and respiratory systems during sleep. Auton Neurosci. 2019;218:54–63.

31. Simon PM, Dempsey JA, Landry DM, Skatrud JB. Effect of sleep on respiratory muscle activity during mechanical ventilation. Am Rev Respir Dis. 1993;147(1):32–7.

32. Henke KG, Arias A, Skatrud JB, Dempsey JA. Inhibition of inspiratory muscle activity during sleep. Chemical and nonchemical influences. Am Rev Respir Dis. 1988;138(1):8–15.

33. Dubois M, Chenivesse C, Raux M, Morales-Robles A, Nierat MC, Garcia G, et al. Neurophysiological evidence for a cortical contribution to the wakefulness-related drive to breathe explaining hypocapnia-resistant ventilation in humans. J Neurosci. 2016;36(41):10673–82.

34. Henke KG, Badr MS, Skatrud JB, Dempsey JA. Load compensation and respiratory muscle function during sleep. J Appl Physiol (1985). 1992;72(4):1221–34.

35. Nakayama H, Smith CA, Rodman JR, Skatrud JB, Dempsey JA. Carotid body denervation eliminates apnea in response to transient hypocapnia. J Appl Physiol (1985). 2003;94(1):155–64.

36. Chow CM, Xi L, Smith CA, Saupe KW, Dempsey JA. A volume-dependent apneic threshold during NREM sleep in the dog. J Appl Physiol (1985). 1994;76(6):2315–25.

37. Smith CA, Blain GM, Henderson KS, Dempsey JA. Peripheral chemoreceptors determine the respiratory sensitivity of central chemoreceptors to CO_2: role of carotid body CO_2. J Physiol. 2015;593(18):4225–43.

38. Badr MS, Toiber F, Skatrud JB, Dempsey J. Pharyngeal narrowing/occlusion during central sleep apnea. J Appl Physiol (1985). 1995;78(5):1806–15.

39. Leevers AM, Simon PM, Xi L, Dempsey JA. Apnoea following normocapnic mechanical ventilation in awake mammals: a demonstration of control system inertia. J Physiol. 1993;472:749–68.

40. Xi L, Smith CA, Saupe KW, Henderson KS, Dempsey JA. Effects of rapid-eye-movement sleep on the apneic threshold in dogs. J Appl Physiol (1985). 1993;75(3):1129–39.

41. Khoo MC. Determinants of ventilatory instability and variability. Respir Physiol. 2000;122(2–3):167–82.

42. Bordier P, Lataste A, Hofmann P, Robert F, Bourenane G. Nocturnal oxygen therapy in patients with chronic heart failure and sleep apnea: a systematic review. Sleep Med. 2016;17:149–57.

43. Marcus NJ, Del Rio R, Schultz EP, Xia XH, Schultz HD. Carotid body denervation improves autonomic and cardiac function and attenuates disordered breathing in congestive heart failure. J Physiol. 2014;592(Pt 2):391–408.

44. Del Rio R, Marcus NJ, Schultz HD. Inhibition of hydrogen sulfide restores normal breathing stability and improves autonomic control during experimental heart failure. J Appl Physiol (1985). 2013;114(9):1141–50.

45. Wang D, Eckert DJ, Grunstein RR. Drug effects on ventilatory control and upper airway physiology related to sleep apnea. Respir Physiol Neurobiol. 2013;188(3):257–66.

46. Javaheri S. Acetazolamide improves central sleep apnea in heart failure: a double-blind, prospective study. Am J Respir Crit Care Med. 2006;173(2):234–7.

47. Berssenbrugge A, Dempsey J, Iber C, Skatrud J, Wilson P. Mechanisms of hypoxia-induced periodic breathing during sleep in humans. J Physiol. 1983;343:507–24.

48. Khayat RN, Xie A, Patel AK, Kaminski A, Skatrud JB. Cardiorespiratory effects of added dead space in patients with heart failure and central sleep apnea. Chest. 2003;123(5):1551–60.

49. Xie A, Teodorescu M, Pegelow DF, Teodorescu MC, Gong Y, Fedie JE, et al. Effects of stabilizing or increasing respiratory motor outputs on obstructive sleep apnea. J Appl Physiol (1985). 2013;115(1):22–33.

50. Charbonneau M, Marin JM, Olha A, Kimoff RJ, Levy RD, Cosio MG. Changes in obstructive sleep apnea characteristics through the night. Chest. 1994;106(6):1695–701.

51. Javaheri S, McKane SW, Cameron N, Germany RE, Malhotra A. In patients with heart failure the burden of central sleep apnea increases in the late sleep hours. Sleep. 2019;42(1): 1–7.

52. El-Chami M, Shaheen D, Ivers B, Syed Z, Badr MS, Lin HS, et al. Time of day affects chemoreflex sensitivity and the carbon dioxide reserve during NREM sleep in participants with sleep apnea. J Appl Physiol (1985). 2014;117(10):1149–56.

53. Spengler CM, Czeisler CA, Shea SA. An endogenous circadian rhythm of respiratory control in humans. J Physiol. 2000;526(Pt 3):683–94.

54. Stephenson R, Mohan RM, Duffin J, Jarsky TM. Circadian rhythms in the chemoreflex control of breathing. Am J Physiol Regul Integr Comp Physiol. 2000;278(1):R282–6.

55. Montserrat JM, Kosmas EN, Cosio MG, Kimoff RJ. Mechanism of apnea lengthening across the night in obstructive sleep apnea. Am J Respir Crit Care Med. 1996;154(4 Pt 1):988–93.

56. Kasai T, Motwani SS, Elias RM, Gabriel JM, Taranto Montemurro L, Yanagisawa N, et al. Influence of rostral fluid shift on upper airway size and mucosal water content. J Clin Sleep Med. 2014;10(10):1069–74.

57. White LH, Bradley TD. Role of nocturnal rostral fluid shift in the pathogenesis of obstructive and central sleep apnoea. J Physiol. 2013;591(5):1179–93.

58. Hering D, Zdrojewski Z, Król E, Kara T, Kucharska W, Somers VK, et al. Tonic chemoreflex activation contributes to the elevated muscle sympathetic nerve activity in patients with chronic renal failure. J Hypertens. 2007;25(1):157–61.

59. Di Vanna A, Braga AM, Laterza MC, Ueno LM, Rondon MU, Barretto AC, et al. Blunted muscle vasodilatation during chemoreceptor stimulation in patients with heart failure. Am J Physiol Heart Circ Physiol. 2007;293(1):H846–52.

60. Heindl S, Lehnert M, Criée CP, Hasenfuss G, Andreas S. Marked sympathetic activation in patients with chronic respiratory failure. Am J Respir Crit Care Med. 2001;164(4):597–601.

61. Phillips DB, Steinback CD, Collins S, Fuhr DP, Bryan TL, Wong EYL, et al. The carotid chemoreceptor contributes to the elevated arterial stiffness and vasoconstrictor outflow in chronic obstructive pulmonary disease. J Physiol. 2018;596(15):3233–44.

62. Siński M, Lewandowski J, Przybylski J, Bidiuk J, Abramczyk P, Ciarka A, et al. Tonic activity of carotid body chemoreceptors contributes to the increased sympathetic drive in essential hypertension. Hypertens Res. 2012;35(5):487–91.

63. Narkiewicz K, van de Borne PJ, Montano N, Dyken ME, Phillips BG, Somers VK. Contribution of tonic chemoreflex activation to sympathetic activity and blood pressure in patients with obstructive sleep apnea. Circulation. 1998;97(10):943–5.

64. Sacramento JF, Andrzejewski K, Melo BF, Ribeiro MJ, Obeso A, Conde SV. Exploring the Mediators that promote carotid body dysfunction in type 2 diabetes and obesity related syndromes. Int J Mol Sci. 2020;21(15):5545.

65. Del Rio R, Andrade DC, Lucero C, Arias P, Iturriaga R. Carotid body ablation abrogates hypertension and autonomic alterations induced by intermittent hypoxia in rats. Hypertension. 2016;68(2):436–45.

66. Marcus NJ, Li YL, Bird CE, Schultz HD, Morgan BJ. Chronic intermittent hypoxia augments chemoreflex control of sympathetic activity: role of the angiotensin II type 1 receptor. Respir Physiol Neurobiol. 2010;171(1):36–45.

67. Morgan BJ, Adrian R, Wang ZY, Bates ML, Dopp JM. Chronic intermittent hypoxia alters ventilatory and metabolic responses to acute hypoxia in rats. J Appl Physiol (1985). 2016;120(10):1186–95.

68. Fletcher EC, Lesske J, Behm R, Miller CC, Stauss H, Unger T. Carotid chemoreceptors, systemic blood pressure, and chronic episodic hypoxia mimicking sleep apnea. J Appl Physiol (1985). 1992;72(5):1978–84.

69. Fletcher EC, Lesske J, Qian W, Miller CC, Unger T. Repetitive, episodic hypoxia causes diurnal elevation of blood pressure in rats. Hypertension. 1992;19(6 Pt 1): 555–61.

70. Fletcher EC, Orolinova N, Bader M. Blood pressure response to chronic episodic hypoxia: the renin-angiotensin system. J Appl Physiol (1985). 2002;92(2):627–33.

71. da Silva AQ, Fontes MA, Kanagy NL. Chronic infusion of angiotensin receptor antagonists in the hypothalamic paraventricular nucleus prevents hypertension in a rat model of sleep apnea. Brain Res. 2011;1368:231–8.

72. Semenza GL, Prabhakar NR. Neural regulation of hypoxia-inducible factors and redox state drives the pathogenesis of hypertension in a rodent model of sleep apnea. J Appl Physiol (1985). 2015;119(10):1152–56.

73. Peng YJ, Prabhakar NR. Reactive oxygen species in the plasticity of respiratory behavior elicited by chronic intermittent hypoxia. J Appl Physiol (1985). 2003;94(6):2342–9.

74. Peng YJ, Yuan G, Khan S, Nanduri J, Makarenko VV, Reddy VD, et al. Regulation of hypoxia-inducible factor-α isoforms and redox state by carotid body neural activity in rats. J Physiol. 2014;592(Pt 17):3841–58.

75. Peng YJ, Nanduri J, Yuan G, Wang N, Deneris E, Pendyala S, et al. NADPH oxidase is required for the sensory plasticity of the carotid body by chronic intermittent hypoxia. J Neurosci. 2009;29(15):4903–10.

76. Nanduri J, Vaddi DR, Khan SA, Wang N, Makerenko V, Prabhakar NR. Xanthine oxidase mediates hypoxia-inducible factor-2α degradation by intermittent hypoxia. PLoS One. 2013;8(10):e75838.

77. Nanduri J, Vaddi DR, Khan SA, Wang N, Makarenko V, Semenza GL, et al. HIF-1α activation by intermittent hypoxia requires NADPH oxidase stimulation by xanthine oxidase. PLoS One. 2015;10(3):e0119762.

78. Peng YJ, Yuan G, Ramakrishnan D, Sharma SD, Bosch-Marce M, Kumar GK, et al. Heterozygous HIF-1alpha deficiency impairs carotid body-mediated systemic responses and reactive oxygen species generation in mice exposed to intermittent hypoxia. J Physiol. 2006;577(Pt 2):705–16.

79. Morgan BJ, Bates ML, Rio RD, Wang Z, Dopp JM. Oxidative stress augments chemoreflex sensitivity in rats exposed to chronic intermittent hypoxia. Respir Physiol Neurobiol. 2016;234:47–59.

80. Tafil-Klawe M, Trzebski A, Klawe J, Pałko T. Augmented chemoreceptor reflex tonic drive in early human hypertension and in normotensive subjects with family background of hypertension. Acta Physiol Pol. 1985;36(1):51–8.

81. Abdala AP, McBryde FD, Marina N, Hendy EB, Engelman ZJ, Fudim M, et al. Hypertension is critically dependent on the carotid body input in the spontaneously hypertensive rat. J Physiol. 2012;590(17):4269–77.

82. Brognara F, Felippe ISA, Salgado HC, Paton JFR. Autonomic innervation of the carotid body as a determinant of its sensitivity—implications for cardiovascular physiology and pathology. Cardiovasc Res. 2020;117(4):1015–1032.

83. Eyzaguirre C, Lewin J. The effect of sympathetic stimulation on carotid nerve activity. J Physiol. 1961;159:251–67.

84. Acker H, O'Regan RG. The effects of stimulation of autonomic nerves on carotid body blood flow in the cat. J Physiol. 1981;315:99–110.

85. Marina N, Ang R, Machhada A, Kasymov V, Karagiannis A, Hosford PS, et al. Brainstem hypoxia contributes to the development of hypertension in the spontaneously hypertensive rat. Hypertension. 2015;65(4):775–83.

86. Ponikowski P, Banasiak W. Chemosensitivity in chronic heart failure. Heart Fail Monit. 2001;1(4):126–31.

87. Schultz HD, Sun SY. Chemoreflex function in heart failure. Heart Fail Rev. 2000;5(1):45–56.

88. Stickland MK, Miller JD, Smith CA, Dempsey JA. Carotid chemoreceptor modulation of regional blood flow distribution during exercise in health and chronic heart failure. Circ Res. 2007;100(9):1371–8.

89. Schultz HD, Marcus NJ, Del Rio R. Role of the carotid body chemoreflex in the pathophysiology of heart failure: a perspective from animal studies. Adv Exp Med Biol. 2015;860:167–85.

90. Ding Y, Li YL, Schultz HD. Role of blood flow in carotid body chemoreflex function in heart failure. J Physiol. 2011;589(Pt 1):245–58.

91. Marcus NJ, Del Rio R, Ding Y, Schultz HD. KLF2 mediates enhanced chemoreflex sensitivity, disordered breathing and autonomic dysregulation in heart failure. J Physiol. 2018;596(15):3171–85.

92. Andreas S, Haarmann H, Klarner S, Hasenfuss G, Raupach T. Increased sympathetic nerve activity in COPD is associated with morbidity and mortality. Lung. 2014;192(2):235–41.

93. Stickland MK, Fuhr DP, Edgell H, Byers BW, Bhutani M, Wong EY, et al. Chemosensitivity, cardiovascular risk, and the ventilatory response to exercise in COPD. PLoS One. 2016;11(6):e0158341.

94. Hansen J, Sander M. Sympathetic neural overactivity in healthy humans after prolonged exposure to hypobaric hypoxia. J Physiol. 2003;546(Pt 3):921–9.

95. Chen TK, Knicely DH, Grams ME. Chronic kidney disease diagnosis and management: a review. JAMA. 2019;322(13):1294–304.

96. Franchitto N, Despas F, Labrunee M, Vaccaro A, Lambert E, Lambert G, et al. Cardiorenal anemia syndrome in chronic heart failure contributes to increased sympathetic nerve activity. Int J Cardiol. 2013;168(3):2352–7.

97. Converse RL, Jacobsen TN, Toto RD, Jost CM, Cosentino F, Fouad-Tarazi F, et al. Sympathetic overactivity in patients with chronic renal failure. N Engl J Med. 1992;327(27):1912–8.

98. Masuo K, Mikami H, Ogihara T, Tuck M. Hormonal mechanisms in blood pressure reduction during hemodialysis in patients with chronic renal failure. Hypertens Res. 1995;18(Suppl 1):S201–3.

99. Despas F, Detis N, Dumonteil N, Labrunee M, Bellon B, Franchitto N, et al. Excessive sympathetic activation in heart failure with chronic renal failure: role of chemoreflex activation. J Hypertens. 2009;27(9):1849–54.

100. Ye C, Qiu Y, Zhang F, Chen AD, Zhou H, Wang JJ, et al. Chemical stimulation of renal tissue induces sympathetic activation and a pressor response via the paraventricular nucleus in rats. Neurosci Bull. 2020;36(2):143–52.

101. Tuncel M, Augustyniak R, Zhang W, Toto RD, Victor RG. Sympathetic nervous system function in renal hypertension. Curr Hypertens Rep. 2002;4(3):229–36.

102. Ksiazek A, Załuska W. Sympathetic overactivity in uremia. J Ren Nutr. 2008;18(1):118–21.

103. Dempsey JA, Smith CA. Update on chemoreception: influence on cardiorespiratory regulation and pathophysiology. Clin Chest Med. 2019;40(2):269–83.

104. Ponikowski P, Chua TP, Anker SD, Francis DP, Doehner W, Banasiak W, et al. Peripheral chemoreceptor hypersensitivity: an ominous sign in patients with chronic heart failure. Circulation. 2001;104(5):544–9.

105. Grassi G, Quarti-Trevano F, Esler MD. Sympathetic activation in congestive heart failure: an updated overview. Heart Fail Rev. 2021;26(1):173–182.

106. Grassi G, Ram VS. Evidence for a critical role of the sympathetic nervous system in hypertension. J Am Soc Hypertens. 2016;10(5):457–66.

107. Masuo K, Lambert GW, Esler MD, Rakugi H, Ogihara T, Schlaich MP. The role of sympathetic nervous activity in renal injury and end-stage renal disease. Hypertens Res. 2010;33(6):521–8.

108. Andreas S, Anker SD, Scanlon PD, Somers VK. Neurohumoral activation as a link to systemic manifestations of chronic lung disease. Chest. 2005;128(5):3618–24.

109. Del Rio R, Andrade DC, Marcus NJ, Schultz HD. Selective carotid body ablation in experimental heart failure: a new therapeutic tool to improve cardiorespiratory control. Exp Physiol. 2015;100(2):136–42.

110. Andrade DC, Arce-Alvarez A, Toledo C, Díaz HS, Lucero C, Quintanilla RA, et al. Revisiting the physiological effects of exercise training on autonomic regulation and chemoreflex control in heart failure: does ejection fraction matter? Am J Physiol Heart Circ Physiol. 2018;314(3):H464–H74.

111. McBryde FD, Abdala AP, Hendy EB, Pijacka W, Marvar P, Moraes DJ, et al. The carotid body as a putative therapeutic target for the treatment of neurogenic hypertension. Nat Commun. 2013;4:2395.

112. Li YL, Ding Y, Agnew C, Schultz HD. Exercise training improves peripheral chemoreflex function in heart failure rabbits. J Appl Physiol (1985). 2008;105(3):782–90.

113. Haack KK, Marcus NJ, Del Rio R, Zucker IH, Schultz HD. Simvastatin treatment attenuates increased respiratory variability and apnea/hypopnea index in rats with chronic heart failure. Hypertension. 2014;63(5):1041–9.

114. Niewinski P, Ponikowski P. The story of carotid body resection for HF: how an intriguing pathophysiology concept became a valid target for intervention. Eur Heart J. 2017;38(47):3481–2.

115. Narkiewicz K, Ratcliffe LE, Hart EC, Briant LJ, Chrostowska M, Wolf J, et al. Unilateral carotid body resection in resistant hypertension: a safety and feasibility trial. JACC Basic Transl Sci. 2016;1(5):313–24.

116. Nakayama K. Surgical removal of the carotid body for bronchial asthma. Dis Chest. 1961;40:595–604.

117. Honda Y. Respiratory and circulatory activities in carotid body-resected humans. J Appl Physiol (1985). 1992;73(1):1–8.

118. Gielen S, Laughlin MH, O'Conner C, Duncker DJ. Exercise training in patients with heart disease: review of beneficial effects and clinical recommendations. Prog Cardiovasc Dis. 2015;57(4):347–55.

119. Pearson MJ, Smart NA. Effect of exercise training on endothelial function in heart failure patients: a systematic review meta-analysis. Int J Cardiol. 2017;231:234–43.

120. Powell FL. Lake Louise consensus methods for measuring the hypoxic ventilatory response. Adv Exp Med Biol. 2006;588:271–6.

121. Duffin J. Measuring the ventilatory response to hypoxia. J Physiol. 2007;584(Pt 1):285–93.

122. Teppema LJ, Dahan A. The ventilatory response to hypoxia in mammals: mechanisms, measurement, and analysis. Physiol Rev. 2010;90(2):675–754.

123. Wellman A, Malhotra A, Jordan AS, Stevenson KE, Gautam S, White DP. Effect of oxygen in obstructive sleep apnea: role of loop gain. Respir Physiol Neurobiol. 2008;162(2):144–51.

124. Nielsen M, Smith H. Studies on the regulation of respiration in acute hypoxia; with a appendix on respiratory control during prolonged hypoxia. Acta Physiol Scand. 1952;24(4):293–313.

125. Hornbein TF, Griffo ZJ, Roos A. Quantitation of chemoreceptor activity: interrelation of hypoxia and hypercapnia. J Neurophysiol. 1961;24:561–8.

126. Dahan A, DeGoede J, Berkenbosch A, Olievier IC. The influence of oxygen on the ventilatory response to carbon dioxide in man. J Physiol. 1990;428:485–99.

127. Lahiri S, DeLaney RG. Stimulus interaction in the responses of carotid body chemoreceptor single afferent fibers. Respir Physiol. 1975;24(3):249–66.

128. Pedersen ME, Fatemian M, Robbins PA. Identification of fast and slow ventilatory responses to carbon dioxide under hypoxic and hyperoxic conditions in humans. J Physiol. 1999;521 Pt 1:273–87.

129. Dahan A, Nieuwenhuijs D, Teppema L. Plasticity of central chemoreceptors: effect of bilateral carotid body resection on central CO_2 sensitivity. PLoS Med. 2007;4(7):e239.

130. Rodman JR, Curran AK, Henderson KS, Dempsey JA, Smith CA. Carotid body denervation in dogs: eupnea and the ventilatory response to hyperoxic hypercapnia. J Appl Physiol (1985). 2001;91(1):328–35.

131. Blain GM, Smith CA, Henderson KS, Dempsey JA. Peripheral chemoreceptors determine the respiratory sensitivity of central chemoreceptors to CO(2). J Physiol. 2010;588(Pt 13):2455–71.

132. Dejours P. Control of respiration by arterial chemoreceptors. Ann N Y Acad Sci. 1963;109:682–95.

133. Prasad B, Morgan BJ, Gupta A, Pegelow DF, Teodorescu M, Dopp JM, et al. The need for specificity in quantifying neurocirculatory vs. respiratory effects of eucapnic hypoxia and transient hyperoxia. J Physiol. 2020;598(21):4803–19.

134. Ciarka A, Cuylits N, Vachiery JL, Lamotte M, Degaute JP, Naeije R, et al. Increased peripheral chemoreceptors sensitivity and exercise ventilation in heart transplant recipients. Circulation. 2006;113(2):252–7.

135. Trombetta IC, Maki-Nunes C, Toschi-Dias E, Alves MJ, Rondon MU, Cepeda FX, et al. Obstructive sleep apnea is associated with increased chemoreflex sensitivity in patients with metabolic syndrome. Sleep. 2013;36(1):41–9.

136. Narkiewicz K, van de Borne PJ, Pesek CA, Dyken ME, Montano N, Somers VK. Selective potentiation of peripheral chemoreflex sensitivity in obstructive sleep apnea. Circulation. 1999;99(9):1183–9.

137. Fernandes IA, Rocha MP, Campos MO, Mattos JD, Mansur DE, Rocha HNM, et al. Reduced arterial vasodilatation in response to hypoxia impairs cerebral and peripheral oxygen delivery in hypertensive men. J Physiol. 2018;596(7):1167–79.

138. Somers VK, Mark AL, Abboud FM. Potentiation of sympathetic nerve responses to hypoxia in borderline hypertensive subjects. Hypertension. 1988;11(6 Pt 2):608–12.

139. Keir DA, Duffin J, Millar PJ, Floras JS. Simultaneous assessment of central and peripheral chemoreflex regulation of muscle sympathetic nerve activity and ventilation in healthy young men. J Physiol. 2019;597(13):3281–96.

140. Olson EB, Vidruk EH, Dempsey JA. Carotid body excision significantly changes ventilatory control in awake rats. J Appl Physiol (1985). 1988;64(2):666–71.

141. Mortola JP, Rezzonico R, Lanthier C. Ventilation and oxygen consumption during acute hypoxia in newborn mammals: a comparative analysis. Respir Physiol. 1989;78(1):31–43.

142. Morgan BJ, Adrian R, Bates ML, Dopp JM, Dempsey JA. Quantifying hypoxia-induced chemoreceptor sensitivity in the awake rodent. J Appl Physiol (1985). 2014;117(7):816–24.

143. Cannon B, Nedergaard J. Brown adipose tissue: function and physiological significance. Physiol Rev. 2004;84(1):277–359.

144. Morrison SF. Central pathways controlling brown adipose tissue thermogenesis. News Physiol Sci. 2004;19:67–74.

145. Matsuoka T, Dotta A, Mortola JP. Metabolic response to ambient temperature and hypoxia in sinoaortic-denervated rats. Am J Physiol. 1994;266 (2 Pt 2):R387–91.

146. Kolobow T, Gattinoni L, Tomlinson TA, Pierce JE. Control of breathing using an extracorporeal membrane lung. Anesthesiology. 1977;46(2):138–41.

147. Phillipson EA, Bowes G, Townsend ER, Duffin J, Cooper JD. Role of metabolic CO_2 production in ventilatory response to steady-state exercise. J Clin Invest. 1981;68(3):768–74.

148. Marcus NJ, Olson EB, Bird CE, Philippi NR, Morgan BJ. Time-dependent adaptation in the hemodynamic response to hypoxia. Respir Physiol Neurobiol. 2009;165(1):90–6.

149. Stornetta RL, Moreira TS, Takakura AC, Kang BJ, Chang DA, West GH, et al. Expression of Phox2b by brainstem neurons involved in chemosensory integration in the adult rat. J Neurosci. 2006;26(40):10305–14.

150. Takakura AC, Moreira TS, Colombari E, West GH, Stornetta RL, Guyenet PG. Peripheral chemoreceptor inputs to retrotrapezoid nucleus (RTN) CO_2-sensitive neurons in rats. J Physiol. 2006;572(Pt 2):503–23.

151. Duffin J, Mateika JH. Cross-Talk opposing view: peripheral and central chemoreflexes have additive effects on ventilation in humans. J Physiol. 2013;591(18):4351–3.

152. Wilson RJ, Day TA. CrossTalk opposing view: peripheral and central chemoreceptors have hypoadditive effects on respiratory motor output. J Physiol. 2013;591(18):4355–7.

153. Curran AK, Rodman JR, Eastwood PR, Henderson KS, Dempsey JA, Smith CA. Ventilatory responses to specific CNS hypoxia in sleeping dogs. J Appl Physiol (1985). 2000;88(5):1840–52.

154. Gourine AV, Funk GD. On the existence of a central respiratory oxygen sensor. J Appl Physiol (1985). 2017;123(5):1344–9.

155. Xie A, Skatrud JB, Barczi SR, Reichmuth K, Morgan BJ, Mont S, et al. Influence of cerebral blood flow on breathing stability. J Appl Physiol (1985). 2009;106(3):850–6.

156. Deacon-Diaz NL, Sands SA, McEvoy RD, Catcheside PG. Daytime loop gain is elevated in obstructive sleep apnea but not reduced by CPAP treatment. J Appl Physiol (1985). 2018;125(5):1490–7.

157. Dempsey JA. Central sleep apnea: misunderstood and mistreated! F1000Res. 2019;8. doi: 10.12688/f1000research.18358.1

3 Developmental Changes in the Respiratory System of the Neonate-Child

Ahuva Brown, Liran Tamir Hostovsky, and Estelle B Gauda

INTRODUCTION

Breathing is an essential autonomic function that is critical to extrauterine life with the specific goals of providing oxygen to cells and tissues and removing carbon dioxide. Breathing must be automatic, reliable, and nimble, able to adjust seamlessly to different activity levels (asleep/awake, resting/exercising), the environment (hot/cold), and emotions (anxious/calm). The cells that initiate rhythmogenesis and the nerves that innervate the diaphragm and upper airway muscles are localized in the spinal cord and lower brainstem, respectively. However, the duration, intensity, and frequency of the activation of these cells and nerves are modulated by input from higher brain centers, the brainstem, and the periphery. Breathing movements are detected as early as 10-weeks' gestation in the human fetus (1). Prior to birth, fetal breathing movements are essential for normal lung development but not gas exchange; thus, fetal breathing is punctuated with periods of long pauses. With fetal maturation, breathing becomes more regular and sustained, but for those infants who are born at ≤34 weeks of gestation, unstable breathing is common. Because of these frequent and at times long respiratory pauses of ≥20 seconds, interventions are often required to sustain life in infants who are born at ≤26 weeks of gestation. Even for infants born at term, the central respiratory network and the peripheral inputs that modulate it are not completely developed (2). In this chapter, we will describe the major components of the central respiratory network in the brainstem and its major afferent inputs from mechanoreceptors and chemoreceptors and how they contribute to a versatile autonomic system that sustains life during development. Much of what we know about the central respiratory network is derived from experiments performed in newborn animals using reduced *in vitro* preparations. When available, we discuss relevant findings in human infants with breathing disorders.

NEUROANATOMY OF THE CENTRAL RESPIRATORY NETWORK

Respiratory movements are produced by a semi-autonomous neuronal network called a central pattern generator (CPG) found in the brainstem. Within this type of network are excitatory and inhibitory clusters of interneurons that interact to generate rhythmic patterns of activity. The CPG responsible for respiration transmits a coordinated output to the motoneurons that innervate the muscles of respiration (3) which include the pump muscles (diaphragm, intercostals, and abdominal muscles) and muscles of the upper airway (alae nares, pharyngeal, and laryngeal muscles). Activity of clusters of neurons in specific regions in the brainstem corresponds with the activity (contraction or relaxation) of the muscles involved in the three phases of respiration (inspiration, post inspiration, and expiration) (Figure 3.1). In the triple-oscillator hypothesis, the three phases of respiration are controlled by alternating activity between three regions of the brainstem (4, 5) (Figure 3.2).

Mapping the Respiratory Network

The cells that generate rhythm and the neurons that transmit activity are located in three anatomical areas of the brainstem: the **ventral respiratory column (VRC)** in the ventral medulla, the **dorsal respiratory group (DRG)** in the dorsal medulla, and specialized cells in the dorsal lateral pons that form the **pontine respiratory group (PRG).**

Ventral Respiratory Column (VRC)

The VRC is composed of clusters of neurons and neuronal projections that form columns on the ventral side of the medulla bilaterally (Figure 3.3). It is subdivided into the **rostral VRC** and the **caudal VRC** that contain neurons involved in rhythmogenesis and pattern formation, respectively.

The **rostral VRC** is comprised of the rostral ventral respiratory group (**rVRGroup**), the caudal ventral respiratory group (**cVRGroup**), the pre-Bötzinger complex (PBC), and the Bötzinger complex.

The **rVRGroup** contains inspiratory bulbospinal neurons, which are neurons that originate in the brainstem and synapse with motoneurons in the spinal cord such as phrenic motoneurons, external intercostal motoneurons, and expiratory neurons in the **cVRGroup**. The **cVRGroup** is comprised of expiratory bulbospinal neurons that project to abdominal and internal intercostal motoneurons.

DOI: 10.1201/9781003000631-4

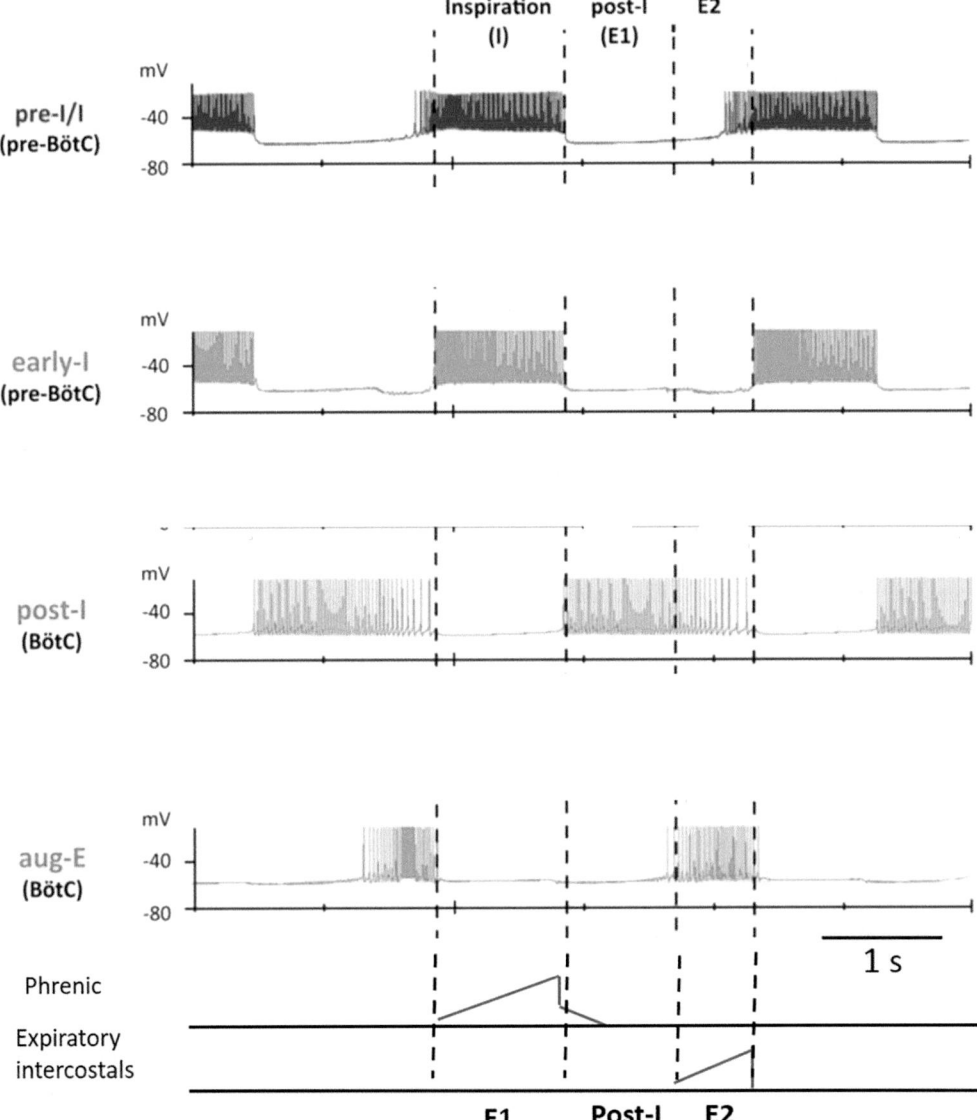

Figure 3.1 Three-phase organization of neuronal spike activity and motor output patterns during the respiratory cycle. Illustration showing spiking patterns in single representative neurons from the four main neuronal populations in the pre-Bötzinger (pre-BötC) and Bötzinger complex (BötC), as well as the motor output of the phrenic and expiratory intercostal nerves. **Pre-inspiratory/inspiratory** (pre-I/I) neurons in the pre-BötC start firing before inspiration and continue into inspiration, corresponding to phrenic nerve activity. **Early-inspiratory** (early-I) neurons in the pre-BötC have a peak spiking pattern early in inspiration and then slow. **Post-inspiratory** (post-I) neurons in the BötC that augment the first phase of expiration (E1) have a decrementing firing pattern and inhibit inspiratory neurons associated with silencing of the phrenic nerve. **Augmenting-expiratory** (aug-E) neurons in the BötC have a ramp firing pattern during E2 associated with the activation of expiratory intercostal muscles. During E2, pre-I/I neurons are initially weakly inhibited by aug-E neurons and receive a high level of excitatory drive, thereby allowing the pre-I/I neurons to escape from inhibition and start to fire. Activation of pre-I/I neurons provides strong excitation of early-I inhibitory neurons. The rapid onset of the early-I spiking initiates a wave of inhibition of post-I and aug-E neurons that completes the E-to-I transition. These phases are not strictly sequential but exhibit considerable temporal overlap. (Adapted and reprinted from Smith et al. Brainstem respiratory networks: building blocks and microcircuits. Trends Neurosci. 2013;152–62.)

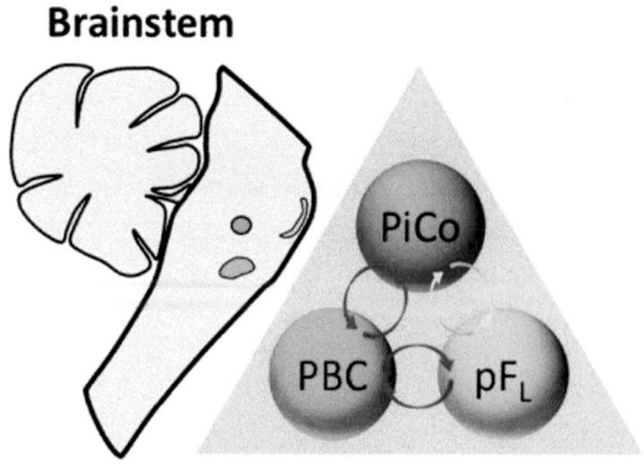

Brainstem

Figure 3.2 Illustration of the triple-oscillator hypothesis of respiratory rhythmogenesis. Respiratory rhythm is generated by three oscillators located in discrete regions of the brainstem—the pre-Bötzinger complex (PBC, green) for inspiration, the lateral parafacial region (pFL, turquoise, also known as the Bötzinger complex) for active expiration, and the post-inspiratory complex (PiCo, blue) for the post-inspiratory phase of breathing. (Adapted with permission from Jensen, Alilain and Crone. Role of propriospinal neurons in control of respiratory muscles and recovery of breathing following injury. Front Syst. Neurosci. 2019;13:84.)

The **pre-Bötzinger complex** (PBC) contains pacemaker cells that are essential to maintaining respiratory rhythm (6) and are neurochemically identified by their expression of neurokinin-1 receptors and activation by the neuromodulator substance P (7). In newborn rats, the appearance of respiratory activity coincides with the expression of neurokinin receptors in this cluster of primary inspiratory cells that initiates rhythmogenesis (8). Destruction of the PBC disrupts rhythmogenesis and therefore results in death in animals (9). A decreased number of neurons in the PBC has been found at autopsy in adults with neurodegenerative diseases with deficits in central respiratory control (10).

The **Bötzinger complex** contains propriobulbar inhibitory neurons that originate in the brainstem and send projections to inspiratory and expiratory bulbospinal neurons in the VRC.

Dorsal Respiratory Group (DRG)

Located within the nucleus tractus solitarii (NTS) in the medulla, the DRG contains mainly inspiratory neurons. It receives sensory input from mechanoreceptors and peripheral arterial chemoreceptors and sends output projections that innervate the diaphragm and intercostal muscles through motoneurons.

Pontine Respiratory Group (PRG)

The PRG is located in the parabrachial complex and consists of neurons that are involved in phase transition between inspiration and expiration, essentially functioning as the inspiratory off-switch via the Hering-Breur reflex. The parabrachial complex is comprised of the lateral and medial parabrachial nuclei and the Kölliker-Fuse nucleus (KFN). The PRG is important in coordinating upper airway activity with breathing during other behavioral activities such as swallowing, coughing, and speaking and mediates protective reflexes in the airway (11, 12).

Neurons in the KFN are exquisitely sensitive to hypoxia during fetal life. Via inhibitory projections to inspiratory and spinal neurons, the KFN is responsible for the decrease in fetal breathing and limb movements (postural atonia) during fetal hypoxia (13). After birth, this inhibitory reflex is deactivated, however, some have postulated that reactivation of this reflex after birth during hypoxia may cause early sudden infant death syndrome (SIDS) (14). Abnormalities in the neurochemical composition of the KFN have been identified in the brains of some infants born to mothers who smoked during pregnancy that subsequently died of SIDS (12).

Retrotrapezoid nucleus (RTN)

The RTN is another major anatomic region in the brainstem that is involved in the rhythm and pattern of diaphragmatic activity. The RTN contains CO_2/H^+-chemosensitive cells that depolarize in response to an increased concentration of CO_2 and H^+ ions, thereby decreasing the pH, leading to enhanced expiratory activity of abdominal muscles (15, 16). These chemosensitive cells express the *PHOX2B* gene that regulates the development of the neural crest cells; genetic mutations in the *PHOX2B* cause a constellation of findings affecting the autonomic nervous system and are pathognomonic for congenital central hypoventilation syndrome (CCHS). Lack of CO_2 chemosensitivity is the hallmark of infants who have CCHS (17).

Postinspiratory Complex (PiCo)

A newly discovered area, the PiCo, located medial to the nucleus ambiguous and caudal to the nucleus of cranial nerve VII, controls postinspiratory activity through semi-autonomous rhythm-generating properties (18).

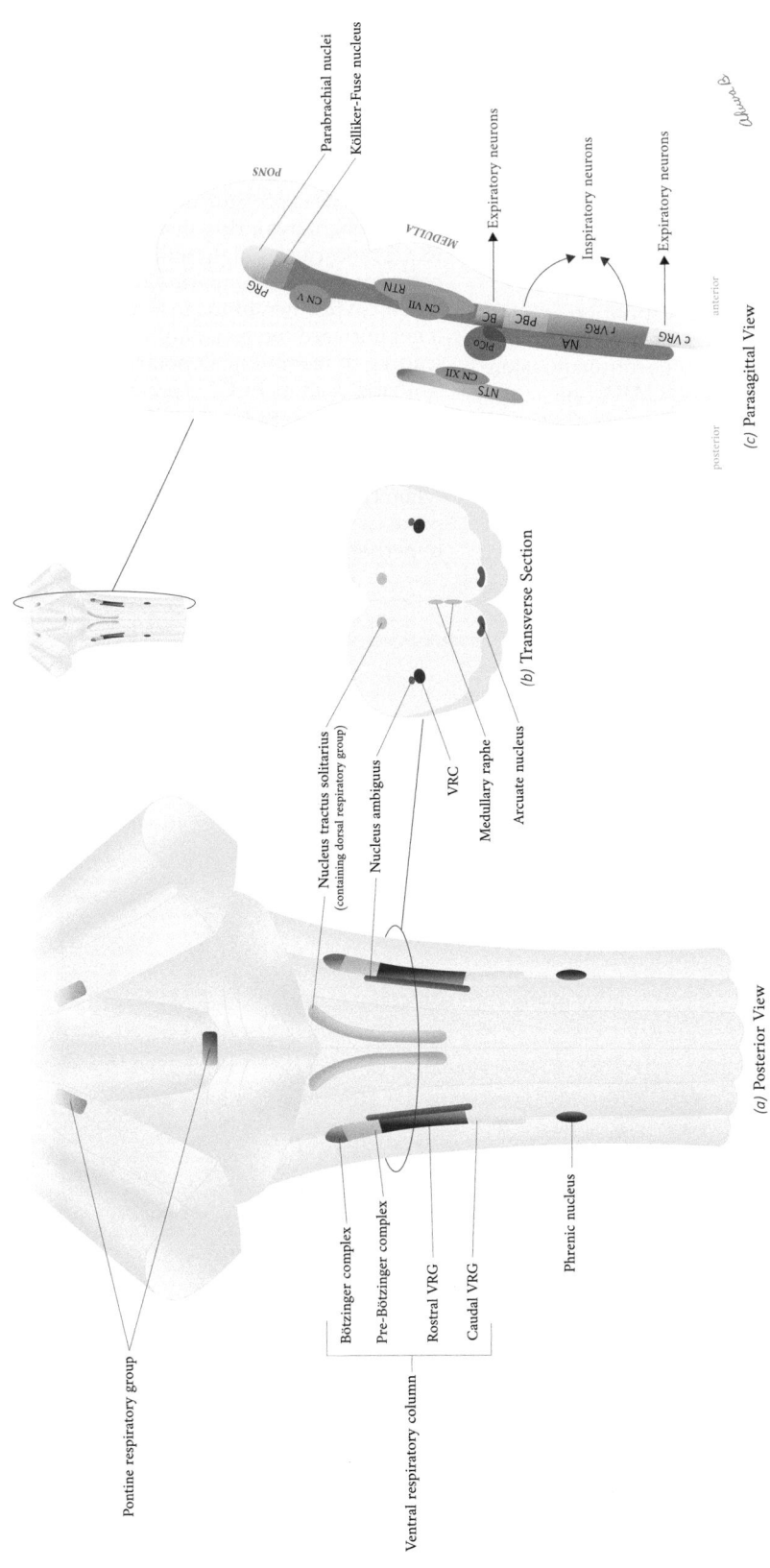

Figure 3.3 Mapping the respiratory network in the brainstem from (A) a posterior view, (B) a transverse section, and (C) a parasagittal view.

Abbreviations: BC, Bötzinger complex; cVRG, Caudal ventral respiratory group; NA, Nucleus ambiguous; NTS, Nucleus tractus solitarii; PiCo, Postinspiratory complex; PRG, Pontine respiratory group; PBC, Pre-Bötzinger complex; RTN, Retrotrapezoid nucleus; rVRG, Rostral ventral respiratory group; VRC, Ventral respiratory column; VRG, Ventral respiratory group.

45

NEUROTRANSMITTERS: THE MESSENGERS THAT REGULATE BREATHING (GABA AND GLUTAMATE)

In the brain, gamma-aminobutyric acid (GABA) and glycine are the major inhibitory neurotransmitters, while the major excitatory neurotransmitter is glutamate. They bind to inotropic receptors that are fast-acting ligand-gated ion channels and to metabotropic receptors that initiate intracellular signaling by G-proteins activation (Figure 3.4).

The different phases of respiration and its precise timing depend on the balance of excitatory and inhibitory neurotransmission in the respiratory network. GABA (via $GABA_A$ receptors) and glycine (via glycine receptors) mediate fast synaptic inhibition in the respiratory network by activating chloride channels that are part of the receptor (19). However, in early development, GABA and glycine are not always inhibitory and can, in

fact, be excitatory in many neuronal circuits (20–22), including the respiratory network (23). Whether glycine and GABA cause excitation or inhibition of postsynaptic neurons depends on the ratio of the (Na^+)-sodium (K^+)-potassium (Cl^-)-chloride cotransporter 1 (NKCC1) to the potassium-chloride cotransporter (KCC2) on the cell. Low expression of KCC2 during early development, resulting in a high NKCC1/KCC2 ratio, causes high intracellular chloride concentrations in immature neurons. Thus, when GABA then binds to $GABA_A$ receptors, a net outward movement of Cl^- ions occurs, leading to membrane depolarization (24). With maturation, KCC2 expression increases, reversing the NKCC1/KCC2 ratio and lowering intracellular Cl^- ions in rodents (25) (Figure 3.5) and human infants (26). Now when GABA binds to $GABA_A$ receptors, more Cl^- ions come into the cell leading to hyperpolarization. Clinically, the high NKCC1/

(a) LIGAND-GATED ION CHANNELS

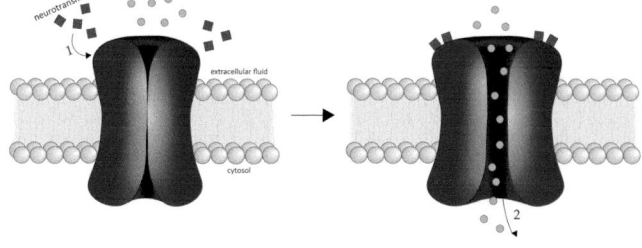

(b) G-PROTEIN-COUPLED RECEPTORS

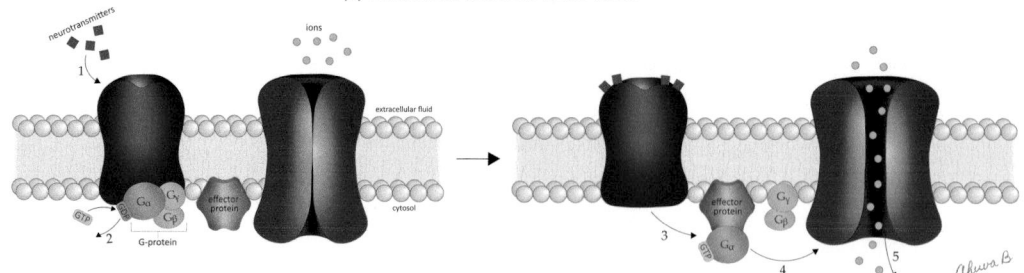

Figure 3.4 Neurotransmitters use two different kinds of receptors to transmit a signal. **(A) Ligand-gated ion channels**, also known as inotropic receptors, contain the receptor and ion channel in one protein complex and regulate the ion channel through the following process: (1) Neurotransmitter (the ligand) binds to the receptor site. (2) The channel opens, allowing ions to flow across. **(B) G-protein-coupled receptors**, also known as metabotropic receptors, activate G-proteins to regulate the ion channel through the following process: (1) Neurotransmitter binds to the receptor site. (2) GDP is replaced by GTP. (3) The α-subunit of the G-protein separates and binds to an effector protein (ex. adenylyl cyclase) which stimulates a second messenger system. (4) Second messenger systems (e.g. cAMP) then trigger a response (e.g. phosphorylation of the ion channel receptor). (5) The channel opens, allowing ions to flow across.

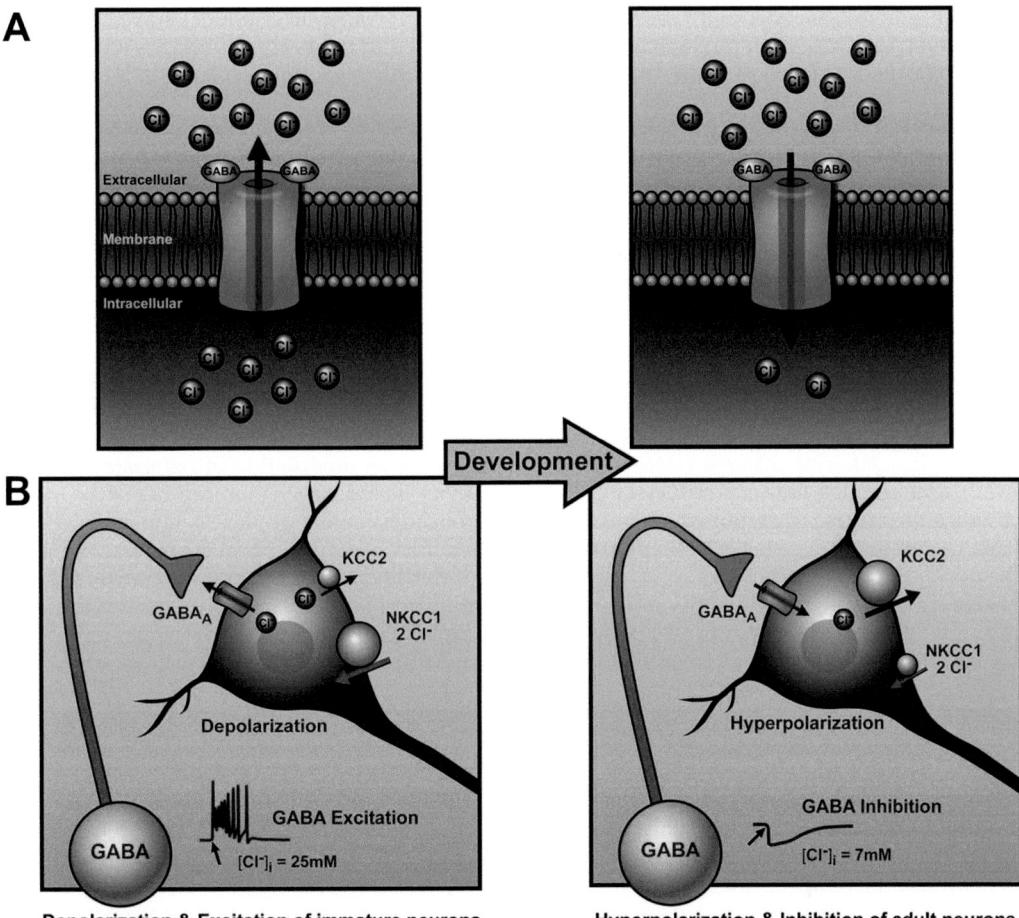

Figure 3.5 Schematic diagram showing the changes in intracellular chloride $[Cl\text{-}]_i$ levels and the polarity of the actions of GABA and chloride cotransporters. (A) The baseline intracellular $[Cl\text{-}]_i$ levels are higher in immature neurons than in adult neurons. (B) GABA depolarizes and excites immature neurons and inhibits adult ones. The chloride exporter KCC2 is minimally active, whereas the NKCC1 importer is highly active in immature neurons, resulting in high intracellular $[Cl\text{-}]_i$ levels. Thus, with the opening of the chloride channel, when GABA binds to the $GABA_A$ receptor, chloride flows out of the cell against the concentration gradient bringing the cell closer to its action potential, thereby mediating depolarization. With maturation, the KCC2 chloride exporter becomes more active resulting in lower intracellular $[Cl\text{-}]_i$ levels. Thus, when GABA binds to the $GABA_A$ receptor, chloride flows into the cell bringing it further from its action potential and resulting in hyperpolarization. (Reprinted from Ben-Ari. The GABA excitatory/inhibitory developmental sequence: A personal journey. Neuroscience. 2014).

KCC2 ratio is responsible for the myoclonic jerks and neuronal excitation associated with midazolam use in premature infants and is why midazolam may be ineffective in treating seizures in premature infants (27). Reduced GABAergic transmission from sensory input to the NTS can lead to the disordered breathing often observed in children with RETT syndrome because of a genetic mutation in the X-linked methyl-CpG binding protein 2 (Mecp2) gene (28).

Fast excitatory transmission is mediated by glutamate binding to the ligand-gated ion receptors N-methyl-D-aspartate (NMDA) and the non-NMDA AMPA (alpha-amino-3-hydroxy-5-methyl-4-isoxazolepropionic acid) and kainate receptors. The generation of respiratory rhythm within the central respiratory network and transmission to the phrenic and upper airway motoneurons is mediated by glutamate binding to AMPA and kainate receptors. Increased glutamate transmission is associated with increased ventilatory response to hypoxia in adults (29). However, a marked increase in AMPA receptor expression in the NTS during early development in rodents is not directly associated with an increase in ventilatory response to hypoxia (30).

NEUROMODULATORS: FINE TUNING GABAERGIC AND GLUTAMATERGIC NEUROTRANSMISSION

While glutamate and GABA/glycine may be the major excitatory and inhibitory neurotransmitters, respectively, in the brain and respiratory network, numerous neuromodulators such as serotonin, substance P, neurokinin, adenosine, adenosine triphosphate (ATP), and acetylcholine can reduce or enhance the release of glutamate and GABA from respiratory neurons (7, 31). Exploiting the power of neuromodulators is how many pharmaceuticals alter the activity of neurons throughout the brain. For example, premature infants who have apnea of prematurity are routinely given caffeine which enhances breathing and decreases the frequency of apnea (32). Caffeine and methyxanthines non-specifically block adenosine receptors (A1 and A2) on cells and neurons (33, 34). Adenosine binding to A1 receptors hyperpolarizes the neuron, while binding to A2 receptors depolarizes the neuron. Adenosine binding to the inhibitory A1 receptors on respiratory-related glutamatergic neurons depresses respiration (35); thus, blocking the binding of adenosine to A1-adenosine receptors by caffeine on excitatory (glutamatergic) respiratory neurons will increase neuronal excitation, decreasing apnea. Caffeine also blocks excitatory A2-adenosine receptors, which are heteroreceptors on GABAergic neurons, and decreases the release of GABA, again leading to excitation (36). In addition to stimulating breathing at baseline, caffeine also increases chemosensitivity to CO_2, likely at central chemoreceptors as opposed to peripheral (37), thereby stabilizing breathing in premature infants (38).

Serotonin can function either as a neurotransmitter or neuromodulator (39) but appears to have a primary neuromodulatory role in the respiratory network (40). Serotonin receptors are expressed in the brainstem (specifically the dorsal and median raphe) and are central to respiratory and cardiovascular homeostasis and arousal (41). Differences in the level of expression of some classes of serotonin receptors, the vesicular monoamine transporters (VMAT and VMAT2) and the serotonin transporter (SERT), have been identified in the brains of infants who have died of SIDS (for review see (41)). Increased frequency of specific polymorphisms in the promoter region of the SLC6A4 gene that encodes the serotonin transporter, resulting in a relative deficiency of serotonin levels, has also been found in the brains of infants who died of SIDS (42). A more recent finding suggests that the neurokinin-1 receptor in key respiratory brainstem nuclei is altered in premature infants who have died of SIDS (43).

PERIPHERAL INPUTS THAT MODULATE THE CENTRAL RESPIRATORY NETWORK

The peripheral inputs that have the greatest influence on modulation of respiratory activity include mechanoreceptors in the lung (bronchopulmonary reflexes), upper airway chemoreceptors (laryngeal chemoreceptors), and peripheral arterial chemoreceptors in the carotid body. The RTN integrates these peripheral inputs to send messages to the diaphragm and upper airway muscles. The central chemoreceptors in the RTN are responsive to changes in CO_2/pH and form synapses with neurons in the VRC including the PBC (44).

Bronchopulmonary Reflexes

Bronchopulmonary reflexes arising from the lung modulate the depth and duration of inspiration and expiration and are mediated through the vagal nerve (45) (for review see (46)). The vagal nerve has both myelinated and unmyelinated fibers that are activated by different stimuli (Figure 3.6).

Slowly Adapting Stretch Receptors (SARs): The Hering-Breuer (H-B) Reflex

Changes in lung volume activate the **H-B reflex** that mediates the duration of inspiration and expiration by activating SARs in the smooth muscle of the lung parenchyma. This reflex avoids lung overinflation and lung collapse. Lung expansion activates the SARs that lead to termination of inspiration, while lung deflation activates the H-B deflation reflex that terminates expiration and prolongs inspiration. The strength of the H-B reflex is greater at birth and decreases with maturation. Increased strength of the reflex is associated with premature birth (47), prone sleeping (48), active sleep (49), and acute respiratory distress syndrome (50). The decrease in respiratory rate that often occurs with lung inflation from continuous positive airway pressure in premature infants is

(a) **MYELINATED VAGUS NERVE**

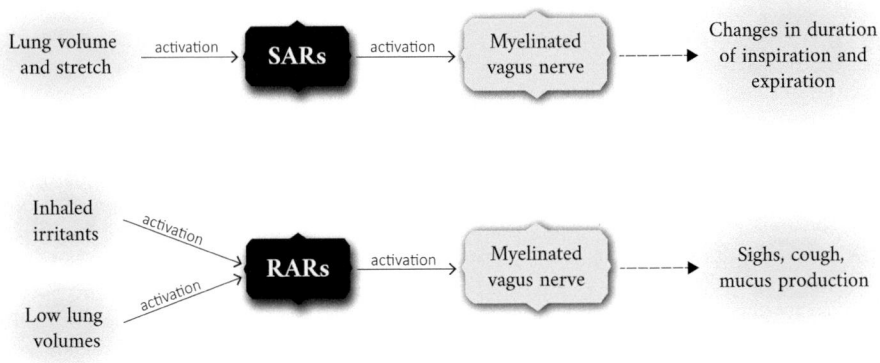

(b) **UNMYELINATED VAGUS NERVE (C-FIBERS)**

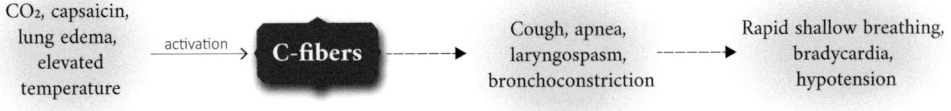

Figure 3.6 Schematic showing the vagally mediated bronchopulmonary reflexes in the airway and lung.

Reflex responses transmitted by myelinated nerve fibers fall into two categories: slowly adapting stretch receptors (SARs) and rapidly adapting stretch receptors (RARs). SARs mediate the duration of inspiration and expiration and are activated by lung stretch, while RARs are responsible for cough and augmented breaths (sighs) and are activated by airway irritants and low lung volumes. Sighs are commonly observed in premature infants and are important in restoring lung volume. Reflex responses transmitted by unmyelinated fibers of the vagus nerve (C-fibers) are classically activated by capsaicin and airway CO_2 (85); when activated, they increase the respiratory rate.

in part mediated by the H-B reflex. Vagal afferents mediating the H-B reflex synapse onto second-order neurons in parabrachial complex subnuclei in the PRG, inhibiting inspiratory neurons in the DRG (11).

Rapidly Adapting Receptors (RARs)

Low lung volume (lung deflation) also activates RARs located throughout the airways and lungs, prompting augmented breaths (sighs) and restoring functional residual capacity (FRC). Because excessively compliant chest walls in premature infants result in lung volumes less than FRC at the end of expiration, augmented breaths occur frequently. RARs are also activated by chemical irritants and airway CO_2 and mediate coughing, augmented breaths, and mucus production (51).

C-Fiber Receptors

Bronchial and pulmonary C-fiber receptors are unmyelinated vagal fibers that are found throughout the airway from the nose to the alveoli. The bronchial C-fibers are activated by stimuli in the bronchial circulation, while pulmonary C-fibers are activated by stimuli in the pulmonary circulation. Both are identified via their activation by capsaicin, found in hot peppers. They are both responsive to and activated by inflammatory mediators (52). The reflex response to C-fiber activation can include cough, apnea, broncho- and laryngospasm, rapid shallow breathing, and hypotension. Lung edema activates C fibers called Juxtacapillary receptors in the alveolar wall, which causes rapid shallow breathing (53). However, in infants, prolonged expiratory apnea is the most common response to C-fiber activation. Apnea is often an early sign of inflammation in infants that can be induced by C-fiber activation (54) and viral infections (55). Of interest, C-fibers can be sensitized by prenatal exposure to nicotine (56), explaining the association between increased incidence of SIDS in infants with upper airway infection who have also been exposed prenatally to cigarette smoke (reviewed in (57)).

Vagally Mediated Mechano- and Chemoreceptors in the Larynx

Mechano- and chemoreceptors are found in the upper airway. Activation of SARs, RARs, and C-fibers in the upper airway elicits a variety of physiological responses with the aim of preventing aspiration and modulating activity of the upper airway muscles and diaphragm. The most well described and extensively studied vagally mediated reflex in the upper airway is the laryngeal chemoreflex (LCR)

mediated by the superior laryngeal nerve (58). It is activated by solutions that are hypo-osmolar or have low chloride content and elicits a constellation of physiological responses that differs with maturation. Coughing, swallowing, arousal, and short apnea characterize the response seen in children and adults. In contrast, in term and premature infants and immature animals, this reflex may cause prolonged and profound apnea, bradycardia, hypoxemia, swallowing, and laryngeal closure that can be life threatening (59–61). The physiological responses to water in the upper airway may also differ between premature and term infants (Figure 3.7) (62).

The LCR is a complex reflex mediated through the superior laryngeal branch of the vagus nerve. C-fiber activation may also contribute to the response. The afferent fibers synapse onto neurons in the NTS, which sends (1) excitatory projections to motoneurons of the recurrent laryngeal nerve, causing contraction

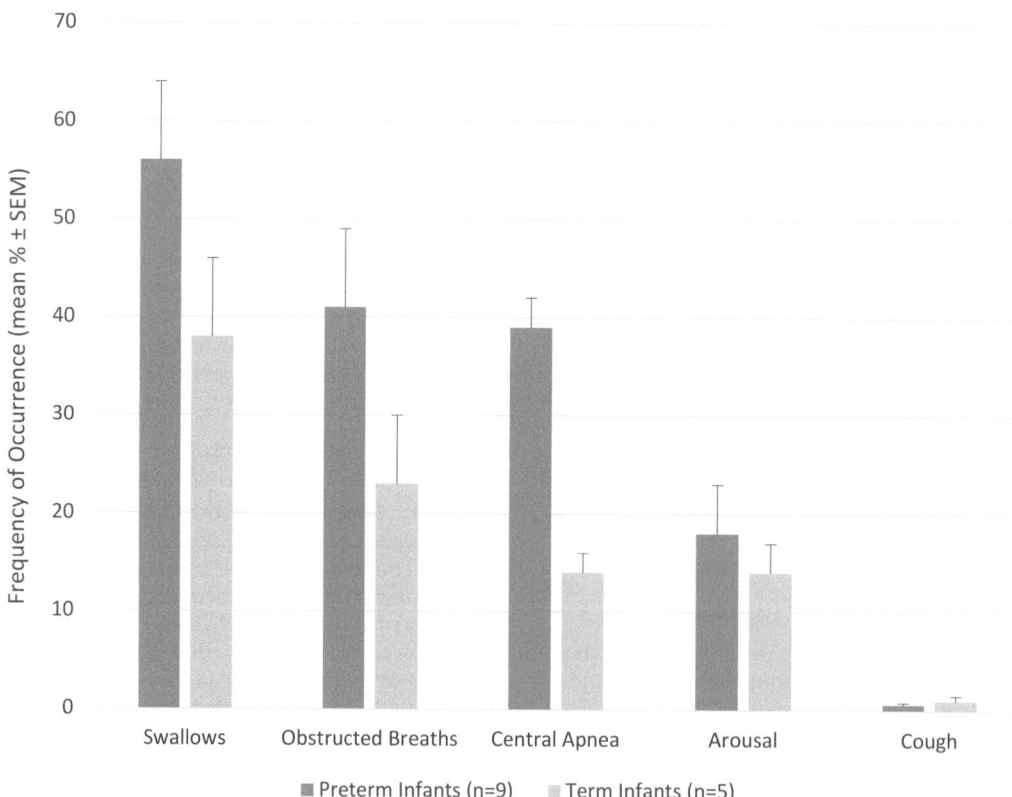

Figure 3.7 Bar graph showing the frequency of the responses when a small bolus of saline was introduced into the pharynx of sleeping term and preterm infants. (Reproduced from Thach BT. Maturation of cough and other reflexes that protect the fetal and neonatal airway. Pulm Pharmacol Ther. 2007;20:365–70.)

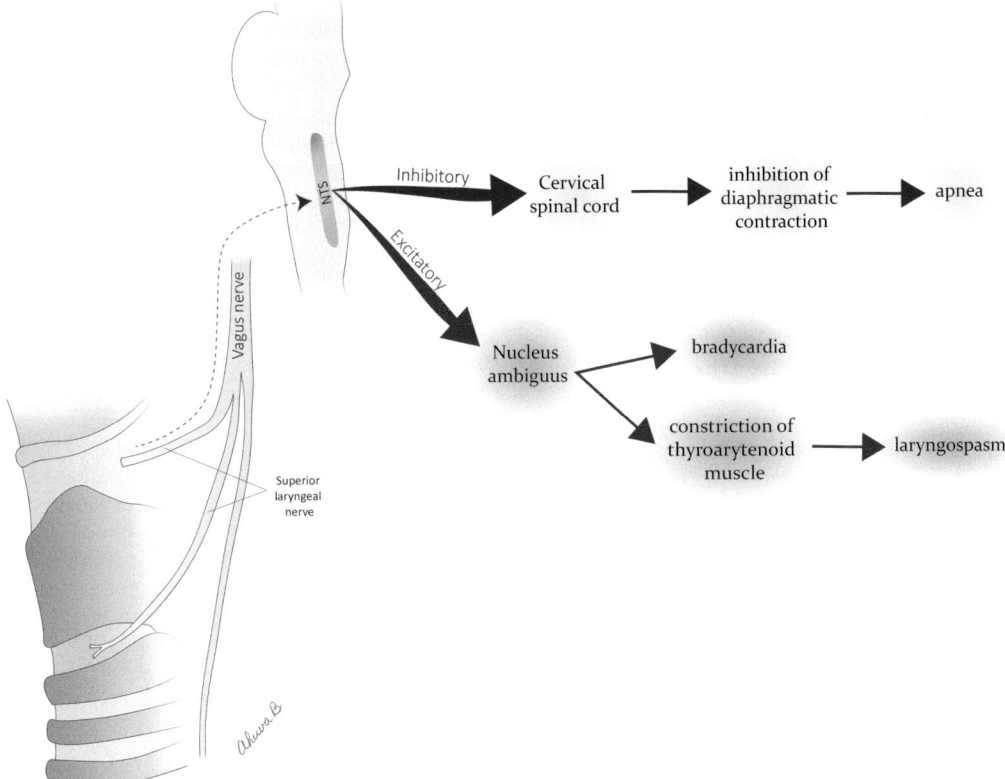

Figure 3.8 Schematic diagram illustrating the physiological components of the LCR. When receptors in the larynx are activated the signal is transmitted by the superior laryngeal nerve, a sensory branch of the vagus nerve that synapses on to neurons in the nucleus tractus solitarii (NTS) with neuronal projections that (1) activate motoneurons of the recurrent laryngeal nerve, causing laryngospasm, (2) inhibit phrenic motoneurons, causing apnea, and (3) activate cardiac vagal neurons in the nucleus ambiguous, causing bradycardia.

of the thyroarytenoid muscle that closes the larynx, (2) inhibitory projections to the phrenic motoneurons, inhibiting diaphragmatic activity, and (3) excitatory projections to cardiac vagal neurons in the nucleus ambiguous, causing bradycardia. (Figure 3.8).

Activation of the LCR in newborn infants can have significant adverse consequences and is thought to be causative in some cases of SIDS (63). Concurrent hypoxia accentuates the LCR in human infants who presented with acute life-threatening events (64).

Secretions in the upper airway associated with viral infections and dysfunctional swallowing, or severe gastroesophageal reflux to the level of the larynx, will activate this reflex and may be the cause of intermittent apneic and hypoxic episodes in premature infants with dysregulated swallow or infants with bronchopulmonary dysplasia (for review see (65)). Data from a recent preclinical study in newborn rodents showed that intermittent

hypoxia in the pregnant dam sensitized the LCR in rat pups and was associated with reduced expression of serotonin receptor binding in the NTS (66). Decreased expression of serotonin receptor binding has been found in infants who have died of SIDS (41), as outlined above in the section on neuromodulators.

Proprioceptors

Limb movements also stimulate respiration via activation of proprioceptors in the muscles with locomotion and exercise being the most common examples of this reflex (67). The reflex pathway involves afferents synapsing onto pattern generators in the spinal cord or a monosynaptic pathway to neurons in the central respiratory network (68, 69). Sustained low-level vibratory stimulation of proprioceptors in the palms and soles of premature infants decreased the frequency of apnea (70).

Peripheral Arterial Chemoreceptors

The peripheral arterial chemoreceptors in the carotid body, located in the bifurcation of the carotid artery, are the principal chemoreceptors responsible for reflex ventilatory responses to changes in oxygen tension, although they are also responsive to changes in blood CO_2/H^+ levels. Hypoxia and hypercapnia increase ventilation, while hyperoxia and hypocapnia decrease ventilation. The carotid body consists of nerve fibers, blood vessels, and two types of glomus cells, type I that are chemosensitive and type II that are glial-like, i.e. supportive. In response to hypoxia, the type I cell depolarizes and releases excitatory and inhibitory neurotransmitters/neuromodulators that then bind to postsynaptic receptors on the carotid sinus nerve, a branch of cranial nerve IX, and to autoreceptors on the type I cell that alters further release of the neurotransmitter/neuromodulator (Figure 3.9) (71). Although multiple neurotransmitters have been identified in the carotid body, dopamine is the most abundant. Dopamine binding to postsynaptic D2 dopamine receptors inhibits carotid sinus nerve activity while ATP

binding to postsynaptic purinergic receptors increases carotid sinus nerve activity (71). The intrinsic properties of the chemosensitive cells and the balance of excitatory/inhibitory neurotransmission in the carotid body change during early development (72). Chronic and intermittent hypoxia, hyperoxic exposure, and inflammation during early development can change the transmitter profile in the carotid body and alter hypoxic chemosensitivity (reviewed in (57)).

The peripheral arterial chemoreceptors are responsive to hypoxia in fetal life but are silenced immediately after birth because of the higher oxygen tension. Within several days after birth, the peripheral arterial chemoreceptors again become responsive to oxygen at a higher threshold. Hypoxic chemosensitivity of the peripheral arterial chemoreceptors progressively increases during the first 2–3 weeks of postnatal life, which is similar for infants born at preterm or at term gestation (73). Activation of the carotid body is not necessary for spontaneous breathing at birth, but activity from the carotid body during the first several weeks after birth appears essential for maturation of the stable central

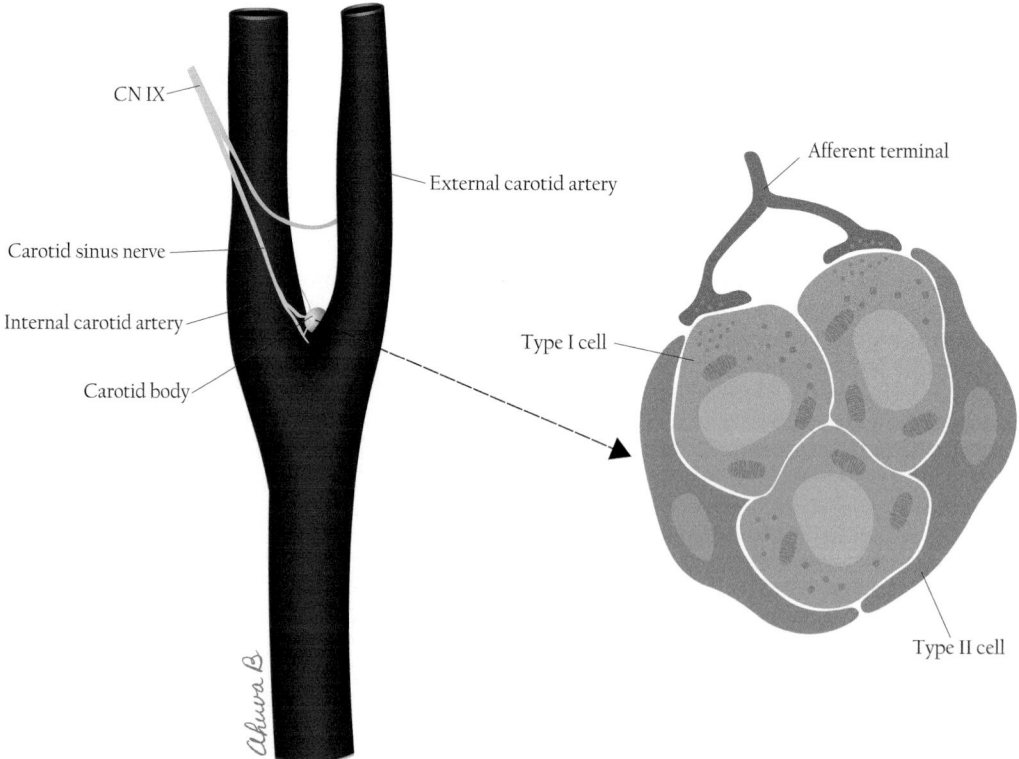

Figure 3.9 Illustration of the cellular organization and innervation of the carotid body. Type I cell clusters are closely associated with glial-like type II cells. Type I cells contain dense-core granules and receive afferent innervation from the carotid sinus nerve and cranial nerve IX.

respiratory network (65). Newborn rodents raised in 60% oxygen from birth through the first 7–14 days of life and who are then returned to room air have underdeveloped carotid bodies and absent hypoxic chemosensitivity throughout adulthood (74–76) and are intolerant to asphyxia (77). Moreover, in several mammalian species, resection of the carotid sinus nerve, the afferent output from the carotid body, during the first week of life leads to spontaneous death several weeks later (reviewed in (65)).

While the hypoxic chemosensitivity of the carotid body *increases* with development, the influence of tonic input from the carotid body on baseline breathing *decreases* with development. Periodic breathing is characterized by cycles of hyperventilation followed by a short 3–4 second apnea; it is a normal breathing pattern that occurs in premature infants and is mediated by the carotid body (78). As outlined above, the carotid body is highly sensitive to low oxygen tension and hypoxia will induce periodic breathing. Lower oxygen tension often occurs in premature infants at baseline and is therefore likely the stimulus activating the carotid body and causing periodic breathing. Supplemental oxygen decreases the frequency of periodic breathing and stabilizes respiration (79). However, type I cells are also exquisitely sensitive to changes in CO_2; the drop in pCO_2

that occurs during the hyperventilation phase markedly reduces the excitatory output from the carotid body to the central respiratory network. With the subsequent increase in CO_2 (by only a few torr), output from the carotid body will increase, initiating the hyperventilation phase of periodic breathing. The levels of pCO_2 that activate and silence the carotid body differ by only 2–4 torr in premature infants. This narrow difference substantially contributes to the increased incidence of periodic breathing in premature infants (80–82). The location of the carotid body and its size are two key features that allow it to respond rapidly to changes in arterial CO_2/H^+ and O_2: it is in the bifurcation of the carotid artery, and it has the highest level of blood flow per gram of tissue than any other organ in the body (83). These features, combined with the small size of the infant, create the perfect storm for cyclic breathing in premature infants. In those infants who also have a low FRC, these short apneas can be associated with intermittent hypoxia and untoward effects on developing organs (84).

SUMMARY

Breathing is an intricate, nimble process that is vital to extrauterine life (Figure 3.10). All components involved in the process of breathing are undergoing significant changes

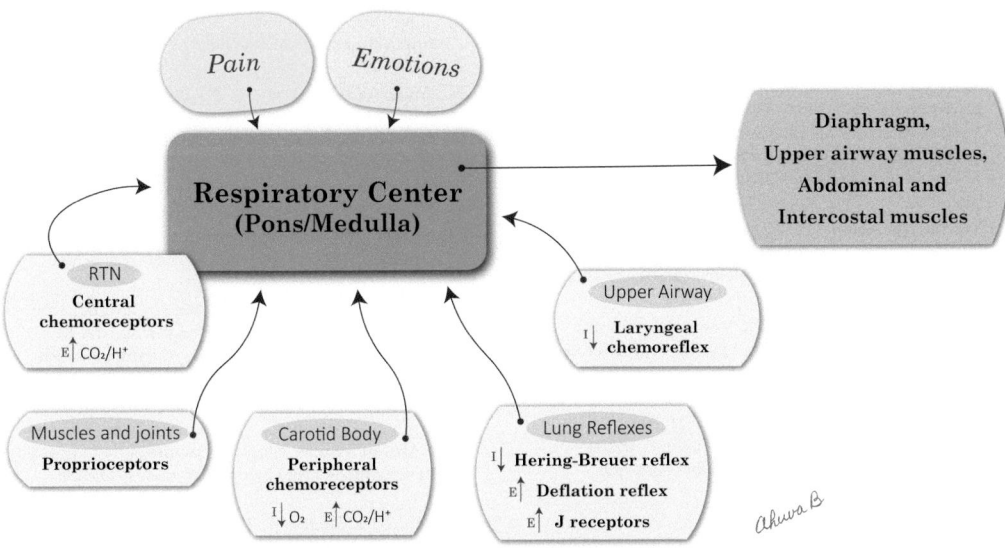

Figure 3.10 Schematic summarizing the integration of peripheral reflexes, central chemoreceptors, and inputs from higher brain structures controlling pain and emotions to the central respiratory network and corresponding output to the muscles of respiration. Small blue up arrows represent excitatory input and down arrows represent inhibitory influence on the central respiratory network.

during development and are therefore vulnerable to adverse stimuli such as nicotine exposure, intermittent or chronic hypoxia and/or hyperoxia, and prenatal and postnatal inflammation. Plasticity-induced changes from adverse stimuli lead to a less agile respiratory network often failing in response to stressors during a critical period, leading to SIDS. Genetic and epigenetic modifications of neurotransmitters and neuromodulators or developmental disruption of specific neuronal groups can permanently disrupt normal breathing with significant consequences such as what occurs in Rett syndrome, congenital central hypoventilation syndrome, and some cases of SIDS. Other patterns of breathing instability, such as periodic breathing or apnea of prematurity, are examples of an immature respiratory network that put it at risk for failure during the first 2–6 months of life. Thus, it is important to understand the neuroanatomy, intrinsic and extrinsic factors that are involved in the maturation of respiration, and factors that adversely affect the normal development of the respiratory network. This knowledge increases the opportunity to find therapeutic targets to stabilize breathing during development and strategies to mitigate early exposures that may compromise normal development leading to increased risk of respiratory failure during infancy.

REFERENCES

1. Koos BJ, Rajaee A. Fetal breathing movements and changes at birth. Adv Exp Med Biol. 2014;814:89–101.

2. Wong-Riley MT, Liu Q, Gao XP. Peripheral-central chemoreceptor interaction and the significance of a critical period in the development of respiratory control. Respir Physiol Neurobiol. 2013;185(1):156–69.

3. Smith JC, Abdala AP, Borgmann A, Rybak IA, Paton JF. Brainstem respiratory networks: building blocks and microcircuits. Trends Neurosci. 2013;36(3):152–62.

4. Anderson TM, Ramirez JM. Respiratory rhythm generation: triple oscillator hypothesis. F1000Res. 2017;6:139.

5. Carroll MS, Viemari JC, Ramirez JM. Patterns of inspiratory phase-dependent activity in the in vitro respiratory network. J Neurophysiol. 2013;109(2):285–95.

6. Smith JC, Ellenberger HH, Ballanyi K, Richter DW, Feldman JL. Pre-Bötzinger complex: a brainstem region that may generate respiratory rhythm in mammals. Science. 1991;254(5032):726–9.

7. Doi A, Ramirez JM. Neuromodulation and the orchestration of the respiratory rhythm. Respir Physiol Neurobiol. 2008;164(1–2):96–104.

8. Bonham AC. Neurotransmitters in the CNS control of breathing. Respir Physiol. 1995;101(3):219–30.

9. Ramirez JM, Schwarzacher SW, Pierrefiche O, Olivera BM, Richter DW. Selective lesioning of the cat pre-Bötzinger complex in vivo eliminates breathing but not gasping. J Physiol. 1998;507 (Pt 3):895–907.

10. Schwarzacher SW, Rüb U, Deller T. Neuroanatomical characteristics of the human pre-Bötzinger complex and its involvement in neurodegenerative brainstem diseases. Brain. 2011;134(Pt 1):24–35.

11. Dutschmann M, Dick TE. Pontine mechanisms of respiratory control. Compr Physiol. 2012;2(4):2443–69.

12. Varga AG, Maletz SN, Bateman JT, Reid BT, Levitt ES. Neurochemistry of the Kölliker-Fuse nucleus from a respiratory perspective. J Neurochem. 2021;156(1):16–37.

13. Walker DW. Hypoxic inhibition of breathing and motor activity in the foetus and newborn. Clin Exp Pharmacol Physiol. 1995;22(8):533–6.

14. Lavezzi AM. A new theory to explain the underlying pathogenetic mechanism of sudden infant death syndrome. Front Neurol. 2015;6:220.

15. Guyenet PG, Stornetta RL, Bayliss DA. Retrotrapezoid nucleus and central chemoreception. J Physiol. 2008;586(8):2043–8.

16. Abbott SB, Stornetta RL, Coates MB, Guyenet PG. Phox2b-expressing neurons of the parafacial region regulate breathing rate, inspiration, and expiration in conscious rats. J Neurosci. 2011;31(45):16410–22.

17. Bishara J, Keens TG, Perez IA. The genetics of congenital central hypoventilation syndrome: clinical implications. Appl Clin Genet. 2018;11:135–44.

18. Anderson TM, Garcia AJ, 3rd, Baertsch NA, Pollak J, Bloom JC, Wei AD, et al. A novel excitatory network for the control of breathing. Nature. 2016;536(7614):76–80.

19. Haji A, Takeda R, Okazaki M. Neuropharmacology of control of respiratory rhythm and pattern in mature mammals. Pharmacol Ther. 2000;86(3):277–304.

20. Rivera C, Voipio J, Payne JA, Ruusuvuori E, Lahtinen H, Lamsa K, et al. The K$^+$/Cl$^-$ co-transporter KCC2 renders GABA hyperpolarizing during neuronal maturation. Nature. 1999;397(6716):251–5.

21. Cellot G, Cherubini E. Functional role of ambient GABA in refining neuronal circuits early in postnatal development. Front Neural Circuits. 2013;7:136.

22. Ben-Ari Y, Gaiarsa JL, Tyzio R, Khazipov R. GABA: a pioneer transmitter that excites immature neurons and generates primitive oscillations. Physiol Rev. 2007;87(4):1215–84.

23. Ritter B, Zhang W. Early postnatal maturation of GABAA-mediated inhibition in the brainstem respiratory rhythm-generating network of the mouse. Eur J Neurosci. 2000;12(8):2975–84.

24. Kaila K, Price TJ, Payne JA, Puskarjov M, Voipio J. Cation-chloride cotransporters in neuronal development, plasticity and disease. Nat Rev Neurosci. 2014;15(10):637–54.

25. Ben-Ari Y. The GABA excitatory/inhibitory developmental sequence: a personal journey. Neuroscience. 2014;279:187–219.

26. Hyde TM, Lipska BK, Ali T, Mathew SV, Law AJ, Metitiri OE, et al. Expression of GABA signaling molecules KCC2, NKCC1, and GAD1 in cortical development and schizophrenia. J Neurosci. 2011;31(30):11088–95.

27. Ozcan B, Kavurt S, Yucel H, Bas AY, Demirel N. Rhythmic myoclonic jerking induced by midazolam in a preterm infant. Pediatr Neurol. 2015;52(6):e9.

28. Chen CY, Di Lucente J, Lin YC, Lien CC, Rogawski MA, Maezawa I, et al. Defective GABAergic neurotransmission in the nucleus tractus solitarius in Mecp2-null mice, a model of Rett syndrome. Neurobiol Dis. 2018;109(Pt A):25–32.

29. Ang RC, Hoop B, Kazemi H. Role of glutamate as the central neurotransmitter in the hypoxic ventilatory response. J Appl Physiol (1985). 1992;72(4):1480–7.

30. Whitney GM, Ohtake PJ, Simakajornboon N, Xue YD, Gozal D. AMPA glutamate receptors and respiratory control in the developing rat: anatomic and pharmacological aspects. Am J Physiol Regul Integr Comp Physiol. 2000;278(2):R520–8.

31. Simakajornboon N, Kuptanon T. Maturational changes in neuromodulation of central pathways underlying hypoxic ventilatory response. Respir Physiol Neurobiol. 2005;149(1–3):273–86.

32. Steer PA, Henderson-Smart DJ. Caffeine versus theophylline for apnea in preterm infants. Cochrane Database Syst Rev. 2000;(2):Cd000273.

33. Fredholm BB. On the mechanism of action of theophylline and caffeine. Acta Med Scand. 1985;217(2):149–53.

34. Biaggioni I, Paul S, Puckett A, Arzubiaga C. Caffeine and theophylline as adenosine receptor antagonists in humans. J Pharmacol Exp Ther. 1991;258(2):588–93.

35. Herlenius E, Lagercrantz H, Yamamoto Y. Adenosine modulates inspiratory neurons and the respiratory pattern in the brainstem of neonatal rats. Pediatr Res. 1997;42(1):46–53.

36. Mayer CA, Haxhiu MA, Martin RJ, Wilson CG. Adenosine A2A receptors mediate GABAergic inhibition of respiration in immature rats. J Appl Physiol (1985). 2006;100(1):91–7.

37. Bairam A, De Grandpré P, Dauphin C, Marchal F. Effects of caffeine on carotid sinus nerve chemosensory discharge in kittens and cats. J Appl Physiol (1985). 1997;82(2):413–8.

38. Rossor T, Bhat R, Ali K, Peacock J, Rafferty GF, Greenough A. The effect of caffeine on the ventilatory response to hypercarbia in preterm infants. Pediatr Res. 2018;83(6):1152–7.

39. Ciranna L. Serotonin as a modulator of glutamate- and GABA-mediated neurotransmission: implications in physiological functions and in pathology. Curr Neuropharmacol. 2006;4(2):101–14.

40. Hodges MR, Richerson GB. Contributions of 5-HT neurons to respiratory control: neuromodulatory and trophic effects. Respir Physiol Neurobiol. 2008;164(1–2):222–32.

41. Kinney HC, Haynes RL. The serotonin brainstem hypothesis for the sudden infant death syndrome. J Neuropathol Exp Neurol. 2019;78(9):765–79.

42. Weese-Mayer DE, Ackerman MJ, Marazita ML, Berry-Kravis EM. Sudden infant death syndrome: review of implicated genetic factors. Am J Med Genet A. 2007;143a(8):771–88.

43. Bright FM, Vink R, Byard RW, Duncan JR, Krous HF, Paterson DS. Abnormalities in substance P neurokinin-1 receptor binding in key brainstem nuclei in sudden infant death syndrome related to prematurity and sex. PLoS One. 2017;12(9):e0184958.

44. Bochorishvili G, Stornetta RL, Coates MB, Guyenet PG. Pre-Bötzinger complex receives glutamatergic innervation from galaninergic and other retrotrapezoid nucleus neurons. J Comp Neurol. 2012;520(5):1047–61.

45. Moreira TS, Takakura AC, Colombari E, West GH, Guyenet PG. Inhibitory input from slowly adapting lung stretch receptors to retrotrapezoid nucleus chemoreceptors. J Physiol. 2007;580(Pt 1):285–300.

46. Widdicombe JG, Sant'Ambrogio G. Mechanoreceptors in Respiratory Systems. In: Ito F, editor. Comparative Aspects of Mechanoreceptor Systems. Berlin, Heidelberg: Springer Berlin Heidelberg; 1992. p. 111–35.

47. Kirkpatrick SM, Olinsky A, Bryan MH, Bryan AC. Effect of premature delivery on the maturation of the Hering-Breuer inspiratory inhibitory reflex in human infants. J Pediatr. 1976;88(6):1010–4.

48. Landolfo F, Saiki T, Peacock J, Hannam S, Rafferty GF, Greenough A. Hering–Breuer reflex, lung volume and position in prematurely born infants. Pediatr Pulmonol. 2008;43(8):767–71.

49. Hand IL, Noble L, Wilks M, Towler E, Kim M, Yoon JJ. Hering-Breuer reflex and sleep state in the preterm infant. Pediatr Pulmonol. 2004;37(1):61–4.

50. Winter JPD, Merth IT, Berkenbosch A, Brand R, Quanjer PH. Strength of the Breuer-Hering inflation reflex in term and preterm infants. J Appl Physiol. 1995;79(6):1986–90.

51. Widdicombe J. Reflexes from the lungs and airways: historical perspective. J Appl Physiol (1985). 2006;101(2):628–34.

52. Carr MJ, Undem BJ. Bronchopulmonary afferent nerves. Respirology. 2003;8(3):291–301.

53. Coleridge JC, Coleridge HM. Afferent vagal C fibre innervation of the lungs and airways and its functional significance. Rev Physiol Biochem Pharmacol. 1984;99:1–110.

54. Eichenwald EC, Aina A, Stark AR. Apnea frequently persists beyond term gestation in infants delivered at 24 to 28 weeks. Pediatrics. 1997;100(3 Pt 1):354–9.

55. Pickens DL, Schefft GL, Storch GA, Thach BT. Characterization of prolonged apneic episodes associated with respiratory syncytial virus infection. Pediatr Pulmonol. 1989;6(3):195–201.

56. Zhao L, Zhuang J, Zang N, Lin Y, Lee LY, Xu F. Prenatal nicotinic exposure upregulates pulmonary C-fiber NK1R expression to prolong pulmonary C-fiber-mediated apneic response. Toxicol Appl Pharmacol. 2016;290:107–15.

57. Gauda EB, McLemore GL. Premature birth, homeostatic plasticity and respiratory consequences of inflammation. Respir Physiol Neurobiol. 2020;274:103337.

58. Harding R, Johnson P, McClelland ME. Liquid-sensitive laryngeal receptors in the developing sheep, cat and monkey. J Physiol. 1978;277:409–22.

59. Boggs DF, Bartlett D, Jr. Chemical specificity of a laryngeal apneic reflex in puppies. J Appl Physiol Respir Environ Exerc Physiol. 1982;53(2):455–62.

60. Thach BT. Maturation and transformation of reflexes that protect the laryngeal airway from liquid aspiration from fetal to adult life. Am J Med. 2001;111(Suppl 8A):69s–77s.

61. Richardson MA, Adams J. Fatal apnea in piglets by way of laryngeal chemoreflex: postmortem findings as anatomic correlates of sudden infant death syndrome in the human infant. Laryngoscope. 2005;115(7):1163–9.

62. Thach BT. Maturation of cough and other reflexes that protect the fetal and neonatal airway. Pulm Pharmacol Ther. 2007;20(4):365–70.

63. Thach BT. The Role of the Upper Airway in SIDS and Sudden Unexpected Infant Deaths and the Importance of External Airway-Protective Behaviors. In: Duncan JR, Byard RW, editors. SIDS Sudden Infant and Early Childhood Death: The Past, the Present and the Future. Adelaide (AU): University of Adelaide Press; 2018. 491–6.

64. Wennergren G, Hertzberg T, Milerad J, Bjure J, Lagercrantz H. Hypoxia reinforces laryngeal reflex bradycardia in infants. Acta Paediatr Scand. 1989;78(1):11–7.

65. Gauda EB, Cristofalo E, Nunez J. Peripheral arterial chemoreceptors and sudden infant death syndrome. Respir Physiol Neurobiol. 2007;157(1):162–70.

66. Donnelly WT, Haynes RL, Commons KG, Erickson DJ, Panzini CM, Xia L, et al. Prenatal intermittent hypoxia sensitizes the laryngeal chemoreflex, blocks serotoninergic shortening of the reflex, and reduces 5-HT(3) receptor binding in the NTS in anesthetized rat pups. Exp Neurol. 2020;326:113166.

67. Gariépy JF, Missaghi K, Dubuc R. The interactions between locomotion and respiration. Prog Brain Res. 2010;187:173–88.

68. Morin D, Viala D. Coordinations of locomotor and respiratory rhythms in vitro are critically dependent on hindlimb sensory inputs. J Neurosci. 2002;22(11):4756–65.

69. Giraudin A, Le Bon-Jégo M, Cabirol MJ, Simmers J, Morin D. Spinal and pontine relay pathways mediating respiratory rhythm entrainment by limb proprioceptive inputs in the neonatal rat. J Neurosci. 2012;32(34):11841–53.

70. Kesavan K, Frank P, Cordero DM, Benharash P, Harper RM. Neuromodulation of limb proprioceptive afferents decreases apnea of prematurity and accompanying intermittent hypoxia and bradycardia. PLoS One. 2016;11(6):e0157349.

71. Nurse CA. Synaptic and paracrine mechanisms at carotid body arterial chemoreceptors. J Physiol. 2014;592(16):3419–26.

72. Gauda EB, Carroll JL, Donnelly DF. Developmental maturation of chemosensitivity to hypoxia of peripheral arterial chemoreceptors–invited article. Adv Exp Med Biol. 2009;648:243–55.

73. Rigatto H, Brady JP, de la Torre Verduzco R. Chemoreceptor reflexes in preterm infants: I. The effect of gestational and postnatal age on the ventilatory response to inhalation of 100% and 15% oxygen. Pediatrics. 1975;55(5):604–13.

74. Erickson JT, Mayer C, Jawa A, Ling L, Olson EB, Jr., Vidruk EH, et al. Chemoafferent degeneration and carotid body hypoplasia following chronic hyperoxia in newborn rats. J Physiol. 1998;509 (Pt 2):519–26.

75. Fuller DD, Bavis RW, Vidruk EH, Wang ZY, Olson EB, Jr., Bisgard GE, et al. Life-long impairment of hypoxic phrenic responses in rats following 1 month of developmental hyperoxia. J Physiol. 2002;538(Pt 3):947–55.

76. Chavez-Valdez R, Mason A, Nunes AR, Northington FJ, Tankersley C, Ahlawat R, et al. Effect of hyperoxic exposure during early development on neurotrophin expression in the carotid body and nucleus tractus solitarii. J Appl Physiol (1985). 2012;112(10):1762–72.

77. Bierman AM, Tankersley CG, Wilson CG, Chavez-Valdez R, Gauda EB. Perinatal hyperoxic exposure reconfigures the central respiratory network contributing to intolerance to anoxia in newborn rat pups. J Appl Physiol (1985). 2014;116(1):47–53.

78. Al-Matary A, Kutbi I, Qurashi M, Khalil M, Alvaro R, Kwiatkowski K, et al. Increased peripheral chemoreceptor activity may be critical in destabilizing breathing in neonates. Semin Perinatol. 2004;28(4):264–72.

79. Weintraub Z, Alvaro R, Kwiatkowski K, Cates D, Rigatto H. Effects of inhaled oxygen (up to 40%) on periodic breathing and apnea in preterm infants. J Appl Physiol (1985). 1992;72(1):116–20.

80. Khan A, Qurashi M, Kwiatkowski K, Cates D, Rigatto H. Measurement of the CO_2 apneic threshold in newborn infants: possible relevance for periodic breathing and apnea. J Appl Physiol (1985). 2005;98(4):1171–6.

81. Durand M, Cabal LA, Gonzalez F, Georgie S, Barberis C, Hoppenbrouwers T, et al. Ventilatory control and carbon dioxide response in preterm infants with idiopathic apnea. Am J Dis Child. 1985;139(7):717–20.

82. Edwards BA, Sands SA, Berger PJ. Postnatal maturation of breathing stability and loop gain: the role of carotid chemoreceptor development. Respir Physiol Neurobiol. 2013;185(1):144–55.

83. Kumar P, Prabhakar NR. Peripheral chemoreceptors: function and plasticity of the carotid body. Compr Physiol. 2012;2(1):141–219.

84. Di Fiore JM, Martin RJ, Gauda EB. Apnea of prematurity–perfect storm. Respir Physiol Neurobiol. 2013;189(2):213–22.

85. Lee LY, Pisarri TE. Afferent properties and reflex functions of bronchopulmonary C-fibers. Respir Physiol. 2001;125(1–2):47–65.

4 Control of Breathing in Older Adults

Susmita Chowdhuri

INTRODUCTION

Aging has a myriad of effects on the respiratory system that may portend disease development or progression. Sleep-disordered breathing (SDB) is one such disease that is highly prevalent in older age groups (1–6). The prevalence of SDB was found to be 3%, 33%, and 39% in 60, 70- and 80-year old adults, respectively (1) and increased with an odds ratio of 2.2 for each 10-year increase in age (7). In older men with apnea hypopnea index (AHI) ≥15/hr age was an independent risk factor for SDB (8). Additionally, the prevalence of central apneas was 1.1% in older adults compared with 0.4% in younger adults (4). This chapter focuses on the pathophysiology of age-related SDB with an emphasis on ventilatory control system mechanisms.

PATHOPHYSIOLOGY OF SDB WITH AGING

The increased risk of age-related SDB can be explained by a multitude of factors. While obesity, upper-airway anatomy, and dilator muscle function (9–11) explain the heterogeneity of SDB, only a portion of the variability in SDB and periodic breathing in older adults can be ascribed to differences in mechanical load. Other mechanisms, including alterations of chemoreceptor ventilatory control, including changes in cerebrovascular blood flow and reactivity may influence breathing stability during sleep in older adults (12–15). In general, the ventilatory control system monitors afferent chemical input (arterial carbon dioxide ($PaCO_2$) and arterial oxygen (PaO_2) through the chemoreceptors to maintain $PaCO_2$ and PaO_2 within a specific range. While the central chemoreceptors modulate ventilation in response to changes in the CO_2/H^+ detected within the brainstem, the faster-acting peripheral chemoreceptors in the carotid body respond to changes in PaO_2 and $PaCO_2$. Evidence pertaining to age-related changes in chemoreceptor mechanisms are derived from experiments performed during wakefulness or sleep as described in Table 4.1.

Chemoreceptor Reactivity and Aging
Wake Chemoresponsivess

Experiments examining the effects of age on chemoreceptor control of breathing during wakefulness have provided conflicting results

(Table 4.1). While a few studies demonstrated decreased hypoxic ventilatory response to acute and sustained hypoxia in older vs. young adults (15–19), others failed to demonstrate differences in ventilatory responsiveness to sustained hypoxia, post-hypoxic ventilatory decline, or chemoresponsiveness to hypercapnia in physically active older adults vs. younger adults (20–24). The variable results from these cross-sectional studies could be attributed to methodological differences, including blunting of the hypercapnic response by background hyperoxia, absence of isocapnia during the hypoxic stimulus, as well as small sample sizes. Conversely, when normal resting $PaCO_2$ was maintained during the experiments, hypoxic ventilatory responsiveness was *higher* among older participants than in young participants (25). In one study, while there was a progressive decline in hypoxic sensitivity until age 75 years, the carbon dioxide (CO_2) threshold was lower in older age groups than in young healthy controls, the latter indicating an increased susceptibility to breathing instability in older adults (18). However, the differences in ventilatory response slopes between young and older adults were less marked or absent when these slopes were corrected for differences in lung capacity.

Notably, in the largest and the only longitudinal study of ventilatory responses during wakefulness with aging (ages 14–85 years, n = 2,789 men, 1,886 women), there was evidence of *increased* ventilatory response to hypoxia, but this was less pronounced in post-menopausal women (26). While the above studies, conducted in a controlled experimental milieu (i.e. isocapnia), may indicate increased ventilatory responsiveness in older vs. young adults, the contradictory experimental data preclude a definitive conclusion regarding age-related differences in chemoresponsiveness during wakefulness.

Chemoresponsiveness during Sleep

A widely held notion is that wake experiments in humans may not reliably predict ventilatory responses to hypoxia and hypercapnia during sleep, because during wakefulness, ventilation is substantially influenced by activities such as swallowing, anxiety, and other behavioral effects, leading to variable results. Skatrud and Dempsey first described that control of breathing becomes critically dependent upon

DOI: 10.1201/9781003000631-5

Table 4.1: Evidence for Age-Related Ventilatory Responses to Hypoxia and Hypercapnia

Study First Author, Year	Age Groups (Sample Size)	Intervention	Physiologic Responses
Acute Hypoxia during Wakefulness			
Decreased Hypoxic Ventilatory Response with Older Age			
Kronenberg & Drage, 1973 (16)	22–30 yr (8 men) 64–73 yr (8 men)	Hypoxia	Ventilatory responses to hypoxia were reduced by 51 ± 6% in older adults vs. young
Peterson (17)	65–79 yr (10) 19–30 yr (9)	Hypercapnia	Ventilatory responses to hypoxia were reduced in older adults by ~50%
Garcia-Rio (18)	20–40 yr (47) 65–69, 70–74, 75–79 and 80–84 yr (65)	Isocapnic progressive hypoxia	Hypoxic ventilatory response decreased till age 70–74yr, then unchanged after age 75 yr
Hartmann (15)	20–39 yr (12) 55–79 yr (14)	Acute isocapnic hypoxia	Hypoxic ventilatory response: old < young; Cerebrovascular sensitivity to hypoxia: old < young
No Age Differences in Hypoxic Ventilatory Response			
Ahmed (20)	Mean age 62 yr (14) Mean age 29 yr (15)	25 min of isocapnic hypoxia	No age differences in ventilatory responses, including minute ventilation, and post-hypoxic ventilatory decline
Smith (21)	30 ± 8 yr (5 men) 73 ± 3 yr (5 men)	Isocapnic sustained hypoxia	No age differences in ventilatory responses, including minute ventilation, timing, and post-hypoxic ventilatory decline
Vovk (22)	Same subjects from Smith, 1996	20 min of eucapnic hypoxia followed by brief hypoxia	No age differences in ventilatory responses: hypoxic ventilatory response, hypoxic ventilatory decline, or recovery
Paleczny (24)	Young, 32 ± 10 yr (38) Old, 61 ± 8 yr (29)	Transient hypoxia	No differences in respiratory response from central and peripheral chemoreceptors between old and young
Increased Ventilatory Response with Older Age			
Chapman (25)	64–76 yr (10) 18–31 yr (10)	Progressive hypoxia at two steady-state levels of CO_2	Ventilatory response to hypoxia at the lower CO_2 level was significantly greater among older adults than among young adults but not significantly different between age groups at higher CO_2 level
Lhuissier (26) (Longitudinal data)	14–85 yr (2,789 men, 1,886 women)	Hypoxic exercise test	Increased ventilatory response to hypoxia; less pronounced in post-menopausal women
Acute Hypercapnia Studies during Wakefulness			
Decreased Hypercapnic Ventilatory Response with Older Age			
Kronenberg & Drage (16)	22–30 yr (8 men) 64–73 yr (8 men)	Hypercapnia	Ventilatory responses to hypercapnia were reduced by 41 ± 7% in older adults vs. young
Peterson (17)	65–79 yr (10) 19–30 yr (9)	Hypercapnia	Ventilatory responses to hypercapnia were reduced in older adults by ~50%
Rubin (99)	>60 yr (10) <30 (18)	Progressive hypercapnia	Ventilation responses to progressively increasing CO_2 were reduced in the older age group, but not significantly
No Age Differences in Hypercapnic Ventilatory Response			
Poulin (23)	28 ± 3 (7) 76 ± 1 (11)	Hypercapnic hyperoxia	No age-related differences in the ventilatory response to CO_2, measured in hyperoxia. Reduced ventilatory response to CO_2, measured in hypoxia in older vs. young (but not in a subsequent study)

(Continued)

Table 4.1: Evidence for Age-Related Ventilatory Responses to Hypoxia and Hypercapnia (Continued)

Study First Author, Year	Age Groups (Sample Size)	Intervention	Physiologic Responses
Davenport (100)	50–64 yr (20) 65–79 yr (19), post-menopausal women	Euoxic hypercapnia	No age-related differences in HCVR
Miller (101)	Young 27 ± 5 yr (22) Old = 60 ± 4 yr (21), habitual exercisers	Stepwise hypercapnia	Cerebrovascular reactivity to CO_2 was not different between young and older adults who habitually exercise
Lower CO_2 Threshold with Older Age			
Garcia-Rio (18)	20–40 yr (47) 65–69, 70–74, 75–79, and 80–84 yr (65)	Hyperoxic progressive hypercapnia	CO_2 threshold was lower in older adults groups than in young healthy controls

Abbreviations: CO_2 carbon dioxide; HCVR Hypercapnic ventilatory response; Yr years.

chemical and mechanical reflex feedback (27) during non-rapid eye movement (NREM) sleep, indicating that the apneic threshold is state dependent. Ventilatory control during sleep operates as a negative–feedback closed-loop cycle to maintain homeostasis of blood gas tensions within a physiologic range. "Loop gain", an engineering term, has been used as a measure of this ventilatory stability (28–30) and represents the overall response of the plant (representing the lung and respiratory muscles), the controller (representing the ventilatory control centers and the chemoreceptors) and the delay, dilution, and diffusion inherent in transferring the signal between the plant and the controller (31). Plant gain is determined by the magnitude of the reduction in $PaCO_2$ resulting from a given change in ventilation $(\dot{V}_I)$, $(\Delta PaCO_2/\Delta\dot{V}_I)$ and is the efficiency with which CO_2 is eliminated (14, 32). Controller gain or chemoresponsiveness is the slope of the ventilatory response to hypercapnia and hypocapnia i.e. $\Delta\dot{V}_I/\Delta PaCO_2$. Hypoxia and hypercapnia initiated chemoreflexes are known to contribute to the regulation of ventilation and a high gain in any of these chemosensory loops could contribute to breathing instabilities. Increased controller gain, for example, due to sustained or episodic hypoxia (EH), or heart failure narrows the CO_2 reserve to increase breathing instability (14, 31). Similarly, an increase in the plant gain due to metabolic alkalosis or due to disorders of hypoventilation narrows the CO_2 reserve to increase breathing instability. Conversely, a reduced controller gain due to hyperoxia or a steady-state reduction of $PaCO_2$ or reduced plant gain with acetazolamide (ACZ) will stabilize breathing by widening the CO_2 reserve (14, 31, 33).

In older adults, a waxing and waning oscillatory breathing pattern during the lighter stages of sleep is prevalent, suggesting ventilatory control mechanisms may be involved that may contribute to a higher propensity of developing periodic breathing (34–36). However, Browne et al. examined and found no age differences in the magnitude of ventilatory response to hypercapnia during NREM sleep (37). Using proportional assist ventilation (PAV), investigators also found no evidence of increased "loop gain" in a group of older obstructive sleep apnea (OSA) subjects (38). However, PAV itself may have altered the loop gain by increasing lung volume and oxygen stores. Edwards et al. found that older patients with OSA had a more collapsible airway with a lower loop gain (5.0 ± 0.7 vs. 2.9 ± 0.5; p <0.05) than young adults, suggesting that upper airway factors were more important in this population with OSA (39). Of note, the study was restricted to participants with a mean age of 64 years, who were adherent to positive airway pressure (PAP) therapy. However, PAP therapy itself reduces breathing instability by decreasing the controller gain (40) (i.e. reduced loop gain); thus, whether the prior use of PAP may have altered the loop gain and its components, thereby altering the outcomes, cannot be determined from this study.

Older patients with congestive heart failure (CHF) have higher chemoresponsiveness than those without CHF, which may explain the prevalence of central sleep apnea (CSA) in these individuals (41). A comprehensive study that included 450 patients with CHF, showed that male gender and age >60 years was a major risk factor for CSA with Cheyne-Stokes respiration (CSR) in CHF patients (42, 43). Left ventricular

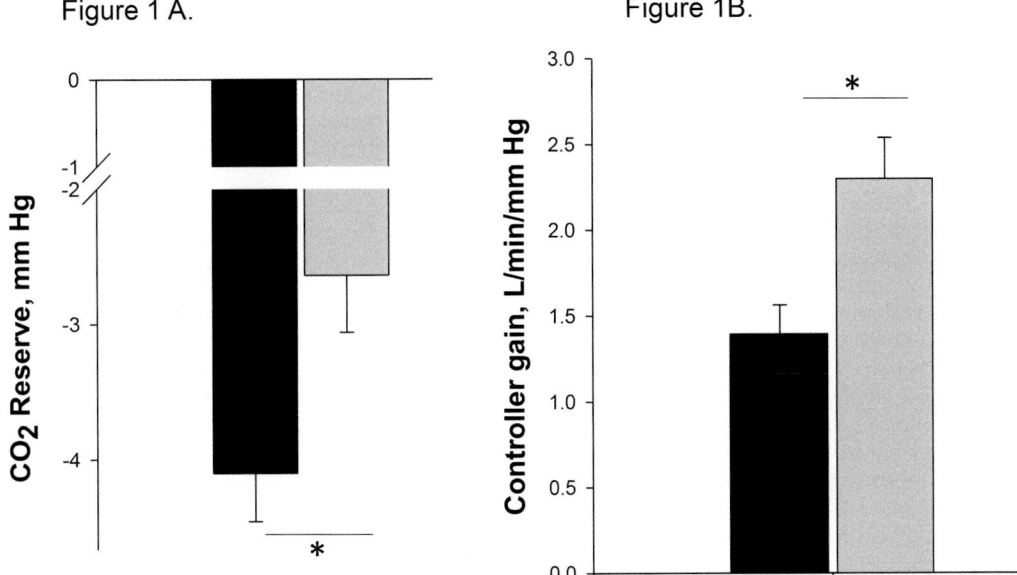

Figure 4.1   **A.** Grouped data of the CO_2 reserve. The CO_2 reserve was reduced in older adults vs. young adults, denoting an increased propensity to central apneas (*p = 0.01). The bars represent averaged data for each age group (black bar = young, n = 15, grey bar = older age, n = 10, respectively). **B.** Grouped data comparing of the controller gain in the two age groups: young and older age. The bars represent averaged data for each age group (black bar = young, grey bar = older age, respectively). The controller gain was significantly higher in older adults compared to young (*p = 0.007). (The figures are adapted with permission from reference (14).)

filling pressures tend to be more elevated in older adults as left ventricle compliance decreases, associated with an increased prevalence of pulmonary venous hypertension. This may lead to hyperventilation and subsequent hypocapnia with increased controller gain during sleep in older adults with CHF (41).

Whether increased chemoventilatory drive during sleep explains the increased prevalence of central SDB in older adults without heart failure was the focus of recent research studies from our lab. During NREM sleep, ventilation in older healthy adults depicted a heightened hyperoxic suppression (Dejours' test) as well as isocapnic hypoxic responsiveness during acute intermittent hypoxia (12). While the ventilatory response to transient exposure to oxygen or to hypercapnia allows one to estimate peripheral chemoresponsiveness (44–47), a prolonged hypoxic and/or hyperoxia-hypercapnic stimulus likely estimates both peripheral-central chemoreceptor response and their interdependence (48). To further delineate ventilatory control mechanisms in healthy older vs. young adults (AHI <10/hr), their apneic thresholds and controller gains were determined using noninvasive positive

pressure ventilation trials during NREM sleep. The controller gain was found to be significantly increased in older (age 66.9 ± 5.4 years) vs. young adults (age 35.9 ± 9.9 years) 2.3 ± 0.2 vs. 1.4 ± 0.2 l/min/mm Hg, p = 0.007 (13) (Figure 4.1 B), indicating increased levels of ventilatory chemoresponsiveness in the older adults Correspondingly, the CO_2 reserve was significantly reduced in older vs. young adults (2.6 ± 0.4 vs. 4.1 ± 0.4 mm Hg, p <0.01) (Figure 4.1 A). The plant gain was not different between the age groups. The higher controller gain in older adults not only enhances the proximity of the apneic threshold $PaCO_2$ to the eupneic $PaCO_2$ (i.e. reduced CO_2 reserve), promoting ventilatory undershoots, but also increases the ventilatory overshoots at the end of an apnea or hypopnea, thereby promoting periodic breathing during sleep. Thus, older adults appear to have a propensity for hypocapnic central apneas and periodic breathing owing to increased chemoresponsiveness during NREM sleep, facilitated by a reduced CO_2 reserve (13).

Age-Related Changes in Plasticity

EH, as seen in recurrent sleep apnea, is associated with a prolonged increase in ventilatory motor output, referred to as long-term facilitation

(LTF), which may stabilize the upper airway to mitigate the recurrence of obstructive apneas (49, 50). Conversely, the propensity to central apnea is increased in the aftermath of EH (51) suggesting that LTF could also promote breathing instability. There is evidence from animal studies, that aging is associated with diminished LTF following EH (52). In humans, EH also elicits LTF of the genioglossus (GG) muscle activity during sleep and the magnitude of the GG LTF during the recovery period appeared to be inversely correlated with age (53), indicating reduced GG plasticity with increasing age. Whereas multiple studies in young adults have demonstrated ventilatory LTF of ventilation (with 108%–122% increase in minute ventilation during post-EH recovery vs. control period), as evidence of plasticity following EH, the same was not apparent in older adults (12). Additionally, there was periodic breathing in the absence of LTF (12). Thus, absence of GG or ventilatory plasticity may contribute to periodic breathing in older adults during NREM sleep. Notably, in *postmenopausal women* respiratory plasticity is also altered. The increased breathing stability and prevalence of SDB in postmenopausal women (3) is likely related to reductions in estradiol and increased testosterone in (54) that in turn modulate chemoresponsiveness (see Chapter 11 for details). Moreover, the lung loses elastic recoil with aging and the distribution of ventilation becomes more non-uniform with increased Vd:Vt. However, minute ventilation increases at any given VCO_2 both at rest and during exercise so that $VA:VCO_2$ stays constant and $PaCO_2$ (at rest and exercise) stays the same across the ages.

The aforementioned mechanisms of increased ventilatory chemoresponsiveness along with reduced respiratory plasticity may explain breathing instability leading to an increased propensity for central apneas and periodic breathing in older adults.

Cerebrovascular Responsiveness with Aging

Cerebrovascular responsiveness to CO_2 (CVR) is an important determinant of breathing stability as it influences eupneic ventilation and hypercapnic ventilatory responsiveness in humans by altering the central chemoreceptor H^+ milieu (55, 56) (also see Chapter 10). Changes in cerebral blood flow (CBF) regulation modify breathing stability in healthy young adults (55–58), where a decrease in CBF allows accumulation of CO_2 that stimulates the medulla. Conversely, an increase in CBF enhances CO_2 removal and depresses ventilation. Thus, reductions in the normal cerebral vascular response to hypocapnia would cause breathing instability

during wakefulness and sleep and an impaired CBF response to hypercapnia contributes to the development of disordered breathing (see Chapter 10). Studies show that age has a significant effect on CBF (59). The cerebral blood vessels' ability to dilate—measured by cerebral vascular reactivity to 5% CO_2 inhalation—was reduced with increasing age (59, 60). Cerebrovascular reactivity in the cerebral cortex of young subjects was significantly higher than that for white matter and significantly higher than in older adults subjects (p <0.001) (61). Cerebrovascular responsiveness to isocapnic hypoxia was also age-related in awake individuals (62). Thus, it is likely that the observed age-related breathing instability during sleep may be mediated, in part, by the age-related reductions in cerebrovascular reactivity (63, 64). In young healthy adults, reduced CBF and cerebrovascular responsiveness to hypocapnia, during both wakefulness and sleep, elevated the apneic threshold and narrowed the CO_2 reserve, i.e. increased ventilatory instability (55, 56). A recent study from our group also demontrated that older age and SDB-related hypoxia are associated with diminished CVR (65). The observed age-related breathing instability during sleep may potentially be mediated, in part, by this impairment in vascular function that occurs with aging.

Upper Airway Mechanics and Function with Aging

Multiple additional factors including pharyngeal cross-sectional area, upper airway mechanics, and upper airway dilator muscle function underpin the pathogenesis of OSA (66). During NREM sleep, the motor output to both the upper airway and respiratory pump muscles is reduced, causing mild to moderate sustained hypoventilation and increased upper airway resistance in most healthy individuals (67, 68). Aging is accompanied by anatomical changes that may decrease upper airway dimensions in both men and women. An increase in pharyngeal airway lumen area with aging at functional residual capacity was noted in one study (69). However, the length of the airway, an important determinant of airway stability, was not greater in older men vs. young adults (9). While a smaller pharyngeal cross-sectional area in older awake adults (10) was noted in one study, in contrast, other studies found no age difference in the pharyngeal luminal volume of men, as measured by magnetic resonance imaging (9) and found a larger airway in older than young adults using computerized scanning of the airway (69, 70).

Thus, the data are inconsistent about changes in airway size with aging.

In one study, there was age-related decrease in upper airway muscle tone and elasticity and an increase in fat deposition promoting upper airway collapsibility (9). Additionally, a decrease in the pharynx dilator reflex and impaired pharyngeal sensory discrimination with aging has been observed (71). However, older age did not seem to influence the respiratory arousal threshold (11). Additionally, age-related changes in motor unit potentials were detected in the GG muscle, suggesting the upper airway in older adults may be compromised due to an overall loss of motoneurons (72) and a reduced GG activity in response to hypoxia was found in older adults (73). The airway may, therefore, be more likely to collapse due to fewer motor units available for recruitment during quiet breathing. However, while a few studies demonstrated increased collapsibility and upper airway resistance in older vs. young adults, others have not (10, 11, 74, 75). For example, increasing age was correlated with both pharyngeal collapsibility (r = 0.69; p <0.01) and an increase in pharyngeal resistance during sleep (r = 0.56; p <0.01) independent of body mass index (BMI) and gender (11) and older OSA patients, compared with young, had a more collapsible airway (39). Additionally, in

a separate study, older age was associated with a higher passive Pcrit only in women but not in men (76). The authors attributed the differential gender effect to increased upper airway mechanical loads secondary to redistribution of body fat. In summary, there are divergent findings from cross-sectional studies in regard to upper airway collapsibility and size with aging, which limit our understanding of the contributions of airway anatomy to the pathogenesis of SDB in older adults.

Studies posit that ventilatory control mechanisms trigger airway collapsibility in humans during sleep (77–79). Conversely, ventilatory control instability may arise from the changes in upper airway collapsibility. Fiberoptic nasopharyngoscopy during NREM sleep revealed that central apneas were associated with pharyngeal narrowing and/or occlusion (79). Thus, any repetitive cycling behavior in airway patency and ventilation is critically dependent upon neuro-chemical control mechanisms and triggers periodic breathing (80). The occurrence of complete pharyngeal collapse during central apnea may impede pharyngeal opening and necessitate a substantial increase in drive that eventually leads to the sequence of events that are responsible for perpetuating breathing instability and periodic breathing (Figure 4.2).

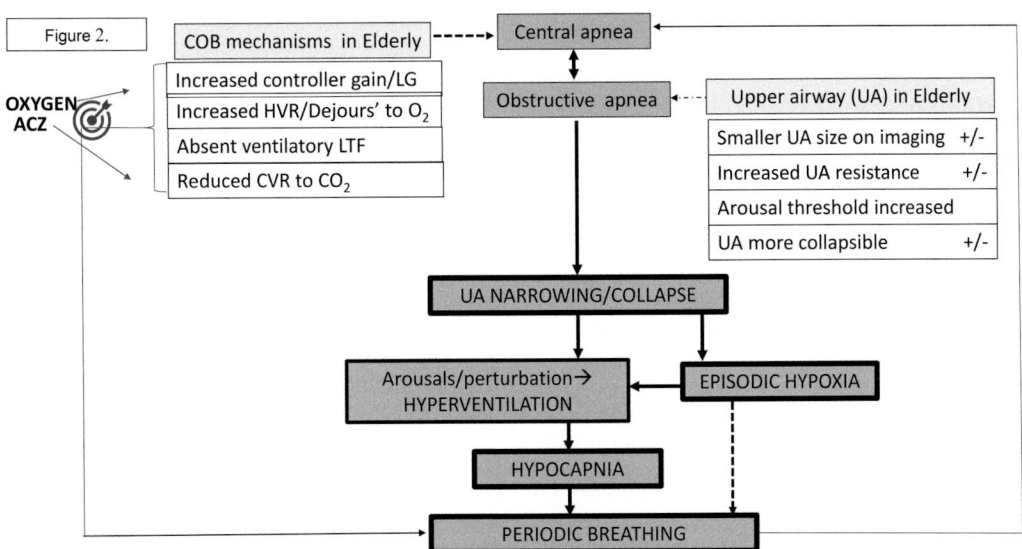

Figure 4.2 Schematic diagram of the potential mechanisms of increased sleep-disordered breathing with periodic breathing in older adults. See the text for a detailed explanation. The red arrows indicate oxygen and ACZ targeting the potential COB mechanism to mitigate SDB. Abbreviations: ACZ acetazolamide; COB control of breathing; CVR to CO_2 cerebrovascular responsiveness to carbon dioxide; HVR hypoxic ventilatory response; LG loop gain; O_2 Brief hyperoxia; LTF long-term facilitation; UA upper airway; +/− indicates conflicting evidence.

Aging and Control of Breathing from Animal Studies

In animal models, aging produces changes in the carotid body (peripheral chemoreceptor), including degenerative changes in the ultrastructure of the carotid body glomus cells (81) and thickening of the connective tissue that surrounds the lobes of the chemoreceptor. However, the peripheral control of ventilation was preserved in aging in rats (82). Thus, a discrepancy was noted between the morphological changes in the carotid body and the ventilatory responses with aging. In adult vs. neonatal rats, responses to chronic intermittent hypoxia varied with the magnitude of sensitization to hypoxia, susceptibility to chronic intermittent hypoxia, induction of sensory LTF, and remodeling of the chemoreceptor tissue (83, 84). Whether similar chronic mechanisms during aging alter carotid chemosensitivity in humans are not known. Additionally, chronic intermittent hypoxia or ablation of the preBötzinger complex (preBötC) in animal models resulted in apneas; it is not known whether a similar mechanism of degeneration of the preBötC neurons contributes to apnea and hypopneas in older adults (85, 86).

Older rats have elevated Pcrit, compared with young and an increase in upper airway collapsibility with age was related to altered neural control rather than to primary alterations in upper airway muscle structure and function (87). A loss of primary dendrites could reduce the number of synaptic inputs and thereby impair GG muscle function (88) and potentially increase upper airway collapsibility. In this study, the hypoglossal motoneuron dendrites decreased significantly with age, however, the study found no changes in the number or size of hypoglossal motoneurons (88) and did not examine any functional impact. Moreover, phrenic LTF was reduced and hypoglossal LTF was almost eliminated in middle-aged (12 mo old) male rats but increased in female rats, suggesting that the expression of LTF may be influenced by both age and gender (52). Additional animal studies on the longitudinal effects of aging on chemoreceptor and GG function may provide insight into the mechanisms of human pathophysiology of SDB.

TRANSLATING PATHOPHYSIOLOGY TO POTENTIAL THERAPY FOR SDB IN OLDER ADULTS

By delineating the mechanisms of age-related SDB, the pathways for developing alternative pathophysiology-directed targeted therapies become possible. For example, a few of these alternative therapies in older adults are underpinned on control of breathing mechanisms, and include supplemental oxygen and ACZ.

Supplemental Oxygen

The high chemoresponsiveness of older adults could be definitively mitigated by interventions that reduced by chemoresponsiveness to eliminate SDB. Authors have demonstrated reduction in loop gain with supplemental oxygen (89, 90) but without altering upper airway collapsibility (91). Moreover, a recent study established that supplemental oxygen, when applied during NREM sleep in older adults with mild-moderate SDB, ameliorated the propensity for breathing instability (i.e. widened the CO_2 reserve) in association with decline in the controller gain to mitigate SDB (92) (Figures 4.3 A–D). The reduced controller gain reduces both the propensity for ventilatory undershoots and overshoots to mitigate SDB. Thus, the level of PaO_2 is an important determinant of chemoreceptor gain and the susceptibility to apnea during sleep in both older and young individuals (92, 93). Supplemental oxygen has also been effectively used to treat CSA with CSR in older adults with heart failure (13).

Acetazolamide

ACZ's effect on ventilatory control has been studied extensively in humans during wakefulness. It improves breathing stability in patients with CSA due to heart failure although the exact mechanism by which it improves CSA is not totally understood. Overall, ACZ produces a metabolic acidosis-induced rise in normoxic ventilation, i.e. reduces plant gain. In rabbits, ACZ reduced the loop gain by 35%; this was driven by a 27% reduction in controller gain and a 12% reduction in plant gain (94). In young and middle-aged humans with OSA, ACZ reduced loop gain by 41% in patients during sleep and was associated with a 51% improvement in the AHI although it did not affect sleep architecture (95). ACZ reduced SDB in younger patients with spinal cord injury (96). ACZ produces a rise in resting cerebral blood flow (CBF) (86) during wakefulness and enhances brain blood flow responses to CO_2 at sea level, while increasing resting minute ventilation (86). Thus, ACZ may improve breathing stability by a reduction in the eupneic PCO_2 (i.e. reduction in plant gain), and via enhancing the cerebrovascular responsiveness to CO_2 (Figure 4.2). The effect of ACZ on breathing stability in older adults with CSA (without heart failure) was studied

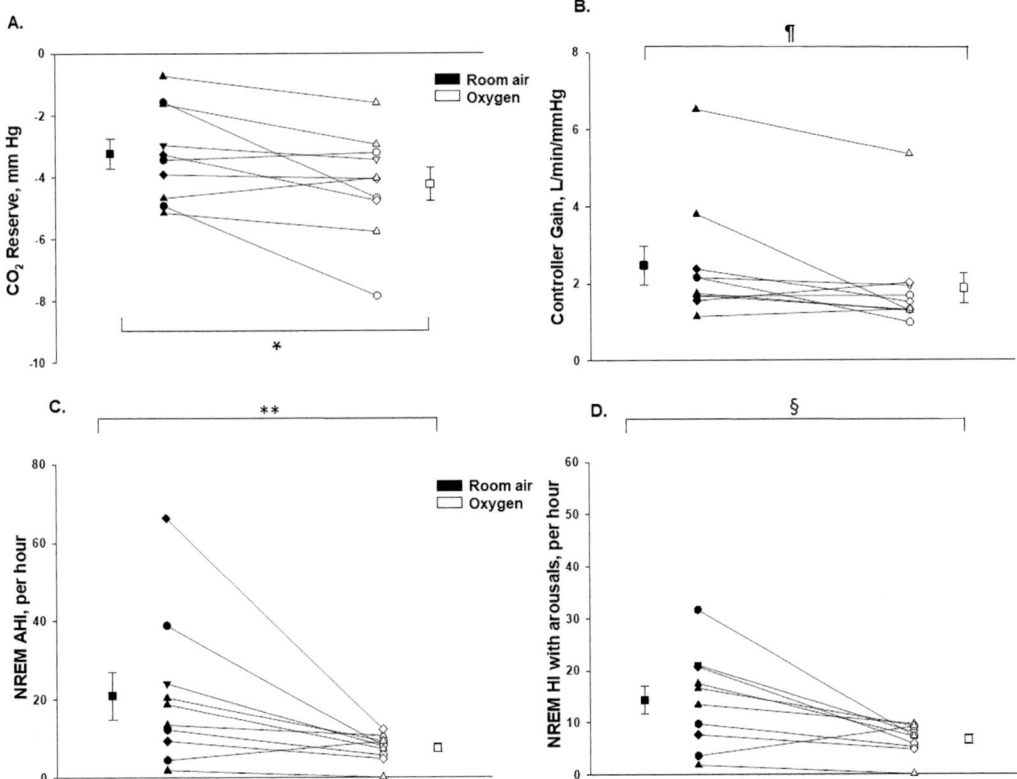

Figure 4.3 **A.** Demonstrates the CO_2 reserve under conditions of oxygen and room air in older adults. The CO_2 reserve was significantly increased (more negative) during oxygen vs. room air exposure, *p = 0.03. **B.** Demonstrates controller gain or hypocapnic ventilatory response under the two conditions of oxygen and room air. The major finding was a significant decline in the hypocapnic ventilatory response during oxygen vs. room air, p = 0.04. **C.** Demonstrates NREM apnea hypopnea index (AHI) under conditions of oxygen and room air. There was a significant decline in the NREM AHI with oxygen vs. room air, **p = 0.01. **D.** Demonstrates NREM hypopnea index (HI) scored with arousals alone (without 3% desaturations) under conditions of oxygen and room air; HI scored with arousals declined significantly with oxygen vs. room air, §p = 0.02. Individual and mean (± SE) data are presented, where black and white symbols represent room air and oxygen trials, respectively. (The figures are adapted with permission from reference (97).)

in a small population of older adults with mild SDB, and observed that the CO_2 reserve was increased with a decline in the plant gain but without a change in the controller gain (97, 98). Ongoing studies will likely elucidate the effects of ACZ on ventilatory control during sleep and its impact on SDB in older adults, and hopefully, present a new line of therapy.

SUMMARY

In summary, we have described the current known pathophysiologic mechanisms of SDB in older adults. Cross-sectional studies during sleep indicate a higher chemoreceptor or controller gain in older adults that can be mitigated by supplemental oxygen to

reduce SDB. Alternatively, ACZ may also stabilize breathing during sleep via reduction in the plant gain and/or via an increase in cerebrovascular CO_2 reactivity. Targeted modifications in control of breathing mechanisms offer new avenues of therapy for SDB in older adults. However, the absence of longitudinal studies hinders our exact understanding of the aging effect on the pathophysiology of SDB. There is a crucial need for longitudinal studies, progressing from young, middle age to older ages, investigating the mechanisms of breathing instability, and of therapeutic interventions that can best mitigate these age-related changes (Table 4.2).

Table 4.2: Research Agenda

Well-Designed Studies Are Needed to Investigate the Following:
1. Longitudinal changes that occur from young to middle age to old age in ventilatory control mechanisms and correlate these with the progression of severity and type of SDB.
2. Age-related longitudinal changes that occur in upper airway function and plasticity and correlate these with the severity and type of SDB, after adjusting for relevant confounders including weight change, medications, sex hormone changes, and other factors.
3. Age-related longitudinal changes in cerebrovascular CO_2 reactivity during sleep and their impact on ventilatory control of breathing and SDB.
4. Determine the mechanisms of effect of alternative therapies that promote ventilatory stability during sleep across a spectrum of age groups.

REFERENCES

1. Hoch C, Reynolds 3rd C, Monk T, Buysse D, Yeager A, Houck P, et al. Comparison of sleep-disordered breathing among healthy elderly in the seventh, eighth, and ninth decades of life. Sleep. 1990;13(6):502–11.

2. Ancoli-Israel S, Kripke DF, Klauber MR, Mason WJ, Fell R, Kaplan O. Sleep-disordered breathing in community-dwelling elderly. Sleep. 1991;14(6):486.

3. Bixler EO, Vgontzas AN, Lin H-M, Ten Have T, Rein J, Vela-Bueno A, et al. Prevalence of sleep-disordered breathing in women: effects of gender. American Journal of Respiratory and Critical Care Medicine. 2001;163(3):608–13.

4. Bixler EO, Vgontzas AN, Ten Have T, Tyson K, Kales A. Effects of age on sleep apnea in men: I. Prevalence and severity. American Journal of Respiratory and Critical Care Medicine. 1998;157(1):144–8.

5. Phillips BA, Berry D, Schmitt FA, Magan LK, Gerhardstein DC, Cook YR. Sleep-disordered breathing in the healthy elderly. Clinically significant? CHEST Journal. 1992;101(2):345–9.

6. Redline S. Epidemiology of sleep-disordered breathing. Seminars in Respiratory and Critical Care Medicine. 1998;9(02):113–22.

7. Durán J, Esnaola S, Rubio R, Iztueta A. Obstructive sleep apnea-hypopnea and related clinical features in a population-based sample of subjects aged 30 to 70 yr. American Journal of Respiratory and Critical Care Medicine. 2001;163(3 Pt 1):685–9.

8. Mehra R, Stone KL, Blackwell T, Ancoli Israel S, Dam T-TL, Stefanick ML, et al. Prevalence and correlates of sleep-disordered breathing in older men: osteoporotic fractures in men sleep study. Journal of the American Geriatrics Society. 2007;55(9):1356–64.

9. Malhotra A, Huang Y, Fogel R, Lazic S, Pillar G, Jakab M, et al. Aging influences on pharyngeal anatomy and physiology: the predisposition to pharyngeal collapse. The American Journal of Medicine. 2006;119(1):72. e9.

10. Martin S, Mathur R, Marshall I, Douglas N. The effect of age, sex, obesity and posture on upper airway size. European Respiratory Journal. 1997;10(9):2087–90.

11. Eikermann M, Jordan AS, Chamberlin NL, Gautam S, Wellman A, Lo Y-L, et al. The influence of aging on pharyngeal collapsibility during sleep. Chest Journal. 2007;131(6):1702–9.

12. Chowdhuri S, Pranathiageswaran S, Franco-Elizondo R, Jayakar A, Hosni A, Nair A, et al. Effect of age on long-term facilitation and chemosensitivity during NREM sleep. Journal of Applied Physiology. 2015;119(10):1088–96.

13. Chowdhuri S, Pranathiageswaran S, Loomis-King H, Salloum A, Badr MS. Aging is associated with increased propensity for central apnea during NREM sleep. Journal of Applied Physiology (Bethesda, MD: 1985). 2018;124(1):83–90.

14. Chowdhuri S, Badr MS. Control of ventilation in health and disease. Chest Journal. 2017;151(4):917–29.

15. Hartmann SE, Waltz X, Kissel CK, Szabo L, Walker BL, Leigh R, et al. Cerebrovascular and ventilatory responses to acute isocapnic hypoxia in healthy aging and lung disease: effect of vitamin C. Journal of Applied Physiology (Bethesda, MD: 1985). 2015;119(4):363–73.

16. Kronenberg RS, Drage CW. Attenuation of the ventilatory and heart rate responses to hypoxia and hypercapnia with aging in normal men. Journal of Clinical Investigation. 1973;52(8):1812.

17. Peterson DD, Pack AI, Silage DA, Fishman AP. Effects of aging on ventilatory and occlusion pressure responses to hypoxia and hypercapnia. American Review of Respiratory Disease. 1981;124(4):387–91.

18. García-Río F, Villamor A, Gómez-Mendieta A, Lores V, Rojo B, Ramírez T, et al. The progressive effects of ageing on chemosensitivity in healthy subjects. Respiratory Medicine. 2007;101(10):2192–8.

19. Poulin MJ, Cunningham DA, Paterson DH. Dynamics of the ventilatory response to step changes in end-tidal PCO_2 in older humans. Canadian Journal of Applied Physiology/Revue canadienne de physiologie appliquee. 1997;22(4):368–83.

20. Ahmed M, Giesbrecht G, Serrette C, Georgopoulos D, Anthonisen N. Ventilatory response to hypoxia in elderly humans. Respiration Physiology. 1991;83(3):343–51.

21. Smith WD, Poulin MJ, Paterson DH, Cunningham DA. Dynamic ventilatory response to acute isocapnic hypoxia in septuagenarians. Experimental Physiology. 2001;86(1):117–26.

22. Vovk A, Smith WDF, Paterson ND, Cunningham DA, Paterson DH. Peripheral chemoreceptor control of ventilation following sustained hypoxia in young and older adult humans. Experimental Physiology. 2004;89(6):647–56.

23. Poulin MJ, Cunningham D, Paterson D, Kowalchuk J, Smith W. Ventilatory sensitivity to CO_2 in hyperoxia and hypoxia in older aged humans. Journal of Applied Physiology. 1993;75(5):2209–16.

24. Paleczny B, Niewiński P, Rydlewska A, Piepoli MF, Borodulin-Nadzieja L, Jankowska EA, et al. Age-related reflex responses from peripheral and central chemoreceptors in healthy men. Clinical Autonomic Research. 2014;24(6):285–96.

25. Chapman KR, Cherniack NS. Aging effects on the interaction of hypercapnia and hypoxia as ventilatory stimuli. Journal of Gerontology. 1987;42(2):202–9.

26. Lhuissier FJ, Canouï-Poitrine F, Richalet JP. Ageing and cardiorespiratory response to hypoxia. The Journal of Physiology. 2012;590(21):5461–74.

27. Skatrud JB, Dempsey JA. Interaction of sleep state and chemical stimuli in sustaining rhythmic ventilation. Journal of Applied Physiology. 1983;55(3):813–22.

28. Khoo MC, Kronauer RE, Strohl KP, Slutsky AS. Factors inducing periodic breathing in humans: a general model. Journal of Applied Physiology: Respiratory, Environmental and Exercise Physiology. 1982;53(3):644–59.

29. Khoo MC. Determinants of ventilatory instability and variability. Respiration Physiology. 2000;122(2):167–82.

30. Cherniack NS, Longobardo GS. Mathematical models of periodic breathing and their usefulness in understanding cardiovascular and respiratory disorders. Experimental Physiology. 2006;91(2):295–305.

31. Dempsey JA. Crossing the apnoeic threshold: causes and consequences. Experimental Physiology. 2005;90(1):13–24.

32. Badr MS, Skatrud JB, Dempsey JA. Determinants of poststimulus potentiation in humans during NREM sleep. Journal of Applied Physiology. 1992;73(5):1958–71.

33. Nakayama H, Smith CA, Rodman JR, Skatrud JB, Dempsey JA. Effect of ventilatory drive on carbon dioxide sensitivity below eupnea during sleep. American Journal of Respiratory and Critical Care Medicine. 2002;165(9):1251–60.

34. Pack A, Cola M, Goldszmidt A, Ogilvie M, Gottschalk A. Correlation between oscillations in ventilation and frequency content of the electroencephalogram. Journal of Applied Physiology. 1992;72(3):985–92.

35. Pack AI, Silage DA, Millman RP, Knight H, Shore ET, Chung D. Spectral analysis of ventilation in elderly subjects awake and asleep. Journal of Applied Physiology. 1988;64(3):1257–67.

36. Hudgel DW, Devadatta P, Hamilton H. Pattern of breathing and upper airway mechanics during wakefulness and sleep in healthy elderly humans. Journal of Applied Physiology (Bethesda, MD: 1985). 1993;74(5):2198–204.

37. Browne HAK, Adams L, Simonds AK, Morrell MJ. Ageing does not influence the sleep-related decrease in the hypercapnic ventilatory response. European Respiratory Journal. 2003;21(3):523–9.

38. Wellman A, Jordan AS, Malhotra A, Fogel RB, Katz ES, Schory K, et al. Ventilatory control and airway anatomy in obstructive sleep apnea. American Journal of Respiratory and Critical Care Medicine. 2004;170(11):1225–32.

39. Edwards BA, Wellman A, Sands SA, Owens RL, Eckert DJ, White DP, et al. Obstructive sleep apnea in older adults is a distinctly different physiological phenotype. Sleep. 2014;37(7): 1227–36.

40. Salloum A, Rowley JA, Mateika JH, Chowdhuri S, Omran Q, Badr MS. Increased propensity for central apnea in patients with obstructive sleep apnea: effect of nasal continuous positive airway pressure. American Journal of Respiratory and Critical Care Medicine. 2010;181(2):189–93.

41. Xie A, Skatrud JB, Puleo DS, Rahko PS, Dempsey JA. Apnea–hypopnea threshold for CO_2 in patients with congestive heart failure. American Journal of Respiratory and Critical Care Medicine. 2002;165(9):1245–50.

42. Sin DD, Fitzgerald F, Parker JD, Newton G, Floras JS, Bradley TD. Risk factors for central and obstructive sleep apnea in 450 men and women with congestive heart failure. American Journal of Respiratory and Critical Care Medicine. 1999;160(4):1101–6.

43. Javaheri S. Central sleep apnea-hypopnea syndrome in heart failure: prevalence, impact, and treatment. Sleep. 1996;19(10 Suppl):S229–31.

44. Dejours P. Control of respiration by arterial chemoreceptors. Annals of the New York Academy of Sciences. 1963;109:682–95.

45. Dejours P, Labrousse Y, Raynaud J, Teillac A. Oxygen chemoreflex stimulus in ventilation at low altitude in man. I. At rest. Journal de physiologie. 1957;49(1):115–20.

46. Gautier H. Hypoxia, hyperoxia and breathing. Journal of Biosciences. 2006;31(2):185–90.

47. Xie A, Skatrud JB, Puleo DS, Dempsey JA. Influence of arterial O_2 on the susceptibility to posthyperventilation apnea during sleep. Journal of Applied Physiology. 2006;100(1):171–7.

48. Dempsey JA, Smith CA, Blain GM, Xie A, Gong Y, Teodorescu M. Role of central/peripheral chemoreceptors and their interdependence in the pathophysiology of sleep apnea. Arterial Chemoreception: Springer; 2012. pp. 343–9.

49. Mateika JH, Narwani G. Intermittent hypoxia and respiratory plasticity in humans and other animals: does exposure to intermittent hypoxia promote or mitigate sleep apnoea? Experimental Physiology. 2009;94(3):279–96.

50. Navarrete-Opazo A, Mitchell GS. Therapeutic potential of intermittent hypoxia: a matter of dose. American Journal of Physiology. Regulatory,

Integrative and Comparative Physiology. 2014;307(10):R1181–R97.

51. Chowdhuri S, Shanidze I, Pierchala L, Belen D, Mateika JH, Badr MS. Effect of episodic hypoxia on the susceptibility to hypocapnic central apnea during NREM sleep. Journal of Applied Physiology. 2010;108(2):369–77.

52. Zabka AG, Behan M, Mitchell GS. Long term facilitation of respiratory motor output decreases with age in male rats. The Journal of Physiology. 2001;531(Pt 2):509–14.

53. Chowdhuri S, Pierchala L, Aboubakr SE, Shkoukani M, Badr MS. Long-term facilitation of genioglossus activity is present in normal humans during NREM sleep. Respiratory Physiology & Neurobiology. 2008;160(1):65–75.

54. Rowley JA, Zhou XS, Diamond MP, Badr MS. The determinants of the apnea threshold during NREM sleep in normal subjects. Sleep. 2006;29(1):95–103.

55. Xie A, Skatrud JB, Morgan B, Chenuel B, Khayat R, Reichmuth K, et al. Influence of cerebrovascular function on the hypercapnic ventilatory response in healthy humans. The Journal of Physiology. 2006;577(1):319–29.

56. Xie A, Skatrud JB, Barczi SR, Reichmuth K, Morgan BJ, Mont S, et al. Influence of cerebral blood flow on breathing stability. Journal of Applied Physiology. 2009;106(3):850–6.

57. Ainslie PN, Duffin J. Integration of cerebrovascular CO_2 reactivity and chemoreflex control of breathing: mechanisms of regulation, measurement, and interpretation. American Journal of Physiology-Regulatory, Integrative and Comparative Physiology. 2009;296(5):R1473–R95.

58. Kety SS, Schmidt CF. The effects of altered arterial tensions of carbon dioxide and oxygen on cerebral blood flow and cerebral oxygen consumption of normal young men. Journal of Clinical Investigation. 1948;27(4):484.

59. Lu H, Xu F, Rodrigue KM, Kennedy KM, Cheng Y, Flicker B, et al. Alterations in cerebral metabolic rate and blood supply across the adult lifespan. Cerebral Cortex. 2011;21(6):1426–34.

60. Peisker T, Bartoš A, Skoda O, Ibrahim I, Kalvach P. Impact of aging on cerebral vasoregulation and parenchymal integrity. Journal of the Neurological Sciences. 2010;299(1–2):112–5.

61. Reich T, Rusinek H. Cerebral cortical and white matter reactivity to carbon dioxide. Stroke. 1989;20(4):453–7.

62. Battisti-Charbonney A, Fisher J, Duffin J. Respiratory, cerebrovascular and cardiovascular responses to isocapnic hypoxia. Respiratory Physiology & Neurobiology. 2011;179(2):259–68.

63. Mayhan WG, Arrick DM, Sharpe GM, Sun H. Age-related alterations in reactivity of cerebral arterioles: role of oxidative stress. Microcirculation. 2008;15(3):225–36.

64. Fu JH, Lu CZ, Hong Z, Dong Q, Ding D, Wong KS. Relationship between cerebral vasomotor reactivity and white matter lesions in elderly subjects without large artery occlusive disease. Journal of Neuroimaging. 2006;16(2):120–5.

65. Rastogi R, Morgan BJ, Badr MS, Chowdhuri S. Hypercapnia-induced vasodilation in the cerebral circulation is reduced in older adults with sleep-disordered breathing. Journal of Applied Physiology. 2022;132(1):14–23.

66. White DP, Lombard RM, Cadieux RJ, Zwillich CW. Pharyngeal resistance in normal humans: influence of gender, age, and obesity. Journal of Applied Physiology (Bethesda, MD: 1985). 1985;58(2):365–71.

67. Issa FG, Edwards P, Szeto E, Lauff D, Sullivan C. Genioglossus and breathing responses to airway occlusion: effect of sleep and route of occlusion. Journal of Applied Physiology (Bethesda, MD: 1985). 1988;64(2):543–9.

68. Horner RL. Motor control of the pharyngeal musculature and implications for the pathogenesis of obstructive sleep apnea. Sleep. 1996;19(10):827–53.

69. Burger CD, Stanson AW, Sheedy PF, 2nd, Daniels BK, Shepard JW, Jr. Fast-computed tomography evaluation of age-related changes in upper airway structure and function in normal men. The American Review of Respiratory Disease. 1992;145(4 Pt 1):846–52.

70. Mayer P, Pépin JL, Bettega G, Veale D, Ferretti G, Deschaux C, et al. Relationship between body mass index, age and upper airway measurements in snorers and sleep apnoea patients. The European Respiratory Journal. 1996;9(9):1801–9.

71. Aviv JE, Martin JH, Jones ME, Wee TA, Diamond B, Keen MS, et al. Age-related changes in pharyngeal and supraglottic sensation. Annals of Otology, Rhinology and Laryngology. 1994;103(10):749–52.

72. Saboisky JP, Stashuk DW, Hamilton-Wright A, Trinder J, Nandedkar S, Malhotra A. Effects of aging on genioglossus motor units in humans. PLOS One. 2014;9(8):e104572.

73. Klawe JJ, Tafil-Klawe M. Age-related response of the genioglossus muscle EMG-activity to hypoxia in humans. Journal of Physiology and Pharmacology: An Official Journal of the Polish Physiological Society. 2003;54(Suppl 1):14–9.

74. Worsnop C, Kay A, Kim Y, Trinder J, Pierce R. Effect of age on sleep onset-related changes in respiratory pump and upper airway muscle function. Journal of Applied Physiology (Bethesda, MD: 1985). 2000;88(5):1831–9.

75. Thurnheer R, Wraith PK, Douglas NJ. Influence of age and gender on upper airway resistance in NREM and REM sleep. Journal of Applied Physiology (Bethesda, MD: 1985). 2001;90(3):981–8.

76. Kirkness JP, Schwartz AR, Schneider H, Punjabi NM, Maly JJ, Laffan AM, et al. Contribution of male sex, age, and obesity to mechanical instability of the upper airway during sleep. Journal of

Applied Physiology (Bethesda, MD: 1985). 2008;104(6):1618–24.

77. Onal E, Burrows DL, Hart RH, Lopata M. Induction of periodic breathing during sleep causes upper airway obstruction in humans. Journal of Applied Physiology. 1986;61(4):1438–43.

78. Warner G, Skatrud JB, Dempsey JA. Effect of hypoxia-induced periodic breathing on upper airway obstruction during sleep. Journal of Applied Physiology. 1987;62(6):2201–11.

79. Badr MS, Toiber F, Skatrud JB, Dempsey J. Pharyngeal narrowing/occlusion during central sleep apnea. Journal of Applied Physiology. 1995;78(5):1806–15.

80. Badr MS. Effect of ventilatory drive on upper airway patency in humans during NREM sleep. Respiration Physiology. 1996;103(1):1–10.

81. Pokorski M, Walski M, Dymecka A, Marczak M. The aging carotid body. Journal of Physiology and Pharmacology: An Official Journal of the Polish Physiological Society. 2004;55(Suppl 3):107–13.

82. Monteiro TC, Batuca JR, Obeso A, González C, Monteiro EC. Carotid body function in aged rats: responses to hypoxia, ischemia, dopamine, and adenosine. Age (Dordrecht, Netherlands). 2011;33(3):337–50.

83. Pawar A, Peng YJ, Jacono FJ, Prabhakar NR. Comparative analysis of neonatal and adult rat carotid body responses to chronic intermittent hypoxia. Journal of Applied Physiology (Bethesda, MD: 1985). 2008;104(5):1287–94.

84. Prabhakar N, Peng Y-J, Kumar G, Nanduri J, Di Giulio C, Lahiri S. Long-term regulation of carotid body function: acclimatization and adaptation–invited article. Arterial Chemoreceptors: Springer; 2009. pp. 307–17.

85. Garcia AJ, Zanella S, Dashevskiy T, Khan SA, Khuu MA, Prabhakar NR, et al. Chronic intermittent hypoxia alters local respiratory circuit function at the level of the preBötzinger complex. Frontiers in Neuroscience. 2016;10(4).

86. Montandon G, Qin W, Liu H, Ren J, Greer JJ, Horner RL. PreBötzinger complex neurokinin-1 receptor-expressing neurons mediate opioid-induced respiratory depression. The Journal of Neuroscience. 2011;31(4):1292–301.

87. Ray AD, Ogasa T, Magalang UJ, Krasney JA, Farkas GA. Aging increases upper airway collapsibility in Fischer 344 rats. Journal of Applied Physiology. 2008;105(5):1471–6.

88. Schwarz EC, Thompson JM, Connor NP, Behan M. The effects of aging on hypoglossal motoneurons in rats. Dysphagia. 2009;24(1):40–8.

89. Edwards BA, Sands SA, Owens RL, Eckert DJ, Landry S, White DP, et al. The Combination of supplemental oxygen and a hypnotic markedly improves obstructive sleep apnea in patients with a mild to moderate upper airway collapsibility. Sleep. 2016;39(11):1973–83.

90. Wellman A, Malhotra A, Jordan AS, Stevenson KE, Gautam S, White DP. Effect of oxygen in obstructive sleep apnea: role of loop gain. Respiratory Physiology & Neurobiology. 2008;162(2):144–51.

91. Xie A, Teodorescu M, Pegelow DF, Teodorescu MC, Gong Y, Fedie JE, et al. Effects of stabilizing or increasing respiratory motor outputs on obstructive sleep apnea. Journal of Applied Physiology (Bethesda, MD: 1985). 2013;115(1):22–33.

92. Rastogi R, Badr MS, Ahmed A, Chowdhuri S. Amelioration of sleep disordered breathing with supplemental oxygen in older adults. Journal of Applied Physiology (Bethesda, MD: 1985). 2020;129(6):1441–50.

93. Chowdhuri S, Sinha P, Pranathiageswaran S, Badr MS. Sustained hyperoxia stabilizes breathing in healthy individuals during NREM sleep. Journal of Applied Physiology (Bethesda, MD: 1985). 2010;109(5):1378–83.

94. Kiwull-Schöne H, Teppema L, Wiemann M, Kiwull P. Loop gain of respiratory control upon reduced activity of carbonic anhydrase or Na$^+$/H$^+$ exchange. The Arterial Chemoreceptors: Springer; 2006. pp. 239–44.

95. Edwards BA, Sands SA, Eckert DJ, White DP, Butler JP, Owens RL, et al. Acetazolamide improves loop gain but not the other physiological traits causing obstructive sleep apnoea. The Journal of Physiology. 2012;590(5):1199–211.

96. Ginter G, Sankari A, Eshraghi M, Obiakor H, Yarandi H, Chowdhuri S, et al. Effect of acetazolamide on susceptibility to central sleep apnea in chronic spinal cord injury. Journal of Applied Physiology (Bethesda, MD: 1985). 2020;128(4):960–6.

97. R. Rastogi KAB, M.S. Badr, S. Chowdhuri. Effect of acetazolamide on pathophysiology of sleep disordered breathing in older adults. American Journal of Respiratory and Critical Care Medicine 2020;201:A6454.

98. Pranathiageswaran S, Badr MS, Chowdhuri S. Acetazolamide Stabilizes Breathing in Healthy Older Adults during NREM Sleep. B110 Upper Airway and Respiratory Control during Sleep. American Thoracic Society International Conference Abstracts: American Thoracic Society; 2014. p. A3903–A.

99. Rubin S, Tack M, Cherniack NS. Effect of aging on respiratory responses to CO_2 and inspiratory resistive loads. Journal of Gerontology. 1982;37(3):306–12.

100. Davenport MH, Beaudin AE, Brown AD, Leigh R, Poulin MJ. Ventilatory responses to exercise and CO_2 after menopause in healthy women: effects of age and fitness. Respiratory Physiology & Neurobiology. 2012;184(1):1–8.

101. Miller KB, Howery AJ, Rivera-Rivera LA, Johnson SC, Rowley HA, Wieben O, et al. Age-related reductions in cerebrovascular reactivity using 4D flow MRI. Frontiers in Aging Neuroscience. 2019;11:281.

5 Breathing Control in Exercise

Philippe Haouzi

INTRODUCTION

This chapter addresses one of the most controversial and long-debated topics in the field of breathing control, which is the control of respiration during a muscular exercise. We will here only consider the question of breathing regulation during a dynamic exercise, i.e. an exercise consisting of rhythmic muscle contractions and relaxations, such as walking, running, or cycling, and which results in an increase in metabolic rate. The ventilatory responses to static or isometric contractions of a group of muscles (1) will not be discussed in this chapter (2, 3).

WHAT ARE THE QUESTIONS?

During a muscular exercise, transferring molecules of oxygen from the atmosphere to the mitochondrial electron chain of the contracting muscle cells while removing the molecules of CO_2 produced by the Krebs cycle, requires a constant adjustment of the respiratory control system (4, 5).

What is the magnitude of such an adjustment? Oxygen consumption ($\dot{V}O_2$) and CO_2 production ($\dot{V}CO_2$) can increase up to 15–20-fold during high-intensity muscle exercise (4, 6), leading to a rise in body $\dot{V}O_2$ from a resting value of a 250–300 mL of O_2 per min to up to 4 l/min in very fit subjects, with even higher levels of $\dot{V}CO_2$. Since the variations in pulmonary gas exchange mirror those occurring in the peripheral tissues, the convection of gas in the regions of the lungs wherein gas exchange takes place, i.e. the alveolar regions, must increase in proportion to the rate at which peripheral gas exchanges, or rather pulmonary gas exchanges, increase in order to prevent alveolar (and thus arterial) PCO_2 ($PACO_2$ and $PaCO_2$) to rise and alveolar and arterial PO_2 (PAO_2 and PaO_2) to drop. The relationship between $PACO_2$ (or PAO_2), pulmonary gas exchange rate, and alveolar ventilation is dictated by the alveolar equation: $PAO_2 = PIO_2 - k\dot{V}O_2/\dot{V}A$ and $PACO_2 = k\dot{V}CO_2/\dot{V}A$ (Equation 1). Consequently, it is the ratio between pulmonary gas exchange rate and alveolar ventilation that dictates the level of mean $PACO_2$ and PAO_2. As an example, for a 15-fold increase in $\dot{V}CO_2$, a 15-fold increase in $\dot{V}A$ must be produced to maintain $PACO_2$ constant. This requires minute ventilation ($\dot{V}E$) to increase from a resting level of about 8 l/min to well above 100 l/min. Without such

an adjustment, no muscular exercise will be possible without a concomitant hypoxemia and hypercapnia. This remains true even for a light exercise: during a gentle bout of walking, $\dot{V}O_2$ and $\dot{V}CO_2$ increase as much as three-fold. In keeping with Equation 1, $PACO_2$ should increase up to 120 torr and PAO_2 (and PaO_2) would be close to zero, if $\dot{V}A$ did not increase during walking. Conversely, any increase in $\dot{V}A$ in excess to the rise in $\dot{V}CO_2$ will produce a respiratory alkalosis. At this point, it is important to emphasize the view that the rate at which CO_2 is produced in the tissues and exchanged in the lungs (difference in venous and arterial CO_2 volume times the cardiac output) is different from the rate at which CO_2 reaches the lungs, a variable which has often been considered in the literature as the "physiological" surrogate of $\dot{V}CO_2$.

Despite the complexity of the structures that may be involved, the description of the $\dot{V}E$ response to a dynamic exercise of constant intensity or work rate (step exercise) in man appears to be rather simple (7): $\dot{V}E$, after an initial increase of several liters per minute (1), rises exponentially ($\dot{V}E$ phase II) toward a steady state, which is reached within about 3 minutes. When exercise stops, ventilation returns to baseline with a time course that appears to track the changes in pulmonary gas exchange rate (8). What we have learnt over more than a century of research on the description of the ventilatory response to exercise, is that not only does minute ventilation increase in proportion to the pulmonary gas exchange rate, but this ventilatory adjustment has kinetics that seems to "follow" changes in $\dot{V}O_2$ or $\dot{V}CO_2$ measured at the lungs (9). As a result, until heavy levels of exercise are reached, the response to exercise remains isocapnic in humans. As illustrated in Figure 5.1, if a ramp-like exercise is performed until exhaustion, and $PaCO_2$ is measured at different intensities, the $PaCO_2$-$\dot{V}E$ relationship remains vertical (ventilation rises with no increase in $PaCO_2$). Such a relationship is therefore different from the expected $PaCO_2$-$\dot{V}E$ relationship produced by CO_2 inhalation or CO_2 loading or unloading of the venous blood returning to the central circulation (10). In other words, the absence of significant increasing in $PaCO_2$ during muscular exercise has been regarded as a proof that chemical control of breathing, at least as we understand it, cannot explain by itself the isocapnic response to exercise hyperpnea; since the ventilatory

DOI: 10.1201/9781003000631-6

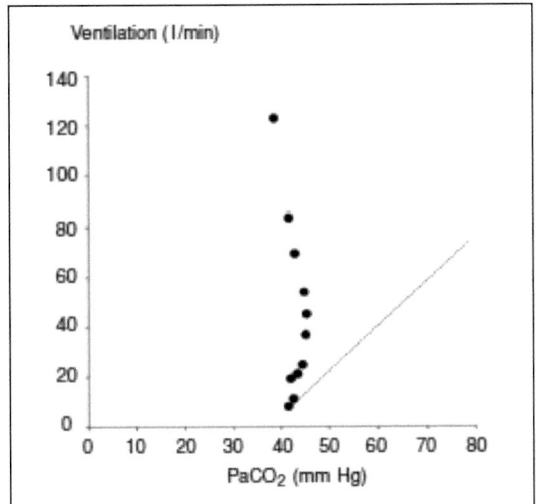
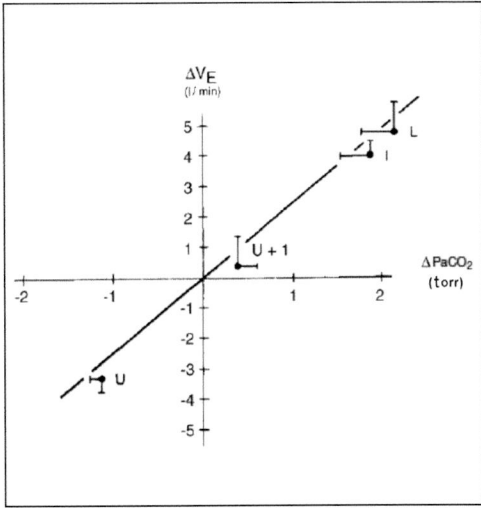

Figure 5.1 **Left panel:** Relationship between arterial PCO_2 and minute ventilation during a ramp-like increase in workload in humans (92). Note that ventilation increases with no increase in $PaCO_2$ during a moderate level of exercise, while hypocapnia develops at a higher level of work rate and breathing. The relationship is very different (*black line*) from the response to inhaled CO_2, which requires hypercapnia for ventilation to increase (with a "gain" of 1–3 l/min/torr). **Right panel:** Delta VE-Delta $PaCO_2$ relationship in awake dogs during venous CO_2 unloading (U) via a venous-venous ECMO, simultaneous unloading and CO_2 inhalation (U+I), CO_2 loading (L), and CO_2 inhalation (I) (46). The slopes of all these relationships are identical whether CO_2 was loaded into the venous blood or through the airways in marked contrast to the physiological response to exercise.

response to CO_2 requires an increase in $PaCO_2$ to produce increased breathing (Figure 5.1). This characteristic of the ventilatory response to exercise remains true whether a step, an impulse, or a fluctuating change in workload is applied (11–16). Above 60%–70% of the maximal sustainable $\dot{V}O_2$, a relative hyperventilation occurs, leading to a moderate hypocapnia (Figure 5.1).

How is breathing regulated during a dynamic exercise to produce an increase in alveolar ventilation commensurate to the change in metabolic rate has long puzzled respiratory physiologists (5, 17–30). Of note, as a consequence of the alveolar gas equation, it is alveolar, and not minute, ventilation that controls the alveolar partial pressure of CO_2 and O_2 at any given $\dot{V}CO_2$ and $\dot{V}O_2$. This leads to an even more enigmatic question: how could *alveolar* ventilation be regulated—in keeping with the level of metabolism—while it is minute ventilation (a tidal volume at a given frequency) that is generated by the respiratory neurons? This certainly adds another level of complexity to the search of the putative mechanisms of exercise-induced hyperpnea. Extensive and numerous reviews have been written on the many proposed theories proposed to account for such a regulation (5, 22, 31, 32), including the most recent version of the handbook of

physiology (23); the reader will find in these reviews all the appropriate references on the different concepts and their history along with the fascinating debates on blood gas homeostasis during exercise. This subject also has major practical interests since many patients suffering from dyspnea on exertion would benefit from a better understanding of the structures involved in the ventilatory response to exercise.

THE CONTROL OF BREATHING DURING EXERCISE IN A NUTSHELL

A dynamic exercise is a complex situation which, as a first approximation, combines an increase in metabolic rate and a motor activity. The motor act requires the voluntary and automatic control of movements and produces muscle contraction-related information transmitted through the spinal cord. The mechanical consequences of the contractions have long been shown to stimulate breathing and the sensing mechanisms mostly involve populations of groups III and IV muscle afferent fibers (33–39). At the central nervous system level, various structures have been shown to be able to increase, via a primarily descending pathway, breathing along with the motor/locomotor activity through "a parallel central" activation of the 2 "systems": for instance, the sub-thalamic locomotor regions (40)—studied exclusively in animals—during real or fictive walking, and the motor cortex, (41, 42) which role has been investigated in humans, (43) have been suggested to be key players in the ventilatory response to exercise. The fact that various central motor or locomotor-related efferent signals appear to be capable of increasing ventilation is undisputable; however, it is difficult to imagine a system deprived from any information on the magnitude or the kinetics of the variations in the gas exchange rate in the tissues or at the lung level that could account for the coupling between metabolism and ventilation. Indeed, whenever the motor act is dissociated from metabolic or gas exchange rate (11, 44), the strategy adopted by the ventilatory control system is not to follow factors related to the motor activity but to follow factors proportional or related to some of the changes associated with the rate at which CO_2 eliminated from the tissues and exchanged in the lungs (14). This is illustrated in Figure 5.2,

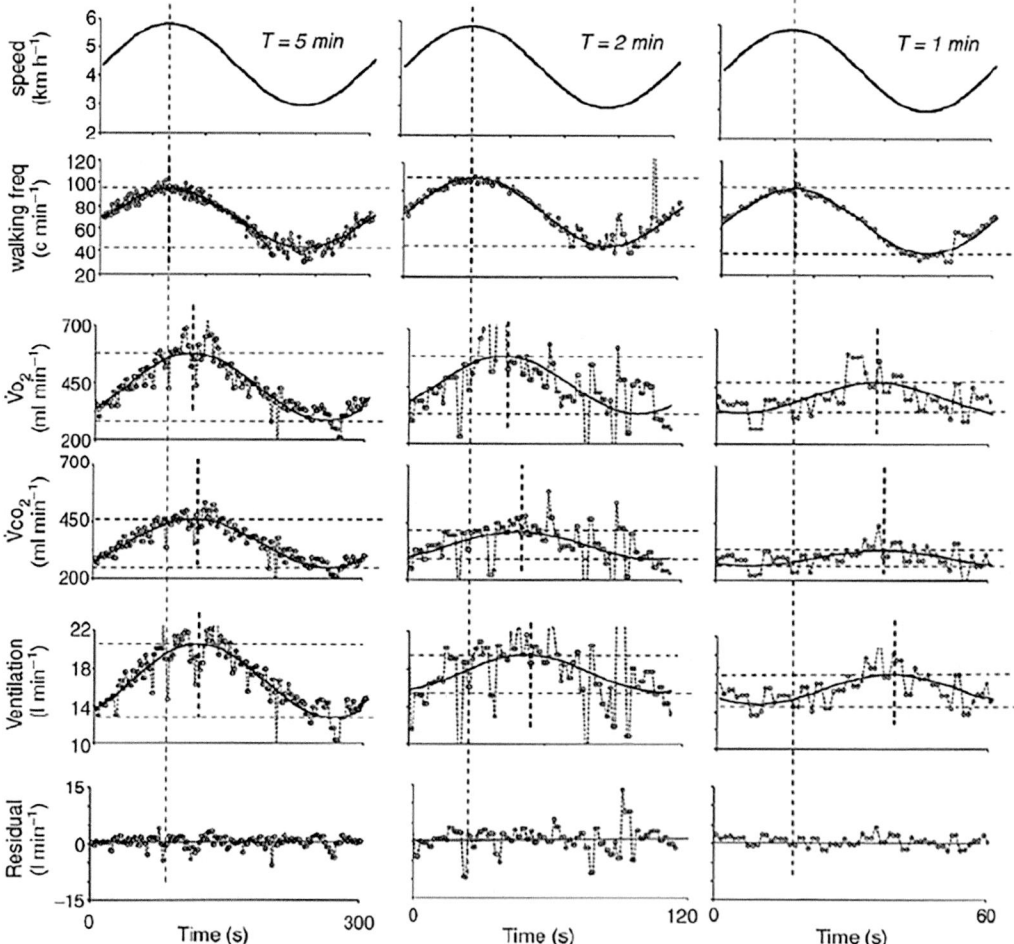

Figure 5.2 Example of the pulmonary gas exchange and ventilatory responses to a sinusoidal change in work rate during walking exercise in a sheep (14). The period of sinusoidal changes in treadmill speed are shown for periods of 5, 2, and 1 min. Note that the changes in walking frequency are in phase with the sinusoidal changes in the speed of the treadmill and that there is no reduction in amplitude when the frequency of oscillations of the treadmill speed increases. In contrast, as the period of the oscillations in work rate decreased, the pulmonary gas exchange response became more and more dissociated from the motor activity, due to their longer time constant response (about 1 min). Minute ventilation follows the change in pulmonary gas exchange, with a reduction in amplitude and an increase in phase lag despite unchanged motor control and work rate intensity.

wherein the pulmonary gas exchange rate and ventilatory responses to a sinusoidal change in work rate (treadmill speed) in a sheep are shown (14). Similar results have been reported during cycling exercise in humans (11). The amplitude of the work rate actually performed is the same at any period of oscillation in work rate; in contrast, due to the slow kinetics of the pulmonary gas exchange rate (time constant response of about 1 min), the amplitude of the $\dot{V}CO_2$ and $\dot{V}O_2$ response decreases as the period of oscillation in work rate decreases. Meanwhile, the phase increases as the periods of oscillations in work rate become shorter, and the pulmonary gas exchange rate variations become more and more dissociated from the motor activity. Minute ventilation follows the change in pulmonary gas exchange, with a reduction in amplitude and an increase in phase when the period of oscillation in work rate decreases, despite unchanged motor control and work rate intensity. Any proposed theory (10, 45) that neglects this crucial observation cannot account for the fundamental mechanism of $\dot{V}E$ control during exercise (28).

If the answer to the challenging question of blood gas homeostasis during exercise is not to be found in the mechanical effects of contractions or the primary production of a locomotor or motor activity, could the change in metabolic rate directly and indirectly control breathing during exercise? The metabolic changes during exercise can produce a large variety of inputs to the medullary neurons that have all been shown to be able to increase breathing, when considered separately. These include, and are not limited to (1) the increase in CO_2 venous content (46, 47) and a decrease in the mixed venous O_2 content (48); (2) the change in the chemical composition in the muscles (49, 50) also affecting the Group III and IV muscle afferents; (3) the increase in local and systemic temperature (51–53); or (4) the increase in systemic and muscle blood flow potentially stimulating receptors located in the central (54–57) as well as peripheral circulation (14, 34, 58). The confrontations of the different theories that were developed over many decades have taught us that neither signals related to the pulmonary gas exchange per se—via receptors in the lungs or in the heart—nor the changes in arterial blood composition can prevent the rise in $PaCO_2$ (and decrease in PaO_2), when $\dot{V}CO_2$ (and $\dot{V}O_2$) increase, in a manner similar to what is produced during a muscular exercise. Despite the fact that these inputs, with their different magnitude and time constants, can" reach" the CNS in an almost infinite number of combinations and can all increase breathing separately, there is no evidence that any of these inputs taken in isolation or

association can provide a good explanation to the observation that the ventilatory response follows the "metabolism" in a perfectly predictive manner (16, 59).

HOW TO UNDERSTAND THE APPARENT MATCHING BETWEEN ALVEOLAR VENTILATION AND PULMONARY GAS EXCHANGE RATE DURING EXERCISE?

How the medullary and supra-medullary structures including the motor, premotor and limbic cortex involved in breathing control process the multitude of available sources of information reaching the central nervous system to produce a very simple response, as presented in the first paragraph, is unknown (60–64). The strategy used by the "respiratory neurons" to maintain blood gas homeostasis, when rapid and very large change in metabolism are produced, seems to rely on properties that have more to do with the *selection* of information rather than using the sum/integration of individual inputs (61). In other words, not all of the signals produced by exercise are important in generating a ventilatory output in the context of an exercise (23). Accordingly, the central nervous system does not respond in proportion to (or as a function of) the response of any individual stimulus, which could be predicted by, for instance, the elementary $\dot{V}E$ response to CO_2, hypoxia, muscle contractions or a change in blood flow. The respiratory control system seems to use various sources of information to determine that an exercise is actually being performed and to select the most relevant information for adjusting breathing to the gas exchange rate. It is quite puzzling that any physiological mechanism which seems to play a significant role to control exercise hyperpnea, almost always loses its relevance when the "integrated" response is considered (8, 65, 66). Certainty methodological limitations must be considered. For instance, data obtained in animals or in reduced/altered preparation (fictive locomotion, spinal cord section, sedation) may or may not be transferable to humans. Yet, despite a very predictable overall ventilatory pattern, the potential mechanisms controlling breathing during exercise seem to produce profoundly non-linear responses (67). This property could explain why some very convincing published studies, which support a given theory, are contradicted by experiments apparently as convincing, causing perplexity to any serious reader. Figure 5.3 is an attempt to illustrate this conundrum by juxtaposing different experimental conditions. In Figure 5.3A, a total obstruction of blood flow to and

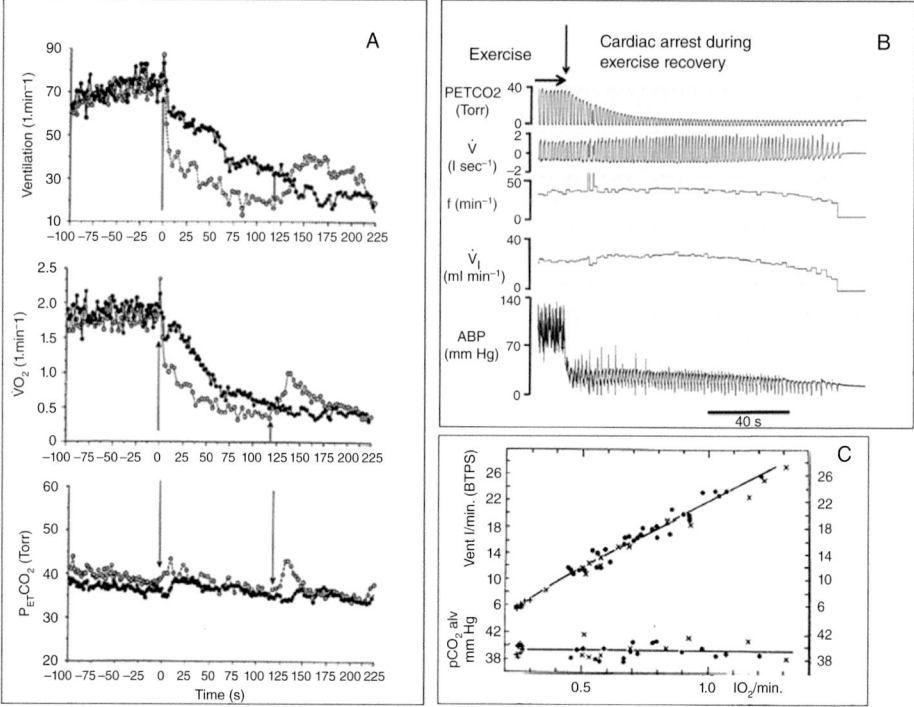

Figure 5.3 **Panel A:** Minute ventilation ($\dot{V}E$), O_2 uptake ($\dot{V}O_2$), and end-tidal PCO_2 ($PETCO_2$) during recovery (*closed symbols*) from a constant work rate cyclo-ergometer exercise performed above the lactate threshold and during recovery with cuffs inflated for 2 min around the upper thigh after the cessation of all contractions (*open symbols*) (69). The first arrow indicates the cessation of exercise and cuff inflation; the second arrow indicates the moment of occlusion release. The normal ventilatory decline was sped up during cuff occlusion, resulting in a large ventilatory deficit, despite expected accumulation of metabolites in the muscle circulation. **Panel B:** Ventricular fibrillation-induced cardiac arrest after electrically induced exercise in one sedated sheep (75). This example shows a long period of "eupneic" breathing during cardiac arrest (CA) at the cessation of muscle contractions. Breath-by-breath respired CO_2, respiratory flow ($\dot{V}$), respiratory rate (f), minute ventilation ($\dot{V}I$), and arterial carotid blood pressure (ABP) are displayed. Horizontal arrow represents the end of the period of exercise, which lasted 4 min (*not shown*). Vertical arrow is the moment when the heart was fibrillated. Note that breathing averaged 30–35 l/min by the end of the period of exercise; ventilation increases modestly thereafter, before stopping 2 min or so later. Breathing pattern and minute ventilation were unchanged at the onset of the cardiac arrest. Note the swings in ABP during CA caused by persistent breathing activity. The responses shown in this panel is difficult to reconcile with the responses presented in panels A and B, since ventilation is maintained at a level commensurate to the gas exchange prior to exercise recovery, while no muscular activity is performed anymore and circulation has stopped. **Panel C:** Effect of voluntary (*circles*) and electrically (x) induced exercise on minute ventilation and alveolar PCO_2 relative to metabolic rate (17). Responses to electrically induced exercise and "voluntary" exercise were the same, contradicting the theory supporting an important role of "central command" in the ventilatory response to exercise.

from the post exercising limbs is performed using a cuff placed around the upper thighs in a group of subjects, at the cessation of dynamic exercise. Breathing is not stimulated, but its normal decline (recovery from exercise) is actually sped up toward resting levels in humans (68–71). Similarly, impeding, by intravascular occluders, the circulation to the hindlimbs (acute aortic obstruction) during

electrically induced muscle contractions (69, 72) leads to a reduction in ventilation along with a reduction in the pulmonary exchange rate (73, 74). Incidentally, this observation initiated a series of studies which led to the theory that the level of muscle perfusion in the skeletal muscles, proportional to the level of muscle peripheral metabolic rate, could represent a significant source of ventilatory stimulation via group III and IV muscle afferent fibers (58). However, during a complete interruption of circulation at the end of an exercise, such as produced by a cardiac arrest (Figure 5.3B), minute ventilation is maintained at the same level as prior to the phase of asystole (75), despite no contraction being performed and no blood going to or leaving the post-exercising muscles. As previously argued (75), it is difficult to reconcile these two observations.

Similarly, the stimulation of supra-pontine structure increases the phrenic activity along with the efferent signal sent to the skeletal muscle in paralyzed cats (fictive locomotion)—an effect refereed as central command by Eldridge et al. (76). However, as shown in Figure 5.3B, the increase in ventilation produced by electrically contracting muscles (no central command) is indistinguishable from that of voluntary exercise, keeping alveolar PCO_2 constant (77–79). This last observation strongly suggests that a "central command" is not obligatory for ventilatory response to exercise, akin to the data obtained following the spinal cord section, when all information coming from the contracting muscles are suppressed. This effect was best illustrated by Kao (80–82) who studied the $\dot{V}E$ response in dogs in which the circulatory systems were connected in such a way that the blood leaving the exercising muscles of one dog (the neural dog) was infused into the venous system of another animal (the humoral dog). Electrically induced muscle contractions provoked an

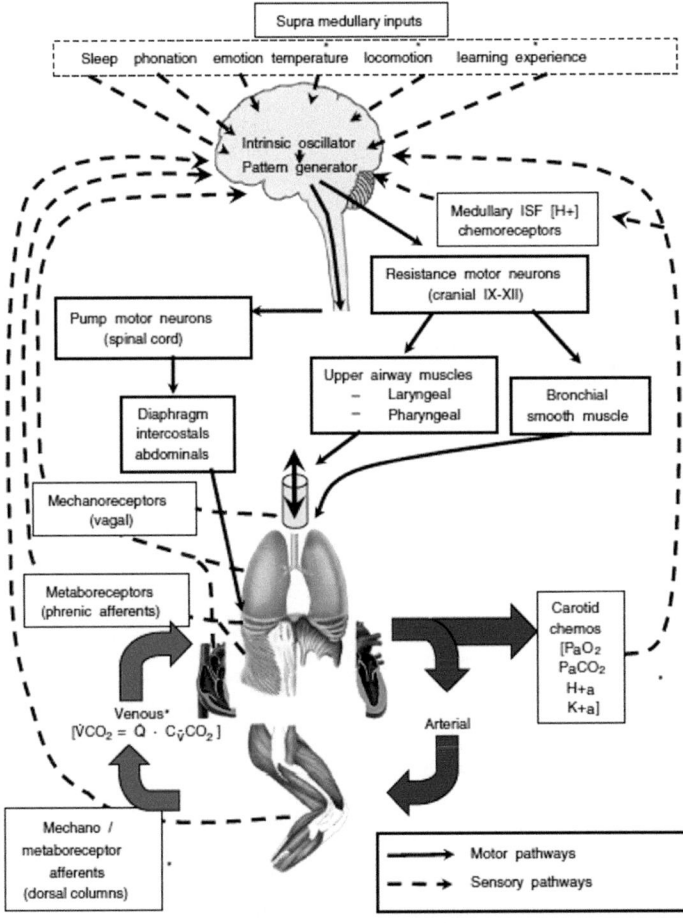

Figure 5.4 Schematic representation of the structures (peripheral and central) which have been shown to contribute to the control of breathing in exercise (from (23)). The results of all these interactions is a complex system wherein any element taken individually is not able to provide—or explain—the essential characteristic of the integrated response, i.e. a ventilatory-gas exchange coupling, but allows novel properties to emerge. This behavior can be mimicked by a Rube-Goldberg machine (61). The mechanisms leading to such an emerging property are not known.

isocapnic hyperpnoea in the neural dog prior to the circulatory diversions. After "connection" of the "neural" dog to the "humoral" dog, the exercise stimulated ventilation in the "neural" dog with a profound hypocapnia. In the "humoral" dog, however, $PaCO_2$ rose in the same way as during CO_2 inhalation. Following the destruction of the antero-lateral system, i.e. the pathway followed by the projections of the unmyelinated and small myelinated fibers, the response was abolished. Details of these theories and the debate over the effects of loading and unloading CO_2 in the venous system can be found in several reviews (7, 23).

It remains quite difficult to reconcile all these studies using a single theory. How pieces of information are processed by the medullary and supra-medullary structures involved in respiration during exercise is therefore largely unknown. The neurophysiological basis of intriguing and somehow unreconcilable observations may well remain difficult to uncover due to the Rube-Goldberg machine-like features (Figure 5.4) of the respiratory control system (61). Plasticity (60, 83, 84), optimization (63), short-term potentiation (85, 86), after discharge (87), reconfiguration (88), redundancy (66, 89), or degeneracy (90, 91) are some of the properties that have been proposed to render comprehensible the operational modalities of the respiratory control system. Although very original attempts have been made to offer theories that could explain blood homeostasis during increase in metabolic rate, based, for instance, on optimization (63), novel experimental approaches aimed at identifying and characterizing such fundamental properties of the central nervous system are warranted.

CONCLUSIONS

The matching between alveolar ventilation and pulmonary gas exchange observed during exercise is the result of a complex process wherein the ventilatory strategy "chosen" by the central nervous system is determined by (1) the magnitude and kinetics of the feedback inputs, which are the direct or indirect, but still poorly understood, consequences of the changes in gas exchange or one of its surrogates, (2) central mechanisms selecting, filtering or favoring certain of these inputs. These interactions lead to an apparently very simple ventilatory response that follows the gas exchange rate, preserving arterial blood gas homeostasis. The enormous body of literature generated over one century to understand this question has not brought a definitive answer to this challenging question. As a result, one must consider the rather pessimist conclusion that no conceptual framework can currently be used to understand how $\dot{V}A$ can increase in proportion to a rise in the pulmonary gas exchange rate.

REFERENCES

1. Dejours P. La regulation de la ventilation au cours de l'exercise musculaire chez l'homme. *Journal of Physiology* 51: 163, 1959.

2. Imms FJ and Mehta D. Respiratory responses to sustained isometric muscle contractions in man: the effect of muscle mass. *Journal of Physiology* 419: 1–14, 1989.

3. Poole DC, Ward SA, Whipp BJ. Control of blood-gas and acid-base status during isometric exercise in humans. *Journal of Physiology* 396: 365–377, 1988.

4. Astrand and Rodahl. *Textbook of Work Physiology.* Toronto: McGraw-Hill, 1977.

5. Dejours P. Control of respiration in muscular exercise. In: *Handbook of Physiology, Section 3, Volume I, Chapter 25*, edited by Fenn WO and Rahn H. Washington DC: American Physiological Society, 1964, pp. 631–648.

6. Dejours P. Comparative aspects of maximal oxygen consumption. *Respiration Physiology* 80: 155–162, 1990.

7. Haouzi P. Theories on the nature of the coupling between ventilation and gas exchange during exercise. *Respiratory Physiology & Neurobiology* 151: 267–279, 2006.

8. Haouzi P. Tracking pulmonary gas exchange by breathing control during exercise: role of muscle blood flow. *The Journal of Physiology* 592: 453–461, 2014.

9. Whipp BJ, Lamarra N, Ward SA, Davis JA, Wasserman K. Estimating arterial PCO_2 from flow-weighted and time-average alveolar PCO_2 during exercise. In: *Respiratory Control: A Modelling Perspective*, edited by Swanson GD, Grodins FS and Hughson RL. New York: Plenum Press, 1989, pp. 91–99.

10. Whipp BJ, Lamarra N, Griffiths TL, Wasserman K. Model implications of ventilatory dynamics during exercise. In: *Modelling and Control of Breathing*, edited by Whipp BJ, Weiberg DM, Bellville JW, Ward SA. New York: Elsevier Biomedical, 1983, pp. 229–236.

11. Casaburi R, Whipp BJ, Wasserman K, Beaver WL, Koyal SN. Ventilatory and gas exchange dynamics in response to sinusoidal work. *Journal of Applied Physiology* 42: 300–311, 1977.

12. Fujihara Y, Hildebrandt J, Hildebrandt JR. Cardiorespiratory transients in exercising man. ll. Linear models. *Journal of Applied Physiology* 35: 68–76, 1973.

13. Fujihara Y, Hildebrandt JR, Hildebrandt J. Cardiorespiratory transients in exercising man. I. Tests of superposition. *Journal of Applied Physiology* 35: 58–67, 1973.

14. Haouzi P, Chenuel B, Chalon B. The control of ventilation is dissociated from locomotion during walking in sheep. *Journal of Physiology* 559: 315–325, 2004.

15. Whipp BJ. *The Control of Exercise Hyperpnea*. New York: Marcel Dekker, 1981, pp. 1069–1139.

16. Whipp BJ. Tenets of the exercise hyperpnea and their degree of corroboration. *Chest* 73: 274–277, 1978.

17. Asmussen E. Exercise and the regulation of ventilation. In: *Physiology of Muscular Exercise*, edited by American Heart Association. New York: American Heart Association, 1967, pp. 132–145.

18. Comroe JH and Schmidt CF. Reflexes from the limbs as a factor in the hyperpnea of muscular exercise. *American Journal of Physiology* 138: 536–547, 1943.

19. Dejours P. Existance de deux groups de facteurs dans la regulation ventilatoire de l'exercise musculaire. *Journal of Physiology (Paris)* 48: 484–488, 1956.

20. Dejours P. The regulation of breathing during muscular exercise in man: A neuro-humoral theory. In: *The Regulation of Human Respiration*, edited by Cunningham DJC and Lloyd BB. Oxford: Blackwell Scientific, 1963, pp. 535–547.

21. Dempsey JA. Exercise hyperpnea. Chairman's introduction. *Advances in Experimental Medicine and Biology* 393: 133–136, 1995.

22. Dempsey JA, Mitchell GS, Smith CA. Exercise and chemoreception. *American Review of Respiratory Disease* 129: S31–S34, 1984.

23. Forster HV, Haouzi P, Dempsey JA. Control of breathing during exercise. *Comprehensive Physiology* 2: 743–777, 2012.

24. Geppert J and Zuntz N. Ueber die Regulation der Atmung. *Arch Ges Physiol* 42: 189–245, 1888.

25. Grodins FS. Analysis of factors concerned in the regulation of breathing in exercise. *Physiology Reviews* 30: 220–239, 1950.

26. Harrison TR, Harrison WG, Calhoun JA, Marsh JP. Congestive heart failure. The mechanism of dyspnea on exertion. *Archives of Internal Medicine* 50: 690–720, 1932.

27. Krogh A, Lindhard J. The regulation of respiration and circulation during the initial stages of muscular work. *Journal of Physiology* 47: 112–136, 1913.

28. Whipp BJ, Ward SA. Coupling of ventilation to pulmonary gas exchange during exercise. In: *Exercise: Pulmonary Physiology and Pathophysiology*, edited by Whipp BJ and Wasserman K. New York: Marcel Dekker, 1991, pp. 271–307.

29. Whipp BJ, Ward SA. Determinants and control of breathing during muscular exercise. *British Journal of Sports Medicine* 32: 199–211, 1998.

30. Zuntz N, Geppert J. Uber die Natur der normalen Atemreize und den ort ihrer Wirkung. *Arch Ges Physiol* 38: 337–338, 1886.

31. Wasserman K, Whipp B, Casaburi R. Respiratory control during exercise. *In: Handbook of Physiology the Respiratory System*, edited by Macklem P and Mead J. Bethesda: American Physiology Society, 1986, pp. 595–619.

32. Whipp B, Ward S. Coupling of ventilation to pulmonary gas exchange during exercise. In: *Exercise Pulmonary Physiology and Pathophysiology, Lung Biology in Health and Disease*, edited by Whipp B and Wasserman K. New York: Marcel Dekker, 1991, pp. 271–307.

33. Adreani CM, Hill JM and Kaufman MP. Responses of group III and IV muscle afferents to dynamic exercise. *Journal of Applied Physiology* 82: 1811–1817, 1997.

34. Haouzi P, Hill JM, Lewis BK, Kaufman MP. Responses of group III and IV muscle afferents to distension of the peripheral vascular bed. *Journal of Applied Physiology* 87: 545–553, 1999.

35. Kaufman MP. Afferents from limb skeletal muscle. In: *Lung Biology in Health & Disease. Regulation of Breathing*, edited by Dempsey JA and Pack AI. New York: Dekker, 1995, pp. 583–616.

36. Kaufman MP, Forster HV. Reflexes controlling circulatory, ventilatory and airway responses to exercise. In: *Handbook of Physiology, Section 12, Chapter 10*, edited by Rowell LB and Shepherd JT. Oxford: Oxford University Press, 1996, pp. 381–447.

37. Kniffki K-D, Mense S, Schmidt RF. Responses of group IV afferent units from skeletal muscle to stretch, contraction and chemical stimulation. *Experimental Brain Research* 31: 511–522, 1978.

38. Mense S. Group III and IV receptors in skeletal muscle: are they specific or polymodal? *Progress in Brain Research* 113: 83–100, 1996.

39. Pickar JG, Hill JM, Kaufman MP. Dynamic exercise stimulates group III muscle afferents. *Journal of Neurophysiology* 71: 753–760, 1994.

40. Eldridge FL, Millhorn DE, Waldrop TG. Exercise hyperpnea and locomotion: Parallel activation from the hypothalamus. *Science* 211: 844–846, 1981.

41. Fink GR, Adams L, Watson JD, Innes JA, Wuyam B, Kobayashi I, Corfield DR, Murphy K, Jones T, Frackowiak RS, et al. Hyperpnoea during and immediately after exercise in man: evidence of motor cortical involvement. *The Journal of Physiology* 489: 663–675, 1995.

42. Thornton J, Guz A, Murphy K, Griffith A, Pedersen D, Kardos A, Leff A, Adams L, Casadei B, Paterson D. Identification of higher brain centres that may encode the cardiorespiratory response to exercise in humans. *The Journal of Physiology* 533: 823–836, 2001.

43. Haouzi P. Initiating inspiration outside the medulla does produce eupneic breathing. *Journal of Applied Physiology* 110: 854–856, 2011.

44. Casaburi R, Whipp BJ, Wasserman K, Koyal SN. Ventilatory and gas exchange responses to cycling with sinusoidally varying pedal rate. *Journal of Applied Physiology* 44: 97–103, 1978.

45. Duffin J, Greszczuk RF. *A Mathematical Model Investigating the Control of Breathing during Exercise.* New York: Elsevier, 1983, pp. 353–360.

46. Bennett FM, Tallman RD, Jr. and Grodins FS. Role of VCO_2 in control of breathing of awake exercising dogs. *Journal of Applied Physiology* 56: 1335–1339, 1984.

47. Greco EC, Jr., Fordyce WE, Gonzalez F, Jr., Reischl P, Grodins FS. Respiratory responses to intravenous and intrapulmonary CO_2 in awake dogs. *Journal of Applied Physiology* 45: 109–114, 1978.

48. Phillipson EA, Duffin J, Cooper JD. Critical dependence of respiratory rhythmicity on metabolic CO2 load. *Journal of Applied Physiology* 50: 45–54, 1981.

49. Kaufman MP, Rybicki KJ. Discharge properties of group III and IV muscle afferents: their responses to mechanical and metabolic stimuli. *Circulation Research* 61: I60–I65, 1987.

50. Mense S, Stahnke M. Responses in muscle afferent fibres of slow conduction velocity to contractions and ischaemia in the cat. *Journal of Physiology* 342: 383–397, 1983.

51. Budzinska K. Effects of hyperthermia and stimulation of the hypothalamus on the activity of the phrenic nerve in hypo- normo- and hypercapnic rabbits. *Acta Neurobiologiae Experimentalis* 35: 227–240, 1975.

52. Dejours P, Teillac A, Girard F, Lacaisse A. Study of the role of moderate central hyperthermia in the regulation of ventilation during muscular exercise in man. *Revue Francaise d'Etudes Cliniques et Biologiques* 3: 755–761, 1958.

53. Hertel HC, Howaldt B, Mense S. Responses of group IV and group III muscle afferents to thermal stimuli. *Brain Research* 113: 201–205, 1976.

54. Huszczuk A, Jones P, Oren A, Shors E, Nery L, Whipp B, Wasserman K. Venous return and ventilatory control. In: *Modelling and Control of Breathing*, edited by Whipp B and Wiberg D. New-York: Elsevier, 1983, pp. 78–85.

55. Jones PW, Huszczuk A and Wasserman K. Cardiac output as a controller of ventilation through changes in right ventricular load. *Journal of Applied Physiology* 53: 218–224, 1982.

56. Wasserman K, Whipp BJ, Castagna J. Cardiodynamic hyperpnea: hyperpnea secondary to cardiac output increase. *Journal of Applied Physiology* 36: 457–464, 1974.

57. Haouzi P. Venous pressure and dyspnea on exertion in cardiac failure: was Tinsley Randolph Harrison right? *Respiratory Physiology & Neurobiology* 167: 101–106, 2009.

58. Haouzi P, Chenuel B, Huszczuk A. Sensing vascular distension in skeletal muscle by slow conducting afferent fibers: neurophysiological basis and implication for respiratory control. *Journal of Applied Physiology* 96: 407–418, 2004.

59. Whipp B, Ward S, Lamarra N, Davis J, Wasserman K. Parameters of ventilatory and gas exchange dynamics during exercise. *Journal of Applied Physiology* 52: 1506–1513, 1982.

60. Feldman JL, Mitchell GS, Nattie EE. Breathing: rhythmicity, plasticity, chemosensitivity. *Annual Review of Neuroscience* 26: 239–266, 2003.

61. Haouzi P. Precedence and autocracy in breathing control. *Journal of Applied Physiology* 118(12): 1553–6, 2015.

62. Poon C-S, Lin S-L, Knudson OB. Optimization character of inspiratory neural drive. *Journal of Applied Physiology* 72: 2005–2017, 1992.

63. Poon CS. Ventilatory control in hypercapnia and exercise: optimization hypothesis. *Journal of Applied Physiology* 62: 2447–2459, 1987.

64. Poon CS, Greene JG. Control of exercise hyperpnea during hypercapnia in humans. *Journal of Applied Physiology* 59: 792–797, 1985.

65. Haouzi P. Counterpoint: supraspinal locomotor centers do not contribute significantly to the hyperpnea of dynamic exercise. *Journal of Applied Physiology* 100: 1079–1082; discussion 1082-1073, 2006.

66. Pan LG, Forster HV, Wurster RD, Murphy CL, Brice AG, Lowry TF. Effect of partial spinal cord ablation on exercise hyperpnea in ponies. *Journal of Applied Physiology* 69: 1821–1827, 1990.

67. Haouzi P. The ventilatory component of the muscle metaboreflex: catch me if you can! *Experimental Physiology* 2020.

68. Dejours P, Mithoefer JC and Raynaud J. Evidence against the existence of specific ventilatory chemoreceptors in the legs. *Journal of Applied Physiology* 10: 367–371, 1957.

69. Haouzi P, Huszczuk A, Porszasz J, Chalon B, Wasserman K, Whipp BJ. Femoral vascular occlusion and ventilation during recovery from heavy exercise. *Respiration Physiology* 94: 137–150, 1993.

70. Innes JA, Solarte A, Huszczuk E, Whipp BJ, Wasserman K. Respiration during recovery from exercise: effects of trapping and release of femoral blood flow. *Journal of Applied Physiology* 67: 2608–2613, 1989.

71. Rowell LB, Hermansen L, Blackmon JR. Human cardiovascular and respiratory responses to graded muscle ischemia. *Journal of Applied Physiology* 41: 693–701, 1976.

72. Huszczuk A, Yeh E, Innes JA, Solarte I, Wasserman K, Whipp BJ. Role of muscle perfusion and baroreception in the hyperpnea following muscle contraction in dog. *Respiration Physiology* 91: 207–226, 1993.

73. Haouzi P, Huszczuk A, Gille JP, Chalon B, Marchal F, Crance JP, Whipp BJ. Vascular distension in muscles contributes to respiratory control in sheep. *Respiration Physiology* 99: 41–50, 1995.

74. Haouzi P, Marchal F, Huszczuk A. Muscle perfusion and control of breathing. Is there a neural link? *Advances in Experimental Medicine and Biology* 393: 363–368, 1995.

75. Haouzi P, Van De Louw A, Haouzi A. Breathing during cardiac arrest following exercise: a new function of the respiratory system? *Respiratory Physiology & Neurobiology* 181: 220–227, 2012.

76. Eldridge FL. Central integration of mechanisms in exercise hyperpnea. *Medicine and Science in Sports and Exercise* 26: 319–327, 1994.

77. Asmussen E, Johansen SH, Jorgenson, Nielsen M. On the nervous factors controlling respiration and circulation during exercise: Experiments with curarization. *Acta Physiologica Scandinavica* 63: 343–350, 1965.

78. Asmussen E and Nielsen M. Studies on the initial changes in respiration at the transition from rest to work and from work to rest. *Acta Physiologica Scandinavica* 16: 270–285, 1948.

79. Huszczuk A, Whipp BJ, Oren A, Shors EC, Pokorski M, Nery LE, Wasserman K. Ventilatory responses to partial cardiopulmonary bypass at rest and exercise in dogs. *Journal of Applied Physiology* 61: 575–583, 1986.

80. Kao F. An experimental study of the pathways involved in exercise hyperpnoea employing cross-circulation techniques. In: *The Regulation of Human Respiration*, edited by Cunningham D and BB L. Oxford: Blackwell Sci, 1963, pp. 461–502.

81. Kao FF. *An Experimental Study of the Pathways Involved in Exercise Hyperpnea, Employing Cross-Circulation Techniques*. Oxford: Blackwell Scientific, 1963, pp. 461–502.

82. Kao FF. The peripheral neurogenic drive: an experimental study. In: *Muscular Exercise and the Lung*, edited by Dempsey JA and Deed CE. Madison: University of Wisconsin Press, 1977, pp. 71–85.

83. Ling L, Olson EB, Jr., Vidruk EH, Mitchell GS. Developmental plasticity of the hypoxic ventilatory response. *Respiration Physiology* 110: 261–268, 1997.

84. Poon C, Siniaia MS. Plasticity of cardiorespiratory neural processing: classification and computational functions. *Respiration Physiology* 122: 83–109, 2000.

85. Eldridge FL, Waldrop TG. Neural control of breathing during exercise. In: *Exercise: Pulmonary Physiology and Pathophysiology*, edited by Whipp BJ and Wasserman K. New York: Marcel Dekker, 1991.

86. Wagner PG, Eldridge FL. Development of short-term potentiation of respiration. *Respiration Physiology* 83: 129–140, 1991.

87. Eldridge FL, Gill-Kumar P. Central neural respiratory drive and afterdischarge. *Respiration Physiology* 40: 49–63, 1980.

88. Lindsey BG, Hernandez YM, Morris KF, Shannon R, Gerstein GL. Dynamic reconfiguration of brain stem neural assemblies: Respiratory phase-dependent synchrony versus modulation of firing rates. *Journal of Neurophysiology* 67: 923–930, 1992.

89. Pan LG, Forster HV, Bisgard GE, Kaminski RP, Dorsey SM, Busch MA. Hyperventilation in ponies at the onset of and during steady-state exercise. *Journal of Applied Physiology* 54: 1394–1402, 1983.

90. Haouzi P, Bell HJ. Control of breathing and volitional respiratory rhythm in humans. *Journal of Applied Physiology* 106: 904–910, 2009.

91. Mellen NM. Degeneracy as a substrate for respiratory regulation. *Respiratory Physiology & Neurobiology* 172: 1–7, 2010.

92. Sun XG, Hansen JE, Stringer WW, Ting H, Wasserman K. Carbon dioxide pressure-concentration relationship in arterial and mixed venous blood during exercise. *Journal of Applied Physiology* 90: 1798–1810, 2001.

6 Control of the Upper Airway during Sleep

Leszek Kubin

INTRODUCTION

Motor innervation of upper airway muscles originates in the trigeminal, facial, glossopharyngeal, ambiguous, and hypoglossal (XII) cranial motor nuclei. The contribution of upper airway muscles to the maintenance of airway patency for breathing varies from accessory to essential depending on the physiologic and pathophysiologic conditions. The high prevalence of the obstructive apnea/hypopnea syndrome (OSA), and its association with major cardiovascular, metabolic and cognitive consequences, stimulate tremendous interest in the regulatory mechanisms that operate in association with OSA. The focus of this chapter is on those aspects of the regulation of upper airway muscle activity that help reduce excessive upper airway resistance.

The following reviews are recommended for complementary coverage of: central respiratory neurons during sleep (1); chemical control of breathing and its contribution to respiratory instability (2–4); neuromechanical control of the upper airway (5, 6); and state-dependent neural control of upper airway motoneurons (7, 8).

BIOMECHANICAL ENVIRONMENT IN THE UPPER AIRWAY VULNERABLE TO COLLAPSE AND ITS MODELS

The upper airway includes the nasal passages, the pharynx, and the larynx. The pharyngeal segment is the most compliant and most vulnerable to obstruction under the negative transmural pressure generated during inspiration. The structural features of the pharynx may critically predispose to OSA, and the compliance of this part of the upper airway is particularly dependent on neuromuscular support. The nasal and laryngeal portions of the upper airway are unlikely to collapse, but their resistance to airflow varies as a result of local tissue swelling, secretions, and neuromuscular activation, all of which ultimately determine the pressure gradient along the upper airway.

The notion that, in OSA patients, the pharyngeal airway is in a critical need of neuromuscular support inspired important concepts and models of the control of the size and compliance of the upper airway. One of them, referred to as the "balance of forces model", emphasized the opposing actions exerted on pharyngeal patency by negative intraluminar pressure secondary to the suction force generated by inspiratory pump muscles and the airway-dilating forces generated by upper airway muscles, with both being driven by the central respiratory network (9, 10). Reflex effects from respiratory chemoreceptors and upper and lower airway mechanoreceptors were incorporated in some of these models (11, 12) (Figure 6.1).

The model incorporating the opposing interaction between the pharyngeal transmural pressure and neuromuscular dilating force was then transformed to include the pressure exerted by the surrounding tissue (13), which allowed it to be subjected to the analysis developed in the field of fluid mechanics and referred to as the Starling resistor model. With this approach, one could quantify the collapsibility of the upper airway across individuals and in the presence or absence of neural drive to upper airway muscles by measuring one clinically relevant variable—the critical closing pressure (Pcrit)—defined as the nasal pressure at which the airway collapses under the eupneic inspiratory pressure (14–18). Depending on the conditions of the measurements, a passive Pcrit or an active Pcrit could be determined, with upper airway muscle tone largely eliminated or significantly present, respectively. For measurements of passive Pcrit, a sufficiently high steady positive pressure is applied to the airway of a sleeping or anesthetized subject prior to measurement to inhibit all upper airway muscle activity. Under such condition, a sudden drop of the elevated pressure to a less positive (or negative) value may elicit a complete obstruction of the airway during the first inspiratory period after the drop. The highest nasal pressure at which this occurs is defined as the passive Pcrit. Although individual passive Pcrit values vary, the mean population Pcrit measured during non-rapid eye movement (non-REM) sleep consistently shifts from about −15 cm H_2O in healthy individuals, to −6 cm in snorers, −3 cm in persons with predominantly hypopneas (rather than full obstructions), and +3 cm in patients with predominantly obstructive apneas (14). In contrast to passive Pcrit, active Pcrit is measured with some upper airway muscle tone present. In awake OSA patients who typically exhibit a significant level of upper airway muscle tone, active Pcrit values can be in excess of −40 cm H_2O (19). This indicates that the awake state allows one to mount a powerful

DOI: 10.1201/9781003000631-7

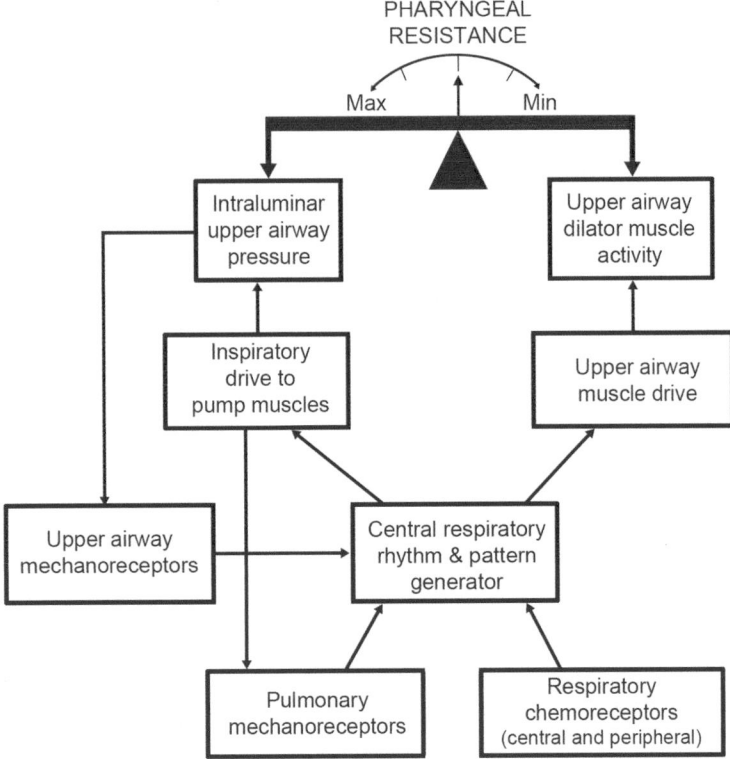

Figure 6.1 The "balance of forces" model emphasized the interplay between collapse-preventing neuromuscular control of the upper airway and the collapse-promoting intraluminar airway pressure generated during inspiration by the respiratory pump muscles. Effects exerted on the respiratory pump and upper airway motor systems by the neural networks responsible for the generation of sleep-wake states were not incorporated in the balance of forces models.

neuromuscular defense against airway collapse.

SLEEP-WAKE PATTERNS OF UPPER AIRWAY MUSCLE ACTIVITY, WITH EMPHASIS ON THE GENIOGLOSSUS

The size, stiffness, and resistance of the upper airway are determined by its passive anatomy and contraction of the muscles that line up the upper airway walls. Many EMG studies were conducted in both healthy humans and OSA patients, and during both wakefulness and sleep, with the goal to elucidate activity patterns and respiratory functions of these muscles (reviewed in (6–8, 20)). Most upper airway muscles consistently act as either dilators or constrictors but some contribute to changes in stiffness of airway walls more than to the airway cross-sectional area (21).

The recognition of a key role of upper airway muscles in protecting upper airway patency in OSA was based on recordings of EMG activity of the genioglossus (GG) muscle in humans (9, 10, 22). Subsequent studies of the relative contributions of different muscles to the maintenance of upper airway patency confirmed a major role of GG but also revealed that sleep may exert different effects on different upper airway muscles and that the effectiveness of the muscles of the tongue to protect the airway against collapse depends on properly timed coactivation of other muscles (21, 23–25). Nevertheless, control of the tongue across sleep-wake states is a major target for basic and clinical research due to the ease of access to its muscles for recording, technical feasibility to monitor tongue position, and the XII cranial nucleus being relatively accessible for invasive animal studies (see (26) for a focused review).

Upper Airway EMG at Sleep Onset and during Non-REM Sleep

Although it is frequently stated that upper airway EMG declines at sleep onset, this is not a uniform finding. In the original study of Sauerland and Harper with healthy subjects, GG EMG did not change much at sleep onset or during the progression into deeper stages of non-REM sleep (22). Similar to GG, inspiratory cricothyroid activity in healthy humans does not change as non-REM sleep progresses from stages N1–N2 to N3–N4 (27). Other studies of GG in healthy humans report a decrease at sleep onset and further decrease thereafter (28, 29). In healthy persons, moderate declines occur in the palatoglossus and levator palatini, but both activities return to the pre-sleep levels with the progression of non-REM sleep or even increase above that level (30–32). This secondary increase has been attributed to combined effects of reflex activation originating from upper airway negative pressure mechanoreceptors and respiratory chemoreceptors (32, 33).

In contrast to GG and cricothyroid, arytenoideus and alea nasi EMGs drop precipitously at sleep onset and remain depressed (34, 35). It has been proposed that muscles with mostly tonic activity (with no respiratory modulation), such as tensor palatini or masseter, exhibit large declines, whereas those with a prominent inspiratory component, such as GG, show small declines or no change (36), but there are many exceptions to this pattern (34, 35, 37).

The elevated baseline upper airway muscle tone during wakefulness in OSA subjects when compared to healthy persons (38, 39) creates more favorable conditions for the assessment of the effect of sleep onset because the reference activity is clearly above the noise level. Indeed, most measurements in OSA patients conducted without continuous positive airway pressure (CPAP) reveal a decline of GG activity at sleep onset (40–42).

Effects of REM Sleep

Quantitative data for upper airway muscle activity during REM sleep in humans are limited. This is likely due to difficulties with attaining fully developed episodes of REM sleep under laboratory conditions. The onset of REM sleep is relatively uniformly associated with a reduction of GG EMG (28, 43). In one study in healthy men, both GG and alea nasi exhibited prominent declines in association with periods of REM sleep with eye movements but not during REM sleep segments without eye movements (44). In a study of arytenoideus activity in healthy adults, only two out of six subjects generated REM sleep episodes of sufficient duration to allow reliable examination; in both persons, activity was absent during non-REM sleep but reappeared during REM sleep in the form of large, non-respiratory bursts (34). Similar non-respiratory

bursting occurs in thyroarytenoid, critothyroid, pharyngeal constrictor, and GG (27, 37, 45, 46).

Recordings of upper airway EMG during REM sleep in OSA patients are even less complete than for healthy persons. In one study with eight OSA patients, the average levels of GG EMG did not differ between non-REM sleep and REM sleep (43), whereas in another study in six OSA patients, both tonic and inspiratory-modulated components of GG activity were lower in REM sleep than in non-REM sleep (47). OSA patients on CPAP had qualitatively similar non-respiratory bursts of activity during REM sleep in their pharyngeal constrictors to those generated by this muscle in healthy subjects (37, 48).

Additional Insights from Studies of Single Motor Units

Fine wire EMG recordings allow one to extract from the compound EMG activity action potentials generated by individual motor units. With this approach, one can distinguish motor units of different types, such as those with and without respiratory-modulated activity patterns, and gain insight into the extent to which state-dependent changes in multiunit activity occur as a result of firing rate changes in active motor units vs. recruitment/de-recruitment (49, 50).

About half of spontaneously active during quiet wakefulness GG motor units in healthy humans had a degree of inspiratory modulation. The remaining half were roughly evenly distributed between expiratory-modulated and entirely tonic units (50–53). Data indicate that human GG motor units operate within a relatively narrow range of peak firing rates (12–22 Hz); when there is a need for increased activity, it is achieved primarily through recruitment of previously silent units (53, 54).

At sleep onset, inspiratory-modulated GG motor units reduce their activity or fall silent, whereas expiratory-modulated and tonic units show small changes (52, 55). In multiunit recordings, the tensor palatini activity had no respiratory modulation during quiet wakefulness (28, 36). However, in a single motor unit study, around 40% of tensor palatini units were inspiratory-modulated, nearly 30% were expiratory-modulated, and only about 30% had tonic activity (56). Thus, single motor unit data provide a new basis for the interpretation of changes in activity previously documented in multiunit studies.

In a population of mild OSA subjects, sleep-related changes in the activity of GG motor units were consistent with the findings based on compound GG muscle activity (57). When single GG motor unit data were compared between healthy persons and OSA patients, the latter had slightly elevated peak inspiratory activity in inspiratory phasic units but relatively lower peak activity in inspiratory tonic units (58). Additionally, action potentials of motor units recorded from OSA patients were wider, possibly in connection with complex neuromuscular morphologic changes observed in GG in this population (59, 60). In a study comparing the activity of single GG motor units in 19 healthy subjects and 10 OSA patients during REM sleep, only 5 of the former but all of the latter yielded single-unit data (61).

Comparison to Findings in Experimental Animals

The relative elongation of the pharynx and the "floating" attachment of the hyoid bone represent the two unique features of the human upper airway seen as key for the generation of speech. The cost of this evolutionary development is the increased propensity of the human upper airway to collapse. While the English bulldog has been identified as a "natural" model of OSA (62), nearly all other animal models of sleep-related upper airway problems are "induced models" in which experimental interventions trigger a propensity for upper airway obstructions (reviewed in (7)). This includes studies in mice in which diet-induced or genetically mediated obesity impairs both sleep and ventilation (see Fraire et al. in this volume).

The activity of GG and other upper airway muscles has been recorded in multiple animal species. The focus here is limited to data from rats because they have been most extensively investigated due to their exceptional suitability for complex experiments combining electrophysiological, anatomical, and genetic levels of analysis.

Compared to quiet wakefulness, rat GG activity is significantly reduced during non-REM sleep and further reduced during REM sleep. Some studies report prominent inspiratory modulation of GG activity during wakefulness and a partial attenuation of this modulation during non-REM sleep (63–67). In one series of studies, the presence of inspiratory modulation in GG, as well as the sternohyoid and inferior pharyngeal constrictor, was associated with the animal sleeping in a curled-up posture (64, 68). In more recent studies, respiratory modulation of GG activity was rare regardless of the behavioral state and the magnitude of activity decrease on entry into non-REM sleep was such that it often resulted in abolition of all activities (69–71) (Figure 6.2).

The onset of REM sleep is associated with a profound attenuation or abolition of GG, posterior cricoarytenoid, and cricothyroid activities (if present during the preceding non-REM sleep) (63–67, 72). In all studies, GG exhibits prominent non-respiratory bursts of activity (63, 64, 67–69, 73) (Figure 6.2). When analyzed in a quantitative manner, these bursts occur with a progressively increasing frequency and amplitudes with the duration of REM sleep episodes to reach over 60% of the average level of activity measured during wakefulness at 90–120 s into the episode (69, 70, 74–76). The magnitude of this change is larger during the lights-on (rest), than during the lights-off, period of the circadian cycle (77).

REFLEX CONTROL FROM UPPER AIRWAY NEGATIVE PRESSURE MECHANORECEPTORS

Reflex activation of upper airway dilator muscles elicited by negative upper airway pressure receptors located in the peripharyngeal region provides the upper airway with the first line of defense against upper airway collapse promoted by negative intraluminal pressure. As such, these reflex effects play a fundamental protective and regulatory role for the upper airway analogous to that played by pulmonary slowly adapting stretch receptors in the regulation of the depth and rate of breathing.

The reflex pathway activated by upper airway negative pressure originates in superficial mucosal receptors. The receptor locations, mechanical properties, and central connections have been worked out in considerable detail in animal studies (78–80). Based on this information, experiments were then conducted in humans with various waveforms of negative pressure applied to the airway while reflex effects were recorded from upper airway muscles (10, 81–88).

Reflexes from Upper Airway Negative Pressure Receptors Awake and Asleep

Negative pressure swings in the upper airway, whether those occurring naturally during inspiration or those applied as a matter of experimental intervention, produce a reflex increase of GG activity; the activation is much weaker for the tensor palatini (89, 90). Spontaneous GG activity is reduced following the elimination of afferent inflow from superficial airway receptors, which shows that tonic reflexes from these receptors help maintain baseline GG activity (88, 91). Of

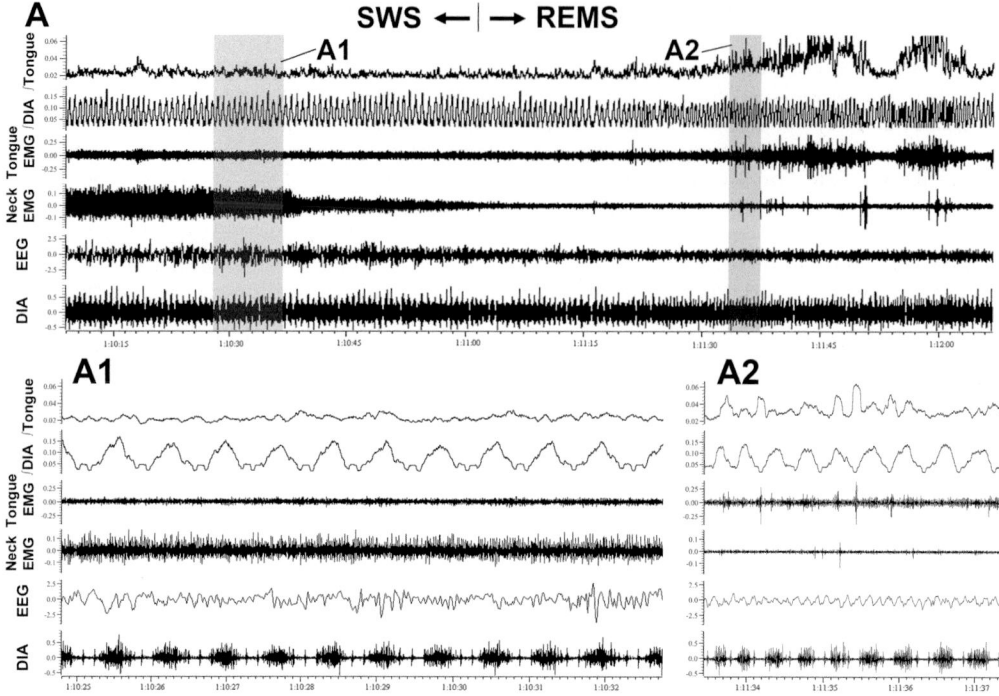

Figure 6.2 Typical activity of the GG muscles of the tongue during sleep states in rats. A: transition from slow-wave sleep (SWS) to REM sleep (REMS). The following features of GG EMG are typical: (i) no, or minimal, level of activity during SWS so that no further change is noticeable during transition into REMS; (ii) gradual appearance of intense phasic bursts of activity that start with a delay after REMS onset; (iii) absence of respiratory modulation during either sleep state. These features are illustrated in detail in the expanded parts of the record in A shown in panels A1 and A2. The signals listed from the top are: integrated tongue EMG, integrated EMG of the diaphragm (DIA), raw tongue EMG, dorsal neck muscle EMG, cortical EEG, and raw DIA EMG. In A2, note that the bursts of tongue EMG, albeit semi-rhythmic, occur independently of the respiratory rhythm in DIA, and the presence of theta rhythm in cortical EEG as a hallmark of REMS. (Data from Lu and Kubin (70).)

special relevance to OSA are those studies in which the effects of airway pressure oscillations on upper airway muscle activity were investigated as a model of the conditions akin to snoring (92–94). The key finding was that oscillatory pressure stimulus has a powerful excitatory effect on upper airway muscle tone, which suggests that the relevant receptors have a high dynamic sensitivity.

In healthy awake humans, negative swings of upper airway pressure associated with inspiration contribute to reflex enhancement of upper airway muscle tone (84, 90). In OSA patients and snorers who have larger amplitudes of respiratory swings of upper airway pressure than healthy persons, this effect is expected to be more prominent (95). However, in severe OSA patients, a blunting of the airway protecting upper airway reflexes

was reported in one (5), but not in another (96), study.

Compared to wakefulness, non-REM sleep is associated with a reduced magnitude of reflexes from negative pressure receptors (33, 90). For example, GG activation in response to resistive loads of moderate amplitude (5–15 cm H_2O) was difficult to elicit during non-REM sleep, but additional stimulation of breathing by inspiratory CO_2 unveiled a distinct excitatory component related to activation of negative airway pressure receptors (97). In addition to the reduced magnitude, the sleep-related attenuation of the response to inspiratory resistive load is reflected in the delayed occurrence of GG response (98). Of potential clinical significance are the measurements obtained during sleep suggesting that reflex activation of GG by negative airway pressure receptors is less effective in OSA patients than in healthy persons (99, but see 100, 101).

In addition to the investigation of upper airway reflexes elicited by naturally occurring or experimentally imposed steady changes in upper airway pressure, numerous studies explored short-latency responses elicited in upper airway muscles by rapid pulses of negative pressure. Advantages of this approach include the ability to: (i) obtain multiple replications within and across subjects and generate average responses; (ii) apply stimuli with a precise timing relative to the phase of the respiratory cycle; (iii) determine response latencies; and (iv) generate strength-response characteristics. Such studies, conducted both awake and asleep, were recently reviewed elsewhere (6).

NEUROCHEMISTRY OF CENTRAL STATE-DEPENDENT PATHWAYS CONVERGING ON UPPER AIRWAY MOTONEURONS

Sleep-related hypopneic and apneic events of OSA are causally associated with a decline of upper airway muscle tone. Since, in OSA patients, wake-related activity of many upper airway muscles includes a phasic inspiratory component, it appeared plausible that an important part of the sleep-dependent decline in upper airway EMG was due to a reduction of respiratory-modulated inputs to motoneurons. An alternative, or complementary, concept would be that sleep-related changes are caused by non-respiratory pathways whose one function is to mediate decrements of upper airway muscle tone during sleep. Data accumulated during the last two decades strongly support the latter concept. There is currently a considerable list of candidate transmitters and modulators that can uniquely contribute to sleep-related decrements of upper airway muscle tone either by means of a sleep-dependent withdrawal of excitation or sleep-specific active inhibition. These modulators are released from highly divergent neuronal networks and affect activity at multiple levels, including respiratory motoneurons, respiratory premotor pathways, and the central respiratory rhythm generator. Among these distinct sites of action, information about state-dependent modulation at the motoneuronal level is most comprehensive.

Wakefulness Stimulus for Breathing and Its Substrates

Recordings from central respiratory neurons across sleep-wake states revealed that those that drive respiratory pump muscles show small sleep-related changes that closely follow the magnitude and pattern of the effects of non-REM and REM sleep on inspiratory activity of the diaphragm (102–104). Recordings also revealed the presence in the medulla, pons, and midbrain of the weakly respiratory-modulated cell whose activity strongly declined during sleep (105–107). Such mildly respiratory-modulated reticular formation cells were considered as a possible substrate for the concept of the "wakefulness stimulus for breathing" (108). The essence of this concept was that distinct neurons with predictable changes of activity in association with sleep are functionally connected with upper airway motoneurons. Initially, such neurons were hypothesized to be an important source of inspiratory drive to upper airway muscles, as this could explain the sleep-related loss of respiratory modulation of upper airway muscle activity. Ultimately the evidence for such neurons being responsible for sleep-related upper airway hypotonia proved to be weak due to the absence of evidence that such cells have appropriate efferent connections. Still, the concept proved important for the search for other sources of state-dependent regulation of upper airway muscle tone.

Currently, four neurochemically distinct cell groups have properties that fit the definition of the wakefulness stimulus for breathing. They are the norepinephrine (NE)-containing (noradrenergic) neurons located mainly in the pons (66, 109–111), serotonin (5-hydroxytryptamine—5HT)-containing neurons located in the medulla (112–114), posterior hypothalamic neurons that synthesize the excitatory peptides orexins (ORX, a.k.a. hypocretins) (115–117), and histamine (HI)-containing neurons also located in the posterior hypothalamus (118, 119).

Animal studies provide extensive evidence that NE and 5-HT release onto motoneurons contributes to the maintenance of upper airway muscle tone during wakefulness. The activity of NE and 5-HT cells declines on transition from wakefulness to non-REM sleep and ceases during REM sleep. The α_1-adrenergic and 5-HT_2 receptors are the main mediators of NE and 5-HT excitatory effects in motoneurons (120–123). Importantly, the depression of XII nerve activity elicited as a pharmacological analog of REM sleep is functionally equivalent to the decline of XII nerve activity produced by a combined antagonism of the excitations mediated within the XII nucleus by just two transmitters, NE and 5-HT (109) (Figure 6.3). The magnitudes of endogenous activations of XII motoneurons by NE and 5-HT at the

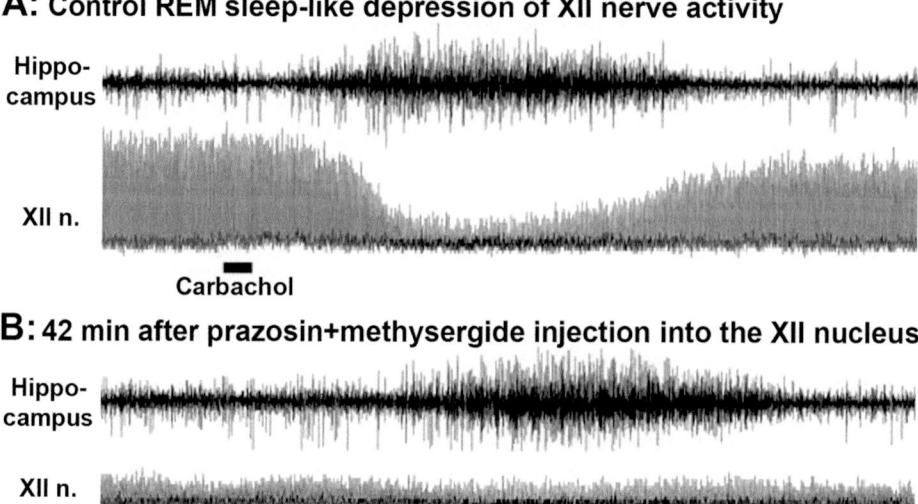

A: Control REM sleep-like depression of XII nerve activity

Hippo-campus

XII n.

Carbachol

B: 42 min after prazosin+methysergide injection into the XII nucleus

Hippo-campus

XII n.

Carbachol

1 min

Figure 6.3 Withdrawal of excitation mediated by NE and 5-HT by combined microinjections of the excitatory α_1-adrenergic receptor antagonist, prazosin, and a broad-spectrum 5-HT receptor antagonist, methysergide, into the XII nucleus reduces spontaneous XII nerve (XII n.) activity to the same level as the depression attained during the REM sleep-like state. The equivalence demonstrates that, at least in this pharmacological model, the depression of upper airway muscle tone is caused by a withdrawal from motoneurons of the endogenous excitatory effects mediated by only two transmitters, NE and 5-HT. In both panels, the top trace shows raw hippocampal signal (Hippocampus) and the bottom trace the moving average of XII n. activity. Each peak in the XII n. signal represents one inspiratory burst. REM sleep-like state-triggering carbachol injections were made at the markers. A: control (pre-prazosin/pre-methysergide) REM sleep-like episode with the characteristic hippocampal activation and a coincident XII n. depression. B: another REM sleep-like episode elicited 42 min after microinjection of prazosin and methysergide into the XII nucleus; the pre-carbachol XII n. activity is now reduced to a level similar to that observed at the time of maximal depression during the control REM sleep-like episode (in A) and no further depression occurs while hippocampal activation provides evidence that the REM sleep-like episode occurred at the systemic level. (Data from Fenik *et al.* (109) obtained from an anesthetized rat model of REM sleep in which microinjections of a cholinergic agonist, carbachol, into the dorsomedial pons can repeatedly elicit 3–5 min-long episodes of REM sleep-like state characterized by hippocampal activation and suppression of XII n. activity.)

motor nucleus level vary among species. In cats, endogenous excitatory effects of 5-HT are stronger than those of NE (113, 119, 124). In rats, NE contribution to spontaneous activity of XII motoneurons is more prominent than that of 5-HT (65, 66, 109, 125).

ORX-containing terminals and ORX type 2 receptors are present in the XII nucleus (115, 126, 127). ORX facilitates respiratory activation under conditions of stress or chemical stimulation of breathing with little evidence for the presence of an endogenous ORX-dependent drive to XII motoneurons under the baseline conditions (128). As with ORX, while there is evidence for excitatory effects of HI on XII motoneurons (119, 129), HI does not exert

endogenous excitatory effects within the rat XII motor nucleus (118).

Additional potential wake-related activators of upper airway motoneurons include at least two peptides, substance P and thyrotropin-releasing hormone (TRH). Both these peptides activate XII motoneurons when administered into the XII nucleus (130–132) and both are frequently co-localized within 5-HT-containing terminals (133–135). At this time, it is not clear under what conditions spontaneous activity of upper airway motoneurons depends on endogenous effects mediated by substance P or TRH. Figure 6.4 shows a scheme of all established and tentative sources of wake-related excitation that converge on upper airway motoneurons.

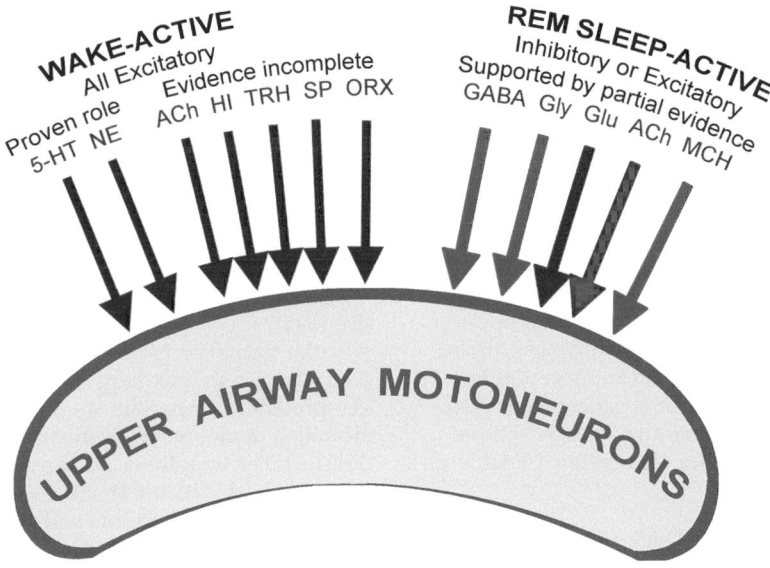

Figure 6.4 Established and putative neurotransmitters released onto upper airway motoneurons from neurochemically distinct central neurons with state-dependent activity patterns. Of the many wake-active premotor inputs, only serotonin (5-HT) and norepinephrine (NE) have proven endogenous excitatory effects; acetylcholine (ACh), histamine (HI), thyrotropin-releasing hormone (TRH), substance P (SP), and orexins (ORX) meet some, but not all, criteria for being involved in providing endogenous wake-related drive to upper airway motoneurons. Appropriate receptors and/or afferent pathways for these candidates exist but it is not clear under what conditions they exert their effects. The REM sleep-active premotor pathways may release both inhibitory (gamma aminobutyric acid (GABA), glycine (Gly), melanin-concentrating hormone (MCH), and ACh acting through muscarinic receptors), as well as excitatory (glutamate (Glu), or ACh acting on nicotinic receptors), transmitters but evidence is incomplete because definite premotor cells with required axonal projections to upper airway motoneurons, appropriate transmitters, or appropriate state-dependence activity have not been ascertained. There are no known sources of active, non-REM sleep-related effects exerted directly onto upper airway motoneurons.

Suppression of motoneuronal excitability caused by a reduced release (withdrawal) of 5-HT, NE, ORX, TRH, and substance P occurs through the opening of potassium ion (K^+) channels (136, 137). The considerable molecular diversity of these channels makes them potentially attractive targets for pharmacological interventions that aim to increase upper airway muscle tone during sleep. Recently, Grace *et al.* (67) investigated the effects of microdialysis perfusion of the XII nucleus region with various K^+ channel blockers in chronically instrumented, behaving rats. Their main observations were that: (a) perfusion with a solution containing barium ions (blockers of inwardly rectifying K^+ channels) elevated tongue EMG in all sleep-wake states, with the effect being most prominent during wakefulness and REM sleep with muscle twitches; (b) perfusion with methanandamide (antagonist of the tandem pore domain (TASK) channels) produced activation limited to wakefulness; and (c) perfusion with either 4-aminopyridine or tetraethylammonium (blockers of different voltage-dependent K^+ channels) increased GG activity across all sleep-wake states but most prominently during REM sleep with twitches. Collectively, closure of certain K^+ channels elevated tongue EMG during sleep to the levels comparable to those during wakefulness. In normal rats, the effects mediated by TASK channels appear detectable during wakefulness only (138), but following exposure to chronic intermittent hypoxia (CIH), at least TASK-1 channels are upregulated in the XII nucleus (139).

A few additional recent studies explored the impact of CIH on the control of upper airway muscles. Exposure to CIH for 35 days increased the density of NE and 5-HT axon terminals in the XII nucleus (139–142), as well as the immunostaining of XII motoneurons for the excitatory α_1-adrenoceptors (140). Consistent with these anatomical findings, rats subjected to CIH had larger decrements of XII nerve activity in response to microinjections into the XII nucleus of the α_1-adrenoceptor antagonist, prazosin, than sham-treated animals (143). Collectively, these findings show that CIH increases endogenous excitatory effects of NE and 5-HT in XII motoneurons. Extrapolation of this data to OSA suggests that CIH may be one of the causes of the elevated upper airway muscle tone seen during wakefulness in OSA patients (38, 39). In support of this, experimental CIH in OSA patients may have increased their upper airway muscle tone because it reduced the therapeutic CPAP level (144, 145).

Active Sleep-Dependent Effects

At least seven distinct groups of sleep-active neurons have been identified but, in contrast to those active in wakefulness, it is uncertain whether any of the sleep-active ones make direct connections with upper airway motoneurons (Figure 6.4). Two of the sleep-active groups increase their activity during non-REM sleep only and use gamma-aminobutyric acid (GABA) as their main transmitter. The larger of these two groups is located in the anterior hypothalamus and the smaller one in the parafacial region of the rostral medulla (146–148; reviewed in 149).

The remaining five groups of sleep-active neurons are all associated with REM sleep. Among those, a subset of acetylcholine (ACh)-containing neurons of the pedunculopontine and lateral tegmental regions of the pons have activity that distinctly increases during REM sleep only. They are intermixed among other ACh neurons that are activated during both wakefulness and REM sleep (150, 151). Additional ACh cells with activity related to REM sleep are scattered in the medullary reticular formation (152). Some of the pontomedullary ACh cells have efferent projections to the orofacial motor nuclei (153–155) but it remains to be determined whether ACh cells with connections to motoneurons are REM sleep-active.

The second REM sleep-related group comprises the cells located in the posterior lateral hypothalamus that synthesize melanin-concentrating hormone (MCH) (156). MCH cells have extensive axonal projections that extend to the pontomedullary reticular formation but their specific targets need studies (157). Although MCH is their unique neurochemical marker, they also use GABA as

their transmitter (158). Thus, their enhanced activity during REM sleep would inhibit their postsynaptic targets. Another GABAergic group of REM sleep-active cells is located in a small subregion of the anterior hypothalamus called the extended ventrolateral preoptic nucleus (eVLPO). These cells facilitate the generation of REM sleep through their extensive ascending and descending projections (159).

A potentially important collection of REM sleep-active cells is located in the ventromedial reticular formation of the rostral medulla (160). These cells have long been hypothesized to represent an important source of active inhibition of motoneurons during REM sleep (161, 162). The hypothesis has been supported by anatomical evidence that the same medial medullary region contains cells that use the inhibitory amino acid glycine (possibly co-localized with GABA) (163–165), and that glycine mediates a portion of inhibitory effects of REM sleep on spinal motoneurons (166). However, to date, there has been no demonstration that the same glycinergic cell located in the ventromedial medulla is REM sleep-active and sends axonal projections to an orofacial motor nucleus, which would be required as evidence that suppression of activity in upper airway motoneurons during REM sleep has a component caused by active glycinergic inhibition that originates in the ventromedial medullary reticular formation. Against this hypothesis, several studies have demonstrated that antagonism of glycinergic or GABA-ergic inhibition does not cause any major attenuation of REM sleep-related decrements of activity in either XII or trigeminal motoneurons (63, 109, 167–169).

The adrenergic neurons located in the rostral ventrolateral medulla (C1 group) are important for the regulation of sympathetic tone, especially under the hypoxic and hypercapnic conditions and under stress (170–172). To date, little is known about any contribution of these cells to the regulation of cardiorespiratory changes with sleep-wake states, but recent data indicate that at least the caudal cohort of C1 cells is activated during pharmacologically induced REM sleep-like state (173), and activation of these cells is associated with the termination of non-REM sleep (174).

Recent experiments in rats implicate ACh cells with axonal projections to the XII nucleus in active suppression of activity in XII motoneurons during REM sleep. Specifically, microperfusion of the XII nucleus region with Tertiapin-Q, a blocker of certain K^+ channels, increased tongue EMG in a similar pattern to that obtained with perfusion of the XII nucleus with the muscarinic (M) cholinergic receptor antagonist, scopolamine (175). Scopolamine is a broad-spectrum M receptor antagonist; based on the distribution of different M receptors in the brainstem, it was proposed that scopolamine enhanced tongue EMG due to its antagonistic action on M_2 receptors (175, 176).

CIRCADIAN EFFECTS

Among the many adverse consequences of OSA is its disruptive effect on sleep continuity. OSA patients do not obtain sufficient amounts of sleep during the night and then tend to compensate by naps and sleep bouts during the day. This misalignment between the time of sleep and the rest phase of the circadian cycle may affect OSA pattern and severity. To date, circadian effects on ventilation and upper airway muscle tone received little attention (177, 178).

Relevant for the focus of this review, at least in rats, important components of the molecular circadian clock reside within motor nuclei for XII and phrenic motoneurons. At the transcriptional level, mRNAs for such key circadian proteins as Bmal1, Clock, and Per are expressed in XII and phrenic motoneurons and oscillate with the 24 hr cycle (77, 179). Furthermore, mRNA levels for the excitatory $5\text{-}HT_2$ receptors are higher in the XII and phrenic motor nuclei during the active period than during the rest period of circadian cycle (127, 179), and $5\text{-}HT_{2A}$ receptor-like protein in the XII nucleus follows the same pattern (127). These changes are functional because antagonism of $5\text{-}HT_2$ receptors in the XII nucleus causes a more profound decline of tongue EMG during nighttime wakefulness than during the day (114). Indeed, tongue EMG level measured during wakefulness is more intense during the active phase than during the rest phase of circadian cycle (77). While such circadian rhythmicity may be more robust in rodents than in humans, there is also a "time of the day" effect on respiratory chemosensitivity, the frequency and duration of "respiratory events", and propensity for upper airway obstructions in OSA patients (180, 181). These observations indicate that the activity of upper airway muscles is regulated in a manner that aligns muscle effort with the rest-activity cycle.

CONCLUDING REMARK

The focus of this review has been on the effects of sleep-wake states on the activity of upper airway muscles. EMG activity is quantifiable and its examination offers an invaluable insight into the mechanisms of the neural control of the upper airway in humans. Indeed, there is probably no substitute for monitoring of upper airway EMG in mechanistic studies and those exploring therapeutic interventions.

ACKNOWLEDGMENTS

The author's research discussed in this review was supported by the following grants from the Heart, Lung and Blood Institute of the National Institutes of Health: HL-047600, HL-071097, HL-060287, HL-074385, HL-092962, HL-116506.

REFERENCES

1. Orem J, Kubin L. Respiratory physiology: central neural control. In: Kryger MH, Roth T, Dement WC, eds. *Principles and Practice of Sleep Medicine, 4th ed.* Philadelphia: Elsevier-Saunders; 2005. pp. 213–223.

2. Dempsey JA, Veasey SC, Morgan BJ, O'Donnell CP. Pathophysiology of sleep apnea. *Physiol Rev* 2010;**90**:47–112.

3. Javaheri S, Dempsey JA. Central sleep apnea. *Compr Physiol* 2013;**3**:141–163. [https://doi.org/10.1002/cphy.c110057]

4. Deacon-Diaz N, Malhotra A. Inherent vs. induced loop gain abnormalities in obstructive sleep apnea. *Front Neurol* 2018;**9**:896. [https://doi.org/10.3389/fneur.2018.00896]

5. Patil SP, Schneider H, Marx JJ, Gladmon E, Schwartz AR, Smith PL. Neuromechanical control of upper airway patency during sleep. *J Appl Physiol* 2007;**102**:547–556.

6. Horner RL. Neural control of the upper airway: integrative physiological mechanisms and relevance for sleep disordered breathing. *Compr Physiol* 2012;**2**:479–535. [https://doi.org/10.1002/cphy.c110023]

7. Kubin L. Neural control of the upper airway: respiratory and state-dependent mechanisms. *Compr Physiol* 2016;**6**:1801–1850. [https://doi.org/10.1002/cphy.c160002]

8. Horner RL, Hughes SW, Malhotra A. State-dependent and reflex drives to the upper airway: basic physiology with clinical implications. *J Appl Physiol* 2014;**116**:325–336.

9. Remmers JE, DeGroot WJ, Sauerland EK, Anch AM. Pathogenesis of upper airway occlusion during sleep. *J Appl Physiol* 1978;**44**:931–938.

10. Brouillette RT, Thach BT. A neuromuscular mechanism maintaining extrathoracic airway patency. *J Appl Physiol* 1979;**46**:772–779.

11. Cistulli PA, Sullivan CE. Pathophysiology of sleep apnea. In: Saunders NA, Sullivan CE, eds. *Sleep and Breathing, 2nd ed.* New York: Marcel Dekker; 1994. pp. 405–448.

12. Kuna S, Remmers JE. Anatomy and physiology of upper airway obstruction. In: Kryger MH, Roth T,

Dement WC, eds. *Principles and Practice of Sleep Medicine, 3rd ed.* Philadelphia: Saunders; 2000. pp. 840–858.

13. Isono S, Remmers JE. Anatomy and physiology of upper airway obstruction. In: Kryger MH, Roth T, Dement WC, eds. *Principles and Practice of Sleep Medicine.* Philadelphia: Saunders; 1994. pp. 642–656.

14. Gleadhill IC, Schwartz AR, Schubert N, Wise RA, Permutt S, Smith PL. Upper airway collapsibility in snorers and in patients with obstructive hypopnea and apnea. *Am Rev Respir Dis* 1991;**143**:1300–1303.

15. Issa FG, Sullivan CE. Upper airway closing pressures in obstructive sleep apnea. *J Appl Physiol* 1984;**57**:520–527.

16. Issa FG, Sullivan CE. Upper airway closing pressure in snorers. *J Appl Physiol* 1984;**57**:528–535.

17. Schwartz AR, Smith PL, Gold AR, Wise RA, Permutt S. Induction of upper airway occlusion in sleeping individuals with subatmospheric nasal pressure. *J Appl Physiol* 1988;**64**:535–542.

18. Morrison DL, Launois SH, Isono S, Feroah TR, Whitelaw WA, Remmers JE. Pharyngeal narrowing and closing pressures in patients with obstructive sleep apnea. *Am Rev Respir Dis* 1993;**148**:606–611.

19. Suratt PM, Wilhoit SC, Cooper K. Induction of airway collapse with subatmospheric pressure in awake patients with sleep apnea. *J Appl Physiol* 1984;**57**:140–146.

20. Pilarski JQ, Leiter JC, Fregosi RF. Muscles of breathing: development, function, and patterns of activation. *Compr Physiol* 2019;**9**:1025–1080. [https://doi.org/10.1002/cphy.c180008]

21. Kuna ST. Respiratory-related activation and mechanical effects of the pharyngeal constrictor muscles. *Respir Physiol* 2000;**119**:155–161.

22. Sauerland EK, Harper RM. The human tongue during sleep: electromyographic activity of the genioglossus muscle. *Exp Neurol* 1976;**51**:160–170.

23. Bilston LE, Gandevia SC. Biomechanical properties of the human upper airway and their effect on its behavior during breathing and in obstructive sleep apnea. *J Appl Physiol* 2014;**116**:314–324.

24. Dotan Y, Pillar G, Schwartz AR, Oliven A. Asynchrony of lingual muscle recruitment during sleep in obstructive sleep apnea. *J Appl Physiol* 2015;**118**:1516–1524.

25. Oliven R, Cohen G, Dotan Y, Somri M, Schwartz AR, Oliven A. Alteration in upper airway dilator muscle coactivation during sleep: comparison of patients with obstructive sleep apnea and healthy subjects. *J Appl Physiol* 2018;**124**:421–429.

26. Cori JM, O'Donoghue FJ, Jordan AS. Sleeping tongue: current perspectives of genioglossus control in healthy individuals and patients with obstructive sleep apnea. *Nat Sci Sleep* 2018;**10**:169–179.

27. Kuna ST, Smickley JS, Vanoye CR, McMillan TH. Cricothyroid muscle activity during sleep in normal adult humans. *J Appl Physiol* 1994;**76**:2326–2332.

28. Carberry JC, Jordan AS, White DP, Wellman A, Eckert DJ. Upper airway collapsibility (Pcrit) and pharyngeal dilator muscle activity are sleep stage dependent. *Sleep* 2016;**39**:511–521.

29. Worsnop C, Kay A, Pierce R, Kim Y, Trinder J. Activity of respiratory pump and upper airway muscles during sleep onset. *J Appl Physiol* 1998;**85**:908–920.

30. Tangel DJ, Mezzanotte WS, White DP. Influences of NREM sleep on activity of palatoglossus and levator palatini muscles in normal men. *J Appl Physiol* 1995;**78**:689–695.

31. Basner RC, Ringler J, Schwartzstein RM, Weinberger SE, Weiss JW. Phasic electromyographic activity of the genioglossus increases in normals during slow-wave sleep. *Respir Physiol* 1991;**83**:189–200.

32. Hicks A, Cori JM, Jordan AS, Nicholas CL, Kubin L, Semmler JG, Malhotra A, McSharry DGP, Trinder JA. Mechanisms of the deep, slow-wave, sleep-related increase of upper airway muscle tone in healthy humans. *J Appl Physiol* 2017;**122**:1304–1312.

33. Fogel RB, Trinder J, Malhotra A, Stanchina M, Edwards JK, Schory KE, White DP. Within-breath control of genioglossal muscle activation in humans: effect of sleep-wake state. *J Physiol* 2003;**550**:3–910.

34. Kuna ST, Insalaco G, Villeponteaux RD. Arytenoideus muscle activity in normal adult humans during wakefulness and sleep. *J Appl Physiol* 1991;**70**:1655–1664.

35. Wheatley JR, Tangel DJ, Mezzanotte WS, White DP. Influence of sleep on alae nasi EMG and nasal resistance in normal men. *J Appl Physiol* 1993;**75**:626–632.

36. Tangel DJ, Mezzanotte WS, Sandberg EJ, White DP. Influences of NREM sleep on the activity of tonic vs. inspiratory phasic muscles in normal men. *J Appl Physiol* 1992;**73**:1058–1066.

37. Kuna ST, Smickley JS, Vanoye CR. Respiratory-related pharyngeal constrictor muscle activity in normal human adults. *Am J Respir Crit Care Med* 1997;**155**:1991–1999.

38. Suratt PM, McTier RF, Wilhoit SC. Upper airway muscle activation is augmented in patients with obstructive sleep apnea compared with that in normal subjects. *Am Rev Respir Dis* 1988;**137**:889–894.

39. Mezzanotte WS, Tangel DJ, White DP. Waking genioglossal electromyogram in sleep apnea patients versus normal controls (a neuromuscular compensatory mechanism). *J Clin Invest* 1992;**89**:1571–1579.

40. Fogel RB, Trinder J, White DP, Malhotra A, Raneri J, Schory K, Kleverlaan D, Pierce RJ. The effect of

sleep onset on upper airway muscle activity in patients with sleep apnoea versus controls. *J Physiol* 2005;**564**:2–62.

41. Okabe S, Hida W, Kikuchi Y, Taguchi O, Takishima T, Shirato K. Upper airway muscle activity during REM and non-REM sleep of patients with obstructive apnea. *Chest* 1994;**106**:767–773.

42. Katz ES, White DP. Genioglossus activity in children with obstructive sleep apnea during wakefulness and sleep onset. *Am J Respir Crit Care Med* 2003;**168**:664–670.

43. Eckert DJ, Malhotra A, Lo YL, White DP, Jordan AS. The influence of obstructive sleep apnea and gender on genioglossus activity during rapid eye movement sleep. *Chest* 2009;**135**:957–964.

44. Wiegand L, Zwillich CW, Wiegand D, White DP. Changes in upper airway muscle activation and ventilation during phasic REM sleep in normal men. *J Appl Physiol* 1991;**71**:488–497.

45. Kuna ST, Insalaco G, Woodson GE. Thyroarytenoid muscle activity during wakefulness and sleep in normal adults. *J Appl Physiol* 1988;**65**:1332–1339.

46. Chokroverty S. Phasic tongue movements in human rapid-eye-movement sleep. *Neurology* 1980;**30**:665–668.

48. Kuna ST, Smickley JS. Superior pharyngeal constrictor activation in obstructive sleep apnea. *Am J Respir Crit Care Med* 1997;**156**:874–880.

47. Schwartz AR, O'Donnell CP, Baron J, Schubert N, Alam D, Samadi SD, Smith PL. The hypotonic upper airway in obstructive sleep apnea: role of structures and neuromuscular activity. *Am J Respir Crit Care Med* 1998;**157**:1051–1057.

49. Trinder J, Woods M, Nicholas CL, Chan JK, Jordan AS, Semmler JG. Trinder J, Woods M, Nicholas CL, Chan JK, Jordan AS, Semmler JG. Motor unit activity in upper airway muscles genioglossus and tensor palatini. *Respir Physiol Neurobiol* 2013;**188**:362–369.

50. Trinder J, Jordan AS, Nicholas CL. Discharge properties of upper airway motor units during wakefulness and sleep. *Progr Brain Res* 2014;**212**:59–75.

51. Saboisky JP, Butler JE, Fogel RB, Taylor JL, Trinder JA, White DP, Gandevia SC. Tonic and phasic respiratory drives to human genioglossus motoneurons during breathing. *J Neurophysiol* 2006;**95**:2213–2221.

52. Bailey EF, Fridel KW, Rice AD. Sleep/wake firing patterns of human genioglossus motor units. *J Neurophysiol* 2007;**98**:3284–3291.

53. Nicholas CL, Bei B, Worsnop C, Malhotra A, Jordan AS, Saboisky JP, Chan JK, Duckworth E, White DP, Trinder J. Motor unit recruitment in human genioglossus muscle in response to hypercapnia. *Sleep* 2010;**33**:1529–1538.

54. Saboisky JP, Jordan AS, Eckert DJ, White DP, Trinder JA, Nicholas CL, Gautam S, Malhotra A. Recruitment and rate-coding strategies of the human genioglossus muscle. *J Appl Physiol* 2010;**109**:1939–1949.

55. Wilkinson V, Malhotra A, Nicholas CL, Worsnop C, Jordan AS, Butler JE, Saboisky JP, Gandevia SC, White DP, Trinder J. Discharge patterns of human genioglossus motor units during sleep onset. *Sleep* 2008;**31**:525–533.

56. Nicholas CL, Jordan AS, Heckel L, Worsnop C, Bei B, Saboisky JP, Eckert DJ, White DP, Malhotra A, Trinder J. Discharge patterns of human tensor palatini motor units during sleep onset. *Sleep* 2012;**35**:699–707.

57. McSharry DG, Saboisky JP, DeYoung P, Matteis P, Jordan AS, Trinder J, Smales E, Hess L, Guo M, Malhotra A. A mechanism for upper airway stability during slow wave sleep. *Sleep* 2013;**36**:555–563.

58. Saboisky JP, Butler JE, McKenzie DK, Gorman RB, Trinder JA, White DP, Gandevia SC. Neural drive to human genioglossus in obstructive sleep apnoea. *J Physiol* 2007;**585**:1–46.

59. Series F, Simoneau J-A, St. Pierre S, Marc I. Characteristics of the genioglossus and musculus uvulae in sleep apnea hypopnea syndrome and in snorers. *Am J Respir Crit Care Med* 1996;**153**:1870–1874.

60. Svanborg E. Impact of obstructive apnea syndrome on upper airway respiratory muscles. *Respir Physiol Neurobiol* 2005;**147**:263–272.

61. McSharry DG, Saboisky JP, Deyoung P, Jordan AS, Trinder J, Smales E, Hess L, Chamberlin NL, Malhotra A. Physiological mechanisms of upper airway hypotonia during REM sleep. *Sleep* 2014;**37**:561–569.

62. Hendricks JC, Kline LR, Kovalski RJ, O'Brien JA, Morrison AR, Pack AI. The English bulldog: a natural model of sleep-disordered breathing. *J Appl Physiol* 1987;**63**:1344–1350.

63. Morrison JL, Sood S, Liu H, Park E, Liu X, Nolan P, Horner RL. Role of inhibitory amino acids in control of hypoglossal motor outflow to genioglossus muscle in naturally sleeping rats. *J Physiol* 2003;**552**:975–991.

64. Megirian D, Hinrichsen CFL, Sherrey JH. Respiratory roles of genioglossus, sternothyroid, and sternohyoid muscles during sleep. *Exp Neurol* 1985;**90**:118–128.

65. Sood S, Morrison JL, Liu H, Horner RL. Role of endogenous serotonin in modulating genioglossus muscle activity in awake and sleeping rats. *Am J Respir Crit Care Med* 2005;**172**:1338–1347.

66. Chan E, Steenland HW, Liu H, Horner RL. Endogenous excitatory drive modulating respiratory muscle activity across sleep-wake states. *Am J Respir Crit Care Med* 2006;**174**:1264–1273.

67. Grace KP, Hughes SW, Horner RL. Identification of a pharmacological target for genioglossus reactivation throughout sleep. *Sleep* 2014;**37**:41–50.

68. Sherrey JH, Pollard MJ, Megirian D. Respiratory functions of the inferior pharyngeal constrictor

and sternohyoid muscles during sleep. *Exp Neurol* 1986;**92**:267–277.

69. Lu JW, Mann GL, Ross RJ, Morrison AR, Kubin L. Differential effect of sleep-wake states on lingual and dorsal neck muscle activity in rats. *Respir Physiol Neurobiol* 2005;**147**:191–203.

70. Lu JW, Kubin L. Electromyographic activity at the base and tip of the tongue across sleep-wake states in rats. *Respir Physiol Neurobiol* 2009;**167**:307–315.

71. Stettner GM, Rukhadze I, Mann GL, Lei Y, Kubin L. Respiratory modulation of lingual muscle activity across sleep-wake states in rats. *Respir Physiol Neurobiol* 2013;**188**:308–317.

72. Sherrey JH, Megirian D. Respiratory EMG activity of the posterior cricoarytenoid, cricothyroid and diaphragm muscles during sleep. *Respir Physiol* 1980;**39**:355–365.

73. Megirian D, Cespuglio R, Jouvet M. Rhythmical activity of the rat's tongue in sleep and wakefulness. *EEG Clin Neurophysiol* 1978;**44**:8–13.

74. Fraigne JJ, Orem JM. Phasic motor activity of respiratory and non-respiratory muscles in REM sleep. *Sleep* 2011;**34**:425–434.

75. Rukhadze I, Kalter J, Stettner GM, Kubin L. Lingual muscle activity across sleep-wake States in rats with surgically altered upper airway. *Front Neurol* 2014;**5**:61. [https://doi.org/10.3389/fneur.2014.00061]

76. Rukhadze I, Kamani H, Kubin L. Quantitative differences among EMG activities of muscles innervated by subpopulations of hypoglossal and upper spinal motoneurons during non-REM sleep—REM sleep transitions: a window on neural processes in the sleeping brain. *Arch Ital Biol* 2011;**149**:499–515.

77. Herr KB, Mann GL, Kubin L. Modulation of motoneuronal activity with sleep-wake states and motoneuronal gene expression vary with circadian rest-activity cycle. *Front Integr Neurosci* 2018;**12**:32. [http://dx.doi.org/10.3389/fnint.2018.00032]

78. Sant'Ambrogio G, Mathew OP, Fisher JT, Sant'Ambrogio FB. Laryngeal receptors responding to transmural pressure, airflow and local muscle activity. *Respir Physiol* 1983;**54**:317–330.

79. Mathew OP, Sant'Ambrogio G, Fisher JT, Sant'Ambrogio FB. Laryngeal pressure receptors. *Respir Physiol* 1984;**57**:113–122.

80. van Lunteren E, Van de Graaff WB, Parker DM, Mitra J, Haxhiu MA, Strohl KP, Cherniack NS. Nasal and laryngeal reflex responses to negative upper airway pressure. *J Appl Physiol* 1984;**56**:746–752.

81. Kuna ST, Smickley J. Response of genioglosus muscle activity to nasal airway occlusion in normal sleeping adults. *J Appl Physiol* 1988;**64**:347–353.

82. Henke KG. Upper airway muscle activity and upper airway resistance in young adults during sleep. *J Appl Physiol* 1998;**84**:486–491.

83. Tantucci C, Mehiri S, Duguet A, Similowski T, Arnulf I, Zelter M, Derenne J-P, Milic-Emili J. Application of negative expiratory pressure during expiration and activity of genioglossus in humans. *J Appl Physiol* 1998;**84**:1076–1082.

84. Malhotra A, Pillar G, Fogel RB, Edwards JK, Ayas N, Akahoshi T, Hess D, White DP. Pharyngeal pressure and flow effects on genioglossus activation in normal subjects. *Am J Respir Crit Care Med* 2002;**165**:71–77.

85. Berry RB, White DP, Roper J, Pillar G, Fogel RB, Stanchina M, Malhotra A. Awake negative pressure reflex response of the genioglossus in OSA patients and normal subjects. *J Appl Physiol* 2003;**94**:1875–1882.

86. Horner RL, Innes JA, Holden HB, Guz A. Afferent pathway(s) for pharyngeal dilator reflex to negative pressure in man: a study using upper airway anaesthesia. *J Physiol* 1991;**436**:31–44.

87. White DP, Edwards JK, Shea SA. Local reflex mechanisms: influence on basal genioglossal muscle activation in normal subjects. *Sleep* 1998;**21**:719–728.

88. Carberry JC, Hensen H, Fisher LP, Saboisky JP, Butler JE, Gandevia SC, Eckert DJ. Mechanisms contributing to the response of upper-airway muscles to changes in airway pressure. *J Appl Physiol* 2015;**118**:1221–1228.

89. Philip-Joet F, Marc I, Series F. Effects of genioglossal response to negative airway pressure on upper airway collapsibility during sleep. *J Appl Physiol* 1996;**80**:1466–1474.

90. Malhotra A, Pillar G, Fogel RB, Beauregard J, Edwards JK, Slamowitz DI, Shea SA, White DP. Genioglossal but not palatal muscle activity relates closely to pharyngeal pressure. *Am J Respir Crit Care Med* 2000;**162**:1058–1062.

91. Fogel RB, Malhotra A, Shea SA, Edwards JK, White DP. Reduced genioglossal activity with upper airway anesthesia in awake patients with OSA. *J Appl Physiol* 2000;**88**:1346–1354.

92. Henke KG, Sullivan CE. Effects of high-frequency oscillating pressures on upper airway muscles in humans. *J Appl Physiol* 1993;**75**:856–862.

93. Plowman L, Lauff DC, Berthon-Jones M, Sullivan CE. Waking and genioglossal muscle responses to upper airway pressure oscillation in sleeping dogs. *J Appl Physiol* 1990;**68**:2564–2573.

94. Brancatisano A, Van der Touw T, O'Neill N, Amis TC. Influence of upper airway pressure oscillations on soft palate muscle electromyographic activity. *J Appl Physiol* 1996;**81**:1190–1196.

95. Malhotra A, Fogel RB, Edwards JK, Shea SA, White DP. Local mechanisms drive genioglossus activation in obstructive sleep apnea. *Am J Respir Crit Care Med* 2000;**161**:1746–1749.

96. Ruehland WR, Rochford PD, Pierce RJ, Trinder J, Jordan AS, Cori JM, O'Donoghue FJ. Genioglossus muscle responses to resistive loads in severe OSA patients and healthy control subjects. *J Appl Physiol* 2019;**127**:1586–1598.

97. Stanchina ML, Malhotra A, Fogel RB, Ayas N, Edwards JK, Schory K, White DP. Genioglossus muscle responsiveness to chemical and mechanical stimuli during non-rapid eye movement sleep. *Am J Respir Crit Care Med* 2002;**165**:945–949.

98. Henke KG, Badr MS, Skatrud JB, Dempsey JA. Load compensation and respiratory muscle function during sleep. *J Appl Physiol* 1992;**72**:1221–1234.

99. McGinley BM, Schwartz AR, Schneider H, Kirkness JP, Smith PL, Patil SP. Upper airway neuromuscular compensation during sleep is defective in obstructive sleep apnea. *J Appl Physiol* 2008;**105**:197–205.

100. Fogel RB, Malhotra A, Pillar G, Edwards JK, Beauregard J, Shea SA, White DP. Genioglossal activation in patients with obstructive sleep apnea versus control subjects. Mechanisms of muscle control. *Am J Respir Crit Care Med* 2001;**164**:2025–2030.

101. Hlavac MC, Catcheside PG, Adams A, Eckert DJ, McEvoy RD. The effects of hypoxia on load compensation during sustained incremental resistive loading in patients with obstructive sleep apnea. *J Appl Physiol* 2007;**103**:234–239.

102. Orem J. Medullary respiratory neuron activity: relationship to tonic and phasic REM sleep. *J Appl Physiol* 1980;**48**:54–65.

103. Orem J, Osorio I, Brooks E, Dick TE. Activity of respiratory neurons during NREM sleep. *J Neurophysiol* 1985;**54**:1144–1156.

104. Lovering AT, Fraigne JJ, Dunin-Barkowski WL, Vidruk EH, Orem JM. Medullary respiratory neural activity during hypoxia in NREM and REM sleep in the cat. *J Neurophysiol* 2006;**95**:803–810.

105. Orem J, Montplaisir J, Dement WC. Changes in the activity of respiratory neurons during sleep. *Brain Res* 1974;**82**:309–315.

106. Sieck GC, Harper RM. Pneumotaxic area neuronal discharge during sleep-waking states in the cat. *Exp Neurol* 1980;**67**:79–102.

107. Orem J, Netick A. Characteristics of midbrain respiratory neurons in sleep and wakefulness in the cat. *Brain Res* 1982;**244**:231–241.

108. Orem J. The nature of the wakefulness stimulus for breathing. In: Suratt P, Remmers JE, eds. *Sleep and Respiration.* New York: Wiley-Liss; 1990. pp. 23–31.

109. Fenik VB, Davies RO, Kubin L. REM sleep-like atonia of hypoglossal (XII) motoneurons is caused by loss of noradrenergic and serotonergic inputs. *Am J Respir Crit Care Med* 2005;**172**:1322–1330.

110. Rukhadze I, Kubin L. Differential pontomedullary catecholaminergic projections to hypoglossal motor nucleus and viscerosensory nucleus of the solitary tract. *J Chem Neuroanat* 2007; **33**:23–33.

111. Kubin, L. Sleep-wake control of the upper airway by noradrenergic neurons, with and without intermittent hypoxia. *Progr Brain Res* 2014;**209**:255–274. [http://dx.doi.org/10.1016/B978-0-444-63274-6.00013-8]

112. Kubin L, Tojima H, Reignier C, Pack AI, Davies RO. Interaction of serotonergic excitatory drive to hypoglossal motoneurons with carbachol-induced, REM sleep-like atonia. *Sleep* 1996;**19**:187–195.

113. Woch G, Davies RO, Pack AI, Kubin L. Behavior of raphe cells projecting to the dorsomedial medulla during carbachol-induced atonia in the cat. *J Physiol* 1996;**490**:745–758.

114. Kubin L, Mann GL. Hypoglossal motoneurons are endogenously activated by serotonin during the active period of circadian cycle. *Respir Physiol Neurobiol* 2018;**248**:17–24.

115. Volgin DV, Saghir M, Kubin L. Developmental changes in the orexin 2 receptor mRNA in hypoglossal motoneurons. *NeuroReport* 2002;**13**:433–436.

116. Stettner GM, Kubin L. Antagonism of orexin receptors in the posterior hypothalamus reduces hypoglossal and cardiorespiratory excitation from the perifornical hypothalamus. *J Appl Physiol* 2013;**114**:119–130.

117. Kilduff TS. Hypocretin/orexin: maintenance of wakefulness and a multiplicity of other roles. *Sleep Med Rev* 2005;**9**:227–230.

118. Bastedo T, Chan E, Park E, Liu H, Horner RL. Modulation of genioglossus muscle activity across sleep-wake states by histamine at the hypoglossal motor pool. *Sleep* 2009;**32**:1313–1324.

119. Neuzeret P-C, Sakai K, Gormand F, Petitjean T, Buda C, Sastre J-P, Parrot S, Guidon G, Lin J-S. Application of histamine and serotonin to the hypoglossal nucleus increases genioglossus activity across the wake-sleep cycle. *J Sleep Res* 2009;**18**:113–121.

120. Volgin DV, Mackiewicz M, Kubin L. α_{1B} receptors are the main postsynaptic mediators of adrenergic excitation in brainstem motoneurons, a single-cell RT-PCR study. *J Chem Neuroanat* 2001;**22**:157–166.

121. Okabe S, Mackiewicz M, Kubin L. Serotonin receptor mRNA expression in the hypoglossal motor nucleus. *Respir Physiol* 1997;**110**:151–160.

122. Zhan G, Shaheen F, Mackiewicz M, Fenik P, Veasey SC. Single cell laser dissection with molecular beacon polymerase chain reaction identifies 2A as the predominant serotonin receptor subtype in hypoglossal motoneurons. *Neuroscience* 2002;**113**:145–154.

123. Volgin DV, Fay R, Kubin L. Postnatal development of serotonin 1B, 2A and 2C receptors in brainstem motoneurons. *Eur J Neurosci* 2003;**17**:1179–1188.

124. Kubin L, Tojima H, Davies RO, Pack AI. Serotonergic excitatory drive to hypoglossal motoneurons in the decerebrate cat. *Neurosci Lett* 1992;**139**:243–248.

125. Nie X, Zhou L, Wang A, Jin H, Qin Z, Pang J, Wang W, Kang J. Noradrenergic activation of hypoglossal nucleus modulates the central regulation of genioglossus in chronic intermittent hypoxic rats. *Front Neurol* 2017;**8**:171. [https://doi.org/10.3389/fneur.2017.00171]

126. Fung SJ, Yamuy J, Sampogna S, Morales FR, Chase MH. Hypocretin (orexin) input to trigeminal and hypoglossal motoneurons in the cat: a double-labeling immunohistochemical study. *Brain Res* 2001;**903**:257–262.

127. Volgin DV, Stettner GM, Kubin L. Circadian dependence of receptors that mediate wake-related excitatory drive to hypoglossal motoneurons. *Respir Physiol Neurobiol* 2013;**188**:301–307.

128. Kubin L. Orexinergic tone in cardiorespiratory regulation. In: Sakurai T, Pandi-Perumal SR, Monti JM, eds. *Orexin and Sleep: Molecular, Functional and Clinical Aspects*. Springer International Publishing Switzerland; 2015. pp. 395–410. [http://dx.doi.org/10.1007/978-3-319-23078-8_22]

129. Liu ZL, Wu X, Luo YJ, Wang L, Qu WM, Li SQ, Huang ZL. Signaling mechanism underlying the histamine-modulated action of hypoglossal motoneurons. *J Neurochem* 2016;**137**:277–286.

130. Rekling JC. Excitatory effects of thyrotropin-releasing hormone (TRH) in hypoglossal motoneurons. *Brain Res* 1990;**510**:175–179.

131. Gatti PJ, Llewellyn-Smith IJ, Sun QJ, Chalmers D, Pilowsky P. Substance P-immunoreactive boutons closely appose inspiratory protruder hypoglossal motoneurons in the cat. *Brain Res* 1999;**834**:155–159.

132. Liu WY, Liu H, Aggarwal J, Huang ZL, Horner RL. Differential activating effects of thyrotropin-releasing hormone and its analog taltirelin on motor output to the tongue musculature *in-vivo*. *Sleep* 2020;**43**:1–20. [https://doi.org/10.1093/sleep/zsaa053]

133. Johnson H, Ulfhake B, Dagerlind A, Bennett GW, Fone KCF, Hökfelt T. The serotoninergic bulbospinal system and brainstem-spinal cord content of serotonin-, TRH, and substance P-like immunoreactivity in the aged rat with special reference to the spinal cord motor nucleus. *Synapse* 1993;**15**:63–89.

134. Henry JN, Manaker S. Colocalization of substance P or enkephalin in serotonergic neuronal afferents to the hypoglossal nucleus in the rat. *J Comp Neurol* 1998;**391**:491–505.

135. Hinrichsen CFL, Weston S. Substance P in the hypoglossal nucleus of the rat. *Arch Oral Biol* 1999;**44**:683–691.

136. Funk GD. Neuromodulation: purinergic signaling in respiratory control. *Compr Physiol* 2013;**3**:331–363. [https://doi.org/10.1002/cphy.c120004]

137. Tian C, Zhu R, Zhu L, Qiu T, Cao Z, Kang T. Potassium channels: structures, diseases, and modulators. *Chem Biol Drug Des* 2014;**83**:1–26.

138. Gurges P, Liu H, Horner RL. Modulation of TASK-1/3 Channels at the hypoglossal motoneuron pool and effects on tongue motor output and responses to excitatory inputs *in-vivo*: implications for strategies for obstructive sleep apnea pharmacotherapy. *Sleep* 2020. [https://doi.org/10.1093/sleep/zsaa144]

139. Li WY, Wang A, Jin H, Zou Y, Wang Z, Wang W, Kang J. Transient upregulation of TASK-1 expression in the hypoglossal nucleus during chronic intermittent hypoxia is reduced by serotonin 2A receptor antagonist. *J Cell Physiol* 2019;**234**:17886–17895.

140. Rukhadze I, Fenik VB, Benincasa KE, Price A, Kubin L. Chronic intermittent hypoxia alters density of aminergic terminals and receptors in the hypoglossal motor nucleus. *Am J Respir Crit Care Med* 2010;**182**:1321–1329.

141. Cao R, Zhang MJ, Zhou YT, Liu YJ, Wang HH, Zhang QX, Shi YW, Li JC, Wong TS, Yin M. The dorsal and the ventral side of hypoglossal motor nucleus showed different response to chronic intermittent hypoxia in rats. *Sleep Breath* 2021;**25**:325–330. [https://doi.org/10.1007/s11325-020-02125-x]

142. Baum DM, Saussereau M, Jeton F, Planes C, Voituron N, Cardot P, Fiamma MN, Bodineau L. Effect of gender on chronic intermittent hypoxic *Fosb* expression in cardiorespiratory-related brain structures in mice. *Front Physiol* 2018;**9**:788. [https://doi.org/10.3389/fphys.2018.00788]

143. Stettner GM, Fenik VB, Kubin L. Effect of chronic intermittent hypoxia on noradrenergic activation of hypoglossal motoneurons. *J Appl Physiol* 2012;**112**:305–312.

144. Yokhana SS, Gerst DG, III, Lee DS, Badr MS, Qureshi T, Mateika JH. Impact of repeated daily exposure to intermittent hypoxia and mild sustained hypercapnia on apnea severity. *J Appl Physiol* 2012;**112**:367–377.

145. El-Chami M, Sudan S, Lin HS, Mateika JH. Exposure to intermittent hypoxia and sustained hypercapnia reduces therapeutic CPAP in participants with obstructive sleep apnea. *J Appl Physiol* 2017;**123**:993–1002.

146. Anaclet C, Ferrari L, Arrigoni E, Bass CE, Saper CB, Lu J, Fuller PM. The GABAergic parafacial zone is a medullary slow wave sleep-promoting center. *Nat Neurosci* 2014;**17**:1217–1224.

147. Alam MA, Kostin A, Siegel J, McGinty D, Szymusiak R, Alam MN. Characteristics of sleep-active neurons in the medullary parafacial zone in rats. *Sleep* 2018;**41**:2018.

148. Kroeger D, Absi G, Gagliardi C, Bandaru SS, Madara JC, Ferrari LL, Arrigoni E, Munzberg H, Scammell

TE, Saper CB, Vetrivelan R. Galanin neurons in the ventrolateral preoptic area promote sleep and heat loss in mice. *Nat Comm* 2018;**9**:4129.

149. Brown RE, Basheer R, McKenna JT, Strecker RE, McCarley RW. Control of sleep and wakefulness. *Physiol Rev* 2012;**92**:1087–1187.

150. Boucetta S, Cisse Y, Mainville L, Morales M, Jones BE. Discharge profiles across the sleep-waking cycle of identified cholinergic, GABAergic, and glutamatergic neurons in the pontomesencephalic tegmentum of the rat. *J Neurosci* 2014;**34**:4708–4727.

151. Van Dort CJ, Zachs DP, Kenny JD, Zheng S, Goldblum RR, Gelwan NA, Ramos DM, Nolan MA, Wang K, Weng FJ, Lin Y, Wilson MA, Brown EN. Optogenetic activation of cholinergic neurons in the PPT or LDT induces REM sleep. *Proc Natl Acad Sci USA* 2015;**112**:584–589.

152. Jones BE, Webster HH. Neurotoxic lesions of the dorsolateral pontomesencephalic tegmentum-cholinergic cell area in the cat. I. Effects upon the cholinergic innervation of the brain. *Brain Res* 1988;**451**:13–32.

153. Fort P, Luppi P-H, Sakai K, Salvert D, Jouvet M. Nuclei of origin of monoaminergic, peptidergic, and cholinergic afferents to the cat trigeminal motor nucleus: a double-labeling study with cholera-toxin as a retrograde tracer. *J Comp Neurol* 1990;**301**:262–275.

154. Travers JB, Yoo JE, Chandran R, Herman K, Travers SP. Neurotransmitter phenotypes of intermediate zone reticular formation projections to the motor trigeminal and hypoglossal nuclei in the rat. *J Comp Neurol* 2005;**488**:28–47.

155. Rukhadze I, Kubin L. Mesopontine cholinergic projections to the hypoglossal motor nucleus. *Neurosci Lett* 2007;**413**:121–125.

156. Vetrivelan R, Kong D, Ferrari LL, Arrigoni E, Madara JC, Bandaru SS, Lowell BB, Lu J, Saper CB. Melanin-concentrating hormone neurons specifically promote rapid eye movement sleep in mice. *Neuroscience* 2016;**336**:102–113.

157. Bittencourt JC, Presse F, Arias C, Peto C, Vaughan J, Nahon JL, Vale W, Sawchenko PE. The melanin-concentrating hormone system of the rat brain: an immuno- and hybridization histochemical characterization. *J Comp Neurol* 1992;**319**:218–245.

158. Del Cid-Pellitero E, Jones BE. Immunohistochemical evidence for synaptic release of GABA from melanin-concentrating hormone containing varicosities in the locus coeruleus. *Neuroscience* 2012;**223**:269–276.

159. Lu J, Greco MA, Shiromani P, Saper CB. Effect of lesions of the ventrolateral preoptic nucleus on NREM and REM sleep. *J Neurosci* 2000;**20**:3830–3842.

160. Netick A, Orem J, Dement W. Neuronal activity specific to REM sleep and its relationship to breathing. *Brain Res* 1977;**120**:197–207.

161. Boissard R, Gervasoni D, Schmidt MH, Barbagli B, Fort P, Luppi PH. The rat ponto-medullary network responsible for paradoxical sleep onset and maintenance: a combined microinjection and functional neuroanatomical study. *Eur J Neurosci* 2002;**16**:1959–1973.

162. Vetrivelan R, Fuller PM, Tong Q, Lu J. Medullary circuitry regulating rapid eye movement sleep and motor atonia. *J Neurosci* 2009;**29**:9361–9369.

163. Fort P, Luppi P-H, Jouvet M. Glycine-immunoreactive neurones in the cat brain stem reticular formation. *NeuroReport* 1993;**4**:1123–1126.

164. Rampon C, Peyron C, Petit J-M, Fort P, Gervasoni D, Luppi P-H. Origin of the glycinergic innervation of the rat trigeminal motor nucleus. *NeuroReport* 1996;**7**:3081–3085.

165. Valencia GS, Brischoux F, Clement O, Libourel PA, Arthaud S, Lazarus M, Luppi PH, Fort P. Ventromedial medulla inhibitory neuron inactivation induces REM sleep without atonia and REM sleep behavior disorder. *Nat Comm* 2018;**9**:504.

166. Soja PJ, López-Rodríguez F, Morales FR, Chase MH. The postsynaptic inhibitory control of lumbar motoneurons during the atonia of active sleep: effect of strychnine on motoneuron properties. *J Neurosci* 1991;**11**:2804–2811.

167. Soja PJ, Finch DM, Chase MH. Effect of inhibitory amino acid antagonists on masseteric reflex suppression during active sleep. *Exp Neurol* 1987;**96**:178–193.

168. Kubin L, Kimura H, Tojima H, Davies RO, Pack AI. Suppression of hypoglossal motoneurons during the carbachol-induced atonia of REM sleep is not caused by fast synaptic inhibition. *Brain Res* 1993;**611**:300–312.

169. Brooks PL, Peever JH. Glycinergic and GABA$_A$-mediated inhibition of somatic motoneurons does not mediate rapid eye movement sleep motor atonia. *J Neurosci* 2008;**28**:3535–3545.

170. Wenker IC, Abe C, Viar KE, Stornetta DS, Stornetta RL, Guyenet PG. Blood pressure regulation by the rostral ventrolateral nedulla in conscious rats: effects of hypoxia, hypercapnia, baroreceptor denervation, and anesthesia. *J Neurosci* 2017;**37**:4565–4583.

171. Van Bockstaele EJ, Aston-Jones G. Integration in the ventral medulla and coordination of sympathetic, pain and arousal functions. *Clin Exper Hyperten* 1995;**17**:153–165.

172. Holloway BB, Stornetta RL, Bochorishvili G, Erisir A, Viar KE, Guyenet PG. Monosynaptic glutamatergic activation of locus coeruleus and other lower brainstem noradrenergic neurons by the C1 cells in mice. *J Neurosci* 2013;**33**:18792–18805.

173. Stettner GM, Lei Y, Benincasa HK, Kubin L. Evidence that adrenergic ventrolateral medullary cells are activated whereas precerebellar lateral reticular nucleus neurons are suppressed during REM sleep.

PLoS ONE 2013;**8**:e62410. [https://doi.org/10.1371/journal.pone.0062410]

174. Souza MGPR, Stornetta RL, Stornetta DS, Abbott SBG, Guyenet PG. Differential contribution of the retrotrapezoid nucleus and C1 neurons to active expiration and arousal in rats. *J Neurosci* 2020;**40**:8683–8697.

175. Grace KP, Hughes SW, Horner RL. Identification of the mechanism mediating genioglossus muscle suppression in REM sleep. *Am J Respir Crit Care Med* 2013;**187**:311–319.

176. Grace KP, Hughes SW, Shahabi S, Horner RL. K$^+$ channel modulation causes genioglossus inhibition in REM sleep and is a strategy for reactivation. *Respir Physiol Neurobiol* 2013;**188**:277–288.

177. Stephenson R, Liao KS, Hamrahi H, Horner RL. Circadian rhythms and sleep have additive effects on respiration in the rat. *J Physiol* 2001;**536**:225–235.

178. Fink AM, Topchiy I, Ragozzino M, Amodeo DA, Waxman JA, Radulovacki MG, Carley DW. Brown Norway and Zucker Lean rats demonstrate circadian variation in ventilation and sleep apnea. *Sleep* 2014;**37**:715–721.

179. Kelly MN, Smith DN, Sunshine MD, Ross A, Zhang X, Gumz ML, Esser KA, Mitchell GS. Circadian clock genes and respiratory neuroplasticity genes oscillate in the phrenic motor system. *J Appl Physiol* 2020;**318**:R1058–R1067.

180. El-Chami M, Shaheen D, Ivers B, Syed Z, Badr MS, Lin HS, Mateika JH. Time of day affects chemoreflex sensitivity and the carbon dioxide reserve during NREM sleep in participants with sleep apnea. *J Appl Physiol* 2014;**117**:1149–1156.

181. El-Chami M, Shaheen D, Ivers B, Syed Z, Badr MS, Lin HS, Mateika JH. Time of day affects the frequency and duration of breathing events and the critical closing pressure during NREM sleep in participants with sleep apnea. *J Appl Physiol* 2015;**119**:617–626.

SECTION II

PATHOPHYSIOLOGY OF SLEEP-DISORDERED BREATHING

7 Pathophysiology of Sleep-Disordered Breathing in Children and Neonates

Sofia Konstantinopoulou and Ignacio E Tapia

INTRODUCTION

Sleep and breathing are separate but interdependent processes. Breathing commences in early fetal life and progressively matures through infancy (1). Initial variability in breathing and ventilatory responses progresses to stable ventilation in the first month of life. Respiratory events, including apneas, are more common in infants and decrease in healthy children, plateauing in early childhood such that age-specific normal values are required in order to determine whether respiratory events represent pathology or normal variation. The process of controlling both sleep and breathing is active in early gestation with development after birth. The first few months after birth represent a period of rapid change. Hence, the study of sleep and breathing in early infancy provides an opportunity to understand the mechanisms controlling both processes. It is clear that sleep remains a dynamic process in later life. The most common pathology linking these two processes is OSAS, which is recognized across the lifespan with differences in presentation and effects in different age groups. This chapter will mostly focus on OSAS.

Sleep-Disordered Breathing in Neonates and Children Born Preterm

Periodic breathing (PB) is a normal immature breathing pattern for neonates and occurs in a term as well as preterm infants. It appears the second week after birth, peaks at several weeks of age, then decreases, but it may continue up to 6 months or longer (2). The cause of PB is uncertain but may be related to maturation of receptors. PB may also be seen in infants who are hypoxemic. In these cases, infants may have a combination of chemosensitivity, alterations in arterial O_2 or CO_2, delayed signal transmission between the lung and chemoreceptors, and low lung volumes. These conditions can increase loop gain, resulting in an exacerbated ventilatory response. In infants who are hypoxemic and eucapnic, administration of supplemental oxygen abolishes the PB, suggesting that the carotid body is a primary component responsible for PB (1, 3).

Apnea of prematurity is a well-described condition related to immaturity of the central and autonomic nervous systems and neurotransmitter systems (4). The incidence of apnea is inversely related with the gestational age with the highest incidence occurring in infants <28 weeks of gestation. Apnea may also persist beyond 40 weeks of postmenstrual age in infants born <28 weeks of gestation (5). Physiologic contributors include a blunted ventilatory response to oxygen and carbon dioxide, compromised lung volumes, and small airways that are prone to collapse and obstruction. Apnea of prematurity results from a number of influences (intrinsic and extrinsic) affecting the central respiratory network, the peripheral and central chemoreceptors and the mechanoreceptors, and ultimately leads to a reduction in output to the muscles of respiration. The chest wall and soft tissues of the upper airway, both of which are quite compliant in premature infants, predispose to upper and lower airway collapse and obstruction (6).

Adequate lung volumes at the end of expiration (functional residual capacity (FRC)), normal pulmonary vascular resistance, normal hypoxic pulmonary vasoconstriction and rapid recovery of ventilation mediated by peripheral and central chemoreceptors, are all operative in preventing rapid desaturations from occurring and persisting during apnea. Premature infants are particularly prone to inadequate end-expiratory volumes due to excessive chest wall compliance leading to distal airway closure (7, 8). Activation of chest wall muscles substantially contributes to chest wall stability and maintaining FRC, which is problematic as premature infants spend >80% of their sleep in indeterminate and active sleep, which is a state associated with tonic inhibition of chest wall muscles (9). Prone sleeping position stabilizes the chest wall and increases FRC and oxygen saturation in infants with and without BPD (10, 11). In fact, a prone sleeping position may improve arterial oxygen saturation to a greater extent in infants with chronic lung disease (10), but also by optimizing V/Q match. Vagal-mediated reflexes, particularly the Breuer-Hering (B-H) deflation and inflation reflex, modify inspiratory and expiratory time in infants. Specifically, the deflation reflex is less active in premature than it is in term infants (12). To compensate for these challenges, preterm infants have a high respiratory rate and active rapidly adapting receptors (RARs) during deflation. Stimulating RARs in the lung induces an augmented breath (sigh) of which

DOI: 10.1201/9781003000631-9

premature infants have greater frequency than term infants. These augmented breaths are frequently followed by apnea in premature infants (8). It is important to maintain adequate FRC since it serves as an oxygen buffer that prevents the fall in the oxygen saturation during a respiratory pause. This has been shown in premature infants of 36 weeks postconceptual age with a reduction in FRC during apnea that was inversely correlated with the speed of hemoglobin desaturation (8). In younger premature infants of 32+/− weeks postconceptual age, Adams et al., 1997 found that 14% of apneas were accompanied by severe hypoxemia (<80% for at least 4 sec) and lower expiratory lung volumes (8). Infants at 24–28 weeks' gestation have a progressive increase in chronic intermittent hypoxemia during the first weeks of life (13, 14). These data suggest that premature infants are prone to low expiratory lung volumes predisposing them to a profound and rapid fall in arterial saturation during apnea.

It is easier to understand why premature infants are prone to hypoxemia if the stage of lung development at the time of birth is considered. This is especially true for infants born between 23 and 27 weeks of gestation, as lung development is at the canalicular stage where cellular differentiation gives rise to surfactant producing type II pneumocytes, but the respiratory units are still quite immature (15). At birth, premature infants have reduced alveoli-capillary surface area due to an unformed endothelial/epithelial unit needed for gas exchange. Thus, regardless of the level of surfactant deficiency, the architecture of the lung in premature infants predisposes to impaired gas exchange (16). In addition, the structure and function of all components (sensors, controls, and effectors) of the integrated respiratory network are undergoing significant modification during early development such that ventilation progresses to more sustained breathing as seen in infants born at term (17). The hypothesis states, based on animal models, that respiratory rhythm is generated from the central pattern generator within the ventral brainstem (18). Inspiration is driven by the pre-Botzinger complex an endogenously bursting group of interneurons that project to premotor inspiratory neurons throughout the ventral respiratory column and then project to the diaphragm, external intercostal muscles, and upper airway muscles (pharyngeal and laryngeal (19)). The retrotrapezoid nucleus/

parafacial respiratory group generates active expiration to premotor neurons that project to muscles that are involved in active expiration (19). The intrinsic properties and neurotransmitter profiles of respiratory-related neurons in the brainstem may modify peripheral mechano- and chemoreceptors that synapse on to the respiratory-related neurons. Thus, a stable respiratory pattern is responsive to the metabolic needs depending on the correct balance of excitatory and inhibitory inputs from: (1) higher brain centers (frontal and insular cortex, hypothalamus, reticular activating system, and amygdala); (2) mechanoreceptors in the lungs and upper airways; (3) peripheral chemoreceptors in the carotid body; and (4) central chemoreceptors on the ventral medullary surface (20).

Bronchopulmonary dysplasia (BPD) is a chronic lung disorder of preterm infants associated with long-term respiratory morbidity. Early assessment of both lung structure and ventilatory function may help to detect those children who are more likely to have severe respiratory problems (21). Infants with BDP who are normoxic during wakefulness may desaturate during sleep. In patients with BPD, hypoxemia during sleep has been shown to cause severe central apnea and bradycardia (22). This has been postulated as a mechanism for the increased rate of sudden death in these patients. This central apnea may result from the marked biphasic hypoxic response present during infancy. In addition, it has been shown that infants with BPD have impaired peripheral chemoreceptor response (23).

Furthermore, infants born preterm are at a higher risk for OSAS (24). In childhood, former preterm infants have a 3 to 5 fold elevated risk of developing OSAS compared to those without such a history (25). Evaluation with full overnight polysomnography (PSG) showed a prevalence of 9.6% of OSAS among children born preterm at school age, while the prevalence in the control population was only 1%–4% (24, 26). A number of hypotheses on potential pathogenetic mechanisms may explain the higher prevalence of OSAS in preterm infants (27). Facial asymmetry and elongated head shape can distort the dimensions and growth of the upper airway, resulting in a narrow upper airway (28). In addition, prolonged use of an endotracheal tube and nasal feeding tube may change the shape of the palate and adversely affect upper airway growth. Generalized muscle hypotonia can also predispose preterm born infants to OSAS (29).

PATHOPHYSIOLOGY OF OBSTRUCTIVE SLEEP APNEA SYNDROME

The Importance of Balance of the Upper Airway Anatomy and Upper Airway Muscle Tone

Obstructive sleep apnea syndrome (OSAS) is the most severe form of sleep-disordered breathing in children and is characterized by repetitive partial or complete upper airway obstruction that interrupts normal sleep patterns and ventilation (30). The etiology of childhood OSAS appears to be a dynamic process resulting from a combination of structural and neuromotor abnormalities. These predisposing factors occur as part of a spectrum: in some children with upper airway narrowing due to craniofacial anomalies, structural abnormalities predominate. Whereas in others such as children with hypotonia (e.g. muscular dystrophy (31) or cerebral palsy (32)), neuromuscular factors predominate.

The peak of prevalence of childhood OSAS occurs at 2–8 years, which is the age when the tonsils and adenoids are the largest in relation to the underlying airway size (33). Although childhood OSAS is associated with adenotonsillar hypertrophy, it is not caused by large tonsils and adenoids alone. First, patients with OSAS do not obstruct during wakefulness, showing that structural factors alone cannot be the cause. Second, studies have failed to show a correlation between upper airway or adenotonsillar size and OSAS (34). Third, a small percentage of children with adenotonsillar hypertrophy but no other known risk factors for OSAS are not cured by adenotonsillectomy (AT) (35). Finally, some studies have shown that there is a cohort of children who were cured of their OSAS by AT but developed recurrence during adolescence (36).

Obesity is a recognized risk factor for OSAS in children (37). The prevalence of obesity has tripled since the early 1970s and is presently estimated to be 16%. The risk of OSAS in obese children is high at 36% (38). AT in obese children with OSAS leads to a marked improvement, however, 76% will have the residual disease (39). There is no consistent relationship between pediatric OSAS and measures of fat distribution (40). Although imaging studies specific to obese young children have not been performed, studies in adolescents and adults indicate that increased fat deposition in the pharyngeal fat pads near and within the soft palate contributes to airway obstruction (41, 42). Obese individuals also have lower lung volumes, increasing both collapsibility and gas exchange abnormalities. The finding that both anatomic and structural factors are relevant and synergistic has important therapeutic implications. Based on the findings, it is reasonable to consider AT in adolescents with OSAS, even if obese. However, PSG should be repeated postoperatively to ensure that there is no residual OSAS due to underlying neuromotor deficits.

The imbalance between the structural and neuromuscular factors will lead to an increased upper airway collapsibility and hence result in OSAS. In response to upper airway obstruction, children maintain better patency of the upper airway compared with adults due to increased neuromuscular activation of the upper airway during sleep associated with increased central ventilatory drive (43). Specifically, Marcus et al. studied upper airway dynamics during sleep across the age span, from infancy through adulthood. Upper airway response was tested in several ways including the application of sub-atmospheric pressure administration and administration of carbon dioxide during sleep in a subset of participants. Results showed that adults have more collapsible upper airway during sleep than infants and children. Children have a more vigorous response to both sub-atmospheric pressure administration and hypercapnia during sleep, which indicates the presence of very active upper airway reflexes in young children. Since these reflexes decrease with age, the logical next step was to study adolescents. Studies in this age group showed that puberty is unlikely to contribute to this phenomenon, suggesting that the loss of upper airway protective reflexes is not due to hormonal changes but rather due to the depressant effect of age on the degree of ventilatory drive, which subsequently leads to a decrease in upper airway neuromotor tone (44). Similarly, Ugh et al. demonstrated that obese adolescents without OSAS have a strong compensatory neuromuscular response to sub-atmospheric pressure load during sleep, protecting them from upper airway collapse; whereas those with OSAS have weak protective airway reflexes during sleep. As these reflexes normally decline with age, obese adolescents may develop OSAS as they enter adulthood (45).

Ventilatory Responses during Sleep

It has been shown that children with OSAS have overall normal ventilatory responses to hypoxia and hypercapnia during both wakefulness and sleep, although subtle differences exist in their response to repeated hypercapnic challenges (46). For example, Yuan et al. demonstrated that the ventilatory response to hypercapnia during wakefulness is higher in obese adolescents with or without OSAS compared to lean controls (47). However, obese adolescents with OSAS have blunted ventilatory response to CO_2 during sleep and lack of compensatory prolongation of inspiratory time despite having normal CO_2 responsivity during wakefulness, which indicates that abnormalities in central ventilatory drive may play a role in the pathophysiology of OSAS in this population. Based on this, it is suspected that children with OSAS may have abnormal centrally mediated activation of their upper airway muscles, leading to a more collapsible upper airway (47). However, specific research on apnea threshold during childhood is lacking.

SDB and Arousals

Arousal is a vital protective mechanism against apnea, and it can be spontaneous as part of normal sleep or as a response to apnea, hypopneas, and external stimuli (48). Children with OSAS appear to have a deficit in arousal mechanisms and often do not have arousals following obstructive events. Studies have shown that children have elevated arousal thresholds in response to hypercapnia (49) and increased upper airway resistance (50). However, hypoxia appears to be a weaker stimulus to arousal. Parslow et al. demonstrated that infants are less arousable to mild hypoxia during quiet sleep than during active sleep, and the younger the child, the higher the arousal threshold (51). Ward et al. showed that only 32% of infants had arousals in response to hypoxia (52). Studies have shown that obstructive apneas are associated with EEG arousal in less than half of the apneas in children and only 18% of apneas in infants (53). As a result, sleep architecture is preserved in children with OSAS (54). However, although apnea-related EEG-arousals are uncommon in children, subcortical arousals, as demonstrated by movement (55) or autonomic changes occur frequently (56). It is also possible that subtle disturbances in sleep architecture, which cannot be detected on routine PSG, are present (57). These factors may contribute to neurobehavioral and autonomic complications.

In summary, increased upper airway resistance is an essential component of OSAS, including any combination of anatomical factors, such as narrowing/retropositioning of the maxilla/mandible and/or adenotonsillar hypertrophy. However, in addition to these, the stability of the upper airway depends on neuromuscular activation, ventilatory control, and arousal threshold. At sleep onset, airway muscle activity is reduced, ventilatory variability increases, and an apneic threshold slightly below eupneic levels is observed in non-REM sleep. Airway collapse is offset by pharyngeal dilatator activity in response to hypercapnia and negative luminal pressure. Ventilatory overshoot results in a sudden reduction in airway muscle activation, contributing to obstruction during non-REM sleep. Arousal from sleep exacerbates ventilatory instability and, thus, obstructive cycling. Paroxysmal reductions in pharyngeal dilator activity related to REM sleep processes likely account for the disproportionate severity of OSAS observed during REM sleep. Understanding the pathophysiology of pediatric OSAS may permit more precise clinical phenotyping and therefore improve or target therapies related to anatomy, neuromuscular compensation, ventilatory control, and/or arousal threshold.

Sleep-Disordered Breathing in Children with Chronic Pulmonary Disease

During sleep, normal children experience a small increase in the partial pressure of carbon dioxide ($PaCO_2$) and a small decrease in the arterial oxyhemoglobin saturation (SpO_2) compared to wakefulness (58, 59). It is believed that there is an average drop of 2% for SpO_2 and an average increase of 4 to 6 mm Hg for $PaCO_2$. These sleep-related changes in ventilation, upper airway stability, and gas exchange can be exaggerated in children with an underlying lung disease, thus resulting in increased vulnerability to OSAS (58). Patients with a low FRC have decreased respiratory reserve and are more likely to desaturate as a result of REM-related intercostal muscle hypotonia and increase ventilation-perfusion mismatch. Thus, patients with adequate oxygenation during wakefulness may desaturate during sleep, particularly REM sleep (60). Sleep-related desaturation has been reported in patients with BPD (61), asthma (62), and cystic fibrosis (63), as well as in other causes of chronic obstructive pulmonary disease. Other physiological factors that exacerbate sleep-disordered breathing (SDB) in children with chronic lung disease include increased bronchoconstriction during sleep, reduced mucociliary clearance (64), and decreased cough. During sleep, tracheal irritation is more likely to cause arousal or apnea than cough (65). Thus, sleep architecture is disrupted, and awakenings are frequent. Patients with chronic lung disease may also have abnormalities in ventilatory control that can adversely affect their respiration during sleep. For example, patients with life-threatening episodes of asthma have been shown to have impaired peripheral chemoreceptor function and impaired perception of respiratory loads (66). This could lead to a worsening hypoxemia, as well as abnormal arousal responses to respiratory stimuli.

Special Populations
Central Congenital Hypoventilation Syndrome (CCHS)

This is a rare disorder of respiratory and autonomic regulation, usually presenting in newborns and occasionally in older children and adults due to PHOX2B gene mutation (67). The neonatal presentation is typically associated with larger polyalanine repeat mutation of the PHOX2B gene. Patients with CCHS have intact voluntary control of ventilation but lack automatic control; and hypoventilation occurs either only during sleep or while awake and asleep. Patients usually have a decreased tidal volume and respiratory rate during sleep, thus requiring ventilatory support (68, 69). Although most patients breathe adequately during wakefulness, a subset requires ventilatory support 24 hr/day. However, even those who breathe adequately awake have been shown to have mild hypoventilation in association with increased metabolic demands such as exercise (70). CCHS may be associated with Hirschsprung's disease, autonomic dysfunction (decreased heart rate, hypotension) (71), neural tumors (ganglioneuromas, ganglioneuroblastomas), swallowing dysfunction when young (72), and minor ocular abnormalities (73).

In contrast to almost all types of SDB, children with CCHS breathe slightly better during REM than non-REM sleep, perhaps because hypoventilation during REM sleep is less related to metabolic control (74). Children with CCHS have decreased or absent ventilatory chemosensitivity in response to progressive hypoxia and hypercapnia during wakefulness (75) and sleep (76). However, they do have intact peripheral chemoreceptor responses to acute hypoxia, hypercapnia, and hyperoxia (77). Although they often do not arouse in response to chronic hypercapnia while asleep, they have been demonstrated to arouse when exposed to a superimposed hyperoxic hypercapnic stimulus, albeit at a higher arousal threshold than control subjects (78). These studies suggest that the primary physiological defect in CCHS may be in the area of the brainstem where afferent impulses from the central and peripheral chemoreceptors are integrated (78).

There is a high morbidity and mortality reported in children with CCHS, with death resulting from cor pulmonale, aspiration, or sepsis. Research from centers, however, experienced with CCHS, show prolonged survival with a good quality of life (72). Patients continue to need ventilatory support and do not outgrow their disease. Reversible episodes of pulmonary hypertension may occur with infections or with hypoventilation due to inadequate ventilatory support. Cognitive outcomes appear to be related to the adequacy of control of the hypoventilation.

A form of late-onset central hypoventilation syndrome has been described in the literature (79). Typically, these children present at an older age (2–4 years) and have sleep-related hypoventilation and hypothalamic abnormalities including endocrinopathies and/or obesity. Interestingly, a number of these patients have been reported to have neural tumors such as ganglioneuromas and ganglioneuroblastomas, suggesting an etiological link with CCHS (79).

Myelomeningocele

Central apnea, obstructive apnea, and hypoventilation are relatively common in patients with Arnold-Chiari malformations due to compression and dysplasia of the brainstem. In children, the most common commonly encountered Arnold Chiari malformation is a type II malformation associated with a myelomeningocele. This is indeed the most common cause of central hypoventilation encountered in children. In addition to central hypoventilation, patients may also have OSAS (80) due to collapse at the level of the larynx. Bilateral vocal cord paralysis can occur as a result of traction on the vagal nerve roots (81). Although breathing during wakefulness is usually normal, severe breath-holding spells may occur, indicating further abnormalities of central control of ventilation (81). In addition to SDB, patients with Arnold Chiari malformation type II are predisposed to other pulmonary problems. Patients may have restrictive lung disease, secondary to muscle weakness or scoliosis (82), that may further contribute to significant oxyhemoglobin desaturation following rather short respiratory events during sleep. Studies have shown that children with myelomeningocele have decreased ventilatory and arousal responses to hypercapnia, suggesting an abnormality of central chemoreceptor function or of brainstem processing of central chemoreceptor signals (83). Peripheral chemoreception is depressed in a subset of patients, again suggesting an abnormality of central integration of chemoreception, or perhaps abnormalities of the glossopharyngeal nuclei (which innervate the carotid body) or other chemoreceptive areas. Despite the high prevalence of SDB in infants with myelomeningocele and the known risk for death during sleep or during cyanotic/apneic spells in such infants, the problem remains under recognized.

Prader Willi Syndrome (PWS)

PWS is a congenital disorder typified by hypothalamic obesity, developmental delay, hypotonia, and hypogonadism. The vast majority of patients have abnormalities of chromosome 15 (84). Although patients with PWS do not have classic central hypoventilation, they are included here as physiological testing has shown abnormalities of ventilatory control. OSAS and REM-associated desaturation are seen commonly. Patients tend to have restrictive lung disease based on obesity and muscle weakness (85), which can explain the tendency to desaturate. Excessive daytime sleepiness is common, and it has not been established whether this is due to SDB or also to a CNS component. Patients appear more predisposed to REM-onset sleep, although published studies have not excluded confounding factors such as sleep deprivation or partial upper airway obstruction (86). Physiological studies have shown blunted hypercapnic ventilatory responses secondary to obesity; patients in whom weight has been controlled have a normal hypercapnic drive. However, the ventilatory response to hypoxia (87), as well as other tests of peripheral chemoreceptor function, show a marked decrease in peripheral chemoreceptor function (88). A unifying hypothesis, therefore, is that the abnormalities of ventilatory control are due to the central processing of chemoreceptor input. Interestingly, a recent study shows that baseline ventilation and ventilatory drive increase following growth hormone administration, despite an unchanged body mass index (89).

Trisomy 21 (T21)

T21 is a common disorder, occurring in 1 per 800 births (90–92) which translates to approximately 5,400 children with T21 born in the USA annually (93). Individuals with T21 are predisposed to OSAS due to craniofacial features (midfacial hypoplasia, glossoptosis), hypotonia, comorbid obesity,

and hypothyroidism (94). Studies have shown a prevalence of OSAS in children with T21 between 45 and 55% (95–97). These rates are markedly higher than that of typically developing children (96, 97), in whom the prevalence of OSAS is about 2%–4% (98). However, studies specifically investigating the pathophysiology of SDB in this population are lacking, and much of the knowledge has been extrapolated from research in typically developing children.

REFERENCES

1. MacLean JE, Fitzgerald DA, Waters KA. Developmental changes in sleep and breathing across infancy and childhood. Paediatr Respir Rev. 2015;16(4):276–84.

2. Sharma PB, Baroody F, Gozal D, Lester LA. Obstructive sleep apnea in the formerly preterm infant: an overlooked diagnosis. Front Neurol. 2011;2:73.

3. Kelly DH, Stellwagen LM, Kaitz E, Shannon DC. Apnea and periodic breathing in normal full-term infants during the first twelve months. Pediatr Pulmonol. 1985;1(4):215–9.

4. Zhao J, Gonzalez F, Mu D. Apnea of prematurity: from cause to treatment. Eur J Pediatr. 2011;170(9):1097–105.

5. Eichenwald EC, Aina A, Stark AR. Apnea frequently persists beyond term gestation in infants delivered at 24 to 28 weeks. Pediatrics. 1997;100(3):354–9.

6. Di Fiore JM, Martin RJ, Gauda EB. Apnea of prematurity—perfect storm. Respir Physiol Neurobiol. 2013;189(2):213–22.

7. Poets CF. Apnea of prematurity: what can observational studies tell us about pathophysiology? Sleep Med. 2010;11(7):701–7.

8. Poets CF, Rau GA, Neuber K, Gappa M, Seidenberg J. Determinants of lung volume in spontaneously breathing preterm infants. Am J Respir Crit Care Med. 1997;155(2):649–53.

9. Lopes J, Muller NL, Bryan MH, Bryan AC. Importance of inspiratory muscle tone in maintenance of FRC in the newborn. J Appl Physiol Respir Environ Exerc Physiol. 1981;51(4):830–4.

10. Kassim Z, Donaldson N, Khetriwal B, Rao H, Sylvester K, Rafferty GF, et al. Sleeping position, oxygen saturation and lung volume in convalescent, prematurely born infants. Arch Dis Child Fetal Neonatal Ed. 2007;92(5):F347–50.

11. Saiki T, Rao H, Landolfo F, Smith AP, Hannam S, Rafferty GF, et al. Sleeping position, oxygenation and lung function in prematurely born infants studied post term. Arch Dis Child Fetal Neonatal Ed. 2009;94(2):F133–7.

12. Hannam S, Ingram DM, Milner AD. A possible role for the Hering-Breuer deflation reflex in apnea of prematurity. J Pediatr. 1998;132(1):35–9.

13. Di Fiore J, Arko M, Herynk B, Martin R, Hibbs AM. Characterization of cardiorespiratory events following gastroesophageal reflux in preterm infants. J Perinatol. 2010;30(10):683–7.

14. Di Fiore JM, Bloom JN, Orge F, Schutt A, Schluchter M, Cheruvu VK, et al. A higher incidence of intermittent hypoxemic episodes is associated with severe retinopathy of prematurity. J Pediatr. 2010;157(1):69–73.

15. Hislop A. Developmental biology of the pulmonary circulation. Paediatr Respir Rev. 2005;6(1):35–43.

16. Backstrom E, Hogmalm A, Lappalainen U, Bry K. Developmental stage is a major determinant of lung injury in a murine model of bronchopulmonary dysplasia. Pediatr Res. 2011;69(4):312–8.

17. Givan DC. Physiology of breathing and related pathological processes in infants. Semin Pediatr Neurol. 2003;10(4):271–80.

18. Smith JC, Abdala AP, Koizumi H, Rybak IA, Paton JF. Spatial and functional architecture of the mammalian brain stem respiratory network: a hierarchy of three oscillatory mechanisms. J Neurophysiol. 2007;98(6):3370–87.

19. Feldman JL, Del Negro CA, Gray PA. Understanding the rhythm of breathing: so near, yet so far. Annu Rev Physiol. 2013;75:423–52.

20. Gauda EB, Martin RJ. Apnea of Prematurity—Perfect Storm. In: Gleason CA, Devaskar S, editors. Avery's Diseases of the Newborn. 4th ed. Philadelphia, PA: Saunders; 2012. p. 584–89.

21. Koltsida G, Konstantinopoulou S. Long term outcomes in chronic lung disease requiring tracheostomy and chronic mechanical ventilation. Semin Fetal Neonatal Med. 2019;24(5):101044.

22. Garg M, Kurzner SI, Bautista D, Keens TG. Hypoxic arousal responses in infants with bronchopulmonary dysplasia. Pediatrics. 1988;82(1):59–63.

23. Calder NA, Williams BA, Smyth J, Boon AW, Kumar P, Hanson MA. Absence of ventilatory responses to alternating breaths of mild hypoxia and air in infants who have had bronchopulmonary dysplasia: implications for the risk of sudden infant death. Pediatr Res. 1994;35(6):677–81.

24. Marcus CL, Meltzer LJ, Roberts RS, Traylor J, Dix J, D'Ilario J, et al. Long-term effects of caffeine therapy for apnea of prematurity on sleep at school age. Am J Respir Crit Care Med. 2014;190(7):791–9.

25. Montgomery-Downs HE, Young ME, Ross MA, Polak MJ, Ritchie SK, Lynch SK. Sleep-disordered breathing symptoms frequency and growth among prematurely born infants. Sleep Med. 2010;11(3):263–7.

26. Lumeng JC, Chervin RD. Epidemiology of pediatric obstructive sleep apnea. Proc Am Thorac Soc. 2008;5(2):242–52.

27. Hibbs AM, Johnson NL, Rosen CL, Kirchner HL, Martin R, Storfer-Isser A, et al. Prenatal and neonatal risk factors for sleep disordered breathing in school-aged children born preterm. J Pediatr. 2008;153(2):176–82.

28. Joosten KF, Larramona H, Miano S, Van Waardenburg D, Kaditis AG, Vandenbussche N, et al. How do we recognize the child with OSAS? Pediatr Pulmonol. 2017;52(2):260–71.

29. Greenfeld M, Tauman R, DeRowe A, Sivan Y. Obstructive sleep apnea syndrome due to adenotonsillar hypertrophy in infants. Int J Pediatr Otorhinolaryngol. 2003;67(10):1055–60.

30. Marcus CL, Brooks LJ, Draper KA, Gozal D, Halbower AC, Jones J, et al. Diagnosis and management of childhood obstructive sleep apnea syndrome. Pediatrics. 2012;130(3):576–84.

31. Khan Y, Heckmatt JZ. Obstructive apnoeas in Duchenne muscular dystrophy. Thorax. 1994;49(2):157–61.

32. Kotagal S, Gibbons VP, Stith JA. Sleep abnormalities in patients with severe cerebral palsy. Dev Med Child Neurol. 1994;36(4):304–11.

33. Laurikainen E, Erkinjuntti M, Alihanka J, Rikalainen H, Suonpaa. Radiological parameters of the bony nasopharynx and the adenotonsillar size compared with sleep apnea episodes in children. Int J Pediatr Otorhinolaryngol. 1987;12(3):303–10.

34. Fernbach SK, Brouillette RT, Riggs TW, Hunt CE. Radiologic evaluation of adenoids and tonsils in children with obstructive sleep apnea: plain films and fluoroscopy. Pediatr Radiol. 1983;13(5):258–65.

35. Suen JS, Arnold JE, Brooks LJ. Adenotonsillectomy for treatment of obstructive sleep apnea in children. Arch Otolaryngol Head Neck Surg. 1995;121(5):525–30.

36. Guilleminault C, Partinen M, Praud JP, Quera-Salva MA, Powell N, Riley R. Morphometric facial changes and obstructive sleep apnea in adolescents. J Pediatr. 1989;114(6):997–9.

37. Redline S, Tishler PV, Schluchter M, Aylor J, Clark K, Graham G. Risk factors for sleep-disordered breathing in children. Associations with obesity, race, and respiratory problems. Am J Respir Crit Care Med. 1999;159(5 Pt 1):1527–32.

38. Fryar CD, Carroll MD, Afful J. Prevalence of overweight, obesity, and severe obesity among children and adolescents aged 2–19 years: United States, 1963–1965 through 2017–2018. NCHS Health E-Stats. 2020.

39. Mitchell RB, Kelly J. Outcome of adenotonsillectomy for obstructive sleep apnea in obese and normal-weight children. Otolaryngol Head Neck Surg. 2007;137(1):43–8.

40. Verhulst SL, Schrauwen N, Haentjens D, Suys B, Rooman RP, Van Gaal L, et al. Sleep-disordered breathing in overweight and obese children and adolescents: prevalence, characteristics and the role of fat distribution. Arch Dis Child. 2007;92(3):205–8.

41. Schwab RJ, Pasirstein M, Pierson R, Mackley A, Hachadoorian R, Arens R, et al. Identification of upper airway anatomic risk factors for obstructive sleep apnea with volumetric magnetic resonance imaging. Am J Respir Crit Care Med. 2003;168(5):522–30.

42. Schwab RJ, Kim C, Bagchi S, Keenan BT, Comyn FL, Wang S, et al. Understanding the anatomic basis for obstructive sleep apnea syndrome in adolescents. Am J Respir Crit Care Med. 2015;191(11):1295–309.

43. Marcus CL, Lutz J, Hamer A, Smith PL, Schwartz A. Developmental changes in response to subatmospheric pressure loading of the upper airway. J Appl Physiol (1985). 1999;87(2):626–33.

44. Bandla P, Huang J, Karamessinis L, Kelly A, Pepe M, Samuel J, et al. Puberty and upper airway dynamics during sleep. Sleep. 2008;31(4):534–41.

45. Huang J, Pinto SJ, Yuan H, Katz ES, Karamessinis LR, Bradford RM, et al. Upper airway collapsibility and genioglossus activity in adolescents during sleep. Sleep. 2012;35(10):1345–52.

46. Gozal D, Arens R, Omlin KJ, Ben Ari JH, Aljadeff G, Harper RM, et al. Ventilatory response to consecutive short hypercapnic challenges in children with obstructive sleep apnea. J Appl Physiol. 1995;79(5):1608–14.

47. Yuan H, Pinto SJ, Huang J, McDonough JM, Ward MB, Lee YN, et al. Ventilatory responses to hypercapnia during wakefulness and sleep in obese adolescents with and without obstructive sleep apnea syndrome. Sleep. 2012;35(9):1257–67.

48. Eckert DJ, Younes MK. Arousal from sleep: implications for obstructive sleep apnea pathogenesis and treatment. J Appl Physiol (1985). 2014;116(3):302–13.

49. Marcus CL, Lutz J, Carroll JL, Bamford O. Arousal and ventilatory responses during sleep in children with obstructive sleep apnea. J Appl Physiol (1985). 1998;84(6):1926–36.

50. Marcus CL, Moreira GA, Bamford O, Lutz J. Response to inspiratory resistive loading during sleep in normal children and children with obstructive apnea. J Appl Physiol (1985). 1999;87(4):1448–54.

51. Parslow PM, Harding R, Cranage SM, Adamson TM, Horne RS. Arousal responses to somatosensory and mild hypoxic stimuli are depressed during quiet sleep in healthy term infants. Sleep. 2003;26(6):739–44.

52. Ward SL, Bautista DB, Keens TG. Hypoxic arousal responses in normal infants. Pediatrics. 1992;89(5 Pt 1):860–4.

53. McNamara F, Issa FG, Sullivan CE. Arousal pattern following central and obstructive breathing abnormalities in infants and children. J Appl Physiol (1985). 1996;81(6):2651–7.

54. Marcus CL, Carroll JL, Koerner CB, Hamer A, Lutz J, Loughlin GM. Determinants of growth in children with the obstructive sleep apnea syndrome. J Pediatr. 1994;125(4):556–62.

55. Praud JP, D'Allest AM, Nedelcoux H, Curzi-Dascalova L, Guilleminault C, Gaultier C. Sleep-related abdominal muscle behavior during partial or complete obstructed breathing in prepubertal children. Pediatr Res. 1989;26(4):347–50.

56. Aljadeff G, Gozal D, Schechtman VL, Burrell B, Harper RM, Ward SL. Heart rate variability in children with obstructive sleep apnea. Sleep. 1997;20(2):151–7.

57. Bandla HP, Gozal D. Dynamic changes in EEG spectra during obstructive apnea in children. Pediatr Pulmonol. 2000;29(5):359–65.

58. Poets CF, Stebbens VA, Samuels MP, Southall DP. Oxygen saturation and breathing patterns in children. Pediatrics. 1993;92(5):686–90.

59. Montgomery-Downs HE, O'Brien LM, Gulliver TE, Gozal D. Polysomnographic characteristics in normal preschool and early school-aged children. Pediatrics. 2006;117(3):741–53.

60. Moyer-Mileur LJ, Nielson DW, Pfeffer KD, Witte MK, Chapman DL. Eliminating sleep-associated hypoxemia improves growth in infants with bronchopulmonary dysplasia. Pediatrics. 1996;98(4 Pt 1):779–83.

61. Berthon-Jones M, Lawrence S, Sullivan CE, Grunstein R. Nasal continuous positive airway pressure treatment: current realities and future. Sleep. 1996; 19(9 Suppl):S131–5.

62. Chipps BE, Mak H, Schuberth KC, Talamo JH, Menkes HA, Scherr MS. Nocturnal oxygen saturation in normal and asthmatic children. Pediatrics. 1980;65(6):1157–60.

63. Coffey MJ, FitzGerald MX, McNicholas WT. Comparison of oxygen desaturation during sleep and exercise in patients with cystic fibrosis. Chest. 1991;100(3):659–62.

64. Bateman JR, Pavia D, Clarke SW. The retention of lung secretions during the night in normal subjects. Clin Sci Mol Med Suppl. 1978;55(6):523–7.

65. Sullivan CE, Murphy E, Kozar LF, Phillipson EA. Waking and ventilatory responses to laryngeal stimulation in sleeping dogs. J Appl Physiol Respir Environ Exerc Physiol. 1978;45(5):681–9.

66. Davenport PW, Cruz M, Stecenko AA, Kifle Y. Respiratory-related evoked potentials in children with life-threatening asthma. Am J Respir Crit Care Med. 2000;161(6):1830–5.

67. Berry-Kravis EM, Zhou L, Rand CM, Weese-Mayer DE. Congenital central hypoventilation syndrome: PHOX2B mutations and phenotype. Am J Respir Crit Care Med. 2006;174(10):1139–44.

68. Weese-Mayer DE, Rand CM, Zhou A, Carroll MS, Hunt CE. Congenital central hypoventilation syndrome: a bedside-to-bench success story for advancing early diagnosis and treatment and improved survival and quality of life. Pediatr Res. 2017;81(1–2):192–201.

69. Kerbl R, Litscher H, Grubbauer HM, Reiterer F, Zobel G, Trop M, et al. Congenital central hypoventilation syndrome (Ondine's curse syndrome) in two siblings: delayed diagnosis and successful noninvasive treatment. Eur J Pediatr. 1996;155(11):977–80.

70. Paton JY, Swaminathan S, Sargent CW, Hawksworth A, Keens TG. Ventilatory response to exercise in children with congenital central hypoventilation syndrome. Am Rev Respir Dis. 1993;147(5):1185–91.

71. Woo MS, Woo MA, Gozal D, Jansen MT, Keens TG, Harper RM. Heart rate variability in congenital central hypoventilation syndrome. Pediatr Res. 1992;31(3):291–6.

72. Marcus CL, Jansen MT, Poulsen MK, Keens SE, Nield TA, Lipsker LE, et al. Medical and psychosocial outcome of children with congenital central hypoventilation syndrome. J Pediatr. 1991;119(6):888–95.

73. Goldberg DS, Ludwig IH. Congenital central hypoventilation syndrome: ocular findings in 37 children. J Pediatr Ophthalmol Strabismus. 1996;33(3):175–80.

74. Huang J, Colrain IM, Panitch HB, Tapia IE, Schwartz MS, Samuel J, et al. Effect of sleep stage on breathing in children with central hypoventilation. J Appl Physiol. 2008;105(1):44–53.

75. Paton JY, Swaminathan S, Sargent CW, Keens TG. Hypoxic and hypercapnic ventilatory responses in awake children with congenital central hypoventilation syndrome. Am Rev Respir Dis. 1989;140(2):368–72.

76. Oren J, Newth CJ, Hunt CE, Brouillette RT, Bachand RT, Shannon DC. Ventilatory effects of almitrine bismesylate in congenital central hypoventilation syndrome. Am Rev Respir Dis. 1986;134(5):917–9.

77. Gozal D, Marcus CL, Shoseyov D, Keens TG. Peripheral chemoreceptor function in children with the congenital central hypoventilation syndrome. J Appl Physiol (1985). 1993;74(1):379–87.

78. Marcus CL, Bautista DB, Amihyia A, Ward SL, Keens TG. Hypercapneic arousal responses in children with congenital central hypoventilation syndrome. Pediatrics. 1991;88(5):993–8.

79. Katz ES, McGrath S, Marcus CL. Late-onset central hypoventilation with hypothalamic dysfunction: a distinct clinical syndrome. Pediatr Pulmonol. 2000;29(1):62–8.

80. Waters KA, Forbes P, Morielli A, Hum C, O'Gorman AM, Vernet O, et al. Sleep-disordered breathing in children with myelomeningocele. J Pediatr. 1998;132(4):672–81.

81. Hesz N, Wolraich M. Vocal-cord paralysis and brainstem dysfunction in children with spina bifida. Dev Med Child Neurol. 1985;27(4):528–31.

82. Sherman MS, Kaplan JM, Effgen S, Campbell D, Dold F. Pulmonary dysfunction and reduced exercise capacity in patients with myelomeningocele. J Pediatr. 1997;131(3):413–8.

83. Ward SL, Nickerson BG, van der Hal A, Rodriguez AM, Jacobs RA, Keens TG. Absent hypoxic and hypercapneic arousal responses in children with myelomeningocele and apnea. Pediatrics. 1986;78(1):44–50.

84. Mascari MJ, Gottlieb W, Rogan PK, Butler MG, Waller DA, Armour JA, et al. The frequency of uniparental disomy in Prader-Willi syndrome. Implications for molecular diagnosis. N Engl J Med. 1992;326(24):1599–607.

85. Hakonarson H, Moskovitz J, Daigle KL, Cassidy SB, Cloutier MM. Pulmonary function abnormalities in Prader-Willi syndrome. J Pediatr. 1995;126(4):565–70.

86. Hertz G, Cataletto M, Feinsilver SH, Angulo M. Sleep and breathing patterns in patients with Prader Willi syndrome (PWS): effects of age and gender. Sleep. 1993;16(4):366–71.

87. Arens R, Gozal D, Omlin KJ, Livingston FR, Liu J, Keens TG, et al. Hypoxic and hypercapnic ventilatory responses in Prader-Willi syndrome. J Appl Physiol (1985). 1994;77(5):2224–30.

88. Gozal D, Arens R, Omlin KJ, Ward SL, Keens TG. Absent peripheral chemosensitivity in Prader-Willi syndrome. J Appl Physiol (1985). 1994;77(5):2231–6.

89. Lindgren AC, Hellstrom LG, Ritzen EM, Milerad J. Growth hormone treatment increases CO(2) response, ventilation and central inspiratory drive in children with Prader-Willi syndrome. Eur J Pediatr. 1999;158(11):936–40.

90. Presson AP, Partyka G, Jensen KM, Devine OJ, Rasmussen SA, McCabe LL, et al. Current estimate of Down syndrome population prevalence in the United States. J Pediatr. 2013;163(4):1163–8.

91. Mai CT, Kucik JE, Isenburg J, Feldkamp ML, Marengo LK, Bugenske EM, et al. Selected birth defects data from population-based birth defects surveillance programs in the United States, 2006 to 2010: featuring trisomy conditions. Birth Defects Res A Clin Mol Teratol. 2013;97(11):709–25.

92. de Graaf G, Buckley F, Skotko BG. Estimates of the live births, natural losses, and elective terminations with Down syndrome in the United States. Am J Med Genet A. 2015;167a(4):756–67.

93. Sherman SL, Allen EG, Bean LH, Freeman SB. Epidemiology of Down syndrome. Ment Retard Dev Disabil Res Rev. 2007;13(3):221–7.

94. Rajagopal KR, Abbrecht PH, Derderian SS, Pickett C, Hofeldt F, Tellis CJ, et al. Obstructive sleep apnea in hypothyroidism. Ann Intern Med. 1984;101(4):491–4.

95. Stebbens VA, Dennis J, Samuels MP, Croft CB, Southall DP. Sleep related upper airway obstruction in a cohort with Down's syndrome. Arch Dis Child. 1991;66(11):1333–8.

96. Marcus CL, Keens TG, Bautista DB, von Pechmann WS, Ward SL. Obstructive sleep apnea in children with Down syndrome. Pediatrics. 1991;88(1):132–9.

97. de Miguel-Diez J, Villa-Asensi JR, Alvarez-Sala JL. Prevalence of sleep-disordered breathing in children with Down syndrome: polygraphic findings in 108 children. Sleep. 2003;26(8):1006–9.

98. Marcus CL, Brooks LJ, Draper KA, Gozal D, Halbower AC, Jones J, et al. Diagnosis and management of childhood obstructive sleep apnea syndrome. Pediatrics. 2012;130(3):e714–55.

8 Pathogenesis of Sleep-Disordered Breathing in Adults
Overview

Thomas M Tolbert, Indu Ayappa, and David M Rapoport

INTRODUCTION

This chapter presents an overview of the pathophysiologic mechanisms underlying the respiratory events (apneas and hypopneas) characteristic of obstructive sleep apnea (OSA) and central sleep apnea (CSA). A visual overview of the many systems and processes involved is provided in Figure 8.1. Sleep-disordered breathing (SDB) is a broad term that, according to the International Classification of Sleep Disorders, Third Edition (ICSD-3), includes OSA and CSA as well as sleep hypoventilation disorders (1). For the purposes of this chapter, SDB will refer only to OSA and CSA. Further, this chapter focuses principally on *non-hypercapnic* CSA, in which waking ventilation is preserved (2). Readers interested in the pathophysiology of sleep hypoventilation disorders and hypercapnic CSA are referred elsewhere (for example, see Chapter 15 for obesity hypoventilation syndrome).

SDB is characterized by discrete, self-limited periods during sleep in which ventilation is either near-absent to absent (*apneas*) or reduced (*hypopneas*). These *respiratory events* may be associated with blood gas disturbances, sympathetic nervous system surges in activity, arousals from sleep, or all of these. Broadly, apneas and hypopneas are classified on the basis of their underlying etiology as "obstructive" in the case of increased resistance to airflow through the upper airway, or as "central" in the case of reduced effort by the respiratory muscles, principally the diaphragm (3). By convention, respiratory events are reported in a frequency measure as the apnea-hypopnea index (AHI), or the total number of apneas and hypopneas occurring per hour of sleep. The AHI is generally accepted as indicative of the overall severity of SDB, and may be subdivided into the frequency of obstructive events (obstructive AHI) and the frequency of central events (central AHI). Patients demonstrating a predominance of obstructive events are usually diagnosed with OSA, while patients with a predominance of central events are said to have CSA. However, considerable overlap exists in the mechanisms underlying obstructive and central respiratory events, complicating event classification and thus patient diagnosis (4). An apnea that is apparently completely obstructive may

start with a reduction in effort before effort eventually increases toward the end of the apnea (5, 6). Conversely, an apnea that appears completely central is likely associated with a reduction in upper airway patency (7, 8). It should therefore be kept in mind that many if not most of the mechanisms discussed in this chapter may play a role in any respiratory event observed during sleep. Whether a patient with SDB is ultimately deemed to have predominately OSA or CSA likely depends not only on what mechanisms predominate, but on how those mechanisms interact and influence one another. An overall guiding principle is that CSA tends to occur in the presence of ventilatory control instability, while OSA tends to occur in the presence of both ventilatory control instability and a proclivity for upper airway collapse (see Figure 8.2) (9, 10).

THE VENTILATORY CONTROL SYSTEM

The ventilatory control system—a network of neurological, vascular, respiratory, and muscular structures—continuously monitors blood O_2 and CO_2 levels and maintains or changes ventilation in response (11). Deviations in the partial pressure of arterial CO_2 ($PaCO_2$) from a "set point" of approximately 40 mm Hg during wakefulness and of approximately 2 mm Hg to 8 mm Hg higher during deep sleep in healthy humans are detected, and the system responds with changes in the output to the muscles of inspiration and expiration (12). Though the system is principally attuned to maintenance of CO_2 levels, this typically has the effect of also maintaining homeostatic O_2 levels. All else equal, an increase in ventilation in response to hypercapnia will have the effect of both decreasing $PaCO_2$ and raising PaO_2. For example, during an apnea, the absence of ventilation leads to a rise in $PaCO_2$ and a fall in PaO_2. The rise in $PaCO_2$ is detected by the ventilatory control system, which then signals for an increase in ventilation, which—if successful—will have the effect of decreasing $PaCO_2$ and increasing PaO_2.

THE BRAINSTEM, THE CORTEX, CHEMORECEPTORS, AND CHEMOSENSITIVITY

The brainstem serves as the central controller of the ventilatory system, generating a rhythmic respiratory pattern that dictates the

DOI: 10.1201/9781003000631-10

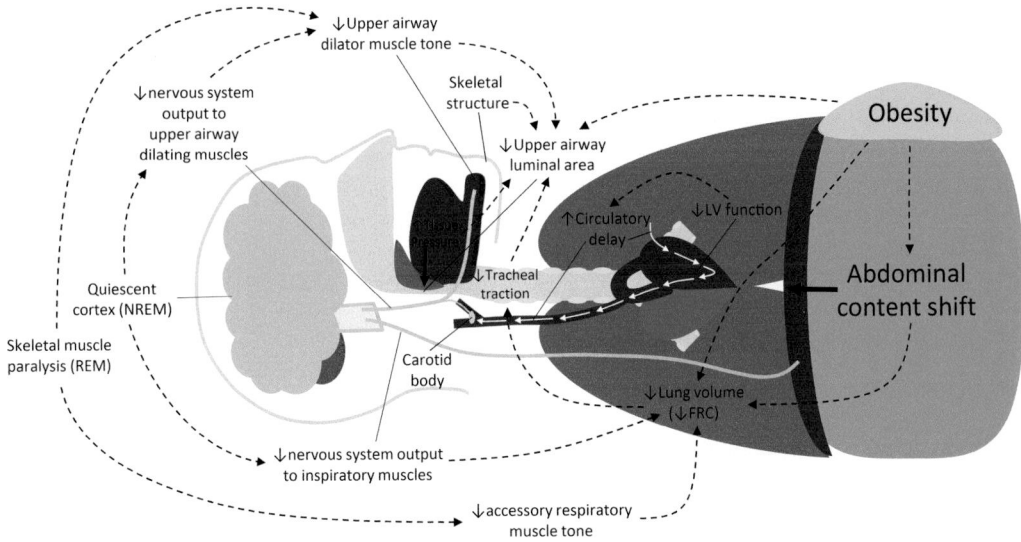

Figure 8.1 Overview of structures and processes involved in sleep-disordered breathing. The complex pathogenesis of sleep-disordered breathing involves multiple interacting systems that undergo changes in the transition from upright to recumbent and from the waking state to sleep. Dashed arrows depict interactions between anatomical structures and processes. For example, obesity can contribute to changes in the upper airway luminal area through multiple pathways: by directly reducing the size of the thoracic cavity (and therefore lung volume and tracheal traction); by augmenting the shift of abdominal contents into the thoracic cavity in the recumbent position, also reducing lung volume and tracheal traction; and by direct effects on the upper airway such as mass effect and fat accumulation in upper airway tissues, both of which contribute to increased tissue pressure surrounding the upper airway lumen.

FRC, functional residual capacity; LV, left ventricle; NREM, non-rapid eye movement sleep; REM, rapid eye movement sleep.

timing, depth, and duration of inspiration and expiration by output to the respiratory muscles, including the diaphragm and the muscles of the upper airway (11, 13, 14). However, during wakefulness, cortical activity can supersede or complement the brainstem control for purposes of speech, eating and drinking, and voluntary breath holding. This cortical contribution to breathing is sometimes termed the "wakefulness drive." In contrast, during NREM sleep, cortical control of breathing is virtually absent so that brainstem control "takes over." The result is that, during NREM sleep, ventilatory control is dependent on the brainstem-driven homeostatic maintenance of blood gas partial pressures, without the cortical-driven modifications for speech, swallowing, emotions, and other high-complexity concerns.

Specialized structures called *chemoreceptors* monitor local O_2 and CO_2 partial pressures (PaO_2 and $PaCO_2$) and provide signals to the brainstem, which integrates these afferent inputs to determine output to the muscles of ventilation, including the respiratory pump (principally the diaphragm) and the muscles of the upper airway. *Central chemoreceptors* are located in the central nervous system, principally in the medulla, and are sensitive to changes in CO_2 and pH. *Peripheral chemoreceptors* are components of the peripheral nervous system, located principally at the bifurcations of the carotid arteries (i.e. the *carotid bodies*) and in the aorta. They mainly respond to local hypoxia, but may also increase their activity in conditions of low pH, elevated $PaCO_2$, or low blood flow (11).

The integration of signals from the central and peripheral chemoreceptors determines the overall *chemosensitivity* of brainstem control, that is, the vigor (or lack thereof) of brainstem signals for changes in ventilation in response to disturbances in PaO_2 and $PaCO_2$. Chemosensitivity affects not only the waking level of $PaCO_2$ but also the magnitude of changes in ventilation: how much to increase ventilation in hypercapnia and how much to decrease ventilation in hypocapnia (and thus the loop gain; see the section "Loop Gain", below). The brainstem therefore largely

109

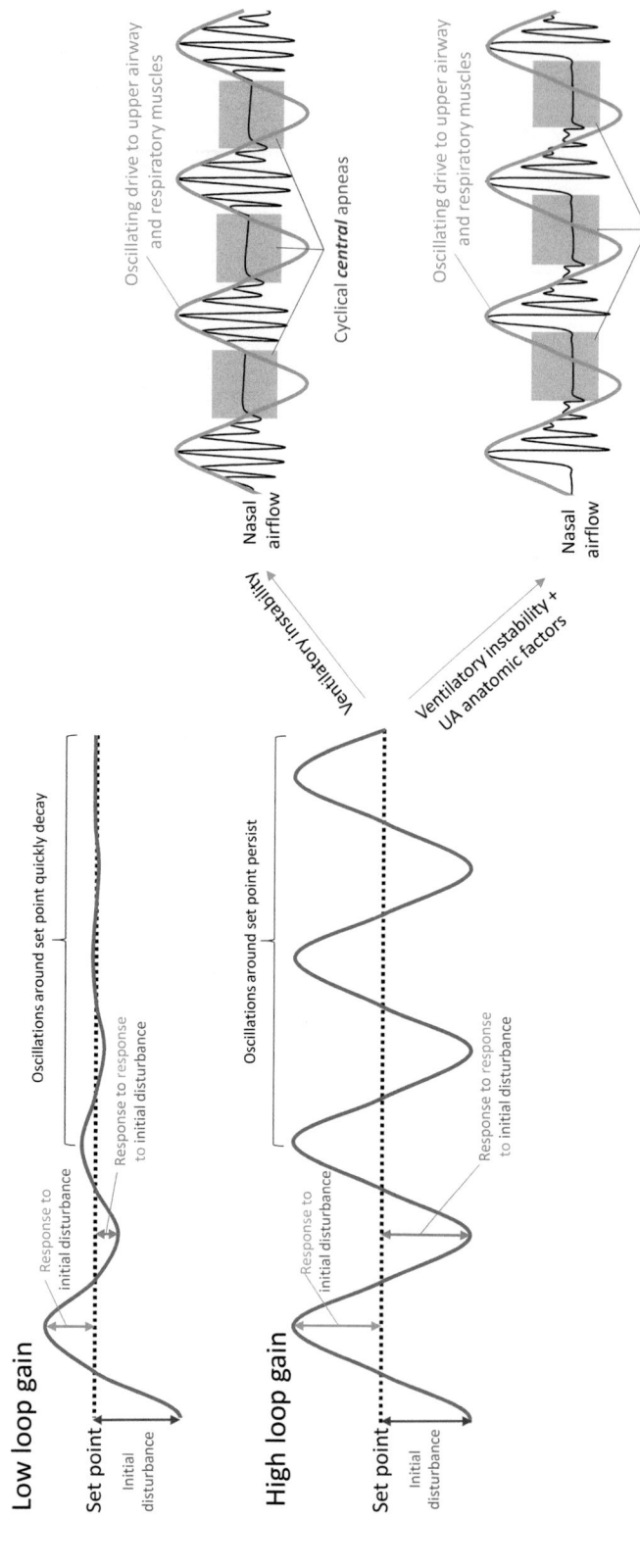

Figure 8.2 Schematic depiction of loop gain and conceptual role in cyclical respiratory events in both central and obstructive sleep apnea. In a negative feedback system such as the ventilatory chemoreflex control system, the system produces a response to any disturbance (or deviation from the set point). Loop gain refers to the ratio of the response to the disturbance. Oscillations around the set point occur when the response leads to an "overshoot" past the set point. That is, the response becomes another disturbance. In low loop gain systems, because each response is less than the disturbance that precedes it, oscillations around the set point quickly decay, and sustained oscillations do not occur. In high loop gain systems, every response approaches, equals, or even exceeds the initial disturbance, and the system oscillates cyclically around the set point. In patients with high loop gain, the "drive" (or neural stimulus) to the upper airway muscles and respiratory muscles may significantly oscillate during NREM sleep. In patients without compromise of the anatomic upper airway, this leads to cyclical central apneas alternating with hyperpneas. In patients with factors contributing to upper airway compromise, ventilatory instability contributes to cyclical obstructive apneas. In both cases, patients may be said to exhibit periodic breathing.

determines the length and magnitude of *hyperpneas*—periods of rigorous inspiration with high tidal volumes—that occur after apneas and hypopneas in sleep. Conditions of hypoxia (for example, high altitude, heart failure) and activation of pulmonary stretch receptors (pulmonary venous congestion) are associated with increased chemosensitivity, while some medications (for example, sedatives, opioids) are associated with decreased chemosensitivity.

The anatomy of the ventilatory control system is further explored in Chapter 1. For greater detail on the structure and function of chemoreceptors, the reader is referred to Chapter 2.

CIRCULATORY DELAY

Gas exchange occurs within the lungs at the interface of the airspace and the alveolar capillaries. Because the carotid and medullary chemoreceptors are not located in the alveolar capillaries themselves, a delay exists between changes in ventilation and detection of the changes by the control system (see Figure 8.1). Blood arriving at the carotid arteries or the medulla is not necessarily representative of the immediate conditions in the alveoli. Rather, the blood sampled by chemoreceptors is representative of the conditions at the time when that blood passed through the alveoli. In health, this *circulatory delay* is short and has a largely negligible effect. In conditions of reduced blood flow, such as left ventricular systolic heart failure, increased circulatory delay may lead to a significant mismatch of the conditions in the alveoli and the conditions at the chemoreceptors. In response to the afferent input from the chemoreceptors, the ventilatory control system may unwittingly alter the activity of the respiratory muscles in a way that does not appropriately match conditions in the lung. The consequent hyperpnea when CO_2 is low in the alveoli and apnea when CO_2 is high in the alveoli will exacerbate hypocapnia and hypercapnia, respectively.

THE APNEIC THRESHOLD AND CO_2 RESERVE

All else equal, a healthy brainstem ventilatory control center will respond to falls in $PaCO_2$ by decreasing the drive to breathe. Brainstem-driven breathing will cease altogether when $PaCO_2$ falls below a certain level, which is termed the *apneic threshold*. The difference between eupneic $PaCO_2$ and the apneic threshold is referred to as CO_2 *reserve*. This difference buffers against the occurrence of apneas. The apneic threshold and the difference between eupneic $PaCO_2$ and the apneic threshold are not fixed; factors that can alter the apneic threshold and CO_2 reserve include chemosensitivity and sleep state and stage (15). Hypoxia (as occurs at high altitude and in patients with heart failure) and pulmonary vascular congestion increase control system chemosensitivity, reducing the CO_2 reserve and increasing the likelihood of apneas and hypopneas during sleep (12). The wakefulness drive appears to prevent apnea when one is awake, even at very low $PaCO_2$ levels, so that no apneic threshold exists during wakefulness.

The apneic threshold is further explored in Chapter 11.

LOOP GAIN

Loop gain is an engineering term used to describe closed-loop control systems, that is, systems that use a controller to maintain a "set point" of some parameter by responding to measured deviations from that set point (i.e. a negative feedback loop). The concept is illustrated in Figure 8.2. A deviation from the set point is a *disturbance*, and the ultimate result of the controller's actions after detecting that disturbance is a *response*. Loop gain, a dimensionless value, is the ratio of the response to the disturbance. A closed-loop control system with a high loop gain is unstable because any disturbance will produce a response equal to or greater than the magnitude of the disturbance. This response "overshoot" is another disturbance, resulting in further response, resulting in further disturbance, etc. This cycle leads to the oscillation of the controlled parameter around the set point. A low loop gain may also produce oscillation around the set level, but the magnitude of oscillations will decay over time, ultimately leading to stability. An analogy is a car with springs for suspension above the wheels; without working shock absorbers, a bump in the road will cause the car to rock up and down repeatedly, oscillating around the car's intended vertical position above the wheels. Working shock absorbers dampen such oscillations, so they decay over time, giving a smoother ride.

The ventilatory control system can be thought of as a closed-loop control system, with the brainstem working to maintain a $PaCO_2$ level in the face of ventilatory disturbances. In the setting of high loop gain, the brainstem-driven ventilation is unstable and will repeatedly "overshoot" with oscillation around the set level, ultimately manifesting in the genesis and maintenance of cyclical respiratory events. The characteristic repetitive, waxing-waning pattern of tidal volumes is termed *periodic breathing*. Cheyne-Stokes breathing (CSB) is the classic example of this phenomenon and is characterized by an apnea followed by breaths with rising, peaking, then falling tidal volumes (a crescendo-decrescendo pattern) followed by another apnea in a repeating cycle. CSB is the pattern of CSA (CSA-CSB) most closely associated with left ventricular systolic heart failure due to the combination of increased chemosensitivity (high loop gain) and circulatory delay (mismatch between conditions in the alveoli and conditions at the chemoreceptors) exacerbating the oscillations.

The combination of high-altitude hypoxia and sleep will cause periodic breathing in most healthy individuals as the hypoxia elevates CO_2 sensitivity (increases loop gain), reducing CO_2 reserve as discussed above. The effect of high altitude on sleep is further explored in Chapter 13.

Though elevated loop gain underlies periodic breathing, the most extreme forms of which are clearly "central" in that apneas are associated with reduced efforts, loop gain should not be misunderstood as a parameter solely relevant to CSA. Even in the absence of overt periodic breathing, loop gain is thought to contribute to the propagation of respiratory events in OSA: Brainstem-driven ventilation affects not only diaphragmatic activity but also upper airway muscle activity. Falls in $PaCO_2$ are associated with less brainstem output to upper airway muscles (see Chapter 6). Therefore, obstructive apneas and hypopneas may also be perpetuated by changes in ventilatory drive caused by preceding respiratory events, and each event may also contribute to subsequent respiratory events. For example, an obstructive apnea is a disturbance that may eventually result in a hyperpnea in response, and the hyperpnea—if it causes overshoot below the $PaCO_2$ set point—creates a further disturbance contributing to another respiratory event, which may be central or obstructive depending on the interacting mechanisms outlined in this chapter.

THE UPPER AIRWAY

The upper airway is a conductive passage for the flow of air from the ambient atmosphere to the trachea. In normal subjects, nasal breathing predominates during sleep, with inspiratory airflow beginning at the nares, passing through the nasal passages, the nasopharynx, velopharynx, oropharynx, and hypopharynx before finally reaching the trachea (16, 17).

The upper airway is not a rigid conduit but has a changing luminal cross-sectional area (patency) and may collapse due to the interaction of a variety of factors. During normal sleep, the ventilatory control system maintains ventilation not only by output to the respiratory pump muscles but also to 20 or more muscles involved in maintaining patency of the upper airway (13, 14). Collapse of the airway is prevented by this muscle tone. However, when this tone is insufficient to maintain patency during sleep, apneas (complete collapse) or hypopneas (partial collapse) may occur. Contributions to this collapse include the intrinsic "collapsibility" of the upper airway, the pressure of the tissues surrounding the airway ("tissue pressure"), and the amount of negative intraluminal airway pressure developed by the respiratory system during a breath.

Flexion of the neck and the supine posture—the tongue and soft palate falling toward the oropharynx—will reduce the upper airway luminal area (18–21). Obesity has both local upper airway effects and more distant effects on the respiratory system (see the section "The Lungs and Chest Wall," below and Chapter 15). Excess fat external to the airway may promote collapse by mass effect (22). Fat accumulation within the structures of the upper airway itself, especially the tongue, appears to contribute to OSA, likely by reducing the upper airway luminal area (23). Upper airway cross-sectional area has been experimentally shown to progressively fall from wakefulness to NREM sleep to REM sleep (24).

The intrinsic collapsibility (the lack of stiffness, compliance, or "floppiness") of the upper airway and tissue pressure reflect the dynamic physical properties of the structures of the head and neck. Skeletal structure, airway mucosal edema brought on by inflammation or fluid shifts, changes in blood flow to cranial structures, and the effects of gravity from positional changes may all influence the pressure in the tissues surrounding the upper airway and the airway's collapsibility. The volume of the lungs contributes to upper airway stiffness by creating a "tug" on the trachea, reducing upper airway collapsibility.

With each effort to take a breath (to inhale), negative intrathoracic pressure generated by the diaphragm during inspiration transmits up the airway, leading to negative intraluminal pressure within the upper airway. In order to prevent airway obstruction, the combined negative intraluminal and tissue pressure must be opposed by the intrinsic recoil of the airway wall, which is augmented by the resting tone and inspiratory contraction of the upper airway musculature (25).

The collapsibility of the upper airway can be assessed either under experimental conditions with anesthesia-induced sleep or by using transient CPAP drops during natural sleep (26, 27). In either case, the "propensity" to collapse is reflected by the increased collapsibility when airway tone is moderately to maximally reduced in sleep compared to airway tone during wakefulness (28). The most common metric of collapsibility is the critical closing pressure (Pcrit) (29). This is the (normally negative) pressure within the airway lumen below which collapse will occur. In healthy individuals, even during sleep, Pcrit is highly negative; airway collapse does not occur as it would require the inspiratory pump muscles to create a very negative intraluminal pressure (30). In patients with OSA, sleeping Pcrit may be close to zero or even positive, implying that collapse will occur at or near atmospheric pressure soon after sleep onset lowers the upper airway muscle tone (31). Emerging therapeutic modalities such as hypoglossal nerve stimulation and various drugs attempt to modify Pcrit by augmenting the neural output to upper airway muscles (see Chapters 19–21). Positive airway pressure (PAP) therapy for OSA is not intended to change Pcrit *per se*, but maintains luminal airway pressure above Pcrit to prevent collapse (see Chapter 17).

Recently, other measures have emerged to describe the patency and collapsibility of the upper airway (26). These anatomic physiologic "traits" include $V_{passive}$, the ventilation during sleep when the upper airway muscles are relaxed, and V_{active}, the ventilation during sleep when the upper airway muscles are active. A low $V_{passive}$ is indicative of a collapsible, obstructed airway and a low V_{active} reflects an inability of the upper airway muscles to counter obstruction. Conversely, a high V_{active} and a large difference between $V_{passive}$ and V_{active} is reflective of upper airway musculature that can effectively open the airway in sleep. Similar to Pcrit, measurement of $V_{passive}$ and V_{active} has required transient CPAP drops in the sleep laboratory, a method that is non-routine and potentially cumbersome. More recently, however, an algorithmic method has emerged which analyzes signals from routine polysomnography in order to calculate $V_{passive}$ and V_{active} (32).

THE LUNGS AND CHEST WALL

The lungs, serving as reserves of gases and having mechanical effects on extrathoracic structures, are relevant to both ventilatory control and upper airway collapsibility. Functional residual capacity (FRC) refers to the volume of the lungs when the muscles of inspiration and of expiration are relaxed. Conceptually, therefore, FRC is the "resting volume" of the lungs, and contains a mix of oxygen, carbon dioxide, and nitrogen reflective of the ambient atmosphere, minute ventilation, metabolic activity, and blood flow to and from the lungs. The oxygen remaining in the lung at FRC serves as a reserve that buffers against desaturation of hemoglobin if ventilation is reduced or absent, while the carbon dioxide in the lung at FRC may buffer against hypocapnia in the setting of hyperpnea (33). Any process which limits the volume of the lungs and FRC will decrease the reserve of oxygen and carbon dioxide, potentially predisposing to desaturation and hypocapnia (34). For example, the combination of a lower FRC and a relatively high metabolic rate in children compared to adults leads to faster desaturation during apneas and hypopneas (35).

Disease processes intrinsic to the lung may alter lung volume, either decreasing FRC (for example, in interstitial lung disease) or increasing FRC (as may occur in chronic obstructive pulmonary disease, COPD). Factors affecting the thoracic cage surrounding the lungs may also reduce lung volume; these include thoracic and abdominal processes, such as scoliosis, obesity, pregnancy, and massive ascites (34, 36). Abdominal factors, in particular, may be associated with significant changes in lung volume with the positional changes from standing to sitting to lying supine.

The volume of the lungs also contributes to traction on the trachea, pulling the trachea caudally toward the thorax with an increase in volume. This has been termed "tracheal tug" on the upper airway (37, 38). The longitudinal traction on the tracheal walls makes them stiffer and therefore less collapsible. A fall in FRC, and thus less tracheal tug, reverses this effect, raising the risk of upper airway collapse. Indeed, increased lung volume has been shown to correlate with falling Pcrit, implying a less collapsible upper airway at greater lung volume (39). Therapies for OSA, including CPAP and nasal resistance valves, may reduce upper airway collapsibility not only by the direct effect of increased pressure within the upper airway lumen but also by the more indirect effect of increased lung volume with greater tracheal traction (37, 40).

AROUSALS

Arousals are transitions from sleep to wakefulness or to a lighter sleep stage, usually evidenced by increased cortical activity on electroencephalography (EEG).

113

During obstructive apneas and hypopneas, disturbances in blood gas levels or inspiratory efforts against a highly resistant or closed upper airway may both contribute to arousal (41, 42). In patients with OSA, an arousal is associated with increased airway patency, effectively terminating any preceding obstructive apnea or hypopnea (43). Historically, therefore, arousal has been thought of as a "survival mechanism" that terminates obstructive events to prevent deleterious hypoxemia and hypercapnia. However, though an arousal is often *sufficient* to terminate an obstructive event, it is not clear that an arousal is *necessary*—that is, obstructive events can end without any apparent arousal (44, 45). Rising ventilatory drive (reflective of rising $PaCO_2$) will increase upper airway muscle activity. Whether arousal occurs before the termination of an event is reflective of the ability of the upper airway to open before reaching the *arousal threshold*—the level of ventilatory drive that results in arousal. In the setting of a high V_{active} (meaning that the upper airway musculature is able to effectively counteract obstruction) and a high arousal threshold, respiratory events may terminate without causing arousal. But if V_{active} and the arousal threshold are both low, respiratory events are likely to disrupt sleep before the airway can open.

In contrast to the pattern seen in obstructive events, arousals related to central apneas and hypopneas tend to occur during the hyperpneic phase *following* the termination of the event. It has been suggested the arousal is consequent to vigorous breathing efforts, rather than its cause.

For both OSA and CSA, it has been suggested that arousals *per se* may have harmful effects. Indeed, arousals are associated with sleep instability, fragmentation, impaired transitions to deeper NREM stages and potentially to REM, and decreased total sleep time. Because arousals resulting from respiratory events are accompanied by an increase in ventilation, arousals themselves may contribute to ventilatory control instability, leading to repetitive respiratory events (45). The overshoots in ventilation that occur after one respiratory event may be augmented by the presence of an arousal, propagating further respiratory events as explained above.

WAKE-SLEEP AND SLEEP STAGE TRANSITIONS

During wakefulness, an upright posture (standing or sitting) is typical; ventilation maintains $PaCO_2$ at a set point of around 40 mm Hg but can be modulated by cortical control to accommodate speaking and eating, and neural stimulus of upper airway musculature maintains a patent airway even in the presence of vigorous inspiratory effort. Typically, a recumbent posture is assumed prior to sleep onset. The fluid accumulated by gravity in the lower extremities and abdomen during wakefulness may now redistribute into the lungs, heart, and the soft tissues of the nasal passages and pharyngeal structures, potentially altering gas exchange, chemosensitivity, and the patency and collapsibility of the upper airway (46, 47). Abdominal contents, pulled out of the thoracic cavity by dint of gravity when upright, may now also redistribute, pushing into the diaphragm and reducing the volume of the thoracic cavity and thus FRC. The fall in FRC may be associated with decreased traction on the trachea, with consequent increased upper airway collapsibility, as well as decreased reserves of O_2, so that any respiratory event will be associated with greater oxygen desaturation or hypocapnia, which may then contribute to repeating respiratory events, arousal, and sleep fragmentation (37).

Even in the presence of these anatomic and positional factors, respiratory events do not occur before sleep onset. Indeed, the change in ventilatory control brought about by falling asleep is an essential condition of the respiratory events that characterize OSA and CSA (notable exceptions include periodic breathing during exercise and late-stage heart failure; see Chapters 5 and 12). This can be appreciated by the observation that OSA patients do not snore while awake. Rather, snoring, a surrogate of obstruction, occurs only after sleep onset brings about changes in upper airway neural control with decreased muscle tone (48).

With the transition from wakefulness to NREM sleep, the centrality of $PaCO_2$ to the control of ventilation by the brainstem and the presence of an apneic threshold portend the possibility of central apneas or hypopneas in association with sleep onset. In the setting of a high loop gain, oscillation of ventilation with apneas or hypopneas interspersed with hyperpneas may occur, causing waxing and waning of the $PaCO_2$ level and thus a waxing and waning ventilatory drive, which leads finally to waxing and waning ventilation in a perpetuating cycle of periodic breathing. Just as output to the diaphragm periodically oscillates with changing $PaCO_2$ levels, output to the upper airway musculature will also wax and wane. In concert, anatomic factors, oscillating output to the diaphragm, and oscillating output to the upper respiratory musculature determine whether respiratory events occur and whether they are primarily central or obstructive in nature.

Recently developed experimental methods attempt to address this complexity by quantifying the physiologic "traits" that contribute to SDB, including anatomic traits ($V_{passive}$ and V_{active}) and non-anatomic traits (loop gain and arousal threshold). Quantification of these traits is a method of "endotyping" a patient's SDB, that is, mechanistically attributing respiratory events to one or more pathophysiologic factors. In principle, quantification of these traits could help in the tailoring of appropriate therapy for a specific patient. For example, acetazolamide has been shown to reduce loop gain in OSA, representing a potential therapy for patients with OSA due to high ventilatory control instability (49). The combination of loop gain and upper airway collapsibility was able to predict the response to dental appliance therapy (50). These methods are limited by their validation largely in NREM sleep without extensive study of REM sleep. Further studies are needed before quantification of physiologic traits is included in the routine assessment and treatment of SDB.

The transition from NREM sleep to REM sleep is associated with a more irregular breathing pattern at a higher respiratory rate. The reasons for this are not completely clear, but it is suspected that during REM, the cortex is involved in ventilatory control similar to wakefulness, rather than leaving ventilatory control entirely to the brainstem as in NREM sleep (51). With cortical input, ventilation is not driven strictly in response to blood gas levels. Even in the total absence of a brainstem drive to breathe, the presence of a cortical drive to breathe in REM makes central apnea rare. Indeed, an apneic threshold, while present in NREM sleep, does not appear to exist in REM sleep (52). Further, the ventilatory response to blood gas disturbances may be reduced in REM relative to NREM, reflective of a reduced chemosensitivity (41, 42, 53). Together, cortical drive and diminished chemosensitivity dampen the ventilatory control system relative to NREM sleep, and periodic breathing and CSB are much less likely. Central events, when they occur at all during REM, tend to be short and irregular without the waxing-waning pattern of periodic breathing.

While central events are relatively unusual in REM sleep, a high frequency of obstructive events during REM sleep may be observed in patients with OSA, even in individuals with no obstructive events during NREM sleep. REM is associated with widespread skeletal muscle paralysis; the extraocular muscles and diaphragm are spared, but the musculature of the upper airway is not (54, 55). The upper airway has been experimentally shown to narrow during REM compared to NREM, and the collapsibility of the upper airway (as measured by Pcrit) also increases in REM sleep compared to NREM sleep (24, 56).

REFERENCES

1. American Academy of Sleep Medicine. *International Classification of Sleep Disorders*. Third ed. Darien, IL: American Academy of Sleep Medicine; 2014.

2. Eckert DJ, Jordan AS, Merchia P, Malhotra A. Central sleep apnea: pathophysiology and treatment. *Chest*. 2007;131(2):595–607.

3. Berry RB, Budhiraja R, Gottlieb DJ, et al. Rules for scoring respiratory events in sleep: update of the 2007 AASM Manual for the Scoring of Sleep and Associated Events. Deliberations of the Sleep Apnea Definitions Task Force of the American Academy of Sleep Medicine. *J Clin Sleep Med*. 2012;8(5):597–619.

4. Orr JE, Malhotra A, Sands SA. Pathogenesis of central and complex sleep apnoea. *Respirology*. 2017;22(1):43–52.

5. Martin RJ, Pennock BE, Orr WC, Sanders MH, Rogers RM. Respiratory mechanics and timing during sleep in occlusive sleep apnea. *J Appl Physiol*. 1980;48(3):432–437.

6. Iber C, Davies SF, Chapman RC, Mahowald MM. A possible mechanism for mixed apnea in obstructive sleep apnea. *Chest*. 1986;89(6):800–805.

7. Badr MS, Toiber F, Skatrud JB, Dempsey J. Pharyngeal narrowing/occlusion during central sleep apnea. *J Appl Physiol*. 1995;78(5):1806–1815.

8. Jobin V, Rigau J, Beauregard J, et al. Evaluation of upper airway patency during Cheyne-Stokes breathing in heart failure patients. *Eur Respir J*. 2012;40(6):1523–1530.

9. Jordan AS, Wellman A, Edwards JK, et al. Respiratory control stability and upper airway collapsibility in men and women with obstructive sleep apnea. *J Appl Physiol (1985)*. 2005;99(5):2020–2027.

10. Eckert DJ, White DP, Jordan AS, Malhotra A, Wellman A. Defining phenotypic causes of obstructive sleep apnea. Identification of novel therapeutic targets. *Am J Respir Crit Care Med*. 2013;188(8):996–1004.

11. Dempsey JA, Smith CA. Pathophysiology of human ventilatory control. *Eur Respir J*. 2014;44(2):495–512.

12. Dempsey JA. Crossing the apnoeic threshold: causes and consequences. *Exp Physiol*. 2005;90(1):13–24.

13. Ayappa I, Rapoport DM. The upper airway in sleep: physiology of the pharynx. *Sleep Med Rev.* 2003;7(1):9–33.

14. Haxhiu MA, Mitra J, van Lunteren E, Prabhakar N, Bruce EN, Cherniack NS. Responses of hypoglossal and phrenic nerves to decreased respiratory drive in cats. *Respiration.* 1986;50(2):130–138.

15. Nakayama H, Smith CA, Rodman JR, Skatrud JB, Dempsey JA. Effect of ventilatory drive on carbon dioxide sensitivity below eupnea during sleep. *Am J Respir Crit Care Med.* 2002;165(9):1251–1260.

16. Fitzpatrick MF, Driver HS, Chatha N, Voduc N, Girard AM. Partitioning of inhaled ventilation between the nasal and oral routes during sleep in normal subjects. *J Appl Physiol.* 2003;94(3):883–890.

17. Fitzpatrick MF, McLean H, Urton AM, Tan A, O'Donnell D, Driver HS. Effect of nasal or oral breathing route on upper airway resistance during sleep. *Eur Respir J.* 2003;22(5):827–832.

18. Wilson SL, Thach BT, Brouillette RT, Abu-Osba YK. Upper airway patency in the human infant: influence of airway pressure and posture. *J Appl Physiol.* 1980;48(3):500–504.

19. Safar P, Escarraga LA, Chang F. Upper airway obstruction in the unconscious patient. *J Appl Physiol.* 1959;14:760–764.

20. Pevernagie DA, Stanson AW, Sheedy PF, Daniels BK, Shepard JW, Jr. Effects of body position on the upper airway of patients with obstructive sleep apnea. *Am J Respir Crit Care Med.* 1995;152(1):179–185.

21. Fouke JM, Strohl KP. Effect of position and lung volume on upper airway geometry. *J Appl Physiol.* 1987;63(1):375–380.

22. Koenig JS, Thach BT. Effects of mass loading on the upper airway. *J Appl Physiol.* 1988;64(6):2294–2299.

23. Wang SH, Keenan BT, Wiemken A, et al. Effect of weight loss on upper airway anatomy and the apnea-hypopnea index. The importance of tongue fat. *Am J Respir Crit Care Med.* 2020;201(6):718–727.

24. Rowley JA, Sanders CS, Zahn BR, Badr MS. Effect of REM sleep on retroglossal cross-sectional area and compliance in normal subjects. *J Appl Physiol (1985).* 2001;91(1):239–248.

25. Isono S, Feroah TR, Hajduk EA, Brant R, Whitelaw WA, Remmers JE. Interaction of cross-sectional area, driving pressure, and airflow of passive velopharynx. *J Appl Physiol.* 1997;83(3):851–859.

26. Wellman A, Edwards BA, Sands SA, et al. A simplified method for determining phenotypic traits in patients with obstructive sleep apnea. *J Appl Physiol (1985).* 2013;114(7):911–922.

27. Croft CB, Pringle M. Sleep nasendoscopy: a technique of assessment in snoring and obstructive sleep apnoea. *Clin Otolaryngol Allied Sci.* 1991;16(5):504–509.

28. Fogel RB, Trinder J, White DP, et al. The effect of sleep onset on upper airway muscle activity in patients with sleep apnoea versus controls. *J Physiol.* 2005;564(Pt 2):549–562.

29. Smith PL, Wise RA, Gold AR, Schwartz AR, Permutt S. Upper airway pressure-flow relationships in obstructive sleep apnea. *J Appl Physiol.* 1988;64(2):789–795.

30. Schwartz AR, Smith PL, Wise RA, Gold AR, Permutt S. Induction of upper airway occlusion in sleeping individuals with subatmospheric nasal pressure. *J Appl Physiol (1985).* 1988;64(2):535–542.

31. Gleadhill IC, Schwartz AR, Schubert N, Wise RA, Permutt S, Smith PL. Upper airway collapsibility in snorers and in patients with obstructive hypopnea and apnea. *Am Rev Respir Dis.* 1991;143(6):1300–1303.

32. Sands SA, Edwards BA, Terrill PI, et al. Phenotyping pharyngeal pathophysiology using polysomnography in patients with obstructive sleep apnea. *Am J Respir Crit Care Med.* 2018;197(9):1187–1197.

33. Series F, Cormier Y, Lampron N, La Forge J. Influence of lung volume in sleep apnoea. *Thorax.* 1989;44(1):52–57.

34. Peppard PE, Ward NR, Morrell MJ. The impact of obesity on oxygen desaturation during sleep-disordered breathing. *Am J Respir Crit Care Med.* 2009;180(8):788–793.

35. Marcus CL. Sleep-disordered breathing in children. *Am J Respir Crit Care Med.* 2001;164(1):16–30.

36. Salome CM, King GG, Berend N. Physiology of obesity and effects on lung function. *J Appl Physiol.* 2010;108(1):206–211.

37. Owens RL, Malhotra A, Eckert DJ, White DP, Jordan AS. The influence of end-expiratory lung volume on measurements of pharyngeal collapsibility. *J Appl Physiol.* 2010;108(2):445–451.

38. Jordan AS, White DP, Owens RL, et al. The effect of increased genioglossus activity and end-expiratory lung volume on pharyngeal collapse. *J Appl Physiol (1985).* 2010;109(2):469–475.

39. Squier SB, Patil SP, Schneider H, Kirkness JP, Smith PL, Schwartz AR. Effect of end-expiratory lung volume on upper airway collapsibility in sleeping men and women. *J Appl Physiol.* 2010;109(4):977–985.

40. Braga CW, Chen Q, Burschtin OE, Rapoport DM, Ayappa I. Changes in lung volume and upper airway using MRI during application of nasal expiratory positive airway pressure in patients with sleep-disordered breathing. *J Appl Physiol (1985).* 2011;111(5):1400–1409.

41. Berthon-Jones M, Sullivan CE. Ventilatory and arousal responses to hypoxia in sleeping humans. *Am Rev Respir Dis.* 1982;125(6):632–639.

42. Berthon-Jones M, Sullivan CE. Ventilation and arousal responses to hypercapnia in normal sleeping

humans. *J Appl Physiol Respir Environ Exerc Physiol.* 1984;57(1):59–67.

43. Khoo MC, Koh SS, Shin JJ, Westbrook PR, Berry RB. Ventilatory dynamics during transient arousal from NREM sleep: implications for respiratory control stability. *J Appl Physiol (1985).* 1996;80(5):1475–1484.

44. Younes M. Role of arousals in the pathogenesis of obstructive sleep apnea. *Am J Respir Crit Care Med.* 2004;169(5):623–633.

45. Younes M. Pathogenesis of obstructive sleep apnea. *Clin Chest Med.* 2019;40(2):317–330.

46. Shepard JW, Jr., Pevernagie DA, Stanson AW, Daniels BK, Sheedy PF. Effects of changes in central venous pressure on upper airway size in patients with obstructive sleep apnea. *Am J Respir Crit Care Med.*153(1):250–254.

47. Yumino D, Redolfi S, Ruttanaumpawan P, et al. Nocturnal rostral fluid shift: a unifying concept for the pathogenesis of obstructive and central sleep apnea in men with heart failure. *Circulation.* 2010;121(14):1598–1605.

48. Mezzanotte WS, Tangel DJ, White DP. Influence of sleep onset on upper-airway muscle activity in apnea patients versus normal controls. *Am J Respir Crit Care Med.* 1996;153(6 Pt 1):1880–1887.

49. Edwards BA, Sands SA, Eckert DJ, et al. Acetazolamide improves loop gain but not the other physiological traits causing obstructive sleep apnoea. *J Physiol.* 2012;590(5):1199–1211.

50. Edwards BA, Andara C, Landry S, et al. Upper-airway collapsibility and loop gain predict the response to oral appliance therapy in patients with obstructive sleep apnea. *Am J Respir Crit Care Med.* 2016;194(11):1413–1422.

51. Oudiette D, Dodet P, Ledard N, et al. Author correction: REM sleep respiratory behaviours match mental content in narcoleptic lucid dreamers. *Sci Rep.* 2018;8(1):6128.

52. Xi L, Chow CM, Smith CA, Dempsey JA. Effects of REM sleep on the ventilatory response to airway occlusion in the dog. *Sleep.* 1994;17(8):674–687.

53. Douglas NJ, White DP, Weil JV, Pickett CK, Zwillich CW. Hypercapnic ventilatory response in sleeping adults. *Am Rev Respir Dis.* 1982;126(5):758–762.

54. Jordan AS, White DP, Lo YL, et al. Airway dilator muscle activity and lung volume during stable breathing in obstructive sleep apnea. *Sleep.* 2009;32(3):361–368.

55. Lo YL, Jordan AS, Malhotra A, et al. Influence of wakefulness on pharyngeal airway muscle activity. *Thorax.* 2007;62(9):799–805.

56. Carberry JC, Jordan AS, White DP, Wellman A, Eckert DJ. Upper airway collapsibility (Pcrit) and pharyngeal dilator muscle activity are sleep stage dependent. *Sleep.* 2016;39(3):511–521.

9 Risk and Causality by Genetics, Gender, and Age

Moshe Y Prero, Nardine Zakhary, Sally Ibrahim, and Kingman P Strohl

INTRODUCTION

Clinically, obstructive sleep apnea hypopnea syndrome (OSAHS) is defined by symptoms of unrefreshing and disturbed sleep, loud snorts and snoring, daytime impairment from sleepiness and/or a fatigue-like state and a certain number (usually >5/hr) of obstructive apneas and hypopnea per hour (apnea-hypopnea index or AHI), and resolution of these features by treatment of upper airway obstruction during sleep. The condition is relieved most directly by tracheostomy (1) or by excellent adherence to continuous positive airway pressure (CPAP) (2), two treatments where substantial evidence for effectiveness exists.

OSAHS is relatively common, as other chapters will detail. The condition is the result of arousals from sleep, falls in oxygen saturation in the presence of a rise in carbon dioxide, and greater negative intrathoracic pressures (3) that produce the symptoms and signs of this illness. The categories of impairment are related to quality of life, including drowsiness and fall asleep crashes and accidents (4), metabolic syndrome (5), and cardiovascular disease—hypertension, stroke, arrhythmia, coronary artery disease, etc. (6, 7). There is also a link to cancer progression and to al-cause death (8, 9). Whether sleep apnea is an active driver or passenger in these associated health conditions or acting in a bidirectional manner is not always clear and there are scenarios where an outcome for a person with a sleep study is predicated based on one or a cluster of features other than AHI itself (10).

Prospectively there appears to be a dose-response association between AHI at baseline and the presence of hypertension 4 years later, independent of known confounding factors (11). If everyone sleeps and has some apneas, how then does one propagate apneas over time to categories of mild >5–<15 (every 4–12 min), moderate >15 <30 (every 2–4 min), severe >30 (one every 2 min or less), or even more >60/hr (>1 every minute). These numbers do matter to some degree. Relative to a reference of an AHI of 0/hr, the presence of hypertension at follow-up for an AHI 1 to <5/hr was 1.42 (CI 1.13–1.78), for 5–14.9/hr 2.03 (CI 1.29–3.17), and for >15/hr 2.89 (CI 1.46–5.64) (11). This finding prompts one to consider how a person arrives as an adult to the AHI severity categories.

A direct but modest trend for increasing AHI is found with increasing obesity (body mass index (BMI)) and with age estimated in 5-year increments above the age of 50 years (12, 13). Yet, many suspect that the origins of adult OSAHS occur earlier. There are few long-term observational studies of individuals spanning the ages of 18 to about 55 years, this age being the most common mean or median age found in many cohorts including the initial reports from the Wisconsin Sleep Cohort (14) and the Sleep Heart Health Study (15, 16). It is difficult to "look back" at the trajectory of disease, and one is left to suppose which causal pathway drove the propagation of sleep apnea, as captured by AHI, over time.

This chapter is intended to address risk and causality for OSAHS in regard to three features—genetics, gender, and age (Figure 9.1). This limited set is chosen to represent reasonable examples in which to address causal pathways. Other chapters will discuss these and other constitutional traits, symptom drivers, and all current and proposed treatments in greater detail, including the need for lifelong chronic care. The emphasis here is on the causes for event rates during sleep in regard to genetics, gender, and age rather than the consequences of these events.

CAUSALITY AND RISK

The causal pathways leading to multiple apneas during sleep are different from risk factors like age, weight, gender, genetics, co-morbidity, etc., which are equally present during wakefulness and sleep. Reviewing the literature on this physiology will set the stage for the discussion of the epidemiology of OSAHS in regard to the clinical definition of personal risk.

Sleep ironically is both a need as well as a risk and cause. If one were not to sleep, one would not have sleep apnea. To be sure, disordered breathing occurs in wakefulness with chest, heart, and neuromuscular disease. While these conditions in wakefulness hardly get better during sleep, the diagnosis of these various conditions does not need sleep in its definition. Some sleep-disordered breathing and specifically sleep apnea/hypopnea is normal in adulthood, most often in the periods of the transition from wakefulness to sleep, after a sigh or arousal, and in REM sleep, particularly during the eye movements and muscle twitches of phasic rather than tonic

DOI: 10.1201/9781003000631-11

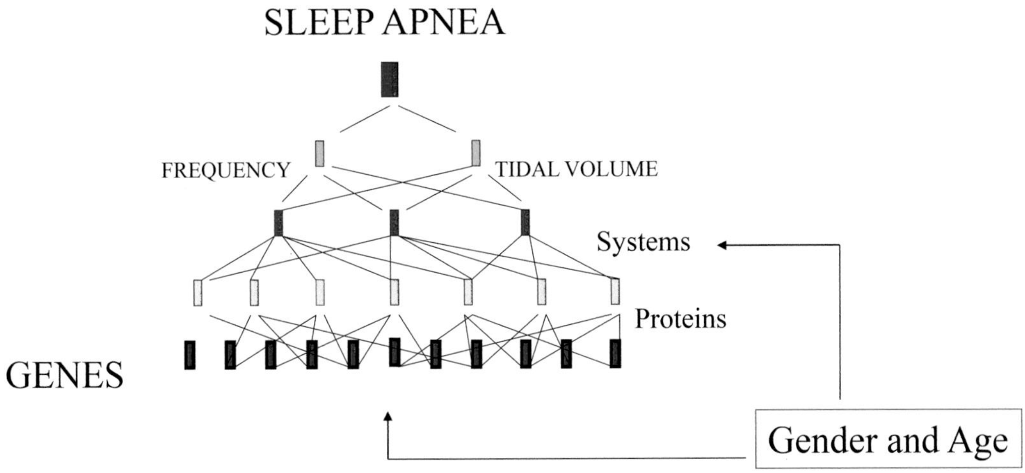

Figure 9.1 This chapter addresses the features of genes, gender and age on the expression of obstructive sleep apnea. This figure illustrates the points of discussion by indicating that the origins of illness are the genetic set and through the biology of the proteins and physiological systems, one creates breathing. Sleep-disordered breathing and specifically obstructive apnea is a disorder of the control of breathing. Gender and age have both genetic and systems influences. Hence, sleep apnea is a complex disease. In the absence of an overwhelming genetic or environmental effect, its expression is the result of common mutations that by themselves are neither necessary nor sufficient but interact to tip the balance toward disease.

REM. As well, there might be some snoring, but transitions across stages are relatively smooth. As for the numbers of events during sleep, the rule of thumb is that health is <5/hr, or 1 every 12 minutes; however, events are usually not evenly spaced but clustered in a vulnerable period (3).

In the past 10 years, we have gained a better sense of how to define causality for the expression of recurrent apneas in patient with a pre-test probability of OSAHS (17, 18). These features cluster into about four categories: the thresholds for arousals from sleep, one anatomic property of closing pressure of the upper airway (Pcrit), the recruitment or gain function of muscles that act to maintain airway patency, and the tendency for a breathing disturbance to "set up" for another apnea, a feature of system gain often called "loop gain" (Figure 9.2).

Sleep is accompanied by a reduction in ventilatory drive, and changes in state and arousals often terminate apneas; both are mechanisms that promote instability in breathing. An arousal can shorten events but also rapidly and suddenly increase "gain." However, a longer time to arousal from sleep might increase the chance chemo-or mechano-reflexes to maintain patency and reduce an abrupt arousal (19, 20). In any event, OSAHS starts with sleep; however, individual variation in the magnitude of these responses plays a

role in the expression of apneas. For instance, in NREM sleep, chemoresponsiveness is lower than in wakefulness, explaining in part the instability in breathing at sleep onset; however, in REM sleep, chemosensitivity falls even furthermore. Nevertheless, the greater the fall in ventilation from wake to NREM sleep, the greater the relative amount of NREM AHI to REM AHI (21). In this way, sleep itself not only gives the disorder its name but the changes in ventilatory control in a given sleep state set up the opportunity for instability.

A physiologic surrogate representing upper airway *anatomy* is its critical closing pressure, also called Pcrit. It is relevant to the expression of obstructive apnea. If drive falls and the transluminal pressure remains above closing pressure, any apnea will be a non-obstructive one, i.e. a central apnea. If, however, the upper airway tube is collapsible (a positive Pcrit), an obstructive apnea will ensue when the drive to stabilize muscles is reduced. There are multiple contributions to Pcrit, but CPAP counteracts the closing tendency (positive Pcrit) (22). Changes in Pcrit are known to be affected by risk factors like obesity and probably by inflammation, edema, trauma to tissues, etc. (3).

Recruitment of muscles is a physiologic term referring to the direct and reflex mechanism for recovery of upper airway patency through muscle activation effects on size and/or compliance. There may be an inherent gain of

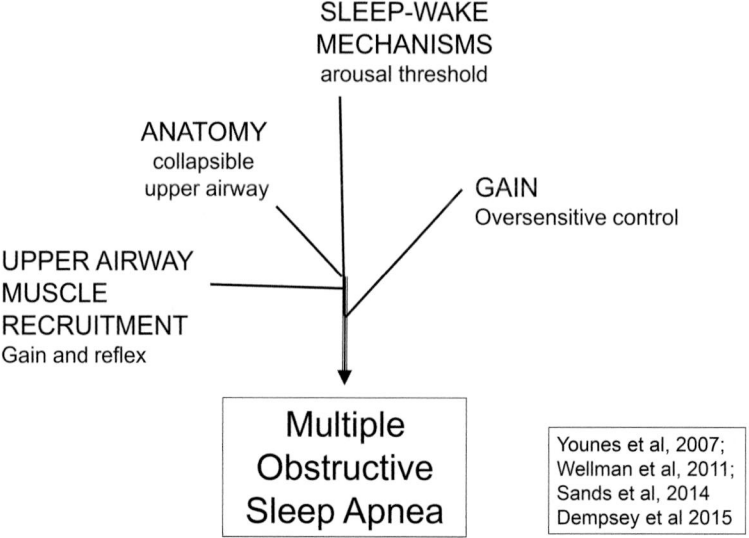

Figure 9.2 Causal pathways in the generation of multiple obstructive apneas are shown as a cascade from sleep and its features, as modified by anatomy, gain of ventilatory controller and the controlled system, and the specific control of upper airway muscle which are needed to keep a vulnerable airway channel open.

recruitment in an individual or deficits might be acquired (23). Impaired reflex recruitment could occur through blunting over time of sensory feedback by vibration injury or by disorders like diabetes (24–26). Furthermore, muscle efferent output must be translated into airway stability, and more muscle tone may be needed in the presence of airway wall edema (27).

The gain of a response to a disturbance like apnea is important. This is referred to as gain or "loop gain," a term encompassing the feedback response of the ventilatory system (the controller and the controlled lungs, chest wall, and upper airway structures, or plant). A high response loop gain can cause the system to oscillate (18, 28, 29). Gain can be quantified as a ratio of the size of a correction or response divided by the size of the prior disturbance.

For example, if ventilation falls for a period of time, ventilation will increase when the event is terminated. A high gain refers to the inability to rapidly return to steady state after a disturbance like an apnea, and a number of studies indicate that high loop gain is a factor for producing recurrent apneas (19, 30) (Figure 9.3).

Sleep is critical. Pcrit, as a marker of anatomy, upper airway muscle recruitment, and loop gain alone or in combination with sleep mechanisms of arousals and sleep stage, contribute to the level of severity and/or development of OSAHS. However, longitudinal studies directed at changes in AHI over time are few, based more on distal risk traits,

namely obesity, age, hypertension, etc., than mechanisms.

GENETIC SET POINTS

The role of inheritance of genetics is invoked as an explanation for a number of paradoxes that confound understanding of clinical cohorts as an individual's risk is a combination of genetic elements, some increasing and some decreasing trait values. First, while sleep apnea can be a normal event during sleep and a numerical marker of a disease state, the number is very loosely correlated to clinical severity. Second, at any given category of numerical severity, there are variable correlations with the sequelae-hypertension, sleepiness, etc. Third, major risk factors for adult sleep apnea such as obesity, cardiovascular disease, etc., have bidirectional effects in that each influences the development of the other. Fourth, our most effective current therapies target anatomic features when the goal is really to maintain some stability of respiratory control during sleep.

Human apnea cohorts contain substantive genetic contributions (~40%) in AHI as a marker for sleep apnea (31, 32); in comparison, these estimates are lower than for apnea of prematurity, ~85% (33). The practical payoffs in the larger and larger gene discovery human cohorts have not occurred in part because common phenotypes are generally apnea number (AHI) captured at one moment in people ascertained by clinical pre-test

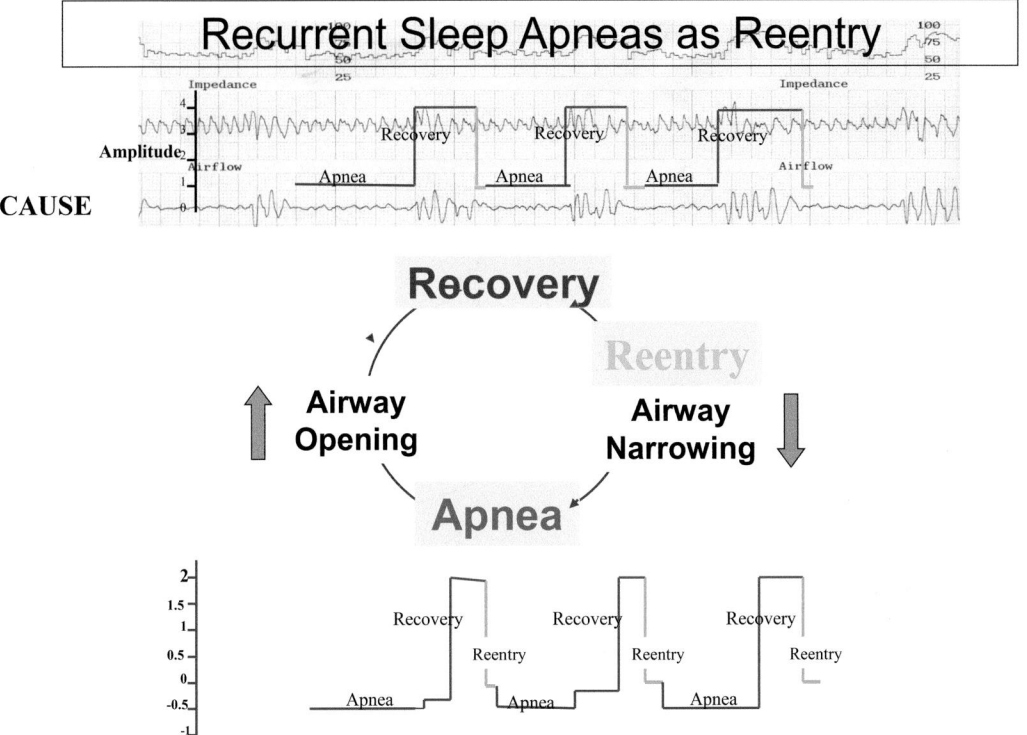

CAUSE

Adapted from Lynn, 1998

Figure 9.3 Recurrent Apnea over time is a cycle of events in which the individual has recurrent apneas. There is a recovery from the first event and the reentry into the next. Airway closure occurs at this point leading to apnea, recovery, and reentry. The extent of recovery is a controller property, influenced by posture, REM-NREM transitions, etc.

or epidemiologic risk. AHI reflects upper airway anatomy, body habitus, state, and respiratory control, each of which has its own set of genes for development, remodeling, and senescence of the organs and communication networks, and features occur both in and out of association with OSA (Figure 9.4). Nevertheless, published candidate markers point to interacting, metabolic regulatory pathways, with associations to diabetes, obesity, and heart disease; however, these analyses often rely on consequences—oxygen saturation or AHI and not the physiologic causal subtypes (34). The reader is directed at representative studies of AHI and oxygenation traits that indicate the complexity of finding and establishing genes in adult OSA (35–38). The *de novo* identification in the adult of strong causal set points for the development of sleep-disordered breathing will be difficult because no one gene contributes a lot (>5%–10%) and polygenes have modifying effects (1%–3%). It is also possible that a causal gene effect size will depend upon aging, length

of illness, or epigenetic modification by OSA consequences.

Identification of risk factor susceptibility in the adult patient with several years of illness is difficult given the multifaceted complexities apparent in the environmental as well as genetic heterogeneity of human populations.

Molecular domains associated with sympathetic activity, oxidative stress, and inflammation are present in some but not all cross-sectional studies (39). Genetics are underpowered, and causal vs. consequential genetic effectors are not distinguished in these studies (40). Presumably, adult OSAHS patients with central or obstructive apneas have other genes and complex pathways which affect rhythmogenesis and loop gain but do so in a subtle and cumulative fashion. Effect size might be small in either promotion or reduction of apneas, but in a given individual, the presence of a major gene with 5%–10% effect might need complementary effect sizes of 10–50 polymorphisms with 2% effect size, leading

121

Shared Genetic Variance

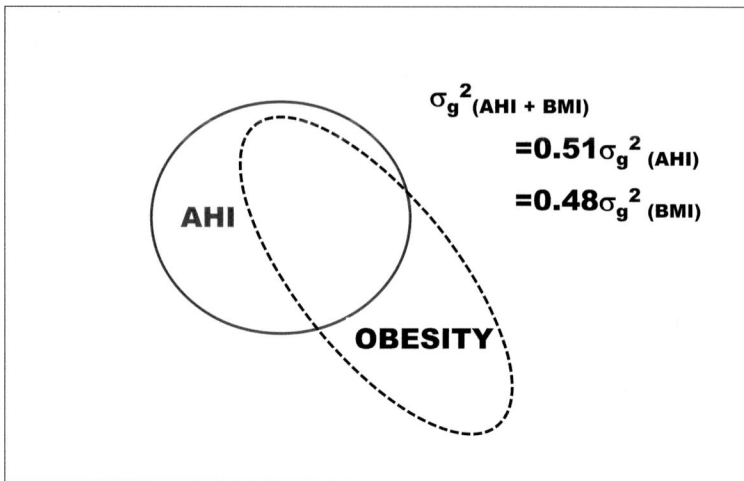

Figure 9.4 Genetic origins for OSA are in all the physiologic systems, some of which can be shared in a given patient. One can have sleep apnea without obesity and obesity without sleep apnea. In a Caucasian/African American population of mild to moderate OSA, the estimates of AHI were about 50% and those for obesity (BMI) about the same (90). In this same cohort, however, there was no significant shared genetic variance with some measures of craniofacial traits.

to an additive inheritance effect of 40% in the general adult OSA population (32, 41).

There are relatively strong genes that can be found in adult OSA cohorts but many were first discovered in childhood congenital disorders and then examined for effect in adult relatives, finding effects with variable or dependent penetrance, or taking some time for its actions to come to clinical attention. Table 9.1 presents some of the known genetic syndromes that could present at birth; however, once identified, some mild childhood conditions appear in adulthood. One pathway, PHOX2b, was identified originally through an unbiased association of genetic polymorphisms to disease traits in childhood and led to the identification of parental phenotypes of sleep apnea and hypoventilation after the diagnosis of the child (42). Now parents of such patients are found to have apneas and hypoventilation with shorter polyalanine repeats. Other genetic syndromes, like Pierre Robin Prader-Willi, and Down syndrome, while recognizable at an early age, can appear with symptomatic sleep-disordered breathing in young adulthood or even later (43, 44). Pompe disease can be noticed in childhood; however, there are those who present in early adulthood, and this condition should be part of the differential diagnosis of adult hypoventilation syndromes. The recognition of Pompe disease is important now that there is enzyme replacement therapy (45,

46). Ehlers-Danlos syndrome, especially in its more mild presentations, may go undiagnosed in childhood (47).

Such clusters of causal genes one estimates form less than 1% of all adult presentations for sleep-disordered breathing.

GENDER AND TRANSGENDER

Women and men differ in the various presentations of sleep apnea. Women are more likely to present with insomnia symptoms when compared with men, and women use higher health care utilization, physician visits, and hospitalization prior to diagnosis (48). Women have higher co-morbid insomnia and Restless Legs syndrome, which may confuse recognition of OSA and management (49). There are also differences in symptom mitigation in which treatment by CPAP in women often reduces symptoms of chronic insomnia disorder more commonly in women vs. men (50). This field of differential presentations and responses probably has its origins in both the biological and behavioral aspects of gender. This chapter is to present the origins and the causes for such OSA differences.

The literature is rather clear in that there is a greater susceptibility in men to snoring, at least up until decades after women experience menopause. The values that are generally cited are on the order of 17% of women and

Table 9.1: Listing of Some Genetic Syndromes Associated with OSA According to Causal Pathways

	Condition	Location	Gene/Locus	OMIM#
Primary Sleep				
	Narcolepsy	17q21.2	HCRT	161400
	Prader-Willi syndrome	15q11.2	SNRPN	176270
Anatomy				
	Recognition at Birth			
	Pfeiffer syndrome	10q26.13	FGFR2	101600
	Crouzon syndrome	10q26.13	FGFR2	123500
	Apert syndrome	10q26.13	FGFR2	101200
	Pierre Robin syndrome	17q24.3-q25.1		261800
	Treacher Collins syndrome	5p32-q33	TCOF1	154500
	Achondroplasia	4p16.3	FGFR3	100800
	Recognition in Second Decade or Later			
	Down syndrome	21q22.3		190685
	Hunter syndrome	Xq28	IDS	309900
	Beckwith-Wiedemann syndrome	11p15.5	ICR1	130650
	Pompe disease	17q25.3	GAA	232300
	Ehlers-Danlos syndrome	9q34.3	COL5A1	130000
	Marfan syndrome	15q21.1	FBN1	154700
Gain				
	Congenital Central Hypoventilation syndrome	4p13	PHOX2B	209880
	Familial Dysautonomia	9q31.3	ELP1	223900
	Rett syndrome	Xq28	MECP2	312750
Muscles				
	Myotonic dystrophy type 1	19q13.32	DMPK	160900
	Myotonic dystrophy type 2	3q21.3	CNBP	602668
	Spinal muscle atrophy	5q13.2	SMN1	253300
	Spinocerebellar Atxia 3	14q32.12	ATXN3	109150
	Charcot-Marie-tooth disease	17p12	PMP22	118220
Sleep, Anatomy, and Gain Pathways				
	Smith-Lemli-Opitz syndrome	11q12.4	DHCR7	270400
	Williams-Beuren syndrome	7q11.23	TMEM270	612547
	Friedreich Ataxia	9q21.11	FXN	229300

22% of men, if the threshold is an AHI of ≥5 (14). Recognition strategies for sleep apnea that include male sex (1 point for male and 0 for female) have a greater positive predictive value, although the relative proportion of risk in a multivariate tool like the STOP-BANG is modest (51). The obvious mechanism is a hormonal one and the potentially protective effects of progesterone and estrogen, as opposed to an enhancing effect of testosterone in males. This is generally the case, although from the point-of-view of this chapter, the considerations of hormones in health are distal factors. Indeed, hormones have genetic and developmental origins, producing acquired characteristics like fat distribution and ventilatory control and temporary states like menstrual cycles or pregnancy (52).

Besides a generally lower prevalence of OSA in women, one Chinese hypertensive population study found that OSA prevalence is related to age in women and BMI in men (53). In a population from two prospective cohort studies, Nurses' Health Study and Nurses' Health Study II, the pooled hazard ratio associated with OSA was 1.27 (CI: 1.17, 1.38) in women who underwent surgical menopause (by means of hysterectomy or oophorectomy) compared with natural menopause. The hazard ratio was essentially unchanged even when

Gender

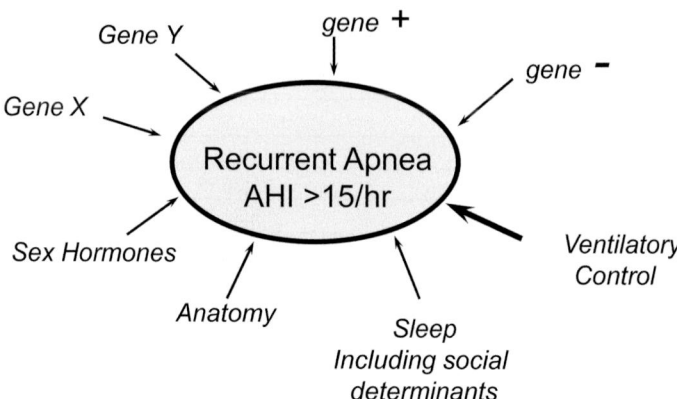

Figure 9.5 In regard to gender, there are a number of "external" factors that will produce a clinical disorder. Some are inherent and some are external to the individual. Some genes or hormones will increase and others will decrease the AHI trait value.

considering age at menopause. Among the surgical menopause group, the OSA risk was higher among non-obese women. Interestingly, among women who never used hormone therapy, AHI and hypertension risk was lower than those who had used hormone therapy. Surgical as compared with natural menopause was independently associated with higher OSA risk in women in the postmenopausal phase of life (52). These cohort studies indicate clinical risk.

Regarding causal pathways for recurrent OSA, there are some general points in the literature concerning the variability among individuals and the lack of measures of pathways in drug trials or interesting case series comparisons (Figure 9.5).

Sleep architecture is different between genders. A progressive decline in N3 sleep occurs earlier and with a steeper decline in men than in women; however, sleep fragmentation and rapid eye movement sleep were both not significantly different when comparing these two age groups (54). Nevertheless, studies examining how the arousal threshold changes with age have found little difference, suggesting that aging does not have a major impact on the threshold. State instability, however, appears more common in the older population, giving opportunity for ventilatory instability.

Known co-morbid chronic diseases can have a substantial impact on sleep length and depth and stability. Sleep architecture is more commonly modified in women compared

with men in certain conditions. For example, young women have a greater delta response to sleep deprivation and more sleep architectural changes associated with depression. Women seem to exhibit and may require more biological flexibility and adaption mechanisms under the challenging conditions of hormonal cycles, pregnancy and childrearing, and menopause (55).

While the prevalence in women of an overall AHI >5 is low on any given night, women have a greater tendency for REM-related OSA, especially evident in those under 50 years of age (56). These results suggest that hormonal changes in women might play some role in REM-related OSA. Perhaps the fall in ventilation with sleep is low and does not trigger apnea-hypopnea events at sleep onset or in unstable breathing periods of state transition in women. Reports from several cohorts suggest that all other things being equal, in women, events are expressed preferentially when muscle tone is lowest (57). Alternatively, it is possible that hormonal status confers differences in REM control of breathing so that in the postmenopausal period, women and men have a more similar tendency to have REM apnea (58). Increased pharyngeal resisting at menopause may affect susceptibility (59).

Muscle recruitment may not play a large role. In a comparison of healthy men and women, no gender difference was present in the resting level of peak inspiratory genioglossal activation, nor a gender or gender-by-time interaction during a hypoxic stimulus (59).

The recruitment was not different during sleep in patients with OSA compared with control subjects (19).However, it is possible that in a given individual, the ability to translate upper airway neural drive to breathe may be important in pathogenesis.

In men and women with severe OSA, *gain* estimates were made during stable supine non-rapid eye movement sleep. In AHI-matched women, there was a higher BMI, but loop gain values were similar between men and women. When matched for BMI, women had less severe OSA during NREM sleep; however, gain values were not different between genders (60). These results do not support an important general effect of this pathway.

RELATED SYNDROMES AND INTERVENTIONS

Polycystic Ovarian Syndrome (PCOS)

This is a within gender difference, as PCOS is a reproductive, endocrine, and metabolic disorder affecting millions of women worldwide. Women with PCOS present with oligomenorrhea, hirsutism, or infertility. The health risks associated with PCOS extend to diabetes mellitus, dyslipidemia, obesity, hypertension, metabolic syndrome, depression, anxiety, nonalcoholic fatty liver disease, endometrial cancer, and cardiovascular disease, in both reproductive-age and older women with PCOS (61, 62). In PCOS, there are bi-directional interactions among the presence and severity of OSA and the metabolic disturbances (63).

Hormone Manipulation

One of the first studies tried progestin and estrogen (medroxyprogesterone acetate, 20 mg tid, and Premarin, 1.25 mg bid) in nine 50-year-old ovariectomized women. This positive report indicated that after 1 wk with placebo (lactose) vs. combined administration, there was a reduction in AHI from 15 +/−4 to 3 +/−1, along with a reduction in event duration (64). However, these results have not been generally replicated. In another placebo-controlled prospective HRT trial in a clinical laboratory (65), estrogen monotherapy was associated with a ~50% reduction in AHI, but estradiol plus progesterone relative to baseline was not statistically different. Total sleep time and non-rapid eye movement sleep time with oxygen saturation less than 90% were no different between baseline and drug conditions. A 6-month study of an estrogen-progesterone combination in premenopausal and late postmenopausal women had only random and marginal effects on sleep and in the direction of mostly unfavorable for EPT (66). In another example, despite a doubling of serum estrogen level, the change is in AHI was small and clinically insignificant and only suggesting a greater number in REM sleep. There was no difference in a group given estrogen plus progesterone group (67). Perhaps longer therapy duration or alternative formulations, a high dose, or engineered drugs that target hormone response elements in the brainstem rather than reproductive organs might have more lasting effects. Another group suppressed in premenopausal women estrogen and progesterone hormones with daily administration of leuprolide acetate (LA), a gonadotropin-releasing hormone. After drug, menses ceased, and plasma concentrations of estrogen and progesterone plummeted. The participants reported snoring; however, polysomnographic arousal index, sleep fragmentation, and AHI (<5/hr), already low at baseline, did not change (68). In summary, there is insufficient data to suggest hormone replacement therapy as a therapeutic option for sleep-disordered breathing.

Transgender Examples

One component that is truly biological is found in genetic mouse models in which a sex chromosome difference will produce sleep differences. Using four core genotypes (phenotypic female, XX; phenotypic male, XX; phenotypic male, XX: phenotypic male, XY), there are differences in effects of sleep deprivation. For example, following a period of sleep deprivation, females with XY compared with XX sleep more and have higher NREM delta power suggesting that sleep recovery may be partially dependent on sex chromosomes (69). However, in the human, one can look for an effect of hormone therapy on sleep-disordered breathing in transgender patients, but this effect has not been well described (70). A case series reported on three patients undergoing gender reassignment and treated with hormone condition replacement(71). One transgender woman (chromosomal male at birth) with severe obstructive sleep apnea experienced resolution of symptoms following treatment with female sex hormones. Two cases of transgender males (chromosomal female at birth) developed OSAHS following initiation of male sex hormones, and both had pretreatment polysomnography documenting the absence of OSA). These descriptions are interesting in that they represent a rather clear argument for the importance of hormone milieu rather than birth and childhood development effects on acquisition and mitigation of sleep-disordered breathing.

AGE AND AGEISM

Aging is inevitable. Ageism is the knowledge that chronological age is not equivalent to aging and that there is no lockstep progression as measured by the calendar in one or more organs and systems, including those comprising ventilatory control or OSA risk and progression (Figure 9.6).

Excluding the apnea of prematurity, the pediatric prevalence of obstructive sleep apnea as expressed by AHI has two time periods for increased sleep-disordered breathing (12). One is in younger children 2–8 years of age and is associated with adenoids and tonsils and with congenital misalignments of the mandible and midface. There is a second adolescence prevalence peak that is currently more related to obesity (72). After the age of 20–25 years, there are little data until about the fourth or fifth decade, and after that, there is a rise until a late-life plateau (12). Perhaps this is a "survivor effect" in which some individuals are more susceptible to the consequences of OSA

than others so that those more susceptible or with certain comorbid conditions are no longer in the older population. Recent analyses do suggest that AHI alone is not the determinant of mortality, at least in the VA population, an older and predominantly male group (10). In the elderly population, obesity and breathing pauses are less sensitive indicators of sleep-disorder breathing (73).

In a healthy 65-year-old a normal median AHI is about 11/hr with an SD of 7/hr (74). Therefore, as a test, the measurement of AHI has in adults could be age adjusted and the normal range could extend to an AHI of 25/hr (the mean plus 2 SDs). In the Sleep Heart Health Study, it is noteworthy that only 20% of subjects aged over 60 years had an RDI ≥15/hr (4). In addition, 26% of older men in a large cohort of almost 3,000 had an RDI ≥15/hr (75).

As well, individuals who are healthy, non-obese, and asymptomatic for OSA demonstrate a marked increase in the respiratory disturbance index with age, especially for men (76).

Therefore, one must be careful about whether this value of what is generally called "moderate OSA" is imperative to treat in the older population. It should be noted that the

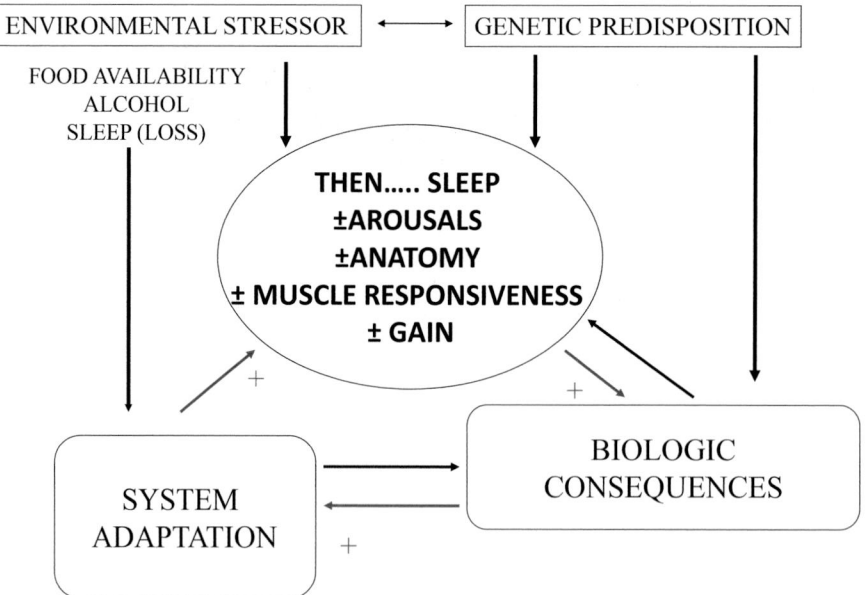

Figure 9.6 The distribution of OSA with aging to adulthood is the sum of environment and its stressors (*left*) and genetic predisposition (*right*). The arrows represent directionality, and most are bidirectional. Genetics in part determines the response to environmental stressors like food availability, alcohol, sleep and its loss, etc. The other elements shown include the causal factors and the biological consequences of OSA on such markers as insulin or inflammatory markers, which affect the individual by adaptation or modification of the systems involved in ventilatory control, for instance, fat accumulation or a change in chemoresponsiveness. These in turn can increase the tendency for recurrent sleep apnea.

Medicare guidelines are for CPAP if the AHI is between 5 and 15 with symptoms, and for an AHI >15, it can be empirically treated without having symptoms. The basis for this recommendation was a function as a convenience guide to approving therapy and is not age-adjusted (77). Good clinical practice remains in that one should not treat a number but a person, and co-morbidity beyond that of sleep-disordered breathing is considered.

The aging process is characterized by cellular and molecular impairments, such as stem cell exhaustion, telomere attrition, and epigenetic changes, that occur with some variation among organs (78) and potentially affect the ventilatory control system at multiple levels of its controller and controlled elements.

OSA potentially modifies functional decline through chronic intermittent hypoxia and sleep fragmentation, and as discussed here and in other chapters in more detail OSA is linked to "lifestyle" diseases like hypertension through these consequences, especially in the older population (79). Two models exist in the extremes when one considers the impact of OSA. One is that OSA is an independent factor, a driver and perhaps a causal one in a process like hypertension or diabetes. The other is that OSA is an amplifier, not affecting per se the origins of the disease but amplifying it so that its expression is earlier, or its severity is greater.

The evidence for OSA being a strong driver comes primarily from studies of interventions, when both are established and causality is implied by an interventional therapy that is directed primarily at the OSA. There are several reviews on these issues and chapters that address the literature. For our purposes, however, one knows that the incidence and prevalence of stroke rise with age, and obstructive sleep apnea, after adjustments, is a moderate and established independent risk factor for stroke (80). However, trials of CPAP for stroke prevention in sleep apnea patients have been largely disappointing. A second chronic disease of aging, dementia, involves a widespread synaptic loss in the neocortex and the hippocampus. Risk factors for dementia including hypertension, hypoperfusion, endothelial dysfunction, inflammation, and oxidative stress, are present in OSA patients. The hippocampus is negatively impacted in both OSA and Alzheimer's disease. OSA promotes hippocampal atrophy, which is associated with memory impairment (81). While there is a recent report that this process is improved by CPAP therapy, there is insufficient evidence that OSA treatment is an effective prevention strategy to reduce risk

for cognitive decline in middle-aged persons and the elderly. The complexity of interactions, however, after a chronic disease like stroke or dementia is present, and the limitations of current OSA therapy are such that new paradigms will be needed, and even then in the end bidirectional interactions may be established at a sub-clinical level.

Sleep-wake pathway. With aging, the total amount of sleep decreases linearly with age with a loss of ~10 minutes per decade (82). The percentage of N3 sleep decreases linearly at 2% per decade. The percentage of REM sleep also slightly diminishes and will plateau after age 60. Sleep efficiency continues to decline due to increasing sleep latency, arousals from sleep, and time awake after sleep onset.

There are more transitions from wake to sleep.

Aging could affect the appearance of OSA by effects on arousal from and reentry into sleep. Indeed, elderly people are known to have an increased number of spontaneous arousals from sleep (83). In late life, men appear to have an increase in time awake and a decrease in light non-REM sleep and REM sleep when compared with midlife men (54), but how this relates to high AHI is not intuitive. In contrast, studies examining directly how the arousal threshold changes with age have found no difference in arousal threshold (84). In addition, even the number of arousals (~20/hr) that are considered pathological is not found in the healthy elderly—~4/hr (83). State length and change could be important, however.

Anatomy Pathway (Pcrit). Upper airway caliber and all dimensions, except at the oropharyngeal junction, decrease modestly with age (85, 86). There may be an increased deposition of parapharyngeal fat in healthy older individuals as compared with younger controls that is independent of BMI (59). Contrasting to static imaging, the published data measuring the effects of aging on pharyngeal resistance and collapsibility are mixed during wakefulness. Thus, it is not surprising that conclusions from the available imaging data about the dynamic predisposition of upper airway toward collapse by dynamic forces or pharyngeal length with age (76).

Muscle Recruitment Pathway. The ability of the genioglossus muscle (the major pharyngeal dilator muscle) to respond to increases in pharyngeal negative pressure is impaired with aging, yielding a more vulnerable airway (87). Although such studies recently reported marked impairment in UA protective reflexes in association with aging, these studies were conducted in healthy subjects during wakefulness. Whether aging influences on pharyngeal airway dilator muscle recruitment are important in mediating a pharyngeal compromise in the elderly is also unclear. One report demonstrated a diminished genioglossus muscle response to hypoxia in association with aging (88), although the mechanistic importance to OSA of this observation is unclear. Nonetheless, UA anatomy and physiology taken in aggregate strongly suggests that susceptibility to OSA appears to worsen with age.

Gain Pathway. There are features in the ventilatory patterning in elderly individuals that suggest that the chemical control of breathing is unstable. For example, an increased proportion of central apneas in elderly patients with sleep apnea have been reported (87). A recent investigation demonstrated that gain values for healthy, elderly patients with or without OSA were quite low (89). The data indicated that ventilatory control is quite stable in the elderly, although the sample size was small. This finding, combined with the uncertainty surrounding the role of changes in the arousal threshold with advancing age, suggests that OSA in the elderly can primarily be attributed to changes in the anatomy and physiology of the upper airway (76).

INTERACTIONS AMONG SET POINTS FOR OSA

Adult OSAHS is a complex disease. This means that no one gene or set of genes or one physiologic process is solely responsible for the closure or near closure of the upper airway during sleep in a sufficient number of patterns that produce an illness. Both being a normal event in healthy sleep and having a fivefold range of values (AHI 20 to >100/hr) considered as representative of clinical concern pose a challenge for those that prefer simple solutions for treatment or policies for prevention. Probably obesity can be called the most common driver or risk, but even then, there are others in which even this measured factor does not work.

REFERENCES

1. Strohl, K. P., N. S. Cherniack and B. Gothe (1986). "Physiologic basis of therapy for sleep apnea." Am Rev Respir Dis **134**(4): 791–802.

2. Schwab, R. J., S. M. Badr, L. J. Epstein, P. C. Gay, D. Gozal, M. Kohler, P. Levy, A. Malhotra, B. A. Phillips, I. M. Rosen, K. P. Strohl, P. J. Strollo, E. M. Weaver and T. E. Weaver (2013). "An official American Thoracic Society statement: continuous positive airway pressure adherence tracking systems. The optimal monitoring strategies and outcome measures in adults." Am J Respir Crit Care Med **188**(5): 613–620.

3. Dempsey, J. A., S. C. Veasey, B. J. Morgan and C. P. O'Donnell (2010). "Pathophysiology of sleep apnea." Physiol Rev **90**(1): 47–112.

4. Baldwin, C. M., K. A. Griffith, F. J. Nieto, G. T. O'Connor, J. A. Walsleben and S. Redline (2001). "The association of sleep-disordered breathing and sleep symptoms with quality of life in the Sleep Heart Health Study." Sleep **24**(1): 96–105.

5. Bonsignore, M. R., C. Esquinas, A. Barcelo, M. Sanchez-de-la-Torre, A. Paterno, J. Duran-Cantolla, J. M. Marin and F. Barbe (2012). "Metabolic syndrome, insulin resistance and sleepiness in real-life obstructive sleep apnoea." Eur Respir J **39**(5): 1136–1143.

6. Kasasbeh, E., D. S. Chi and G. Krishnaswamy (2006). "Inflammatory aspects of sleep apnea and their cardiovascular consequences." South Med J **99**(1): 58–67; quiz 68–59, 81.

7. Kent, B. D., J. F. Garvey, S. Ryan, G. Nolan, J. D. Dodd and W. T. McNicholas (2013). "Severity of obstructive sleep apnoea predicts coronary artery plaque burden: a coronary computed tomographic angiography study." Eur Respir J **42**(5): 1263–1270.

8. Almendros, I., J. M. Montserrat, J. Ramirez, M. Torres, J. Duran-Cantolla, D. Navajas and R. Farre (2012). "Intermittent hypoxia enhances cancer progression in a mouse model of sleep apnoea." Eur Respir J **39**(1): 215–217.

9. Martinez-Garcia, M. A., F. Campos-Rodriguez and R. Farre (2012). "Sleep apnoea and cancer: current insights and future perspectives." Eur Respir J **40**(6): 1315–1317.

10. Zinchuk, A. V., S. Jeon, B. B. Koo, X. Yan, D. M. Bravata, L. Qin, B. J. Selim, K. P. Strohl, N. S. Redeker, J. Concato and H. K. Yaggi (2018). "Polysomnographic phenotypes and their cardiovascular implications in obstructive sleep apnoea." Thorax **73**(5): 472–480.

11. Peppard, P. E., T. Young, M. Palta and J. Skatrud (2000). "Prospective study of the association between sleep-disordered breathing and hypertension." N Engl J Med **342**(19): 1378–1384.

12. Franklin, K. A. and E. Lindberg (2015). "Obstructive sleep apnea is a common disorder in the population-a review on the epidemiology of sleep apnea." J Thorac Dis **7**(8): 1311–1322.

13. Hou, H., Y. Zhao, W. Yu, H. Dong, X. Xue, J. Ding, W. Xing and W. Wang (2018). "Association of obstructive sleep apnea with hypertension: a systematic review and meta-analysis." J Glob Health **8**(1): 010405.

14. Young, T., M. Palta, J. Dempsey, J. Skatrud, S. Weber and S. Bader (1993). "The occurrence of sleep disordered breathing in middle-aged adults." New Engl J Med **328**: 1230–1235.

15. Nieto, F. J., T. B. Young, B. K. Lind, E. Shahar, J. M. Samet, S. Redline, R. B. D'Agostino, A. B. Newman, M. D. Lebowitz and T. G. Pickering (2000). "Association of sleep-disordered breathing, sleep apnea, and hypertension in a large community-based study. Sleep Heart Health Study." JAMA **283**(14): 1829–1836.

16. Shahar, E., C. W. Whitney, S. Redline, E. T. Lee, A. B. Newman, F. J. Nieto, G. T. O'Connor, L. L. Boland, J. E. Schwartz and J. M. Samet (2001). "Sleep-disordered breathing and cardiovascular disease: cross-sectional results of the Sleep Heart Health Study." Am J Respir Crit Care Med **163**(1): 19–25.

17. Wellman, A., D. J. Eckert, A. S. Jordan, B. A. Edwards, C. L. Passaglia, A. C. Jackson, S. Gautam, R. L. Owens, A. Malhotra and D. P. White (2011). "A method for measuring and modeling the physiological traits causing obstructive sleep apnea." J Appl Physiol (1985) **110**(6): 1627–1637.

18. Wellman, A., B. A. Edwards, S. A. Sands, R. L. Owens, S. Nemati, J. Butler, C. L. Passaglia, A. C. Jackson, A. Malhotra and D. P. White (2013). "A simplified method for determining phenotypic traits in patients with obstructive sleep apnea." J Appl Physiol (1985) **114**(7): 911–922.

19. Eckert, D. J., D. P. White, A. S. Jordan, A. Malhotra and A. Wellman (2013). "Defining phenotypic causes of obstructive sleep apnea. Identification of novel therapeutic targets." Am J Respir Crit Care Med **188**(8): 996–1004.

20. Eckert, D. J. and M. K. Younes (2014). "Arousal from sleep: implications for obstructive sleep apnea pathogenesis and treatment." J Appl Physiol 116(3): 302–313.

21. Yamauchi, M., Y. Fujita, M. Kumamoto, M. Yoshikawa, Y. Ohnishi, H. Nakano, K. P. Strohl, and H. Kimura (2015). "Nonrapid eye movement-predominant obstructive sleep apnea: detection and mechanism." J Clin Sleep Med 11(9): 987–993.

22. Oliven, A., E. Kaufman, R. Kaynan, R. Oliven, U. Steinfeld, N. Tov, M. Odeh, L. Gaitini, A. R. Schwartz and E. Kimmel (2010). "Mechanical parameters determining pharyngeal collapsibility in patients with sleep apnea." J Appl Physiol (1985) **109**(4): 1037–1044.

23. Loewen, A., M. Ostrowski, J. Laprairie, R. Atkar, J. Gnitecki, P. Hanly and M. Younes (2009). "Determinants of ventilatory instability in obstructive sleep apnea: inherent or acquired?" Sleep **32**(10): 1355–1365.

24. Kimoff, R. J., E. Sforza, V. Champagne, L. Ofiara and D. Gendron (2001). "Upper airway sensation in snoring and obstructive sleep apnea." Am J Respir Crit Care Med **164**(2): 250–255.

25. Ratnavadivel, R., D. Stadler, S. Windler, J. Bradley, D. Paul, R. D. McEvoy and P. G. Catcheside (2010). "Upper airway function and arousability to ventilatory challenge in slow wave versus stage 2 sleep in obstructive sleep apnoea." Thorax **65**(2): 107–112.

26. Grippo, A., R. Carrai, I. Romagnoli, F. Pinto, F. Fanfulla and A. Sanna (2011). "Blunted respiratory-related evoked potential in awake obstructive sleep apnoea subjects: a NEP technique study." Clin Neurophysiol **122**(8): 1562–1568.

27. Strohl, K. P., J. P. Butler and A. Malhotra (2012). "Mechanical properties of the upper airway." Compr Physiol **2**(3): 1853–1872.

28. Khoo, M. C. (2001). "Using loop gain to assess ventilatory control in obstructive sleep apnea." Am J Respir Crit Care Med **163**(5): 1044–1045.

29. Edwards, B. A., S. A. Sands, D. J. Eckert, D. P. White, J. P. Butler, R. L. Owens, A. Malhotra and A. Wellman (2012). "Acetazolamide improves loop gain but not the other physiological traits causing obstructive sleep apnoea." J Physiol **590**(Pt 5): 1199–1211.

30. Terrill, P. I., B. A. Edwards, S. Nemati, J. P. Butler, R. L. Owens, D. J. Eckert, D. P. White, A. Malhotra, A. Wellman and S. A. Sands (2015). "Quantifying the ventilatory control contribution to sleep apnoea using polysomnography." Eur Respir J **45**(2): 408–418.

31. Strohl, K. P. (1999). "Genetics and the disorders of ventilatory control." Curr Opin Pulm Med **5**(6): 333–334.

32. Palmer, L. J. and S. Redline (2003). "Genomic approaches to understanding obstructive sleep apnea." Respir Physiol Neurobiol **135**(2–3): 187–205.

33. Bloch-Salisbury, E., M. H. Hall, P. Sharma, T. Boyd, F. Bednarek and D. Paydarfar (2010). "Heritability of apnea of prematurity: a retrospective twin study." Pediatrics **126**(4): e779–e787.

34. Edwards, B. A., S. Redline, S. A. Sands and R. L. Owens (2019). "More than the sum of the respiratory events: personalized medicine approaches for obstructive sleep apnea." Am J Respir Crit Care Med **200**(6): 691–703.

35. Wang, H., B. E. Cade, H. Chen, K. J. Gleason, R. Saxena, T. Feng, E. K. Larkin, R. S. Vasan, H. Lin, S. R. Patel, R. P. Tracy, Y. Liu, D. J. Gottlieb, J. E. Below, C. L. Hanis, L. E. Petty, S. R. Sunyaev, A. C. Frazier-Wood, J. I. Rotter, W. Post, X. Lin, S. Redline and X. Zhu (2016). "Variants in angiopoietin-2 (ANGPT2) contribute to variation in nocturnal oxyhaemoglobin saturation level." Hum Mol Genet **25**(23): 5244–5253.

36. Cade, B. E., H. Chen, A. M. Stilp, T. Louie, S. Ancoli-Israel, R. Arens, R. Barfield, J. E. Below, J. Cai, M. P. Conomos, D. S. Evans, A. C. Frazier-Wood, S. A. Gharib, K. J. Gleason, D. J. Gottlieb, D. R. Hillman, W. C. Johnson, D. J. Lederer, J. Lee, J. S. Loredo, H. Mei, S. Mukherjee, S. R. Patel, W. S. Post, S. M. Purcell, A. R. Ramos, K. J. Reid, K. Rice, N. A. Shah, T. Sofer, K. D. Taylor, T. A. Thornton, H. Wang, K. Yaffe, P. C. Zee, C. L. Hanis, L. J. Palmer, J. I. Rotter, K. L. Stone, G. J. Tranah, J. G. Wilson, S. R. Sunyaev, C. C. Laurie, X. Zhu, R. Saxena, X. Lin and S. Redline (2019). "Associations of variants in the hexokinase 1 and interleukin 18 receptor regions with oxyhemoglobin saturation during sleep." PLoS Genet 15(4): e1007739.

37. Dashti, H. S., S. E. Jones, A. R. Wood, J. M. Lane, V. T. van Hees, H. Wang, J. A. Rhodes, Y. Song, K. Patel, S. G. Anderson, R. N. Beaumont, D. A. Bechtold, J. Bowden, B. E. Cade, M. Garaulet, S. D. Kyle, M. A. Little, A. S. Loudon, A. I. Luik, F. Scheer, K. Spiegelhalder, J. Tyrrell, D. J. Gottlieb, H. Tiemeier, D. W. Ray, S. M. Purcell, T. M. Frayling, S. Redline, D. A. Lawlor, M. K. Rutter, M. N. Weedon and R. Saxena (2019). "Genome-wide association study identifies genetic loci for self-reported habitual sleep duration supported by accelerometer-derived estimates." Nat Commun 10(1): 1100.

38. Wang, H., B. E. Cade, T. Sofer, S. A. Sands, H. Chen, S. R. Browning, A. M. Stilp, T. L. Louie, T. A. Thornton, W. C. Johnson, J. E. Below, M. P. Conomos, D. S. Evans, S. A. Gharib, X. Guo, A. C. Wood, H. Mei, K. Yaffe, J. S. Loredo, A. R. Ramos, E. Barrett-Connor, S. Ancoli-Israel, P. C. Zee, R. Arens, N. A. Shah, K. D. Taylor, G. J. Tranah, K. L. Stone, C. L. Hanis, J. G. Wilson, D. J. Gottlieb, S. R. Patel, K. Rice, W. S. Post, J. I. Rotter, S. R. Sunyaev, J. Cai, X. Lin, S. M. Purcell, C. C. Laurie, R. Saxena, S. Redline and X. Zhu (2019). "Admixture mapping identifies novel loci for obstructive sleep apnea in Hispanic/Latino Americans." Hum Mol Genet 28(4): 675–687.

39. Arnardottir, E. S., M. Mackiewicz, T. Gislason, K. L. Teff and A. I. Pack (2009). "Molecular signatures of obstructive sleep apnea in adults: a review and perspective." Sleep 32(4): 447–470.

40. Varvarigou, V., I. J. Dahabreh, A. Malhotra and S. N. Kales (2011). "A review of genetic association studies of obstructive sleep apnea: field synopsis and meta-analysis." Sleep 34(11): 1461–1468.

41. Buxbaum, S. G., R. C. Elston, P. V. Tishler and S. Redline (2002). "Genetics of the apnea hypopnea index in Caucasians and African Americans: I. Segregation analysis." Genet Epidemiol 22(3): 243–253.

42. Weese-Mayer, D. E., E. M. Berry-Kravis, L. Zhou, B. S. Maher, J. M. Silvestri, M. E. Curran and M. L. Marazita (2003). "Idiopathic congenital central hypoventilation syndrome: analysis of genes pertinent to early autonomic nervous system embryologic development and identification of mutations in PHOX2b." Am J Med Genet A 123(3): 267278.

43. Wittig, R. M., F. J. Zorick, T. A. Roehrs, J. M. Sicklesteel and T. Roth (1988). "Familial childhood sleep apnea." Henry Ford Hosp J 36(1): 13–15.

44. Marcus, C. L., T. L. Keens and D. B. Bautista (1991). "Obstructive sleep apnea in children with Down syndrome." Pediatrics 88: 132.

45. Cupler, E. J., K. I. Berger, R. T. Leshner, G. I. Wolfe, J. J. Han, R. J. Barohn and J. T. Kissel (2012). "Consensus treatment recommendations for late-onset Pompe disease." Muscle Nerve 45(3): 319–333.

46. Chan, J., A. K. Desai, Z. B. Kazi, K. Corey, S. Austin, L. D. Hobson-Webb, L. E. Case, H. N. Jones and P. S. Kishnani (2017). "The emerging phenotype of late-onset Pompe disease: A systematic literature review." Mol Genet Metab 120(3): 163–172.

47. Guilleminault, C., M. Primeau, H. Y. Chiu, K. M. Yuen, D. Leger and A. Metlaine (2013). "Sleep-disordered breathing in Ehlers-Danlos syndrome: a genetic model of OSA." Chest 144(5): 1503–1511.

48. Theorell-Haglöw, J., C. B. Miller, D. J. Bartlett, B. J. Yee, H. D. Openshaw and R. R. Grunstein (2018). "Gender differences in obstructive sleep apnoea, insomnia and restless legs syndrome in adults—What do we know? A clinical update." Sleep Med Rev 38: 28–38.

49. Krishnan, V. and N. A. Collop (2006). "Gender differences in sleep disorders." Curr Opin Pulm Med 12(6): 383–389.

50. Loução-de-Amorim, I., C. Bentes and A. R. Peralta (2019). "Men and women with chronic insomnia disorder and OSAS: different responses to CPAP." Sleep Sci 12(3): 190–195.

51. Chung, F., H. R. Abdullah and P. Liao (2016). "STOP-Bang Questionnaire: a practical approach to screen for obstructive sleep apnea." Chest 149(3): 631–638.

52. Huang, T., B. M. Lin, S. Redline, G. C. Curhan, F. B. Hu and S. S. Tworoger (2018). "Type of menopause, age at menopause, and risk of developing obstructive sleep apnea in postmenopausal women." Am J Epidemiol 187(7): 1370–1379.

53. Cai, A., Y. Zhou, J. Zhang, Q. Zhong, R. Wang and L. Wang (2017). "Epidemiological characteristics and gender-specific differences of obstructive sleep apnea in a Chinese hypertensive population: a cross-sectional study." BMC Cardiovasc Disord 17(1): 8.

54. Van Cauter, E., R. Leproult and L. Plat (2000). "Age-related changes in slow wave sleep and REM sleep and relationship with growth hormone and cortisol levels in healthy men." JAMA 284(7): 861–868.

55. Nowakowski, S., J. Meers and E. Heimbach (2013). "Sleep and women's health." Sleep Med Res 4(1): 1–22.

56. Koo, B. B., J. Dostal, O. Ioachimescu and K. Budur (2008). "The effects of gender and age on REM-related sleep-disordered breathing." Sleep Breath 12(3): 259–264.

57. Mano, M., T. Hoshino, R. Sasanabe, K. Murotani, A. Nomura, R. Hori, N. Konishi, M. Baku and T. Shiomi (2019). "Impact of gender and age on rapid eye movement-related obstructive sleep apnea: a clinical study of 3234 Japanese OSA patients." Int J Environ Res Public Health 16(6): 1068.

58. Basoglu, O. K. and M. S. Tasbakan (2018). "Gender differences in clinical and polysomnographic features of obstructive sleep apnea: a clinical study of 2827 patients." Sleep Breath 22(1): 241–249.

59. Eikermann, M., A. S. Jordan, N. L. Chamberlin, S. Gautam, A. Wellman, Y. L. Lo, D. P. White and A. Malhotra (2007). "The influence of aging on pharyngeal collapsibility during sleep." Chest 131(6): 1702–1709.

60. Jordan, A. S., A. Wellman, J. K. Edwards, K. Schory, L. Dover, M. MacDonald, S. R. Patel, R. B. Fogel, A.

Malhotra and D. P. White (2005). "Respiratory control stability and upper airway collapsibility in men and women with obstructive sleep apnea." J Appl Physiol (1985) **99**(5): 2020–2027.

61. Tasali, E., E. Van Cauter and D. A. Ehrmann (2008). "Polycystic ovary syndrome and obstructive sleep apnea." Sleep Med Clin **3**(1): 37–46.

62. Cooney, L. G. and A. Dokras (2018). "Beyond fertility: polycystic ovary syndrome and long-term health." Fertil Steril **110**(5): 794–809.

63. Kahal, H., I. Kyrou, A. A. Tahrani and H. S. Randeva (2017). "Obstructive sleep apnoea and polycystic ovary syndrome: a comprehensive review of clinical interactions and underlying pathophysiology." Clin Endocrinol (Oxf) **87**(4): 313–319.

64. Pickett, C. K., J. G. Regensteiner, W. D. Woodard, D. D. Hagerman, J. V. Weil and L. G. Moore (1989). "Progestin and estrogen reduce sleep-disordered breathing in postmenopausal women." J Appl Physiol (1985) **66**(4): 1656–1661.

65. Manber, R., T. F. Kuo, N. Cataldo and I. M. Colrain (2003). "The effects of hormone replacement therapy on sleep-disordered breathing in postmenopausal women: a pilot study." Sleep **26**(2): 163–168.

66. Kalleinen, N., O. Polo, S. L. Himanen, A. Joutsen and P. Polo-Kantola (2008). "The effect of estrogen plus progestin treatment on sleep: a randomized, placebo-controlled, double-blind trial in premenopausal and late postmenopausal women." Climacteric **11**(3): 233–243.

67. Cistulli, P. A., D. J. Barnes, R. R. Grunstein and C. E. Sullivan (1994). "Effect of short-term hormone replacement in the treatment of obstructive sleep apnoea in postmenopausal women." Thorax **49**(7): 699–702.

68. D'Ambrosio, C., N. S. Stachenfeld, M. Pisani and V. Mohsenin (2005). "Sleep, breathing, and menopause: the effect of fluctuating estrogen and progesterone on sleep and breathing in women." Gend Med **2**(4): 238–245.

69. Mong, J. A. and D. M. Cusmano (2016). "Sex differences in sleep: impact of biological sex and sex steroids." Philos Trans R Soc Lond B Biol Sci **371**(1688): 20150110.

70. Earl, D. C. and L. K. Brown (2019). "On not knowing what we don't know to knowing what we don't know: obstructive sleep apnea in the transgender community." J Clin Sleep Med **15**(10): 1393–1395.

71. Robertson, B. D., B. S. Lerner, J. F. Collen and P. R. Smith (2019). "The effects of transgender hormone therapy on sleep and breathing: a case series." J Clin Sleep Med **15**(10): 1529–1533.

72. Punjabi, N. M. (2008). "The epidemiology of adult obstructive sleep apnea." Proc Am Thorac Soc **5**(2): 136–143.

73. Young, T., P. E. Peppard and D. J. Gottlieb (2002). "Epidemiology of obstructive sleep apnea: a population health perspective." Am J Respir Crit Care Med **165**(9): 1217–1239.

74. Redline, S., B. Briones, K. Spry, P.V. Tishler and D. W. Dockery (1995). "What is a 'normal' respiratory disturbance index?" Am J Respir Crit Care Med **151**: 104.

75. Stone, K. L., T. L. Blackwell, S. Ancoli-Israel, E. Barrett-Connor, D. C. Bauer, J. A. Cauley, K. E. Ensrud, A. R. Hoffman, R. Mehra, M. L. Stefanick, P. D. Varosy, K. Yaffe and S. Redline (2016). "Sleep disordered breathing and risk of stroke in older community-dwelling men." Sleep **39**(3): 531–540.

76. Edwards, B. A., D. M. O'Driscoll, A. Ali, A. S. Jordan, J. Trinder and A. Malhotra (2010). "Aging and sleep: physiology and pathophysiology." Semin Respir Crit Care Med **31**(5): 618–633.

77. Loube, D. I., P. C. Gay, K. P. Strohl, A. I. Pack, D. P. White and N. A. Collop (1999). "Indications for positive airway pressure treatment of adult obstructive sleep apnea patients: a consensus statement." Chest **115**(3): 863–866.

78. Gaspar, L. S., A. R. Álvaro, J. Moita and C. Cavadas (2017). "Obstructive sleep apnea and hallmarks of aging." Trends Mol Med **23**(8): 675–692.

79. Okuro, M. and S. Morimoto (2014). "Sleep apnea in the elderly." Curr Opin Psychiatry **27**(6): 472–477.

80. McDermott, M., D. L. Brown and R. D. Chervin (2018). "Sleep disorders and the risk of stroke." Expert Rev Neurother **18**(7): 523–531.

81. Daulatzai, M. A. (2015). "Evidence of neurodegeneration in obstructive sleep apnea: relationship between obstructive sleep apnea and cognitive dysfunction in the elderly." J Neurosci Res **93**(12): 1778–1794.

82. Ohayon, M. M., M. A. Carskadon, C. Guilleminault and M. V. Vitiello (2004). "Meta-analysis of quantitative sleep parameters from childhood to old age in healthy individuals: developing normative sleep values across the human lifespan." Sleep **27**(7): 1255–1273.

83. Mathur, R. and N. J. Douglas (1995). "Frequency of EEG arousals from nocturnal sleep in normal subjects." Sleep **18**(5): 330–333.

84. Boselli, M., L. Parrino, A. Smerieri and M. G. Terzano (1998). "Effect of age on EEG arousals in normal sleep." Sleep **21**(4): 351–357.

85. Bradley, T. D., I. G. Brown, R. F. Grossman, N. Zamel, D. Martinez, E. A. Phillipson and V. Hoffstein (1986). "Pharyngeal size in snorers, nonsnorers, and patients with obstructive sleep apnea." N Engl J Med. **315**: 1327–1331.

86. Martin, S. E., R. Mathur, I. Marshall and N. J. Douglas (1997). "The effect of age, sex, obesity and posture on upper airway size." Eur Respir J **10**(9): 2087–2090.

87. Edwards, B. A., A. Wellman, S. A. Sands, R. L. Owens, D. J. Eckert, D. P. White and A. Malhotra (2014). "Obstructive sleep apnea in older adults is a distinctly different physiological phenotype." Sleep 37(7): 1227–1236.

88. Klawe, J. J. and M. Tafil-Klawe (2003). "Age-related response of the genioglossus muscle EMG-activity to hypoxia in humans." J Physiol Pharmacol 54(Suppl 1): 14–19.

89. Wellman, A., A. Malhotra, A. S. Jordan, K. Schory, S. Gautam and D. P. White (2007). "Chemical control stability in the elderly." J Physiol 581(Pt 1): 291–298.

90. Patel, S. R., E. K. Larkin and S. Redline (2008). "Shared genetic basis for obstructive sleep apnea and adiposity measures." Int J Obes 32(5): 795–800.

10 The Influence of Cerebral Blood Flow and Cerebrovascular Responsiveness on Ventilatory Control

Jay MJR Carr, Gustavo Vizcardo-Galindo, and Philip N Ainslie

INTRODUCTION

The status of arterial and cerebral tissue partial pressures of CO_2 ($PaCO_2$ and $PbtCO_2$, respectively) and concentrations of H^+ play an intimate role in the regulation of alveolar ventilation ($\dot{V}_A$) and cerebral blood flow (CBF). Ventilation ($\dot{V}_E$) and CBF are entangled due to the role played by the former in determining the magnitude of the latter and vice versa. For example, CBF regulates arterial and brain tissue gas tensions, thereby influencing $\dot{V}_E$, while $\dot{V}_E$ controls arterial gas tensions, which in turn regulate CBF. The relationships between arterial blood gases and CBF are illustrated in Figure 10.1.

Cerebrovascular responsiveness to changes in arterial blood gases also contributes to the stability of breathing rhythm and pattern generation (both during wakefulness and sleep) as a result of the changes in brain tissue PCO_2 that occur due to alterations in CBF. In the following chapter, the vascular regulation of CBF and its role in ventilatory control will be discussed with particular attention to the influence on the central chemoreceptor control of breathing. We begin with a brief overview of the fundamental relationships between $\dot{V}_E$, arterial PCO_2, and CBF regulation. The driving stimuli behind vascular CO_2 regulation and the mechanism(s) of action which define cerebrovascular reactivity will be outlined, as well as the regional heterogeneity of cerebrovascular CO_2 reactivity. Finally, the role of CBF per se and cerebrovascular reactivity in driving central chemoreceptor drive will be summarized.

BRIEF OVERVIEW: CBF REGULATION AND VENTILATORY CONTROL

As mentioned elsewhere in this textbook, the partial pressure of arterial carbon dioxide ($PaCO_2$) is determined by total CO_2 production ($\dot{V}CO_2$) divided by $\dot{V}_A$.

$$PaCO_2 = \frac{\dot{V}CO_2}{\dot{V}_A} \quad (10.1)$$

As such, a reduction or elevation in $\dot{V}_A$ will cause an increase or decrease in $PaCO_2$, respectively. The chemoreflex control of ventilation is determined via $PaCO_2$ and $[H^+]$ (and to a lesser extent PaO_2) at the peripheral chemoreceptors and intracellular $[H^+]$ at the level of the central chemoreceptors

(see Chapter 2 for details). In addition to the concurrent and interwoven roles of the peripheral and central chemoreceptors—which have been well-established—more current hypotheses incorporate newer concepts such as cardioventilatory control based on plasticity of chemosensitivity, multiple sites of hypoxic sensing, interdependence of central and peripheral chemoreceptors, and upregulation of central nervous system neurons comprising respiratory and sympathetic regulatory pathways (reviewed in (1–4) and Chapter 2). Such factors highlight the role of CBF in the broader complexities of chemoreception; however, control of respiratory rhythm and pattern is determined by several mechanisms, the principle command centers for which lie in the brainstem (see Chapter 1 for respiratory network neuroanatomy) and hence may be additionally influenced by the local environment via changes in CBF. In particular, central chemoreceptor tissue PCO_2 ($PbtCO_2$) and $[H^+]$ are determined by the dynamic balance between $PaCO_2$, blood flow across the medulla oblongata, and medullary CO_2 production (and relatedly, extra- and intracellular acid-base status). Since CBF regulates $PaCO_2$ in-flow and medullary CO_2 "washout", as well as changing acid-base balance most rapidly (compared to metabolically induced changes), the main determinant of $PbtCO_2$, at the level of the central chemoreceptors, that alters tissue $[H^+]$ is medullary blood flow. So, for any given cerebral metabolic rate:

$$PbtCO_2 = \frac{PaCO_2}{\text{medullary blood flow}} \quad (10.2)$$

It is known that $PbtCO_2$ is tightly controlled via vascular tonal regulation of blood flow in response to both feedback (e.g. $PaCO_2$, blood pressure) and feed-forward (e.g. neurovascular coupling, autonomic) mechanisms. Since the primary controllers of ventilatory drive reside within the cerebral vascular tree (carotid bodies and ventrolateral medullary tissues), vascular regulation of cerebral $PbtCO_2/[H^+]$ has a direct impact on regulation of ventilation by changes in $PaCO_2$ and changes in CBF. Moreover, whether changes in CBF are pressure-driven, CO_2-driven, or sympathoexcitation-driven— can independently or inter-connectedly influence the milieu at the level of $PbtCO_2$; therefore, such influences can play a

DOI: 10.1201/9781003000631-12

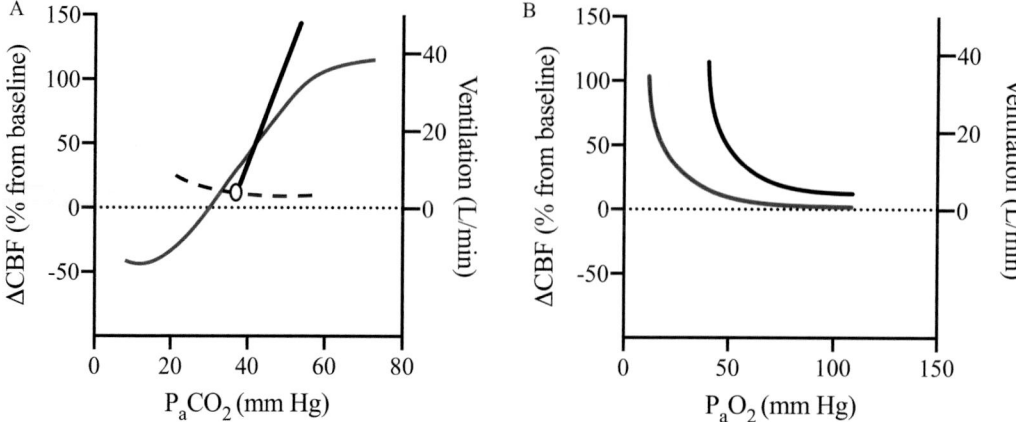

Figure 10.1 Illustration of the relationships between cerebral blood flow and ventilation with changes in arterial blood gases. (A) Relative CBF (red line) and absolute $\dot{V}_E$ (*black line*) changes by $PaCO_2$ (while holding arterial partial pressure of O_2 [PaO_2] constant), and the change in $\dot{V}_A$ concomitant with changes in $\dot{V}_A$ (*dashed line*; metabolic parabola). Normal equilibrium of $PaCO_2$ and $\dot{V}_E$ indicated at the circle. (B) Relative CBF (*red line*) and absolute $\dot{V}_E$ (*black line*) changes by PaO_2 (while holding $PaCO_2$ constant).

contributory (albeit poorly established) role in the chemoreflex control of $\dot{V}_A$.

Hypercapnia causes significant vasodilation and hypocapnia causes constriction throughout the cerebrovascular tree (Figure 10.2; although there likely are significant regional differences, discussed in *Regional CVR Heterogeneity*), via a multitude of mechanisms (see *Vascular CO2 Reactivity: Stimuli Sensing and Mechanisms of Action*; and reviewed in (8)). Regulation of CBF via modulation of vascular resistance in response to these CO_2-induced changes is active at all levels of the cerebral vascular tree, from the large extra-cranial cerebral arteries (7, 9, 10) and intracerebral arteries (6, 11, 12), to the pial vessels (5, 13–17) and capillary pericytes (18, 19).

The magnitude of the blood flow response per unit change in $PaCO_2$ is called *cerebrovascular reactivity* (CVR) for either global CBF or a specified blood flow to a cerebral region.

$$CVR = \frac{\Delta\ CBF}{\Delta\ PaCO_2} \quad (10.3)$$

CVR is often employed as an index of cerebral vasculature health and function, as it represents the effective function of the vasculature. Since CBF is crucial in the determination of intracellular [H^+] at the central chemoreceptors, CVR sensitivity is a relevant factor determining the overall $\dot{V}_E$ response to changes in $PaCO_2$ (ventilatory responses representative of contributions from the entire control loop; $\dot{V}_E$-CO_2) (see Figure 10.3).

CEREBROVASCULAR INFLUENCES ON CHEMORECEPTORS

Driving Stimuli: [H^+]

While $\dot{V}_E$-CO_2 and CVR are commonly said to be driven to $PaCO_2$, more precisely, it is intra- and extra-cellular [H^+] to which they respond. The [H^+] and pH in the intraluminal, interstitial, and intracellular spaces vary according to the equilibrium between CO_2, [HCO_3^-], [H^+], H_2O, and carbonic anhydrase (Equation 10.4) within each compartment.

$$CO_2 + H_2O \leftrightarrow H_2CO_3 \leftrightarrow HCO_3^- + H^+ \quad (10.4)$$

PCO_2 and [HCO_3^-] both alter the pH of these compartments, expressed via the Henderson-Hasselbalch equation (see Equation 10.5). The negative logarithm of the acid dissociation constant (pKa) of 6.1 at 37°C for the equation above gives the following:

$$pH = 6.1 + \log\frac{\left[HCO_3^-\right]}{0.03 \cdot PCO_2} \quad (10.5)$$

The driving stimulus of both vascular responses and ventilatory responses to CO_2 is intracellular pH. Since the transport of CO_2 across the BBB is rapid, and because this movement is dependent on the intraluminal/interstitial CO_2 pressure gradient, $PaCO_2$ and cellular CO_2 production primarily determine [H^+] in any fluid compartment.

Intracellular and interstitial [HCO_3^-] status also fluctuates; [HCO_3^-] is moved transcellularly, but via a series of ionic exchanges rather than diffusion, making its

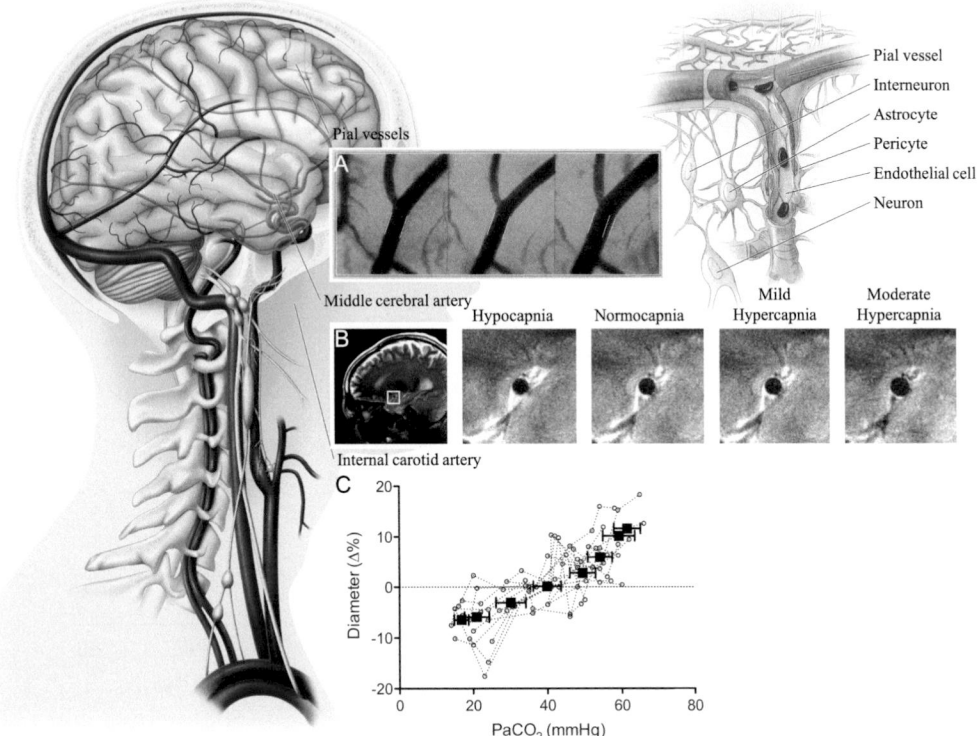

Figure 10.2 Gross and microscopic anatomy of the cerebral circulation and regulation.
Inlay A: photographs of feline pial vessel. Left to right: at normoxic normocapnic rest; minor vasoconstriction with hypoxic hypocapnia; extreme dilation with hypoxic hypercapnia (5). **Inlay B:** high-resolution magnetic resonance images of a human middle cerebral artery. Left to right: white box highlights the area of interest; zoomed images of MCA at ~-7.5, normocapnia, $\sim+7.5$, and $\sim+15$ mm Hg end-tidal partial pressure of CO_2. Note only moderate hypercapnia seems to elicit marked dilation (6). **Inlay C:** Mean (■) and individual (○) duplex ultrasound measurements of internal carotid artery diameter across the vasomotor response to steady state changes in $PaCO_2$ (7), likely predominant mechanisms for which include hypercapnia induced shear stress elevations.

movement slower than CO_2. This means that the concentration of HCO_3^- and other ions within the cerebrospinal and interstitial fluids are remarkably stable over time (21–23). Because $PaCO_2$ changes rapidly and CO_2 is transported readily across cellular membranes, both intra- and extra-cellular brain pH are tightly coupled with $PaCO_2$, dependent on local blood supply. While the predominant view is that pH/[H+] alone is the stimulus for CVR and $\dot{V}_E$-CO_2, there is some evidence for the independent effects of PCO_2, [H+], and $[HCO_3^-]$ (3, 24–28).

Vascular CO_2 Reactivity: Stimuli Sensing and Mechanisms of Action

Vascular regulation of cerebral tissue [H+] through vascular resistance and flow is mediated through a myriad of highly integrated mechanisms, so differentiating the contributions of individual pathways in humans is difficult. Candidate mechanisms from animal *in vitro* as well as progressive human studies are shedding light on the topic. Cerebrovascular reactivity to changes in $PaCO_2$ (Figure 10.1A) is based on the action of intra- and extra-cellular [H+] on vascular smooth muscle cells, astrocytes, pericytes, and endothelial cells in the cerebral tissues. Animal studies indicate that the hypercapnic vasodilator response requires— to some degree—the gaseous signaling molecule nitric oxide (NO), although NO seems permissive rather than obligatory (8, 29–32). In humans, CVR responses are likely driven by pH-mediated neuronal nitric oxide synthase (nNOS) activation (33–35), and acidic disproportionation of nitrites to NO (36–38), as well as acidic (39, 40) and shear-deformation (41) release of adenosine tri-phosphate from red blood cells causing $P2_{Y2}$ receptor activation

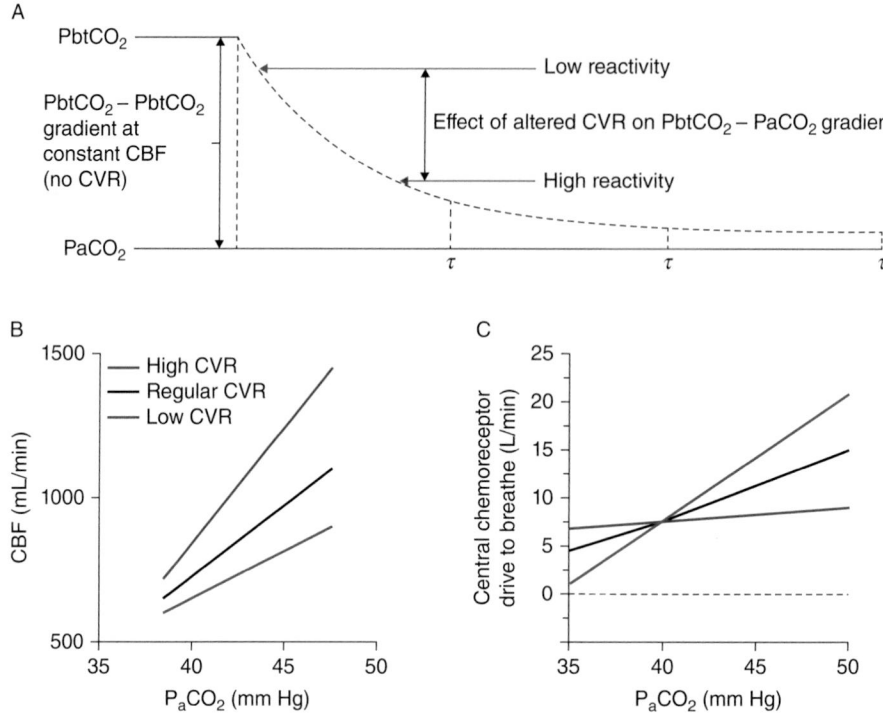

Figure 10.3 Illustration of the relationship between CVR and $\dot{V}_E$-CO_2. (A) Theoretical schematic of the relationship between two adjacent fluid compartments separated by a semipermeable membrane (redrawn (20)). (B) CBF by $PaCO_2$, representative of CVR, with high (red) and low (blue) sensitivity CVR also represented. (C) The implications of both high and low CVR sensitivities on central ventilatory drive. (A) Upon the occurrence of a square-wave change in concentration or pressure of a component substance in one compartment, equilibration up to 95% with the other compartment will occur over three time constants (τ). One τ is the duration required for fluid equal in volume to that of the first compartment to flow through the membrane into the second compartment; as such, if the first compartment is 500 mL, then 95% equilibration would require 1.5 l to move across the membrane. Given the compartmentalization of the cerebrovascular circulation and interstitial fluid compartment of the brain, this model can be applied to understand how changes in CBF and/or CVR can determine prevailing central chemoreceptor PCO_2/[H^+], and therefore, how CVR can inversely alter $\dot{V}_E$-CO_2. This theoretic conception is restricted since tissues are continually producing CO_2 via metabolism, so a constant difference or square wave change is not the case. Yet, for ease, one can assume that the true relationship is such that both compartments reside somewhere on the curved dashed line, based on CBF, prevailing $PaCO_2$, and metabolic CO_2 production. Higher flow across the compartment membrane would result in a right shift down the curved line and a reduced $PaCO_2$—$PbtCO_2$ gradient, as would effectively be the case in an individual with highly sensitive CVR (as noted by the red line). With a very high CVR, the difference between $PaCO_2$ and $PbtCO_2$ would, in theory, remain unchanged regardless of changes in $PaCO_2$, and as such, no changes in the central chemoreceptor drive to breathe would occur (this conception is purely for the purpose of comprehension of the CVR vs. $\dot{V}_E$-CO_2 relationship; this degree of CVR is impossible given the limit of vasodilation within the rigid skull). Conversely, with a low or no CVR response (as noted in the blue line), changes in drive to breathe would occur linearly with changes in $PaCO_2$.

of endothelial nitric oxide synthase (eNOS). These responses all occur within milliseconds to seconds of changes in capillary pH and shear stress and therefore cause the initial pial and parenchymal vessel vasodilation. Furthermore, secondary responses to $PaCO_2$ perturbations, which contribute to CVR steady state blood flow changes occur as far upstream as the large extra-cranial cerebral arteries such as the internal carotid arteries (ICA). Increased blood flow following the above described responses upregulates shear stress mediated eNOS activity and further augments dilation (42–47). See Figure 10.4 for an overview of mechanisms.

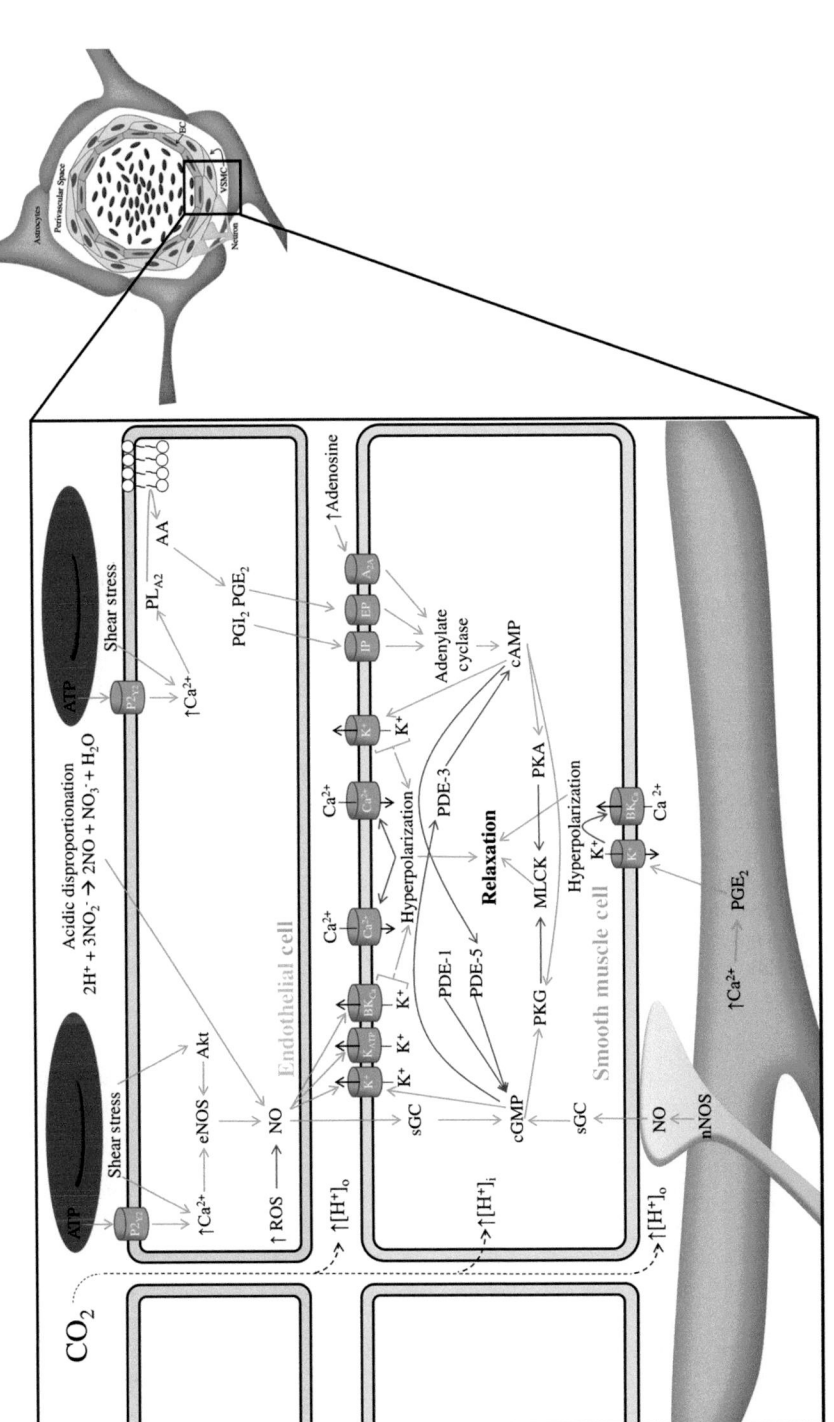

Figure 10.4 Schematic diagram of various CO_2-mediated cerebrovascular reactivity to CO_2. All of the depicted mechanisms induce VSMC relaxation and thereby cause vasodilation. Putative mechanisms of cerebrovascular resistance altering mechanisms. All of the depicted mechanisms induce VSMC relaxation and thereby cause vasodilation, these processes act are initiated in varying locales, at differing rates, and act on VSMCs at different magnitudes. $[H^+]_i$ and $[H^+]_o$ intra- and extra-cellular hydrogen concentration; AA, arachidonic acid; ATP, adenosine triphosphate; Ca_2^+, calcium; cAMP, cyclic adenosine monophosphate; cGMP, cyclic guanosine monophosphate; EC, endothelial cell; Akt, protein kinase; EET, epoxyeicosatrienoic acids; eNOS, endothelial nitric oxide synthase; K^+, potassium; MLCK, myosin light chain kinase; nNOS, neuronal nitric oxide synthase; NO_2^-, nitrite; $P2_{y2}$, purinergic receptor; PGE_2 and PGI_2, prostaglandins (PG); PKA, protein kinase-A; PKG, protein kinase-G; PLA_2, phospholipase-A2; ROS, reactive oxygen species; sGC, soluble guanylate cyclase; VSMC, vascular smooth muscle cells. (Reproduced with permission (8), see for further details.)

137

While ventilatory and vascular regulation are typically determined via the sensing mechanisms briefly outlined above, this is not the comprehensive extent of sensing responsible for each. Indeed, in the respiratory control centers of the brain, endothelial and smooth muscles cells seem to play a contributory role in ventilatory control (48). These important nuances are further explored in sections to follow (see *Regional CVR Heterogeneity*).

Cerebral Blood Flow, Cerebrovascular Reactivity, and Ventilatory Drive

Although, as described above, $PaCO_2$ is integral to the determination of central chemoreceptor PCO_2 and [H^+], it is the arterial "washout" that best represents the degree of acidosis at the tissue level. Both CVR and the central chemoreceptor $\dot{V}_E$-CO_2 response are likely better quantified using either jugular venous PCO_2 or the $PaCO_2$—$PjvCO_2$ gradient. At least in the supine position, since drainage through the jugular veins collect most if not all CBF, these variables more closely relate to central chemoreceptor $PbtCO_2$ and are therefore likely more representative of the true stimulus for CVR and at the central chemoreceptors than $PaCO_2$ *per se* (20, 21, 49–51).

We have seen thus far that in response to elevations in $PaCO_2$/[H^+], there are several mechanisms that cause vasodilation in cerebral vessels to aid cerebral tissue CO_2 washout— or vasoconstriction to promote relative CO_2 retention—both toward appropriate pH maintenance. Just as a change in $PaCO_2$ at the level of the chemoreceptors will influence ventilation (per Equation 10.2), so too, any

change in CBF sensitivity to CO_2 will also result in disturbed $PbtCO_2$ and therefore also affect $\dot{V}_E$-CO_2 responses (see Figure 10.3).

Cerebrovascular and Ventilatory Responses with Acute CBF Reduction

The relationship between acute changes in CVR and acute changes in ventilation during marked but transient reductions in CBF has long been demonstrated in animal models (52–54). Assessment of caprine CVR before and during acute reductions in CBF through arterial ligation (55) showed that slightly reduced CBF to 70% of baseline blunted CVR from 2.45 mL/min/mm Hg to 0.78 mL/min/mm Hg, yet the $\dot{V}_E$-CO_2 response was unaffected (at least when $PjvCO_2$ was taken as the mathematical stimulus) (see Figure 10.5). At 50% of baseline CBF, however, both CVR and $\dot{V}_E$-CO_2 responses were extremely blunted (see Figure 10.5). This differential change in $\dot{V}_E$-CO_2 with decreasing CBF and CVR is potentially suggestive of a threshold below which deteriorating blood supply induces failure of brainstem respiratory control neurons (55). Dampened CVR responses during reduced CBF is possibly representative of the priority of simple perfusion over the maintenance of acid-base balance as well as limitations to cerebrovascular vasodilator reserve enforced by the myogenic response to reduced flow.

In humans, blunted CVR is concomitant with reductions in CBF, and whatever the mechanism(s)—whether induced pharmacologically or by normal diurnal changes—blunted CVR is often reflected by an increased slope of the $\dot{V}_E$-CO_2 response (20, 51, 56–59) (methods of CVR and $\dot{V}_E$-CO_2

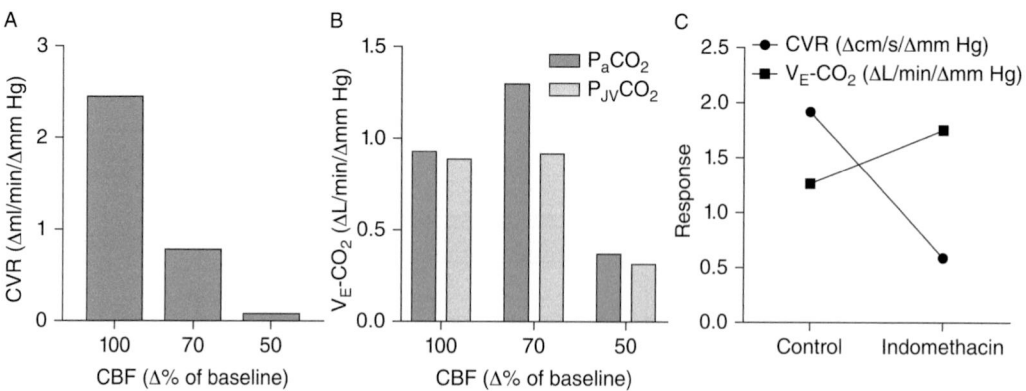

Figure 10.5 Cerebrovascular reactivity and ventilatory sensitivity to carbon dioxide with reductions in cerebral blood flow. Cerebral blood flow (CBF) in goats expressed as 100, 70, and 50% of baseline control (A and B, respectively; $\dot{V}_E$-CO_2 indexed against $PaCO_2$ and $PjvCO_2$, redrawn from (55)); and control baseline vs. post indomethacin ingestion in humans (C; redrawn from (56)).

assessment are crucial in this relationship, see *Reactivity assessment per se*). While CBF certainly contributes to determination of $\dot{V}_E$-CO_2 via modulation of the $PaCO_2$-$PbtCO_2$ gradient at the central chemoreceptors, nonetheless, it seems that *at rest* reductions in basal CBF result in little to no change in resting arterial blood gases or $\dot{V}_E$ (20, 51, 60). Teleologically, increased ventilatory sensitivity as a result of a blunting of CVR serves to systemically rectify the abnormal $PaCO_2$, which the now dulled CVR is insufficient to control at the level of the chemoreceptors. These studies show that reduced washout of H^+ during reductions in baseline CBF—in conjunction with the impairment CVR caused by antecedent vasodilation aimed at re-establishing CBF—causes some degree of agonism of the $\dot{V}_E$-CO_2 response through elevated local central chemoreceptor $PaCO_2$.

Methodological Considerations

While the intertwined nature of CVR and $\dot{V}_E$ sensitivities to CO_2 is unequivocal, there are nevertheless caveats that should be noted along with an interpretation of several of the aforementioned studies. Namely, and discussed below; regional CVR heterogeneity, CVR and $\dot{V}_E$-CO_2 assessment *per se*, and method of CBF reduction.

Regional CVR Heterogeneity

Several studies have shown regional CVR, however, consensus has not been reached whether CVR is superior in the posterior or anterior cerebral areas. Superior CVR in the ICAs over the VAs is well supported (7, 20, 61), likewise for greater middle cerebral artery velocity (MCAv) CVR than the posterior cerebral artery (PCA) (62) and posterior inferior cerebellar artery (63). However, anterior–posterior heterogeneity is minimized when responses are normalized to resting blood flow. Furthermore, equivalent absolute CVR values have been found between MCA and basilar artery (64) and PCA (7). The clinical implications of regional CVR heterogeneity are extensive in stroke and stenosis, including paradigms of arterial steal and asymmetrical CVR (65).

Greater CVR responses through the ICAs than the VAs are readily explained since ~71% of total CBF is directed through the ICAs compared to just ~29% through the VAs. However, as the VAs supply the neuroanatomical structures controlling ventilation (i.e. the brainstem), one could anticipate that these areas may be protected with high priority and, therefore, a superior CVR. In fact, there is recent evidence

in rats that the vessels surrounding the retrotrapezoid nucleus (RTN)—a critical central chemoreceptor area (48)—may even constrict in response to elevated $PaCO_2$ (66, 67) rather than the vasodilation typically expected. These studies suggest that reduced pH causes ATP release and purinergic receptor-mediated vasoconstriction. More human tissue and *in vivo* research need be conducted before application of these findings to human integrative vascular and ventilatory control.

While CVR regulates $PbtCO_2$ and $[H^+]$, $\dot{V}_E$ serves to regulate not only cerebral tissue PCO_2 but PCO_2 of tissues systemically; as such, appropriate $\dot{V}_E$ drive depends on the central chemoreceptor areas receiving input that reflects the requirements between cerebral *and* systemic CO_2/$[H^+]$ status. If the central respiratory center vasculature was regulated with the same efficacy as the rest of the cerebrovascular tree, ventilatory changes may not occur with $PaCO_2$ changes since CVR would reduce the stimulus at the brainstem. $PaCO_2$ reaching the RTN during vasoconstriction would be elevated relative to elsewhere in the brain, and reduced luminal surface area would limit the area available for diffusion of CO_2 across the blood brain barrier, effectively offsetting CVR's increase in global CBF and velocity, resulting in a $PaCO_2$—$PbtCO_2$ gradient at the central chemoreceptors closer to that found in tissues elsewhere in the body that lack CVR mechanisms.

Method of CBF Reduction

As noted above, acutely reduced CBF through indomethacin impairs CVR and enhances $\dot{V}_E$-CO_2 without changing resting $\dot{V}_E$; yet, acutely reduced CBF through direct ligation appears to blunt both CVR and $\dot{V}_E$-CO_2 (at least in goats). As such, the manner with which CVR effects $\dot{V}_E$-CO_2 is dependent on the mechanisms or pathways impaired. While indomethacin reduces CBF and impairs CVR via inhibition of prostaglandin synthesis (68–74), there are marked differences between indomethacin and other cyclooxygenase inhibitors (20, 60, 75–76). Because of these observations, given the varied and complex mechanisms governing CO_2 regulation of CBF, this is indicative that cyclooxygenase plays a permissive rather than obligatory role for CVR. Nonetheless, since indomethacin has little or no effects on metabolic rate, plasma catecholamines, or the peripheral chemoreceptors and ventilation directly, it does provide an ideal pharmacological tool for interrogation of the CVR vs. $\dot{V}_E$-CO_2 relationship. That said, as discussed, any acute changes in CVR impact $\dot{V}_E$ either by quick response peripheral chemoreceptor activity or with steady state changes via the influence on cerebrospinal fluid pH on central chemoreceptor activity. Some anecdotal evidence suggests that indomethacin intravenous infusion may cause immediate changes in $\dot{V}_E$ through rapid reductions in CBF causing changes in interstitial pH balance (Jerry Dempsey, personal communication). This interpretation is complicated via (i) the pharmacokinetics of indomethacin, temporal limits of cerebrovascular responsiveness, and time constants for compartmental equilibrium (see Figure 10.3), further muddied by the consideration of less effective buffering in the interstitial vs. arterial fluids, and (ii), if the above described regional heterogeneity of CVR holds true *in vivo* in humans, then indomethacin may have less impact in those regions where molecular mechanisms controlling vasoconstriction and dilation are differentially regulated.

Reactivity Assessment per se

Additionally, the means through which both CVR and $\dot{V}_E$-CO_2 are assessed (i.e. elevations in fraction of inspired CO_2, vs. rebreathing, vs. dynamic end-tidal forcing) contribute considerably to changes in the $PbtCO_2$—$PaCO_2$ gradient and therefore to the relationship between the two responses. For comprehensive discussion on the nuances of CVR testing, the implications on control of breathing, and the need to standardized guidelines for these assessments across the research and clinical fields, see (8, 20, 77).

CEREBROVASCULAR REACTIVITY AND CENTRAL SLEEP APNEA

Central sleep apnea (CSA) is a substantial and increasing clinical problem common in patients with severe heart failure or stroke. Following ascent to high altitude in otherwise healthy individuals, CSA during sleep is almost universal, occurring in >90% of people above 5,000 m. As detailed elsewhere in this textbook and extensively reviewed (78), the most common trigger to both CSA in heart failure and high-altitude exposure is transient reduction in the partial pressure of $PaCO_2$ below the apneic threshold. The extent of CSA during sleep at high altitude intensifies with duration and severity of exposure and is explained, in part, by elevations in loop gain—an engineering term used to describe the propensity for a feedback loop system to develop unstable behavior. The question arises: is there evidence for a punitive role of CBF and CVR in the etiology of CSA at high altitude or in pathology?

It is well established that CBF is elevated on arrival to high altitude (reviewed in 79), which serves to attenuate the reduction in O_2 delivery in the face of reduced arterial oxygen content (80), and also likely provides a protective effect on CSA (81). In healthy volunteers at 5050 m, an increase in CBF and (for the reasons outlined earlier) $\dot{V}_E$ facilitated an increased removal of locally produced CO_2 from the central chemoreceptors and arterial circulation, respectively, causing a reduction in hypercapnic ventilatory response, and consequently, reduced loop gain (82).

After partial acclimatization, CBF and its reactivity both decline (79). Although the importance of the carotid bodies are clearly established, these reductions in CBF and its reactivity may facilitate the further increases in hyperoxic hypercapnic ventilatory response (HCVR; a proxy of central chemoreflex activity since hyperoxia effectively silences the peripheral chemoreceptors (83) although the degree of hyperoxia often falls far short of complete carotid body shutoff (84, 85)). These elevations, along with further elevations in carotid body sensitivity and hence loop gain result almost universally in severe CSA at altitude (82). As mentioned earlier, however, in addition to the well-established independent roles of the peripheral and central chemoreceptors, more current hypotheses incorporate concepts such as cardioventilatory control based on plasticity of chemosensitivity, multiple sites of hypoxic sensing, the interdependence of central and peripheral chemoreceptors, and upregulation of CNS neurons comprising respiratory and sympathetic regulatory pathways. Changes in cerebrovascular function (i.e. vascular resistance control and related autoregulatory mechanisms) likely also play a contributory role in modifying some of these complex pathways.

During sleep, it seems likely that CBF and its responsiveness become more important in ventilatory control. In the absence of the wakefulness drive to breathe, marked oscillations in CBF occur as a consequence of periodic breathing, similar in nature to that reported in patients who experience sleep apnea at sea level (86, 87)—see Figure 10.7.

While previous studies show there is a decline in CBF from awake to NREM sleep (88, 89), this decline is only a modest predictor of CSA. This relationship between CSA and the sleeping decline in CBF was stronger after 2 weeks at high altitude, when absolute cerebral perfusion was lower (both awake and during sleep), further supporting the idea that insufficient H^+ washout within the brain stimulates further chemoreceptor activation. Moreover, in view of the link between

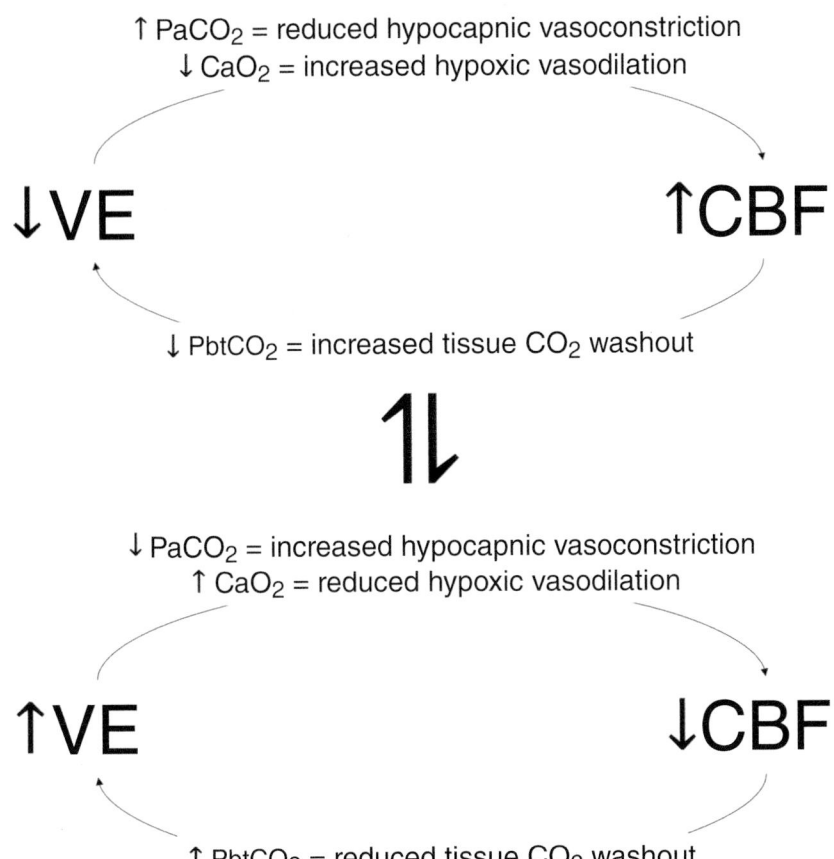

↑ $PaCO_2$ = reduced hypocapnic vasoconstriction
↓ CaO_2 = increased hypoxic vasodilation

↓VE　　　　　　↑CBF

↓ $PbtCO_2$ = increased tissue CO_2 washout

⇅

↓ $PaCO_2$ = increased hypocapnic vasoconstriction
↑ CaO_2 = reduced hypoxic vasodilation

↑VE　　　　　　↓CBF

↑ $PbtCO_2$ = reduced tissue CO_2 washout

Figure 10.6 Model of competing ventilatory and cerebral blood flow influences at high altitude. With ascent to altitude, cerebrovascular responses to hypocapnia and hypoxia and ventilatory responses to hypoxia compete while both serving to optimize O_2 delivery to the brain and whole body, respectively. Ultimately, at least during wakefulness, $\dot{V}_E$ and CBF adjustments should reach a steady state equilibrium determined by individual CVR and $\dot{V}_E$-CO_2 sensitivities; however, in even healthy individuals, the environmental challenges of altitude destabilize this equilibrium, in part via a marked elevation in loop gain resulting in CSA during sleep. Although it seems clear that oscillations in CBF occur secondary to the periodic breathing (Figure 10.7) but nonetheless will lead to further instability in the ventilatory control system as outlined in this model.

breathing pattern and CBF (90, 91), these oscillations in CBF are likely to be important in the pathophysiology of periodic breathing. Indeed, regardless of the causation of the first apneic episode, that is, whether alterations in basal CBF or in $PbtCO_2$ or $PaCO_2$ (or a combination of these and other factors) start the apnea cycle, the large swings in CBF via CVR mechanisms and enhanced loop gain that ensue seem likely to exacerbate the under- and over-shooting of the ventilatory drive that characterizes the CSA disorder (78) (see Figure 10.6 for the competing ventilatory and cerebral blood flow influences on ventilation during sleep at high altitude). Of course, CVR is just one factor among several which can contribute to ventilatory instability.

The potential role for alterations in CBF during sleep at high altitude in the control of breathing has been further supported by the results of pharmacological artificially increasing and reducing CBF during sleep. In a group of 12 healthy volunteers at 5,050 m, oral administration of 100 mg indomethacin reduced CBF by ~23% and increased CSA severity by ~16%. The HCVR also increased by ~66%, suggesting that the reduction in CBF may have mediated, in part, an increase in HCVR, which in turn increased the severity of CSA. Conversely, the combined administration of intravenous acetazolamide and dobutamine, which increased CBF by ~37% without changing $PaCO_2$ in the short term, reduced

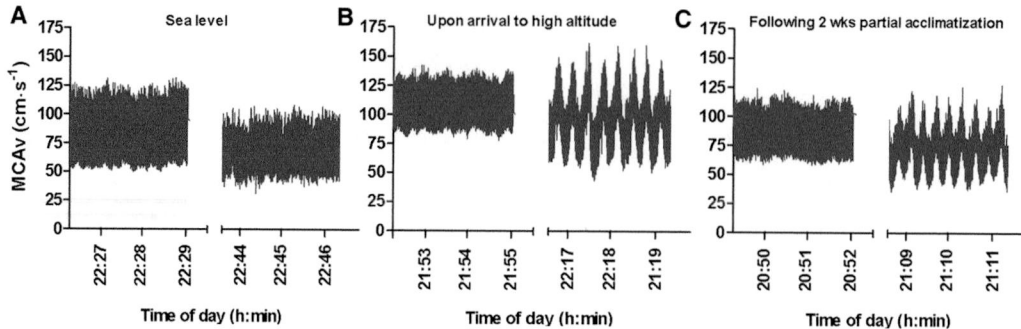

Figure 10.7 A typical profile of the observed changes in cerebral blood flow (as indexed by velocity in the middle cerebral arterial, MCAv) prior to sleep onset (left-hand trace) and during stage 2 sleep (right-hand trace) at sea level (A), then upon arrival to 5,000 m (B) and after 2 wk at high altitude (C) for one participant. Note the elevation in MCAv upon initial arrival, then compared with after 2 wk acclimatization and the marked fluctuations during sleep at high altitude regardless of acclimatization where CSA was >80 events/hr. Note that the oscillations in CBF occur secondary to the periodic breathing but nonetheless will lead to further instability in the ventilatory control system.

the severity of CSA from 140 ± 45 to 48 ± 37 events/hr of sleep (81). These results are consistent with modeling studies and suggest that CBF—through its influence on the central chemoreceptors—not only aids in shaping $\dot{V}_E$-CO_2, but also in stabilizing breathing in challenging environments such as sleeping at altitude. It is important to note, however, that the above-described manipulations of CBF only produced modest changes in CSA. This observation highlights the relative involvement of CBF in the face of other powerful factors that influence loop gain.

Finally, previous reports show that congestive heart failure patients with CSA have a diminished cerebrovascular response to changes in $PaCO_2$ when compared to patients without CSA (90). In the CSA group, the finding of reduced CVR was driven via reductions in only *hypocapnic* responses. Similar to the discussion about high altitude and CSA, it was speculated that compromised CVR might affect breathing pattern stability by causing ventilatory overshoot during hypercapnia and undershoot during hypocapnia. Future studies are needed to extend these findings in awake patients to conditions of sleep. Experimentally reduced CBF and CVR via pharmacological manipulation with indomethacin or by combining multiple inhibitors would shed more light on the clinical implications of the CVR $\dot{V}_E$-CO_2 relationship in congestive heart failure.

REFERENCES

1. Forster H V., Smith CA. Contributions of central and peripheral chemoreceptors to the ventilatory response to CO_2/H^+. J Appl Physiol. 2010;108(4):989–94.

2. Smith CA, Forster H V., Blain GM, Dempsey JA. An interdependent model of central/peripheral chemoreception: evidence and implications for ventilatory control. Respir Physiol Neurobiol. 2010;173(3):288–97.

3. Guyenet PG, Bayliss DA. Neural control of breathing and CO_2 homeostasis. Neuron. 2015;87:946–61.

4. Guyenet PG. Regulation of breathing and autonomic outflows by chemoreceptors. Compr Physiol. 2014;4(4):1511–62.

5. Wolff HG, Lennox WG. Cerebral circulation XII. The effect on pial vessels of variations in the oxygen and carbon dioxide content of the blood. Arch Neurol Psych. 1930;23(6):1097–120.

6. Verbree J, Bronzwaer ASGT, Ghariq E, Versluis MJ, Daemen MJAP, Van Buchem MA, et al. Assessment of middle cerebral artery diameter during hypocapnia and hypercapnia in humans using ultra-high-field MRI. J Appl Physiol. 2014;117(10):1084–9.

7. Willie CK, Macleod DB, Shaw AD, Smith KJ, Tzeng YC, Eves ND, et al. Regional brain blood flow in man during acute changes in arterial blood gases. J Physiol [Internet]. 2012 Apr 18;590(14):3261–75. Available from: https://doi.org/10.1113/jphysiol.2012.228551

8. Hoiland RL, Fisher JA, Ainslie PN. Regulation of the cerebral circulation by arterial carbon dioxide. Compr Physiol. 2019;9(3):1101–54.

9. Carter HH, Atkinson CL, Heinonen IHA, Haynes A, Robey E, Smith KJ, et al. Evidence for shear stress-mediated dilation of the internal carotid artery in humans. Hypertension. 2016;68(5):1217–24.

10. Hoiland RL, Smith KJ, Carter HH, Lewis NCS, Tymko MM, Wildfong KW, et al. Shear-mediated dilation of the internal carotid artery occurs independent of hypercapnia. Am J Physiol Heart Circ Physiol. 2017;313(1):H24–31.

11. Giller CA, Bowman G, Dyer H, Mootz L. Cerebral arterial diameters during changes in blood pressure and carbon dioxide during craniotomy. Neurosurgery. 1993 Jan;32(5):732–7.

12. Coverdale NS, Lalande S, Perrotta A, Shoemaker JK. Heterogeneous patterns of vasoreactivity in the middle cerebral and internal carotid arteries. Am J Physiol Heart Circ Physiol. 2015;308(9):H1030–8.

13. Lennox WG, Gibbs EL. The blood flow in the brain and the leg of man, and the changes induced by alteration of blood gases. J Clin Invest. 1932;11(6):1155–77.

14. Kety SS, Schmidt CF. The effects of altered arterial tensions of carbon dioxide and oxygen on cerebral blood flow and cerebral oxygen consumption of normal young men. J Clin Invest [Internet]. 1948 Jul;27(4):484–92. Available from: https://www.ncbi.nlm.nih.gov/pubmed/16695569

15. Shapiro HM, Stromberg DD, Lee DR, Wiederhielm CA. Dynamic pressures in the pial arterial microcirculation. Am J Physiol. 1971;221(1):279–83.

16. Faraci FM, Mayhan WG, Schmid PG, Heistad DD. Effects of arginine vasopressin on cerebral microvascular pressure. Am J Physiol Heart Circ Physiol. 1988;255(1): H70-H76.

17. Faraci FM, Heistad DD. Regulation of large cerebral arteries and cerebral microvascular pressure. Circ Res. 1990;66(1):8–17.

18. Hall CN, Reynell C, Gesslein B, Hamilton NB, Mishra A, Sutherland BA, et al. Capillary pericytes regulate cerebral blood flow in health and disease. Nature. 2014;508(1):55–60.

19. Gonzales AL, Klug NR, Moshkforoush A, Lee JC, Lee FK, Shui B, et al. Contractile pericytes determine the direction of blood flow at capillary junctions. Proc Natl Acad Sci U S A. 2020;117(43):27022–33.

20. Hoiland RL, Ainslie PN, Wildfong KW, Smith KJ, Bain AR, Willie CK, et al. Indomethacin-induced impairment of regional cerebrovascular reactivity: implications for respiratory control. J Physiol. 2015;593(5):1291–306.

21. Fencl V. Acid-Base Balance in Cerebral Fluids. In: Terjung R, editor, Handbook of Physiology. Bethesda, MD: The Respiratory System II, Control of Breathing; 1986. p. 115–40.

22. Hladky SB, Barrand MA. Fluid and ion transfer across the blood-brain and blood-cerebrospinal fluid barriers; a comparative account of mechanisms and roles. Fluids Barriers CNS. 2016;13:1–69.

23. Siesjö BK. Symposium on acid-base homeostasis. The regulation of cerebrospinal fluid pH. Kidney Int. 1972;1(5):360–74.

24. Shams H. Differential effects of CO_2 and H^+ as central stimuli of respiration in the cat. J Appl Physiol. 1985;58(2):357–64.

25. Nattie E, Li A. Central Chemoreceptors: Locations and Functions. In: Terjung R, editor. Vol. 2, Comprehensive Physiology. Hoboken, NJ: John Wiley & Sons, Inc; 2012. p. 221–54.

26. Gonçalves CM, Mulkey DK. Bicarbonate directly modulates activity of chemosensitive neurons in the retrotrapezoid nucleus. J Physiol. 2018 Sep;596(17):4033–42.

27. Meigh L, Greenhalgh SA, Rodgers TL, Cann MJ, Roper DI, Dale N. CO_2 directly modulates connexin 26 by formation of carbamate bridges between subunits. eLife. 2013;2:e01213.

28. Caldwell HG, Howe CA, Chalifoux CJ, Hoiland RL, Carr JMJR, Brown CV, et al. Arterial carbon dioxide and bicarbonate rather than pH regulate cerebral blood flow in the setting of acute experimental metabolic alkalosis. J Physiol. 2021;599(5):1439–1457.

29. White RP, Deane C, Vallance P, Markus HS. Nitric oxide synthase inhibition in humans reduces cerebral blood flow but not the hyperemic response to hypercapnia. Stroke. 1998;29(2):467–72.

30. Ide K, Worthley M, Anderson T, Poulin MJ. Effects of the nitric oxide synthase inhibitor L-NMMA on cerebrovascular and cardiovascular responses to hypoxia and hypercapnia in humans. J Physiol. 2007;584(1):321–32.

31. Schmetterer L, Findl O, Strenn K, Graselli U, Kastner J, Eichler HG, et al. Role of NO in the O_2 and CO_2 responsiveness of cerebral and ocular circulation in humans. Am J Physiol Regul Integr Comp Physiol. 1997;273(6):42–6.

32. Brian JE. Carbon dioxide and the cerebral circulation. Anesthesiology. 1998;88:1365–86.

33. Iadecola C, Zhang F. Permissive and obligatory roles of NO in cerebrovascular responses to hypercapnia and acetylcholine. Am J Physiol Regul Integr Comp Physiol. 1996;271:990–1001.

34. Okamoto H, Hudetz AG, Roman RJ, Bosnjak ZJ, Kampine JP. Neuronal NOS-derived NO plays permissive role in cerebral blood flow response to hypercapnia. Am J Physiol Circ Physiol [Internet]. 1997 Jan 1;272(1):H559–66. Available from: https://doi.org/10.1152/ajpheart.1997.272.1.H559

35. Wang Q, Pelligrino DA, Baughman VL, Koenig HM, Albrecht RF. The role of neuronal nitric oxide synthase in regulation of cerebral blood flow in normocapnia and hypercapnia in rats. J Cereb Blood Flow Metab. 1995;15:774–8.

36. Modin A, Björne H, Herulf M, Alving K, Weitzberg E, Lundberg JON. Nitrite-derived nitric oxide: a possible mediator of "acidic-metabolic" vasodilation. Acta Physiol Scand. 2001;171(1):9–16.

37. Zweier JL, Wang P, Samouilov A, Kuppusamy P. Enzyme-independent formation of nitric oxide in biological tissues. Nat Med. 1995;1(8):804–9.

38. Weitzberg E, Lundberg JON. Nonenzymatic nitric oxide production in humans. Nitric Oxide Biol Chem. 1998;2(1):1–7.

39. Bergfeld GR, Forrester T. Release of ATP from human erythrocytes in response to a brief period of hypoxia and hypercapnia. Cardiovasc Res. 1992;26:40–7.

40. Ellsworth ML, Forrester T, Ellis CG, Dietrich HH. The erythrocyte as a regulator of vascular tone. Am J Physiol Heart Circ Physiol. 1995;269(6):38–6.

41. Wan J, Ristenpart WD, Stone HA. Dynamics of shear-induced ATP release from red blood cells. Proc Natl Acad Sci U S A. 2008;105(43):16432–7.

42. Mashour GA, Boock RJ. Effects of shear stress on nitric oxide levels of human cerebral endothelial cells cultured in an artificial capillary system. Brain Res. 1999;842(1):233–8.

43. Fujii K, Heistad DD, Faraci FM. Flow-mediated dilatation of the basilar artery in vivo. Circ Res. 1991;69(3):697–705.

44. Fujii K, Heistad DD, Faraci FM. Effect of diabetes mellitus on flow-mediated and endothelium-dependent dilatation of the rat basilar artery. Stroke. 1992;23:1494–8.

45. Rubanyi GM, Freay AD, Kauser K, Johns A, Harder DR. Mechanoreception by the endothelium: mediators and mechanisms of pressure- and flow-induced vascular responses. J Vasc Res. 1990;27(2–5):246–57.

46. Heistad DD, Marcus ML, Abboud FM. Role of large arteries in regulation of cerebral blood flow in dogs. J Clin Investig. 1978;62:761–8.

47. Lee TJ-F. Direct evidence against acetylcholine as the dilator transmitter in the cat cerebral artery. Eur J Pharmacol. 1980;68:393–4.

48. Guyenet PG, Stornetta RL, Souza GMPR, Abbott SBG, Shi Y, Bayliss DA. The retrotrapezoid nucleus: central chemoreceptor and regulator of breathing automaticity. Trends Neurosci [Internet]. 2019;42(11):807–24. Available from: https://doi.org/10.1016/j.tins.2019.09.002

49. Shapiro W, Wasserman AJ, Patterson JL. Mechanism and pattern of human cerebrovascular regulation after rapid changes in blood CO_2 tension. J Clin Invest. 1966;45(6):913–22.

50. Peebles K, Celi L, McGrattan K, Murrell C, Thomas K, Ainslie PN. Human cerebrovascular and ventilatory CO_2 reactivity to end-tidal, arterial and internal jugular vein PCO2. J Physiol. 2007;584(Pt 1):347–57.

51. Fan JL, Burgess KR, Thomas KN, Peebles KC, Lucas SJE, Lucas RAI, et al. Influence of indomethacin on ventilatory and cerebrovascular responsiveness to CO_2 and breathing stability: the influence of PCO2 gradients. Am J Physiol Regul Integr Comp Physiol. 2010;298(6):1648–58.

52. Hill LS. Physiology and Pathology of the Cerebral Circulation. London: J. & A. Churchill; 1896.

53. Hastings AB, Coombs HC, Pike FH. The changes in the concentration of carbon dioxide resulting from changes in the volume of blood flowing through the medulla oblongata. Am J Physiol Content. 1921 Aug 1;57(1):104–9.

54. Pike FH. The Relation of the Rate of Blood Flow through the Medulla Oblongata to the Amplitude and Frequency of Respiratory Movements. In: Vol. 48, Science (American Association for the Advancement of Science). United States: The Science Press; 1918. p. 121–2.

55. Chapman RW, Santiago T V., Edelman NH. Effects of graded reduction of brain blood flow on chemical control of breathing. J Appl Physiol Respir Environ Exerc Physiol. 1979;47(6):1289–94.

56. Xie A, Skatrud JB, Morgan B, Chenuel B, Khayat R, Reichmuth K, et al. Influence of cerebrovascular function on the hypercapnic ventilatory response in healthy humans. J Physiol. 2006;577(1):319–29.

57. Xie A, Skatrud JB, Barczi SR, Reichmuth K, Morgan BJ, Mont S, et al. Influence of cerebral blood flow on breathing stability. J Appl Physiol. 2009;106(3):850–6.

58. Cummings KJ, Swart M, Ainslie PN. Morning attenuation in cerebrovascular CO_2 reactivity in healthy humans is associated with a lowered cerebral oxygenation and an augmented ventilatory response to CO_2. J Appl Physiol. 2007;102(5):1891–8.

59. Fan JL, Burgess KR, Thomas KN, Peebles KC, Lucas SJE, Lucas RAI, et al. Influence of indomethacin on the ventilatory and cerebrovascular responsiveness to hypoxia. Eur J Appl Physiol. 2011;111(4):601–10.

60. Hoiland RL, Tymko MM, Bain AR, Wildfong KW, Monteleone B, Ainslie PN. Carbon dioxide-mediated vasomotion of extra-cranial cerebral arteries in humans: a role for prostaglandins? J Physiol. 2016;594(12):3463–81.

61. Sato K, Sadamoto T, Hirasawa A, Oue A, Subudhi AW, Miyazawa T, et al. Differential blood flow responses to CO_2 in human internal and external carotid and vertebral arteries. J Physiol. 2012;590:3277–90.

62. Skow RJ, MacKay CM, Tymko MM, Willie CK, Smith KJ, Ainslie PN, et al. Differential cerebrovascular CO_2 reactivity in anterior and posterior cerebral circulations. Respir Physiol Neurobiol. 2013;189(1):76–86.

63. Reinhard M, Waldkircher Z, Timmer J, Weiller C, Hetzel A. Cerebellar autoregulation dynamics in humans. J Cereb Blood Flow Metab. 2008 May 21;28(9):1605–12.

64. Ogawa S, Handa N, Matsumoto M, Etani H, Yoneda S, Kimura K, et al. Carbondioxide reactivity of the blood flow in human basilar artery estimated by the transcranial Doppler method in normal men: A comparison with that of the middle cerebral artery. Ultrasound Med Biol. 1988;14(6):479–83.

65. Sobczyk O, Battisti-Charbonney A, Fierstra J, Mandell DM, Poublanc J, Crawley AP, et al. A conceptual model for CO$_2$-induced redistribution of cerebral blood flow with experimental confirmation using BOLD MRI. Neuroimage. 2014;92:56–68.

66. Hawkins VE, Takakura AC, Trinh A, Malheiros-Lima MR, Cleary CM, Wenker IC, et al. Purinergic regulation of vascular tone in the retrotrapezoid nucleus is specialized to support the drive to breathe. Elife. 2017;6:1–16.

67. Cleary CM, Moreira TS, Takakura AC, Nelson MT, Longden TA, Mulkey DK. Vascular control of the CO$_2$/H$^+$ dependent drive to breathe. Elife. 2020;9:1–23.

68. Degiulio PA, Roth RA, Mishra OP, Delivoria-Papadopoulos M, Wagerle LC. Effect of indomethacin on the regulation of cerebral blood flow during respiratory alkalosis in newborn piglets. Pediatr Res. 1989;26(6):593–4.

69. Eriksson S, Hagenfeldt L, Law D, Patrono C, Pinca E, Wennmalm A. Effect of prostaglandin synthesis inhibitors on basal and carbon dioxide stimulated cerebral blood flow in man. Acta Physiol Scand. 1983;117:203.

70. Markus HS, Vallance P, Brown MM. Differential effect of three cyclooxygenase inhibitors on human cerebral blood flow velocity and carbon dioxide reactivity. Stroke (1970). 1994;25:1760–4.

71. St Lawrence KS, Ye FQ, Lewis BK, Weinberger DR, Frank JA, McLaughlin AC. Effects of indomethacin on cerebral blood flow at rest and during hypercapnia: an arterial spin tagging study in humans. J Magn Reson Imaging. 2002;15(6):628–35.

72. Wang Q, Paulson OB, Lassen NA. Indomethacin abolishes cerebral blood flow increase in response to acetazolamide-induced extracellular acidosis: a mechanism for its effect on hypercapnia? J Cereb Blood Flow Metab. 1993;13:724–7.

73. Wennmalm A, Carlsson I, Edlund A, Eriksson S, Kaijser L, Nowak J. Central and peripheral haemodynamic effects of non-steroidal anti-inflammatory drugs in man. Arch Toxicol Suppl. = Archiv fur Toxikologie. Supplement. 1984;7:350.

74. Shoemaker LN, Wilson LC, Lucas SJE, Machado L, Walker RJ, Cotter JD. Indomethacin markedly blunts cerebral perfusion and reactivity, with little cognitive consequence in healthy young and older adults. J Physiol. 2020;0:1–17.

75. Pun M. Indomethacin on extra-cranial cerebral arterial vasomotion: beyond cyclooxygenase–prostaglandin inhibition. J Physiol. 2017;595(11):3671.

76. Hoiland RL, Ainslie PN. Reply from Ryan L. Hoiland and Philip N Ainslie. J Physiol. 2017;595(11):3673–5.

77. Fisher JA. The CO$_2$ stimulus for cerebrovascular reactivity: fixing inspired concentrations vs. targeting end-tidal partial pressures. J Cereb Blood Flow Metab. 2016;36:1004–11.

78. Dempsey JA, Veasey SC, Morgan BJ, O'Donnell CP. Pathophysiology of sleep apnea. Physiological Reviews. 2010;90:47–112.

79. Hoiland RL, Howe CA, Coombs GB, Ainslie PN. Ventilatory and cerebrovascular regulation and integration at high-altitude. Clin Auton Res [Internet]. 2018;28(4):423–35. Available from: https://doi.org/10.1007/s10286-018-0522-2

80. Hoiland RL, Bain AR, Rieger MG, Bailey DM, Ainslie PN. Hypoxemia, oxygen content, and the regulation of cerebral blood flow. Am J Physiol Regul Integr Comp Physiol. 2016;310(5):R398–413.

81. Burgess KR, Lucas SJE, Burgess KME, Sprecher KE, Donnelly J, Basnet AS, et al. Increasing cerebral blood flow reduces the severity of central sleep apnea at high altitude. J Appl Physiol. 2018;124(5):1341–8.

82. Andrews G, Ainslie PN, Shepherd K, Dawson A, Swart M, Lucas SJ, et al. The effect of partial acclimatization to high altitude on loop gain and central sleep apnoea severity. Respirology [Internet]. 2012 Jul 1;17(5):835–40. Available from: https://doi.org/10.1111/j.1440-1843.2012.02170.x

83. Lahiri S, Mulligan E, Andronikou S, Shirahata M, Mokashi A. Carotid body chemosensory function in prolonged normobaric hyperoxia in the cat. J Appl Physiol. 1987;62(5):1924–31.

84. Wilson RJA, Teppema LJ. Integration of central and peripheral respiratory chemoreflexes. Compr Physiol. 2016;6(2):1005–41.

85. Biscoe T, Purves M, Sampson S. The frequency of nerve impulses in single carotid body chemoreceptor afferent fibres recorded in vivo with intact circulation. J Physiol. 1970;208(1):121–31.

86. Hajak G, Klingelhöfer J, Schulz-Varszegi M, Sander D, Rüther E. Sleep apnea syndrome and cerebral hemodynamics. Chest. 1996;110(3):670–9.

87. Klingelhöfer J, Hajak G, Sander D, Schulz-Varszegi M, Rüther E, Conrad B. Assessment of intracranial hemodynamics in sleep apnea syndrome. Stroke. 1992;23(10):1427–33.

88. Burgess KR, Shepherd K, Dawson A, Swart M, Thomas KN, Donnelly J, et al. Worsening of central sleep apnea at high altitude—a role for cerebrovascular function. J Appl Physiol. 2013;114:1021–8.

89. Ainslie PN, Burgess K, Subedi P, Burgess KR. Alterations in cerebral dynamics at high altitude following partial acclimatization in humans: wakefulness and sleep. J Appl Physiol. 2007;102(2):658–64.

90. Xie A, Skatrud JB, Khayat R, Dempsey JA, Morgan B, Russell D. Cerebrovascular response to carbon dioxide in patients with congestive heart failure. Am J Respir Crit Care Med. 2005;172(3):371–8.

91. Topor ZL, Pawlicki M, Remmers JE. A computational model of the human respiratory control system: responses to hypoxia and hypercapnia. Ann Biomed Eng. 2004;32(11):1530–45.

11 Central Apnea

Propensity and Plasticity

M Safwan Badr

INTRODUCTION

Central apnea during sleep is not a single disorder. Rather, it is a manifestation of breathing instability in a variety of clinical conditions. Although our understanding of the specific mechanism(s) of central apnea has grown appreciably, the underlying pathophysiology remains incompletely understood.

The quietude of central apnea has received substantially less attention than the noise of obstructive apnea, despite the adverse consequences of CSA and the contribution of decreased ventilatory motor output to the genesis of sleep-disordered breathing.

DETERMINANTS OF CENTRAL APNEA DURING NREM SLEEP

Initiation of Central Apnea

Central apnea is the result of abolished ventilatory motor output, which represents a balance between excitatory and inhibitory influences (1). Sleep state, hypocapnia, upper airway reflexes, and breathing instability may all have a contributing role in the absence of ventilatory motor output and the development of central apnea.

The sleep state per se underpins the development of post-hyperventilation central apnea. Specifically, NREM sleep removes the wakefulness "drive to breathe" and renders respiration critically dependent on chemical influences, especially $PaCO_2$ (2). Central apnea occurs if arterial PCO_2 is lowered below a highly sensitive hypocapnic "apneic threshold." Experimentally, central apnea in sleeping humans can be induced using nasal mechanical ventilation to decrease arterial PCO_2. The magnitude of hypocapnia required to induce central apnea is referred to as the "CO_2 reserve." Physiologic studies have used this metric to assess the propensity to hypocapnic central apnea in different populations. Studies investigating the determinant of the CO_2 reserve have demonstrated that the propensity to central apnea, as determined by the CO_2 reserve, varies across physiologic and pathologic conditions. For example, the CO_2 reserve is smaller in men compared to premenopausal women (3), in post-menopausal women compared to premenopausal women (4), in older compared to young adults (5), and in patients with obstructive sleep apnea compared to a healthy

comparison group (6). These differences seem to reflect the difference in the prevalence of central apnea in each population (7, 8).

Perpetuation of Central Apnea

Central apnea does not occur as an isolated event but in cycles of apnea or hypopnea, alternating with hyperpnea, a reflection of the negative feedback closed-loop cycle that characterizes ventilatory control (8, 9). Cheyne-Stokes respiration (CSR) is the best-known example of an oscillating respiratory pattern, waxing and waning in a predictable manner (10). This is often described using the engineering concept of "loop gain", combining the response of the ventilatory system to changing $P_{ET}CO_2$, (the *controller*) and the effectiveness of the lung/respiratory system in lowering $P_{ET}CO_2$ in response to hyperventilation (the *plant*). Changes in either parameter would change the requisite magnitude of hypocapnia to reach central apnea (CO_2 reserve). High controller gain is the mechanism underlying central apnea in patients with HFrEF (11); whereas high plant gain is noted in individuals living with cervical spinal cord injury (12). It is of note that *plant factors, expressed by the relationship between ventilation and $PaCO_2$, are critical determinants of susceptibility* to central apnea. Contrary to popular belief, a low $PaCO_2$, for a given metabolic rate, promotes stability by decreasing plant gain; whereas high $PaCO_2$ promotes instability.

Loop Gain: Does It Explain Breathing Instability?

The loop gain construct is a valuable framework to understand the factors predisposing to central apnea. However, this framework is predicated on two considerations: First, the loop gain framework assumes a predictable periodic oscillation in respiration as is seen in CSR. Unfortunately, the typical CSR pattern is rather atypical in real life. Second, this model envisions the occurrence of central apnea as a "closed loop" control system, which relies on feedback to control the final output. However, there are multiple pathways for the development of central apnea that may induce, facilitate, or perpetuate central apnea in a non-periodic fashion. Thus, an open loop construct may represent a more accurate framework to understand the occurrence and recurrence

DOI: 10.1201/9781003000631-13

of central apnea. In fact, the occurrence of central apnea via multiple pathways may be an example of "Equifinality", where a given end state (i.e., central apnea) can be reached via multiple pathways. Examples of non-periodic phenomena that could influence the development of central apnea include:

- Ventilatory instability at sleep onset has been attributed to the oscillation of sleep state and reciprocal oscillation of PCO_2 around the apneic threshold. However, there is evidence that the alpha-theta transition, which characterizes sleep onset, is associated with prolongation of the breath duration and the duration of the expiratory time, independent of chemical stimuli. The morphologic pattern is that of a central apnea, caused by prolongation of expiratory time (13).

- Increased left atrial pressure may be a determinant of central apnea. Acute elevation in left atrial pressure in a canine model is associated with increased chemoreflex sensitivity and narrowing of the CO_2 reserve (14). This phenomenon may explain the increase risk of central apnea in patients with HFpEF.

- Negative pressure may cause a reflex inhibition of respiratory activity. Harms et al. demonstrated that negative pressure applied to the isolated UA in the unanesthetized dog reflexively prolonged expiratory time during both wakefulness and sleep, likely through upper airway receptors that could initiate inhibition of the ventilatory motor output (15). Thus, abrupt resumption of respiratory effort following upper airway obstruction may cause a reflex inhibition of respiration and promote the development of central apnea.

- Sighs are normal physiologic phenomena that occur during wakefulness and sleep in humans. A "pause" of variable duration often follows sighs, many will meet the criteria for central apnea. Typically, respiration returns to normal within 2–3 breaths (16). Similarly, swallowing during sleep is also associated with a respiratory pause, often associated with brief arousal, and may contribute to breathing instability via the combination of arousal and decreased oxygen levels (17). These physiologic events are inconsequential in healthy individuals but may further destabilize respiration in individuals with a high propensity to develop central apnea.

- Once ventilatory motor output completely ceases, rhythmic breathing does not resume at eupneic arterial PCO_2 ($PaCO_2$) due to inertia of the ventilatory control system; an increase in $PaCO_2$ by 4 to 6 mm Hg above eupnea is required for resumption of respiratory effort (18, 19).

- Central apnea is associated with narrowing or occlusion of the pharyngeal airway (20, 21). In fact, upper airway obstruction often follows central apneas upon resumption of respiratory effort, i.e., mixed apnea). Thus, resumption of ventilation requires opening of a narrowed or occluded airway and overcoming tissue adhesion forces and craniofacial gravitational forces.

- Opioid-related CSA does not follow a predictable respiratory pattern, owing to the inhibition of rhythmogenesis. Many patients display either a "cluster" breathing or "ataxic" breathing. Both profiles are irregular and lack predictable periodicity (22).

- The magnitude of the post-apneic overshoot is determined by multiple factors including asphyxia—depending on underlying gas exchange-augmented negative pressure, changes in blood pressure, and transient arousal. While this sequence explains why apnea rarely occurs as a single event (i.e., "apnea begets apnea"), it also underscores the limitation of viewing recurrent central apnea as a predictable respiratory oscillator.

Experimental Induction of Central Apnea

Several interventions are utilized to induce central apnea during sleep. Induction of central apnea requires hypocapnia of sufficient magnitude and duration to induce hypocapnic disfacilitation. There are two broad types of interventions to induce central apnea: hypocapnic hypoxia or mechanical ventilation.

The occurrence of periodic breathing and central apnea upon ascent to high altitude provided a window into the potential mechanisms of central apnea. This has served as the initial model for induction of periodic breathing and recurrent central apnea. Berssenbrugge et al. exposed six healthy males to hypobaric hypoxia during wakefulness and NREM sleep (23). The ensuring hypocapnia was associated with periodic breathing during NREM sleep but not during wakefulness or REM sleep. Periodic breathing manifested as repetitive clusters of breaths in an oscillating fashion, which alternated regularly with central apnea. Restoration of normoxia or the addition of supplemental CO_2 terminated respiratory periodicity and stabilized respiration.

Central apnea can also be induced using nasal mechanical ventilation in a pressure-support mode with a backup rate. Termination of MV results in apnea or hypopnea depending on the magnitude of hypocapnia. Trials are repeated with an increase in the pressure support level until central apnea is induced (4, 24). Alternatively, the pressure support can be applied without a backup rate and increasing the PS level until central apnea occurs spontaneously. The difference between the baseline $P_{ET}CO_2$ and the $P_{ET}CO_2$ that demarcates the apneic threshold is the CO_2 reserve (25).

The mechanical ventilation model of inducing central apnea differs from spontaneously occurring central apnea in multiple ways. Specifically, the pressure gradient is positive in mechanical ventilation and negative in spontaneously occurring central apnea. In addition, mechanical ventilation unloads the respiratory muscles, resulting in decreased work of breathing. Finally, mechanical ventilation is also associated with active neuro-mechanical inhibition, independent of chemical stimuli (19). Therefore, mechanical ventilation may not faithfully mimic spontaneous hyperventilation.

PLASTICITY OF THE APNEIC THRESHOLD

The central nervous system displays high degree of plasticity, a fundamental property of the nervous system, manifesting by the potential of the nervous system to change in response to intrinsic or extrinsic stimuli. Similarly, the propensity to central apnea also demonstrates substantial plasticity in response to clinical or physiologic interventions.

Understanding the determinants of plasticity may inform future therapeutic intervention for central apnea. The plasticity of the apneic threshold provides an opportunity to manipulate the ventilatory control loop to treat central apnea by decreasing the propensity to hypocapnic central apnea.

The Apneic Threshold Across the Clinical Spectrum

The propensity to develop central apnea is best captured by measuring the CO_2 reserve and its response to physiologic perturbations. Variability in the CO_2 reserve across the population appears to mirror the variability in the prevalence of central apnea in different populations. Specifically, central apnea prevalence is higher in men compared to women, in post-menopausal women compared to premenopausal women, and in older adults compared to middle-aged adults. (Figure 11.1). Likewise, patients with heart failure (11) and reduced ejection fraction (HFrEF) and people living with tetraplegia have a higher prevalence of central apnea that is mirrored by a narrow CO_2 reserve and suggesting that the propensity to central apnea is not immutable but is a modifiable trait that can respond to physiologic and pathologic conditions.

Effect of Sex Hormones on the CO_2 Reserve

The difference in CO_2 reserve between men and women was present during the luteal and follicular phase, indicating that differences in the CO_2 reserve could not be explained

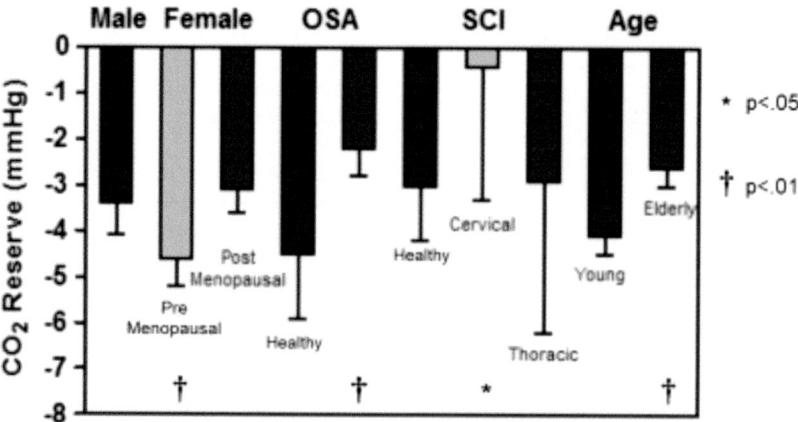

Figure 11.1 The CO_2 reserve across physiologic and pathologic conditions. Values represent the mean CO_2 reserve. A less negative bar indicates a higher propensity to central apnea. Thus, premenopausal women are less susceptible to central apnea compared to men, patients with OSA are more susceptible than the healthy comparator group, older adults are more prone to central apnea, and people living with cervical SCI are exquisitely prone to central apnea.

by e presence of progesterone in women (3). Instead, it implicates testosterone as the primary cause of sex differences in the CO_2 reserve. This notion is supported by a study in adult male rats that exhibited enhanced hypoxic ventilatory response and greater respiratory instability during sleep also exhibited greater expression of androgen receptors in the nucleus tractus solitarius (26). Furthermore, gonadectomy was associated with a significant reduction in the hypoxic ventilatory response. Likewise, Zhou et al. demonstrated that the administration of testosterone to premenopausal women for ten days resulted in narrowing of the CO_2 reserve and increased hypocapnic chemosensitivity (27). Suppression of testosterone with luperomide decreased the chemoreflex ring wakefulness and narrowed the CO_2 reserve during sleep (28). In a randomized double-blind placebo-controlled study, Ahuja et al. demonstrated that testosterone administration to healthy females was associated with increased hypercapnic ventilatory response in the presence of hyperoxia (29). Overall, it appears that testosterone is a destabilizer of respiration during sleep, mainly by increasing the propensity to central apnea. Regarding the specific pathway of testosterone action, Chowdhuri et al. demonstrated that administration of finasteride, which attenuates the conversion to dihydrotestosterone by blocking the 5α-reductase pathway, was associated with a significant widening of the CO_2 reserve in young men (30).

The destabilizing effect of testosterone on the propensity to central apnea does not explain the effect of menopause on the development of central apnea. Epidemiologic studies have shown that central apnea is rare in premenopausal women and increases after menopause (7). Mechanistically, Rowley et al. demonstrated narrowing of the CO_2 reserve in post-menopausal women relative to premenopausal women (4). Administration of hormone replacement therapy was associated with a return of the CO_2 reserve to the values observed in premenopausal women. Thus, the effect of sex hormones on respiration appears to defy simple direct explanations since male and female sex hormones appear to influence ventilation during sleep. Estrogens may be a common mediator of the action of male and female sex hormones since a testosterone is also converted to estrogen levels via aromatase. Alternatively, both sex hormones may influence another—yet to be (31) determined—factor that influence respiration during sleep.

Effect of Pharmacologic Agents on the CO_2 Reserve

Several small studies have investigated the efficacy of several agents that have been approved for other indications. The clinical use of any such agent is "off label." The major targets for pharmacotherapy of CSA are addressing elevated chemoreflex sensitivity, elevated plant gain, and arousal responses. A number of medications have been proposed:

- Acetazolamide is a mild diuretic and a respiratory stimulant that is used to treat periodic breathing at high altitude. Several studies have explored the use of acetazolamide as a treatment for central sleep apnea (31) and for CSR in patients HFrEF (32). It has no effect on peripheral chemo-responsiveness or sympathetic activity and has a strong safety profile in clinical studies. The variable response to this medication may reflect the multiple mechanisms of central apnea. Physiologically, acetazolamide results in widening of the CO_2 reserve by decreasing plant gain via increasing alveolar ventilation (33). Acetazolamide has little effect on CO_2 chemoreflex sensitivity. Acetazolamide may be an attractive option for CSA because of its effect on plant gain.

- Zolpidem, a non-benzodiazepine hypnotic that is being used clinically for the treatment of central apnea based on one open-label study in patients with idiopathic central sleep apnea (34). The biological plausibility is modest and there are no studies addressing safety or effectiveness of this medication for the treatment of central sleep apnea.

- Clonidine, a selective $\alpha2$-adrenergic agonist, has shown a measurable effect on the propensity to central apnea in one study. In a randomized, placebo-control study, Sankri-Tarbichi et al. compared a single dose of either placebo or 0.1 mg/45 Kg of clonidine orally prior to sleep over two separate nights (35). Clonidine use was associated with diminished susceptibility to hypocapnic central apnea as evidenced by a 1 mm Hg widening of the CO_2 reserve without significant effect on ventilation or upper airway mechanics. There are no clinical trials testing the effectiveness of clonidine as an adjunct therapy for the treatment of central apnea.

- Buspirone promotes respiratory rate and a regular breathing pattern in rat models of spinal cord injury (where CSA is common) (36) and of morphine-induced apnea.

Buspirone acutely increases ventilation in rats during wakefulness and NREM sleep (37). There are clinical reports of its benefit. In one child with Rett syndrome treatment with 5 mg of buspirone twice a day stabilized breathing movements and the time below saturation of 90% was reduced by 42.2% (38). A case report showed that buspirone largely abolished the apneustic breathing associated with brainstem infarction (39). Finally, a letter to the editor described an open label, single-dose study of buspirone (20 mg po) taken before a polysomnographic study in five patients (40). The number of apneas and hypopneas per hour (i.e., apnea-hypopnea index; AHI) fell from 31 to 20 events (a drop of ~33%). In four of the five patients, there were substantial decreases in AHI of >40%), along with improvements in overall oxygenation. Other published studies support a potential role for buspirone as having possible clinical benefit. For example, in a B6 animal model, buspirone acutely (41) and after 2-week administration (10 mg/day) (42) reversed the instability of breathing and post-hypoxic pauses. In summary, published studies in humans and animals support a potential role for buspirone in stabilizing respiration and mitigating central apnea.

Effect of PAP and Supplemental Oxygen on the CO_2 Reserve

The majority of patients with central apnea have a number of co-morbid conditions. Obstructive sleep apnea is the most common co-morbid condition associated with central apnea (43, 44). Interestingly, the presence of obstructive sleep apnea is associated with an increased propensity to central apnea, as evidenced by narrow CO_2 reserve, owing to increased CO_2 chemoreflex sensitivity below eupnea (controller gain) in patients with OSA as compared with healthy control subjects (6). Interestingly, PAP therapy resulted in decreased chemoreflex sensitivity and increased CO_2 $resO_2$ reserve to the removal of recurrent apneas.

Several clinical trials have demonstrated a potential therapeutic benefit of supplemental oxygen in the treatment of central sleep apnea. Chowdhuri et al. demonstrated that breathing a hyperoxic gas mixture resulted in widening of the CO_2 reserve and a reduction in the plant gain (45). A similar effect was noted in older adults with sleep-disordered breathing (46). The mechanism underlying the hyperoxic effect is likely a combination of attenuated peripheral chemoreflex sensitivity and increased cerebral tissue PCO_2, likely due to the Haldane effect. In other words, hyperoxia acts as a mild ventilatory stimulant that could be an option for the treatment of central apnea (47, 48).

SUMMARY

Central apnea is a relatively common disorder that is intertwined with obstructive apneas etiologically and clinically. Typically, central apnea occurs in cycles of apnea/hypopnea alternating with hyperpnea. Decreased ventilatory motor output during apnea or hypopnea is often associated with upper airway narrowing or occlusion. Investigating the propensity to develop central apnea by measuring the CO_2 reserve has demonstrated significant variability in the CO_2 reserve across physiologic and pathologic conditions. In addition, these studies demonstrated compelling evidence of the plasticity of the CO_2 reserve, which provides a physiologic basis for pharmacologic therapy for central apnea. In fact, understanding the determinants of central apnea may provide insight into the mechanisms of sleep-disordered breathing and inform the development of targeted interventions to ameliorate the severity of the condition.

REFERENCES

1. Dempsey JA. Crossing the apnoeic threshold: causes and consequences. Exp Physiol. 2005;90(1):13–24.

2. Dempsey JA. Central sleep apnea: misunderstood and mistreated! F1000Res. 2019;8:F1000.

3. Zhou XS, Shahabuddin S, Zahn BR, Babcock MA, Badr MS. Effect of gender on the development of hypocapnic apnea/hypopnea during NREM sleep. J Appl Physiol (1985). 2000;89(1):192–9.

4. Rowley JA, Zhou XS, Diamond MP, Badr MS. The determinants of the apnea threshold during NREM sleep in normal subjects. Sleep. 2006;29(1):95–103.

5. Chowdhuri S, Pranathiageswaran S, Loomis-King H, Salloum A, Badr MS. Aging is associated with increased propensity for central apnea during NREM sleep. J Appl Physiol (1985). 2018;124(1):83–90.

6. Salloum A, Rowley JA, Mateika JH, Chowdhuri S, Omran Q, Badr MS. Increased propensity for central apnea in patients with obstructive sleep apnea: effect of nasal continuous positive airway pressure. Am J Respir Crit Care Med. 2010;181(2):189–93.

7. Bixler EO, Vgontzas AN, Lin HM, Ten Have T, Rein J, Vela-Bueno A, et al. Prevalence of sleep-disordered breathing in women: effects of gender. Am J Respir Crit Care Med. 2001;163(3 Pt 1):608–13.

8. Khoo MC, Gottschalk A, Pack AI. Sleep-induced periodic breathing and apnea: a theoretical study. J Appl Physiol (1985). 1991;70(5):2014–24.

9. Khoo MC. Using loop gain to assess ventilatory control in obstructive sleep apnea. Am J Respir Crit Care Med. 2001;163(5):1044–5.

10. Cherniack NS, Longobardo GS. Cheyne-Stokes breathing. An instability in physiologic control. N Engl J Med. 1973;288(18):952–7.

11. Xie A, Skatrud JB, Puleo DS, Rahko PS, Dempsey JA. Apnea-hypopnea threshold for CO_2 in patients with congestive heart failure. Am J Respir Crit Care Med. 2002;165(9):1245–50.

12. Sankari A, Bascom AT, Chowdhuri S, Badr MS. Tetraplegia is a risk factor for central sleep apnea. J Appl Physiol (1985). 2014;116(3):345–53.

13. Thomson S, Morrell MJ, Cordingley JJ, Semple SJ. Ventilation is unstable during drowsiness before sleep onset. J Appl Physiol (1985). 2005;99(5):2036–44.

14. Chenuel BJ, Smith CA, Skatrud JB, Henderson KS, Dempsey JA. Increased propensity for apnea in response to acute elevations in left atrial pressure during sleep in the dog. J Appl Physiol (1985). 2006;101(1):76–83.

15. Harms CA, Zeng YJ, Smith CA, Vidruk EH, Dempsey JA. Negative pressure-induced deformation of the upper airway causes central apnea in awake and sleeping dogs. J Appl Physiol (1985). 1996;80(5):1528–39.

16. Issa FG, Porostocky S. Effect of sleep on changes in breathing pattern accompanying sigh breaths. Respir Physiol. 1993;93(2):175–87.

17. Rizwan A, Sankari A, Bascom AT, Vaughan S, Badr MS. Nocturnal swallowing and arousal threshold in individuals with chronic spinal cord injury. J Appl Physiol (1985). 2018;125(2):445–52.

18. Dempsey JA, Leevers AM, Wilson CR, Harms CA, Smith CA. Apnea prolongation via short-term inhibition. Sleep. 1996;19(10 Suppl):S160–3.

19. Wilson CR, Satoh M, Skatrud JB, Dempsey JA. Non-chemical inhibition of respiratory motor output during mechanical ventilation in sleeping humans. J Physiol. 1999;518 (Pt 2):605–18.

20. Badr MS, Toiber F, Skatrud JB, Dempsey J. Pharyngeal narrowing/occlusion during central sleep apnea. J Appl Physiol (1985). 1995;78(5):1806–15.

21. Sankri-Tarbichi AG, Rowley JA, Badr MS. Expiratory pharyngeal narrowing during central hypocapnic hypopnea. Am J Respir Crit Care Med. 2009;179(4):313–9.

22. Wang D, Teichtahl H. Opioids, sleep architecture and sleep-disordered breathing. Sleep Med Rev. 2007;11(1):35–46.

23. Berssenbrugge A, Dempsey J, Iber C, Skatrud J, Wilson P. Mechanisms of hypoxia-induced periodic breathing during sleep in humans. J Physiol. 1983;343:507–24.

24. Badr MS, Kawak A. Post-hyperventilation hypopnea in humans during NREM sleep. Respir Physiol. 1996;103(2):137–45.

25. Xie A, Skatrud JB, Dempsey JA. Effect of hypoxia on the hypopnoeic and apnoeic threshold for CO(2) in sleeping humans. J Physiol. 2001;535(Pt 1):269–78.

26. Fournier S, Gulemetova R, Joseph V, Kinkead R. Testosterone potentiates the hypoxic ventilatory response of adult male rats subjected to neonatal stress. Exp Physiol. 2014;99(5):824–34.

27. Zhou XS, Rowley JA, Demirovic F, Diamond MP, Badr MS. Effect of testosterone on the apneic threshold in women during NREM sleep. J Appl Physiol (1985). 2003;94(1):101–7.

28. Mateika JH, Omran Q, Rowley JA, Zhou XS, Diamond MP, Badr MS. Treatment with leuprolide acetate decreases the threshold of the ventilatory response to carbon dioxide in healthy males. J Physiol. 2004;561 (Pt 2):637–46.

29. Ahuja D, Mateika JH, Diamond MP, Badr MS. Ventilatory sensitivity to carbon dioxide before and after episodic hypoxia in women treated with testosterone. J Appl Physiol (1985). 2007;102(5):1832–8.

30. Chowdhuri S, Bascom A, Mohan D, Diamond MP, Badr MS. Testosterone conversion blockade increases breathing stability in healthy men during NREM sleep. Sleep. 2013;36(12):1793–8.

31. DeBacker WA, Verbraecken J, Willemen M, Wittesaele W, DeCock W, Van deHeyning P. Central apnea index decreases after prolonged treatment with acetazolamide. Am J Respir Crit Care Med. 1995;151(1):87–91.

32. Javaheri S. Acetazolamide improves central sleep apnea in heart failure: a double-blind, prospective study. Am J Respir Crit Care Med. 2006;173(2):234–7.

33. Ginter G, Sankari A, Eshraghi M, Obiakor H, Yarandi H, Chowdhuri S, et al. Effect of acetazolamide on susceptibility to central sleep apnea in chronic spinal cord injury. J Appl Physiol (1985). 2020;128(4):960–966.

34. Quadri S, Drake C, Hudgel DW. Improvement of idiopathic central sleep apnea with zolpidem. J Clin Sleep Med. 2009;5(2):122–9.

35. Sankri-Tarbichi AG, Grullon K, Badr MS. Effects of clonidine on breathing during sleep and susceptibility to central apnoea. Respir Physiol Neurobiol. 2013;185(2):356–61.

36. Teng YD, Bingaman M, Taveira-DaSilva AM, Pace PP, Gillis RA, Wrathall JR. Serotonin 1A receptor agonists reverse respiratory abnormalities in spinal cord-injured rats. J Neurosci. 2003;23(10):4182–9.

37. Mendelson WB, Martin JV, Rapoport DM. Effects of buspirone on sleep and respiration. Am Rev Respir Dis. 1990;141(6):1527–30.

38. Andaku DK, Mercadante MT, Schwartzman JS. Buspirone in Rett syndrome respiratory dysfunction. Brain Dev. 2005;27(6):437–8.

39. El-Khatib MF, Kiwan RA, Jamaleddine GW. Buspirone treatment for apneustic breathing in brain stem infarct. Respir Care. 2003;48(10):956–8.

40. Mendelson WB, Maczaj M, Holt J. Buspirone administration to sleep apnea patients. J Clin Psychopharmacol. 1991;11(1):71–2.

41. Yamauchi M, Dostal J, Kimura H, Strohl KP. Effects of buspirone on posthypoxic ventilatory behavior in the C57BL/6J and A/J mouse strains. J Appl Physiol (1985). 2008;105(2):518–26.

42. Moore MW, Chai S, Gillombardo CB, Carlo A, Donovan LM, Netzer N, et al. Two weeks of buspirone protects against posthypoxic ventilatory pauses in the C57BL/6J mouse strain. Respir Physiol Neurobiol. 2012;183(1):35–40.

43. Chowdhuri S, Ghabsha A, Sinha P, Kadri M, Narula S, Badr MS. Treatment of central sleep apnea in U.S. veterans. J Clin Sleep Med. 2012;8(5):555–63.

44. Ratz D, Wiitala W, Badr MS, Burns J, Chowdhuri S. Correlates and consequences central sleep apnea in a national sample of U.S. Veterans. Sleep. 2018;41(9):1-10.

45. Chowdhuri S, Sinha P, Pranathiageswaran S, Badr MS. Sustained hyperoxia stabilizes breathing in healthy individuals during NREM sleep. J Appl Physiol (1985). 2010;109(5):1378–83.

46. Rastogi R, Badr MS, Ahmed A, Chowdhuri S. Amelioration of sleep-disordered breathing with supplemental oxygen in older adults. J Appl Physiol (1985). 2020;129(6):1441–50.

47. Becker H, Polo O, McNamara SG, Berthon-Jones M, Sullivan CE. Ventilatory response to isocapnic hyperoxia. J Appl Physiol (1985). 1995;78(2):696–701.

48. Becker HF, Polo O, McNamara SG, Berthon-Jones M, Sullivan CE. Effect of different levels of hyperoxia on breathing in healthy subjects. J Appl Physiol (1985). 1996;81(4):1683–90.

SECTION III

SLEEP-DISORDERED BREATHING IN DIFFERENT CONDITIONS AND DISEASE STATES

12 Sleep-Disordered Breathing due to Heart Failure

Shahrokh Javaheri and Robin Germany

In spite of recent triumphs in pharmacology for chronic heart failure (HF), it remains a highly prevalent and progressive disorder associated with excessive morbidity, mortality, and tremendous health-related economic cost. According to the American Heart Association 2021 Statistics (1), currently 6.2 million Americans ≥20 years of age have HF, and it is projected that in 2030, more than 8 million people ≥18 years of age will have HF. There are two major phenotypes of HF, HF with reduced ejection fraction (HFrEF) and HF with preserved ejection fraction (HFpEF). Similar to asymptomatic LV systolic dysfunction, which with time leads to HFrEF, asymptomatic LV diastolic dysfunction is also independently associated with incident overt HF and is predictive of all-cause death (2).

The prevalence of SDB and its acute and chronic consequences in HF have been reviewed extensively in previous publications and will be reviewed only briefly in this chapter (3–10).

Both OSA and CSA are common in subjects with LV dysfunction and frequently occur together, although one phenotype is typically predominant. One type of periodic breathing (PB) is Hunter-Cheyne-Stokes Breathing (HCSB) with CSA first described by John Hunter (11, 12), which has a long cycle time (13) and reflects the prolonged circulation time that is a pathologic feature of LV dysfunction (12). Polysomnographic studies have reported a high prevalence of HCSB in ambulatory subjects with LV systolic (3–10) and diastolic dysfunction (14, 15). However, CSA/HCSB is most prevalent in those with systolic dysfunction. Similarly, OSA is highly prevalent in those with obesity, hospitalized patients with decompensated HF and acute cardiogenic pulmonary edema (6, 16, 17). It has been proposed that fluid retention associated with decompensation contributes to the high prevalence of OSA in the supine position as fluid moves cephalad to the pharyngeal area facilitating upper airway collapse (18).

MECHANISMS OF CSA IN HEART FAILURE

Central sleep apnea occurs primarily in non-REM sleep, and is less prevalent in REM sleep. In non-REM sleep, with the removal of wakefulness drive to breathe, normal breathing is driven by metabolic pathways driven primarily by PCO_2. Further, non-REM sleep unmasks a very PCO_2-sensitive apneic threshold, a PCO_2 level below which rhythmic breathing ceases resulting in central apnea. Notably, this apneic threshold PCO_2 is only 2 to 4 mm Hg below the awake level of arterial PCO_2. Thus, a small rise in ventilation could lower the prevailing PCO_2 toward or below apneic threshold PCO_2 causing central hypopnea or apnea, when sleep resumes. As a result of central apnea, PCO_2 rises and after it exceeds the apneic threshold PCO_2, breathing resumes. The rise in PCO_2 elicits a hyperventilatory response, which could be excessive if the system is exquisitely sensitive to PCO_2 (increased controller gain). Hyperventilation decreases PCO_2, leading to another central apnea and the cycle repeats itself. The occurrence of central sleep apneas with repeated cyclic periods of over- and under-ventilation (representing chemo-stimulation and chemo-depression, respectively) is mediated by increased chemosensitivity to hypoxemia and hypercapnia (increased controller gain) related to central apnea. This is an important element of increased loop gain (LG) which defines the ratio of the magnitude of the ventilatory response for a given change in ventilation. When LG is ≥1, the magnitude of the increase in ventilation is greater than or equal to the magnitude of the preceding apnea or hypopnea. Therefore, if, for any reason, a short pause in breathing occurs, the system is so sensitive that it overcorrects increasing ventilation excessively. Consequently, breathing becomes unstable fluctuating between under- and over-ventilation.

The controller gain is the composite sensitivity to PO_2 and PCO_2 of the peripheral arterial and central chemoreceptors, which have been shown to be upregulated in HF, particularly HFrEF with CSA (7–9). Another component of the elevated LG, is prolonged arterial circulation time (increased mixing gain), which delays the transfer of information regarding changes in PO_2 and PCO_2 in the pulmonary capillary bed to the chemoreceptors, converting a negative feedback system to a positive one, perpetuating PB. At the same time, the increased circulation time increases the cycle time of PB observed in sleep studies of patients with HF, particularly those with HFrEF.

The third component of increased LG is the exaggerated physiologic change in blood and chemoreceptor PCO_2, for a given change in ventilation (increased plant gain). With increased plant gain, a small change in

DOI: 10.1201/9781003000631-15

ventilation causes PCO$_2$ to go up and down, crossing apneic threshold facilitating the development of CSA.

MECHANISMS OF OSA IN HEART FAILURE

For mechanical reasons (fat deposition in the upper body, the visceral fat, the tongue, and the throat), obesity remains a major risk factor for OSA in the general population and in those with HF. However, PB predisposes susceptible subjects to develop upper airway occlusion during the nadir of the ventilation. Additionally, pharyngeal venous congestion due to increased right atrial pressure and cephalad movement of fluid from lower extremities could diminish upper airway size in the supine position.

ADVERSE CARDIAC CONSEQUENCES OF SLEEP-RELATED BREATHING DISORDERS IN HF AND RELATED HOSPITALIZATION AND MORTALITY

The cycles of apnea–hypopnea and recovery with hyperpnea are associated with adverse cardiovascular (CV) consequences which include (1) changes in arterial blood gases with intermittent hypoxemia/hypercapnia (during apnea) and reoxygenation/hypocapnia (during recovery) (2), sleep fragmentation characterized by excessive arousals and shift to light sleep stages (3), altered autonomic nervous system activity characterized by increased sympathetic and decreased parasympathetic activity, and (4) large negative swings in intrathoracic pressure (4). The aforementioned neurohormonal and hemodynamic consequences of OSA and CSA cycles are qualitatively similar (but worse in OSA than in CSA) (Figures 12.1 and 12.2) and adversely affect various CV functions. In the long run, these adverse consequences result in excess morbidity, hospital readmission, and mortality of patients with HF (2, 3, 16).

OSA

Observational studies suggest that OSA is independently associated with excess hospital readmission and that treatment of sleep apnea could lower the rate of readmissions (16, 17, 19–21). Specifically, severe OSA has been independently associated with 1.5 times higher readmission of HF patients when compared to those without OSA (17). One clinical trial demonstrated that the use of continuous positive airway pressure (CPAP) was associated with reduced readmission (19). In this study

A 30-second epoch showing polysomnographic features of OSA

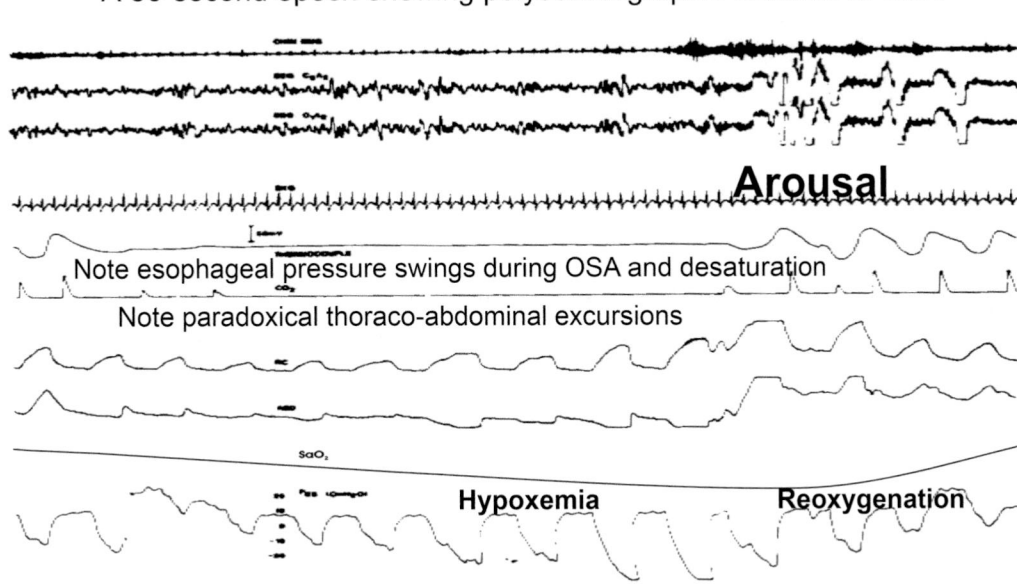

Figure 12.1 Polysomnographic example of OSA. Tracings from top to bottom are: chin electromyogram (1, EMG), electroencephalogram (EEG, and 3), ECG (4), airflow measured by a thermocouple (5) and CO$_2$ (6), rib cage (RC, 7) and abdominal (ABD, 8) excursions, oxyhemoglobin saturation (9) and esophageal pressure (10). Airflow is absent in the face of effort observed on rib cage, abdominal, and esophageal pressure tracings. Breathing resumes with the onset of arousal (increase in chin EMG and EEG α waves) and opening of the upper airway.

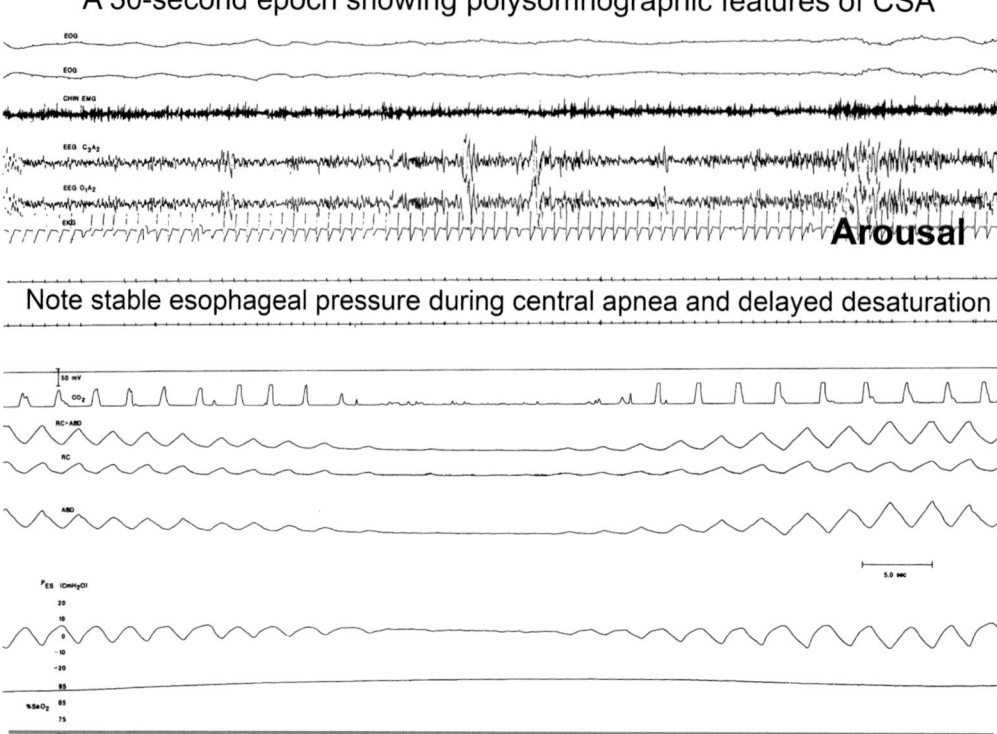

Figure 12.2 Polysomnographic example of CSA. Tracings from top to bottom are: electro-oculogram (EOG, 1st and 2nd), chin electromyogram (EMG, 3rd), electroencephalogram (EEG, 4th and 5th), ECG (7th), airflow measured by a thermocouple (8th) and CO_2 (9th), combined (10th) rib cage (RC) and abdominal (ABD), RC (11th) and ABD (12th) excursions, time in seconds (13th) and esophageal pressure (14th). Airflow is absent in the effort channels observed on rib cage, abdominal and esophageal pressure tracings. Note the smooth and gradual changes in the thoracoabdominal excursions and esophageal pressure in the crescendo and decrescendo arms of the cycle. The arousal occurs at the peak of hyperventilation.

of patients with acute decompensated HF and OSA, treatment began in the hospital. Follow-up at 6 months after discharge revealed a >60% decrease in readmissions for patients who used PAP >3 hr/night compared with those who used it <3 hr/night (P <0.02) and compared with controls (P <0.04).

Observational studies also suggest that in subjects with HF, OSA is independently associated with premature mortality (16, 17, 19, 22, 23), which is attenuated with treatment (19, 24). In the largest study (19) reported to date, among 30,000 Medicare beneficiaries newly diagnosed with HF, treatment of SDB was associated with decreased readmission, health care cost, and mortality (Figure 12.3).

CSA

Similar to OSA, studies have shown that in HFrEF, CSA is an independent predictor of hospital readmission and survival (5, 16, 23,

25–28). We followed 88 HF patients with (n = 56) or without (n = 32) CSA (AHI <15 and 15 or higher per hour of sleep, respectively) with a median follow-up of 51 months (26). After controlling for 24 confounding variables, CSA was associated with excess mortality (hazard ratio, 2.14; P = 0.02; Figure 12.4) (26). The average survival of HF patients without CSA was 90 months compared with 45 months for those with CSA. In the largest study so far reported, 963 well-treated patients with HFrEF were followed for 10 years (5). In this study (5), CSA was independently associated with excess mortality, mediated by the time-dependent desaturation. Among a few variables, time with oxygen saturation <90% was associated with the risk of death in a dose-dependent manner. A similar correlation has been reported in two studies of patients with acute decompensated HF (29, 30) showing that CSA contributes to excess mortality. Further, observational studies

Kaplan-Meier Survival Curves

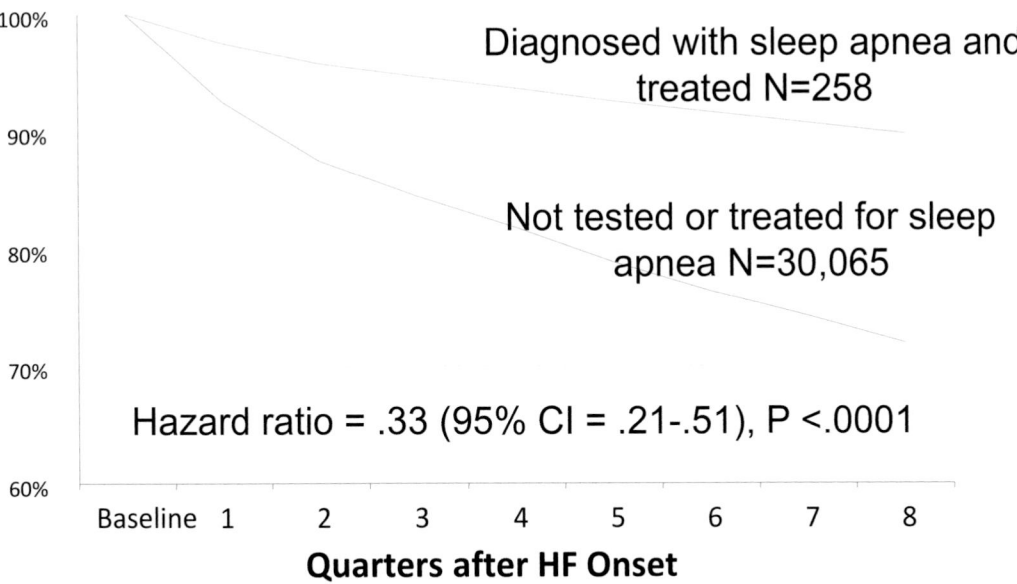

Percent of Cohort Alive

Diagnosed with sleep apnea and treated N=258

Not tested or treated for sleep apnea N=30,065

Hazard ratio = .33 (95% CI = .21-.51), P <.0001

Baseline 1 2 3 4 5 6 7 8

Quarters after HF Onset

Figure 12.3 Survival of the 258 heart failure patients treated for sleep apnea compared to survival of the 30,000 patients who were not tested for sleep apnea. Adjusted by age, gender, and Charlson Comorbidity Index. (Modified from Javaheri, et al., *Am J Respir Crit Care Med*, 2011.)

CSA is a Predictor of Mortality in SHF

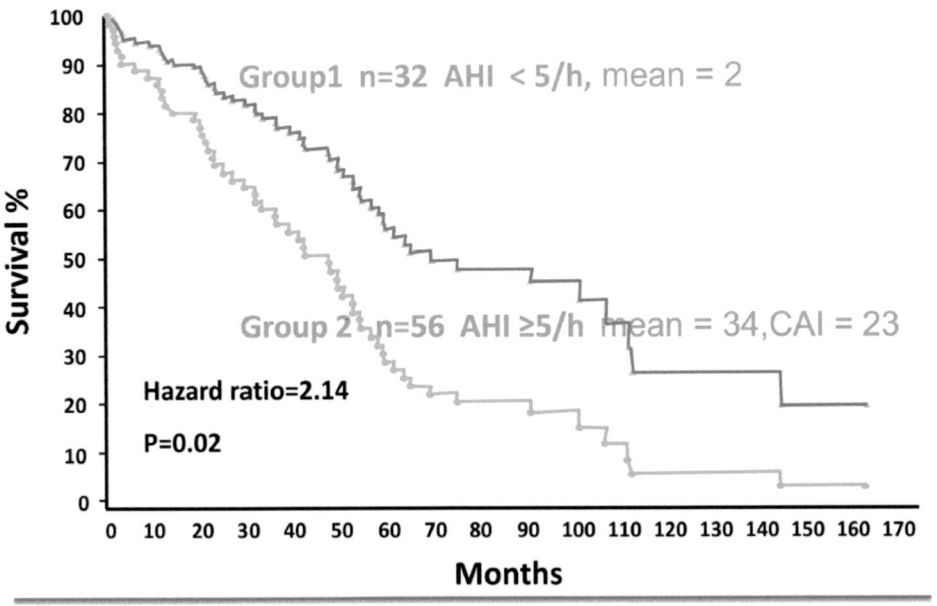

Survival %

Group1 n=32 AHI < 5/h, mean = 2

Group 2 n=56 AHI ≥5/h mean = 34, CAI = 23

Hazard ratio=2.14

P=0.02

Months

Figure 12.4 Probability of survival in patients with systolic heart failure according to the presence or absence of CSA. (Modified from Javaheri, et al. (26).)

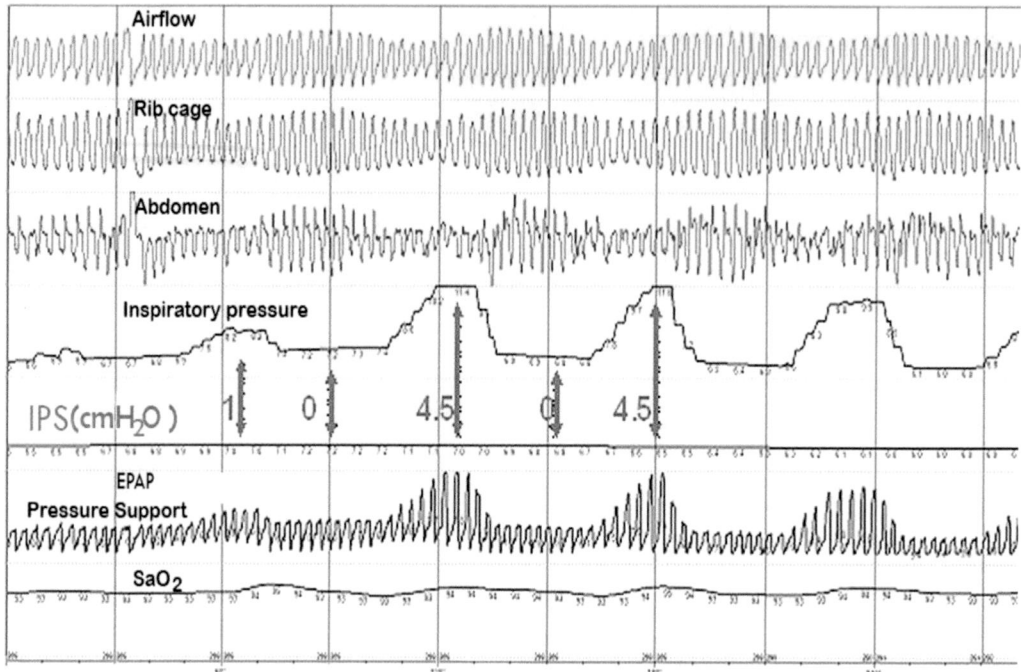

Figure 12.5 This figure depicts the responses of the ASV device to periodic breathing. The top three channels represent the patient's airflow and thoracoabdominal excursions. As the patient's airflow increases (hyperpnea), the pressure delivered by the device decreases (less inspiratory pressure), and when the patient's airflow decreases (hypopnea), the pressure from the device increases (more inspiratory pressure). The device algorithm is anticyclic. (Modified from Javaheri et al, *Chest*, 2014.)

show that effective treatment of CSA with CPAP and adaptive servo-ventilation (ASV) improves survival (27, 28, 31–34). Here, we note that whereas CPAP imposes a constant intrathoracic pressure, ASV algorithms provide an anticyclical pressure support such that when the patient is hypoventilating, the support increases and decreases during hyperventilation (Figure 12.5) (35, 36). In addition, new devices apply automatic EPAP to keep the upper airway open, preventing obstructive events and have been shown to be quite effective in treating CSA (36).

In spite of clear advantages of the ASV algorithm over CPAP devices, surprisingly, the recent ASV trial, SERVE-HF (37) (Treatment of Predominant Central Sleep Apnoea by Adaptive Servo Ventilation in Patients with Heart Failure), designed specifically to treat CSA with ASV, not only did not show a survival benefit, but was associated with excess CV mortality. The latter finding was similar to that of the CANPAP (Canadian Continuous Positive Airway Pressure for Patients with Central Sleep Apnea and Heart Failure) trial, showing

that treatment with CPAP was associated with excess CV mortality early on, and a reason for termination of the trial (38). We suggested (39) that there were two reasons for their findings: (1) there was a subset of patients whose CSA was not suppressed by CPAP as we had previously reported (40), and (2) increased intrathoracic pressure imposed by constant PAP therapy adversely affected the fragile central hemodynamics of HF patients. In regard to the latter suggestion, the SERVE-HF investigators cited this as one of the two reasons for the failure of the ASV device in the clinical trial. The second cited reason was that perhaps CSA serves as a compensatory mechanism with protective effects. In a pro and con debate, we (41–43) scientifically demonstrate that CSA is maladaptive, citing multiple reasons including the associated excess sympathetic activity, which is known to carry a poor prognosis in HF, hence the use of beta-blockers which has been shown to improve survival and remains a mainstay of HF therapy (44). There were also other issues including considerable residual desaturation present throughout the period of the trial (45). Research with newer generation ASV devices is needed, with one in progress (ADVENT-HF [Effect of Adaptive Servo Ventilation (ASV) on Survival and Hospital Admissions in Heart Failure Trial], NCT01128816). However, currently, all ASV devices are contraindicated for use in the treatment of CSA and HFrEF (EF <45%).

WHY IS SDB, PARTICULARLY CSA, UNNOTICED, UNDIAGNOSED, AND UNDER TREATED IN HF PATIENTS?

In the large study of Medicare beneficiaries noted earlier (19), SDB was diagnosed only in the minority of subjects with a diagnosis of HF. The major reason for underdiagnosis is at least in part due to the lack of subjective excessive daytime sleepiness (EDS) in most subjects. In our early study (46), we observed that most subjects did not feel excessively sleepy, in spite of the presence of severe SDB, both in CSA and OSA. Indeed, a minority of the subjects had subjective EDS, both with and without sleep apnea (46) with no difference among them. This observation has been confirmed in later studies using ESS of more than 10 as a criterion (46–49). We found no correlation between subjective ESS and severity of OSA, BMI, age, LVEF, or fatigue severity scale confirming our early observation (46). Notably, when using multiple sleep latency testing (MSLT), studies have consistently shown that many of these subjects may have pathological sleepiness. This is the case for HFrEF patients with either CSA or OSA. In our study of subjects with HFrEF and OSA (47), using both ESS and MSLT, there were patients who scored 10 or less on ESS, but when tested objectively by multiple sleep latency, short sleep latencies, even below 5 minutes were observed (47). Mechanistically, Taranto et al. (50). relate the lack of EDS to increased sympathetic activity. However, this is inconsistent with the pathological sleepiness present when MSLT is performed, and we found no correlation between ESS and mean sleep latency with plasma noradrenaline (47). In contrast, we found a significant correlation with inflammatory markers, consistent with those of Li et al. (51).

We suspect that the main reason for the lack of subjective EDS is related to the overlapping symptoms of two chronic disorders, which are comorbid together for a prolonged period, making it difficult for the subjects to subjectively recognize EDS. It appears that ESS of 10 does not apply to HF, and a lower threshold is more appropriate (52). These overlapping symptoms include sleep-onset and maintenance insomnia, nocturia, waking up with shortness of breath (orthopnea, paroxysmal nocturnal dyspnea,

hyperpnea due to PB), unrefreshed sleep, and daytime fatigue, which are common in both disorders. This is consistent with data showing that when SDB is treated, objective sleepiness improves, but HF subjects do not feel it, because symptoms of HF may persist (48).

It appears that it is easier for cardiologists to suspect OSA, as most of our referrals turn out to have OSA rather than CSA. This is perhaps related to the high presence of obesity and snoring in HF subjects with OSA (2, 6, 32). It has been shown that patients with HFrEF and OSA are significantly heavier and snore habitually, in contrast to those with CSA who are thin and do not snore as much, for which reason we have referred to the presence of SDB in HF as an occult disorder (34).

CURRENT TREATMENT OF SLEEP-RELATED BREATHING DISORDERS IN PATIENTS WITH HEART FAILURE

If mortality and rehospitalization are considered the only outcome to treat SDB in HF, currently, there are no RCTs showing any benefit for treatment for either OSA or CSA. However, given the pitfalls of RCTs and the effects of poor sleep on quality of life, currently, we treat SDB in subjects with HF and the choice of therapy is based on the type of sleep apnea (3, 9).

General recommendations: When applicable, we recommend rules of sleep hygiene, avoidance of alcoholic beverages, benzodiazepines, opioids, and phosphodiesterase-5 inhibitors (particularly at bedtime), smoking cessation, and exercise (3, 9). The use of alcoholic beverages and benzodiazepines may increase the likelihood of upper airway occlusion by promoting the relaxation of the muscles of the upper airway. Opiates may induce CSA and also contribute to OSA, and withdrawal improves both (53). Nicotine, the active chemical in tobacco, increases blood pressure, heart rate, and myocardial oxygen consumption (40). The underlying mechanism is due to increased sympathetic activity via two mechanisms, stimulation of the excitatory nicotinic receptors in the carotid bodies and plasma catecholamine.

Treatment for Obstructive Sleep Apnea in HF

As in the general population, CPAP is the treatment of choice for OSA in patients with HF, although there are some differences. Based on guideline-directed therapy of HF, attempts should be made to optimize cardiopulmonary function, and it has been shown that optimal treatment improves PB by multiple mechanisms (3, 9). One specific issue is related to volume overload present frequently in patients with HF. At least for two reasons,

159

HF may facilitate upper airway narrowing, both the presence of lower extremity edema and the presence of elevated right atrial and central venous pressure can cause pharyngeal congestion and edema (18, 54). In the supine position, fluid from lower extremities is translocated cephalad, resulting in narrowing of the upper airway and measures to decrease the lower extremity edema and venous pressure are advisable (18). Optimal treatment of HF to decrease lung water and pleural effusion could increase lung volumes, which should increase upper airway size, which is dependent on lung volume. Diuretics also improve FEV1, FVC, and FEV1/FVC ratio in normal subjects (55), and should considerably improve airway function in subjects with HF in whom there is increased lung water.

Exercise

In a four-arm RCT in patients with HFrEF, we (56) showed that 3-month supervised aerobic exercise decreased AHI from 28 to 18/hr of sleep (P <0.03) whereas there was no significant change (AHI = 29/hr of sleep vs. 31/hr of sleep) in the control group. The weight change was minimal. Mechanisms could include decreased lower extremity edema (by activating the musculovenous pump), which decreases rostral fluid redistribution in supine position noted earlier, stabilization of chemoreceptor hypersensitivity, improved nasal resistance, strength of pharyngeal dilator muscles, and sleep quality, and weight loss when it occurs (58).

CPAP and Oral Appliance Therapy of OSA

Both CPAP and oral appliances have been used to treat OSA in HF, with the former being the therapy of choice and with most commonly studied, but adherence is a critical factor and remains poor. As noted earlier, two observational studies (19, 22) of patients with HF have shown that effective treatment of OSA with CPAP improves survival, particularly in those who are compliant with CPAP. RCTs are not available and are badly needed. In CPAP-intolerant subjects, custom-made oral appliances are recommended, though limited studies are available in HF (57, 58).

Treatment for Central Sleep Apnea in HF

A pathway for current approach to treat CSA in HF is suggested in Figure 12.6. However, we emphasize that the general measures including

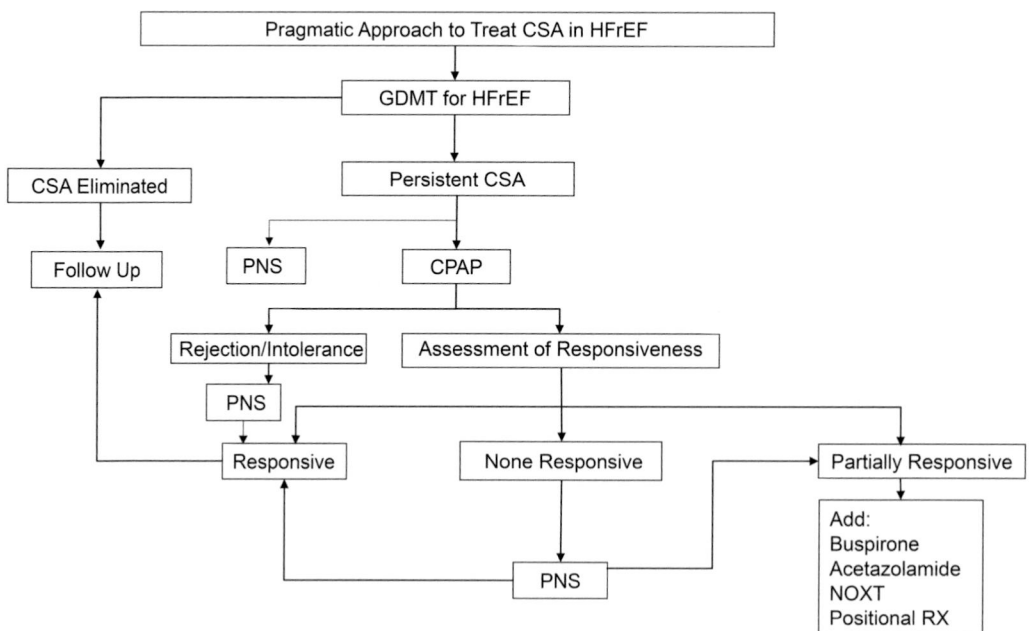

Figure 12.6 A Suggested clinical approach to the treatment of CSA in patients without HFrEF and HFpEF. CSA: Central sleep apnea; HFrEF: Heart failure with reduced ejection fraction; HFpEF: Heart failure with preserved ejection fraction. CPAP: Continuous positive airway pressure device; PNS: Phrenic nerve stimulation; NOXT: nocturnal oxygen therapy. (Modified from Javaheri, et al., *Chest*, 2020.)

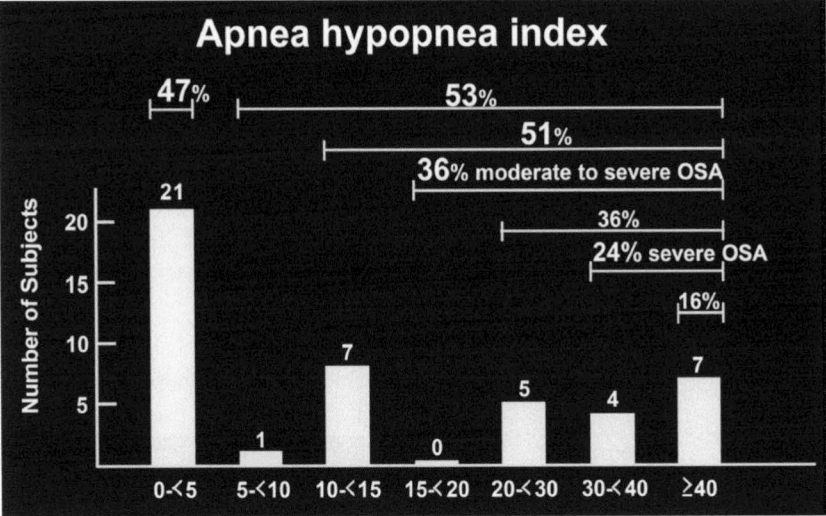

Figure 12.7 Prevalence of obstructive sleep apnea in 45 out of 60 consecutive cardiac transplant recipients. Those who developed sleep apnea had gained the most weight after transplantation. (Modified from Javaheri, et al., *EHJ*, 2004, reference (60).)

recommendation regarding rules of sleep hygiene, optimization of cardiopulmonary function noted for treatment of OSA also apply to the treatment of CSA. Guideline-directed medical therapy (GDMT), intensive pharmacological therapy for HF, and resynchronization therapy (CRT) can improve PB. CRT implanted as part of GDMT improves CSA, particularly in those in whom central hemodynamics improve (59).

Cardiac Transplantation

In the largest and prospective study so far reported after cardiac transplantation (*n* = 60), CSA was virtually eliminated (60), though, with time, a number of recipients develop OSA (Figure 12.7). In this study, 45 of 60 consecutive subjects agreed to undergo full night attended polysomnography. Subjects were at least 5 months post-transplant and were on maintenance dose of prednisone (5 to 10 mg daily), and anti-rejection medications including cyclosporine. OSA developed in those who had gained the most weight after transplantation, and it was associated with habitual snoring, poor quality of life, and systemic hypertension. Development of post-transplant OSA may contribute to rejection, which occurred in one patient in the aforementioned study (60). In this regard, a retrospective study (61) involving 29 consecutive cardiac transplant recipients, 20% with untreated OSA, had a three times higher risk of developing late graft dysfunction than those with treated or no OSA. We, therefore, suggest that cardiac transplant recipients who gain weight, snore, develop hypertension, or rejection should be checked for the development of OSA.

Positive Airway Pressure Devices

As noted earlier, both CPAP and ASV have been used to treat CSA in HF. For now, ASV is contraindicated, though a second trial is ongoing and so far, interim analyses have not reported a signal for excess mortality. CPAP is used to treat CSA in HF, but in a large number of patients, CPAP fails to suppress CSA. Options other than PAP therapies are discussed below.

Transvenous Phrenic Nerve Stimulation (TPNS)

TPNS stabilizes breathing by stimulating a single phrenic nerve using neurostimulation (Figure 12.8). The device activates automatically at night, ensuring compliance. It is implanted in the cardiac suite similar to a cardiac device implant (62). In a multicenter RCT, PNS significantly improved central sleep apnea index, arousal index, and ODI in a varied group of CSA patients (63). Persistent efficacy has been demonstrated up to 5 years with improved Epworth Sleepiness Scale and quality of life (64, 65).

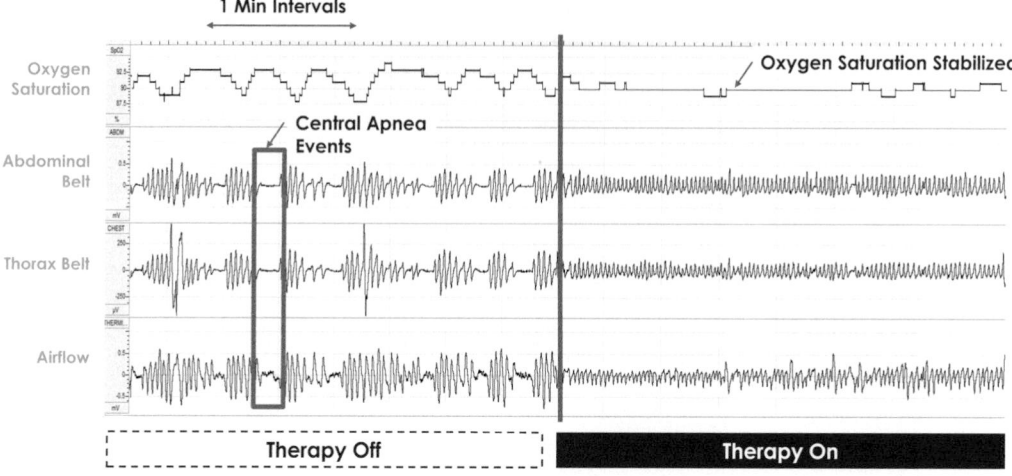

Figure 12.8 Changes in breathing pattern with phrenic nerve stimulation. The left side demonstrates central sleep apnea and the right site demonstrates stabilization of the breathing pattern with phrenic nerve stimulation. (Modified from Costanzo MR, et al., *J Card Fail*, 2015;21:892-902.)

In a post-hoc analysis of the HF cohort (64% of the patients in the trial), improvements were similar to the main cohort including improvements in daytime sleepiness (66). A disease-specific quality of life metric, Minnesota Living with Heart Failure was improved at 12 months (6.8 ± 20, p = 0.005). In addition, there was a non-significant decrease in time to first HF hospitalization at 6 months. In a pooled analysis of the previously discussed RCT and a pilot study, ejection fraction increased at 12 months in patients with HF and ejection fraction ≤45% (67). A recent single-center observational study of HF patients with CSA, improvements were noted in hypoxemic burden and importantly in exercise capacity by 6-minute hall walk distance at 6 months (68).

Safety of the procedure, system, and therapy is similar to cardiac implantable devices. There was 91% freedom from serious adverse events through 12 months in the RCT discussed above (63). Serious adverse events included infection, lead dislodgement, and hematoma. All adverse events were resolved prior to study closure. Safety was monitored closely and there was no difference between therapy and control groups at 6 months (two deaths in each group). Longitudinally, all patients received therapy after 6 months but have been monitored through 5 years without additional safety concerns (65). While the data is encouraging, additional RCTs are needed to determine if TPNS has an impact on CV outcomes. No RCTs

for CV outcomes have been completed with TPNS to date.

Low Flow Nocturnal Oxygen Therapy
Multiple observational studies in patients with systolic HF (3, 9, 69) have shown that low flow nocturnal therapy improves CSA and nocturnal desaturation. Small, randomized, placebo-controlled double-blind studies have shown that short-term (1–4 wk) administration of nocturnal supplemental nasal oxygen improves CSA, nocturnal desaturation, sleep architecture, maximal exercise capacity and decreases overnight urinary norepinephrine excretion (70–72). Three randomized, but open trials (73–75) ranging from 9 to 52 weeks reported that low-flow oxygen therapy improves CSA and desaturation, and significantly increases LVEF and improves the quality of life of patients with HF. Recently, the National Heart, Lung, and Blood Institute (NHLBI) approved a phase III randomized controlled trial evaluating nocturnal oxygen (NOX) for the treatment of central sleep apnea in patients with HFrEF (NCT03745898). This RCT uses nocturnal low-flow oxygen therapy in the active arm and comparable airflow from a concentrator in the control arm. The primary composite outcome is HF-related hospital admissions and all-cause mortality rates. Unfortunately, the trial was terminated because of inadequate enrollment-below the number of expected subjects, during the Covid Sars-2 epidemic.

Supplemental administration of nasal oxygen may decrease PB by several mechanisms. These include an increase in the difference between the prevailing PCO_2 and the PCO_2 at the apneic threshold; a reduction in the ventilatory response to CO_2 and perhaps to hypoxemia; and an increase in body stores (e.g., lung contents) of oxygen, which increases damping. Prospective placebo-controlled long-term studies, however, are necessary to determine whether nocturnal oxygen therapy has the potential to decrease mortality of patients with systolic HF.

Medications

Drugs that decrease plant gain theophylline (76, 77) and acetazolamide (78, 79) have undergone short-term RCTs, but long-term studies have not yet been completed.

Theophylline

In a double-blind randomized placebo-controlled crossover study (76) of 15 patients with treated, stable systolic HF, oral theophylline at therapeutic plasma concentration (11 µg/mL, range 7–15 µg/mL) decreased the AHI by about 50% and improved arterial oxyhemoglobin saturation. At therapeutic serum concentrations, theophylline competes with adenosine at some of its receptor sites. In the central nervous system, adenosine is a respiratory depressant, and theophylline stimulates breathing by competing with adenosine. Conceivably, an increase in ventilation by theophylline decreasing the plant gain could decrease central apnea during sleep.

Potential arrhythmogenic effects and phosphodiesterase inhibition are common concerns with long-term use of theophylline in patients with HF. Therefore, further controlled studies are necessary to ensure its safety. If theophylline is used to treat CSA, frequent and careful follow-ups are necessary.

Acetazolamide

A double-blind placebo-controlled crossover study (78) of 12 patients with HFrEF, showed that acetazolamide, administered at about 3 mg/kg one-half hour before bedtime, decreased the central AHI significantly from about 57/hr (in the placebo arm) to 34/hr. Acetazolamide caused metabolic acidosis by inhibiting renal carbonic anhydrase and decreased PCO_2 significantly. In spite of reduction in PCO_2, CSA improved. With a lower PCO_2, plant gain decreases protecting against developing CSA. Long-term trials are badly needed given the ease of using it as one dose before bedtime.

Buspirone (80, 81)

Buspirone, a presynaptic 5-HT1A receptor agonist used in general anxiety disorder, was shown to decrease the chemosensitivity to hypercapnia and stabilize breathing in a mouse model of hypoxia-induced apneas (80). Therefore, buspirone, by decreasing controller gain, may be effective to treat CSA in HF. A recent double-blind randomized placebo-controlled crossover trial study (81) demonstrated that after 1 week of treatment, buspirone decreased the central chemosensitivity to hypercapnia by 41% and stabilized breathing with a 40 to 80% reduction in the apnea-hypopnea index and amelioration of oxygen desaturation profile compared to placebo, without significant side effects. Long-term trials are badly needed.

PHENOTYPIC TREATMENT OF SLEEP-DISORDERED BREATHING IN HF

In HF, both CSA and OSA are heterogeneous syndrome, with varied pathophysiological mechanisms, clinical presentations, and predisposing factors. Several physiological phenotypes/endotypes exist and each one could become a target of therapy. This approach is in its infancy and has been reviewed in detail elsewhere (82, 83). Large long-term RCTs are needed.

SUMMARY

Because of the increased average life span and improved therapy of ischemic coronary artery disease and hypertension, the prevalence of HF remains high. HF has a significant economic impact and is associated with excess morbidity and mortality.

SDB, both OSA and CSA, are common comorbidities with HF. The pathophysiological consequences of sleep-related breathing disorders have deleterious effects on the CV system and based on multiple observational studies independently are associated with poor quality of life, excess rehospitalization, and premature mortality. Notably, multiple observational studies have demonstrated that effective treatment of both OSA and CSA decreases hospital readmission and improves survival, particularly in those patients who are most adherent to therapy. However, RCTs have been inconclusive. Treatment options should start with evidence-based therapy for HF. If SDB is present, treatment is based on the predominance of OSA or CSA. While it is effective for decreasing AHI, ASV remains contraindicated in patients with EF <45%. Currently, treatment for CSA in HF should be targeted to improve AHI and alleviate patient symptoms until additional RCTs demonstrate improvements in CV outcomes.

REFERENCES

1. Virani SS, Alonso A, Benjamin EJ, et al. Heart Disease and Stroke Statistics-2021 update: a report from the American Heart Association. Circulation 2021;141 (9):e139–e596.

2. Halley CM, Houghtaling PL, Khalil MK, et al. Mortality rate in patients with diastolic dysfunction and normal systolic function. Arch Int Med 2011;171:1082–1087.

3. Javaheri S, Parker TJ, Liming JD, et al. Sleep apnea in 81 ambulatory male patients with stable heart failure. Types and their prevalences, consequences, and presentations. Circulation 1998;97(21):2154–2159.

4. Javaheri S, Barbe F, Campos-Rodriguez F, et al. Sleep apnea: types, mechanisms, and clinical cardiovascular consequences. J Am Coll Cardiol 2017;69(7):841–858.

5. Oldenburg O, Wellmann B, Buchholz A, et al. Nocturnal hypoxaemia is associated with increased mortality in stable heart failure patients. Eur Heart J 2016;37(21):1695–703.

6. Tremel F, Pepin JL, Veale D, et al. High prevalence and persistence of sleep apnoea in patients referred for acute left ventricular failure and medically treated over 2 months. Eur Heart J 1999;20(16):1201–1209.

7. Javaheri S. Sleep disorders in systolic heart failure: a prospective study of 100 male patients. The final report. Int J Cardiol 2006;106(1):21–28.

8. Javaheri S, Dempsey JA. Central sleep apnea. Compr Physiol 2013;3(1):141–163.

9. Javaheri S. Heart Failure. In: Principles and Practices of Sleep Medicine 7/e. Edited by Kryger MH, Roth T, Dement WC; WB Saunders, Philadelphia. 2021.

10. Javaheri S, Elliott M. Central Sleep Apnoea. In: Non-Invasive Ventilation and Weaning: Principles and Practice 2/e. Chapter 43: 408–418. Edited by Mark E, Stefano N, Bernd S; Taylor & Francis Group, Boca Raton, New York, London. 2019.

11. Randerath WJ, Javaheri S. Sleep and Heart. In Oxford textbook of Sleep Disorders. 395–408. Edited by Chokrovery S, Ferini-Strambi L; Oxford University Press, Oxford. 2017.

12. Ward M. Periodic respiration. A short historical note. Ann R Coll Surg Engl 1973;52(5):330–334.

13. Millar TW, Hanly PJ, Hunt B, Frais M, Kryger MH. The entrainment of low frequency breathing periodicity. Chest 1990;98(5):1143–1148.

14. Bitter T, Faber L, Hering D, Langer C, Horstkotte D, Oldenburg O. Sleep-disordered breathing in heart failure with normal left ventricular ejection fraction. Eur J Heart Fail 2009;11(6):602–608.

15. Herrscher TE, Akre H, Overland B, Sandvik L, Westheim AS. High prevalence of sleep apnea in heart failure outpatients: even in patients with preserved systolic function. J Card Fail 2011;17(5):420–425.

16. Khayat R, Abraham W, Patt B, et al. Central sleep apnea is a predictor of cardiac readmission in hospitalized patients with systolic heart failure. J Card Fail 2012;18(7):534–540.

17. Uchoa CHG, Pedrosa RP, Javaheri S, et al. OSA and prognosis after acute cardiogenic pulmonary edema: the OSA-CARE Study. Chest 2017;152(6):1230–1238.

18. Yumino D, Redolfi S, Ruttanaumpawan P, et al. Nocturnal rostral fluid shift: a unifying concept for the pathogenesis of obstructive and central sleep apnea in men with heart failure. Circulation 2010;121(14):1598–1605.

19. Javaheri S, Caref EB, Chen E, Tong KB, Abraham WT. Sleep apnea testing and outcomes in a large cohort of Medicare beneficiaries with newly diagnosed heart failure. Am J Respir Crit Care Med 2011;183(4):539–546.

20. Khayat RN, Javaheri S, Porter K, et al. In-hospital management of sleep apnea during heart failure hospitalization: a randomized, controlled trial. J Cardiac Fail 2020;26:705–712.

21. Kauta SR, Keenan BT, Goldberg L, Schwab RJ. Diagnosis and treatment of sleep disordered breathing in hospitalized cardiac patients: a reduction in 30-day hospital readmission rates. J Clin Sleep Med 2014;10(10):1051–1059.

22. Wang H, Parker JD, Newton GE, et al. Influence of obstructive sleep apnea on mortality in patients with heart failure. J Am Coll Cardiol 2007;49(15):1625–1631.

23. Khayat R, Jarjoura D, Porter K, et al. Sleep disordered breathing and post-discharge mortality in patients with acute heart failure. Eur Heart J 2015;36:1463–9.

24. Kasai T, Narui K, Dohi T, et al. Prognosis of patients with heart failure and obstructive sleep apnea treated with continuous positive airway pressure. Chest 2008;133(3):690–696.

25. Hanly PJ, Zuberi-Khokhar NS. Increased mortality associated with Cheyne-Stokes respiration in patients with congestive heart failure. Am J Respir Crit Care Med 1996;153(1):272–276.

26. Javaheri S, Shukla R, Zeigler H, Wexler L. Central sleep apnea, right ventricular dysfunction, and low diastolic blood pressure are predictors of mortality in systolic heart failure. J Am Coll Cardiol 2007;49(20):2028–2034.

27. Arzt M, Floras JS, Logan AG, et al. Suppression of central sleep apnea by continuous positive airway pressure and transplant-free survival in heart failure: a post hoc analysis of the Canadian Continuous Positive Airway Pressure for Patients with Central Sleep Apnea and Heart Failure Trial (CANPAP). Circulation 2007;115(25):3173–3180.

28. Jilek C, Krenn M, Sebah D, et al. Prognostic impact of sleep disordered breathing and its treatment in heart failure: an observational study. Eur J Heart Fail 2011;13(1):68–75.

29. Huang Y, Wang Y, Huang Y, et al. Prognostic value of sleep apnea and nocturnal hypoxemia in patients with decompensated heart failure. Clin Cardiol 2020;43(4):329–337. doi:10.1002/clc.23319.

30. Azarbarzin A, Sands SA, Stone KL, et al. The hypoxic burden of sleep apnoea predicts cardiovascular disease-related mortality: the Osteoporotic Fractures in Men Study and the Sleep Heart Health Study. Eur Heart J 2019;40:1149–1157.

31. Galetke W, Ghassemi BM, Priegnitz C, et al. Anticyclic modulated ventilation versus continuous positive airway pressure in patients with coexisting obstructive sleep apnea and Cheyne-Stokes respiration: a randomized crossover trial. Sleep Med 2014;15(8):874–879.

32. Kasai T, Usui Y, Yoshioka T, et al. Effect of flow-triggered adaptive servo-ventilation compared with continuous positive airway pressure in patients with chronic heart failure with coexisting obstructive sleep apnea and Cheyne-Stokes respiration. Circ Heart Fail 2010;3(1):140–148.

33. Randerath WJ, Nothofer G, Priegnitz C, et al. Long-term auto-servoventilation or constant positive pressure in heart failure and coexisting central with obstructive sleep apnea. Chest 2012;142(2):440–447.

34. Oldenburg O, Bitter T, Wellmann B, et al. Trilevel adaptive servoventilation for the treatment of central and mixed sleep apnea in chronic heart failure patients. Sleep Med 2013;14(5):422–427.

35. Javaheri S, Brown LK, Randerath WJ. Positive airway pressure therapy with adaptive servoventilation: part 1: operational algorithms. Chest 2014;146(2):514–523.

36. Javaheri S, Goetting MG, Khayat R, et al. The performance of two automatic servo-ventilation devices in the treatment of central sleep apnea. Sleep 2011;34(12):1693–1698.

37. Cowie MR, Woehrle H, Wegscheider K, et al. Adaptive servo-ventilation for central sleep apnea in systolic heart failure. N Engl J Med 2015;373:1095–1105.

38. Bradley TD, Logan AG, Kimoff RJ, et al. Continuous positive airway pressure for central sleep apnea and heart failure. N Engl J Med 2005;353:2025–2033.

39. Javaheri S. CPAP should not be used for central sleep apnea in congestive heart failure patients. J Clin Sleep Med 2006;2(4):399–402.

40. Javaheri S. Effects of continuous positive airway pressure on sleep apnea and ventricular irritability in patients with heart failure. Circulation 2000;101(4):392–397.

41. Javaheri S, Brown LK, Khayat R. CON: persistent central sleep apnea/Hunter-Cheyne-Stokes breathing, despite best guideline-based therapy of heart failure with reduced ejection fraction, is not a compensatory mechanism and should be suppressed. J Clin Sleep Med 2018;14(6):915–921.

42. Naughton M T. PRO: persistent central sleep apnea/Hunter-Cheyne-Stokes Breathing, despite best guideline-based therapy of heart failure with reduced ejection fraction, is a compensatory mechanism and should not be suppressed. J Clin Sleep Med 2018;14:909–913.

43. Javaheri S, Brown LK, Khayat R. Rebuttal to Naughton. J Clin Sleep Med 2018;14(6):923–925.

44. Packer M, Bristow MR, Cohn JN, et al. The effect of carvedilol of morbidity and mortality in patients with chronic heart failure. N Engl J Med 1996;334:1349–1355.

45. Javaheri S, Brown LK, Randerath W, Khayat R. SERVE-HF: more questions than answers. Chest 2016;149(4):900–904.

46. Javaheri S, Parker TJ, Wexler L, et al. Occult sleep-disordered breathing in stable congestive heart failure. Ann Intern Med 1995;122(7):487–492.

47. Hanly P, Zuberi-Khokhar N. Daytime sleepiness in patients with congestive heart failure and Cheyne-Stokes respiration. Chest 1995;107(4):952–958.

48. Pepperell JC, Maskell NA, Jones DR, et al. A randomized controlled trial of adaptive ventilation for Cheyne-Stokes breathing in heart failure. Am J Respir Crit Care Med 2003;168(9):1109–1114.

49. Mehra R, Wang L, Andrews N, et al. Dissociation of objective and subjective daytime sleepiness and biomarkers of systemic inflammation in sleep-disordered breathing and systolic heart failure. J Clin Sleep Med 2017;13(12):1411–1422.

50. Taranto Montemurro L, Floras JS, Millar PJ, et al. Inverse relationship of subjective daytime sleepiness to sympathetic activity in patients with heart failure and obstructive sleep apnea. Chest 2012;142(5):1222–1228.

51. Li Y, Vgontzas AN, Fernandez-Mendoza J, et al. Objective, but not subjective, sleepiness is associated with inflammation in sleep apnea. Sleep 2017;40(2):zsw033.

52. Javaheri S, McKane S, Meyer T, Germany R. Select symptoms from the Epworth Sleepiness Scale questionnaire and response to therapy of central sleep apnea with phrenic nerve stimulation. Sleep 2020;43(S1):A270–A271.

53. Javaheri S, Patel S. Opioids cause central and complex sleep apnea in humans and reversal with discontinuation: a plea for detoxification. J Clin Sleep Med 2017;13(6):829–833.

54. Javaheri S, Bosken CH, Lim SP, Dohn MN, Greene NB, Baughman RP. Effects of hypohydration on lung function in humans. Am Rev Respir Dis 1987; 135:597–599. 56.

55. Iftikhar IH, Kline CE, Youngstedt SD. Effects of exercise training on sleep apnea: a meta-analysis. Lung 2014;192(1):175–118.

56. Servantes DM, Javaheri S, Kravchychyn ACP, et al. Effects of exercise training and CPAP in patients with heart failure and OSA: a preliminary study. Chest 2018;154(4):808–817.

57. Eskafi M, Cline C, Israelsson B, Nilner M. A mandibular advancement device reduces sleep disordered breathing in patients with congestive heart failure. Swed Dent J 2004;28(4):155–163.

58. Eskafi M, Ekberg E, Cline C, Israelsson B, Nilner M. Use of a mandibular advancement device in patients with congestive heart failure and sleep apnoea. Gerodontology 2004;21(2):100–107.

59. Oldenburg O, Faber L, Vogt J, et al. Influence of cardiac resynchronisation therapy on different types of sleep disordered breathing. Eur J Heart Fail 2007;9(8):820–826.

60. Javaheri S, Abraham WT, Brown C, Nishiyama H, Giesting R, Wagoner LE. Prevalence of obstructive sleep apnoea and periodic limb movement in 45 subjects with heart transplantation. Eur Heart J 2004;25(3):260–266.

61. Afzal A, Tecson K M, Jamil AK, et al. The effect of obstructive sleep apnea on 3-year outcomes in patients who underwent orthotopic heart transplantation. Am J Cardiol 2019: 124:51–54. doi:10.1016/j.amjcard.2019.04.005.

62. Costanzo MR, Augostini R, Goldberg LR, et al. Design of the remedē® System Pivotal Trial: a prospective, randomized study in the use of respiratory rhythm management to treat central sleep apnea. J Card Fail 2015;21:892–902.

63. Costanzo MR, Ponikowski P, Javaheri S, et al. Randomised controlled trial of transvenous neurostimulation for central sleep apnoea. The Lancet 2016;388:974–982.

64. Fox H, Oldenburg O, Javaheri S, et al. Long-term efficacy and safety of phrenic nerve stimulation for the treatment of central sleep apnea. Sleep 2019;21;42. 1–8. https://pubmed.ncbi.nlm.nih.gov/31634407/

65. Javaheri S, Schwartz AR, Abraham WT, et al. Effects of transvenous phrenic nerve stimulation on central sleep apnea and sleep architecture: the 5 year analysis. CHEST presentation. October, 2020.

66. Costanzo MR, Ponikowski P, Coats A, et al. Phrenic nerve stimulation to treat patients with central sleep apnoea and heart failure. Eur J Heart Fail 2018;12:1746–1754.

67. Fudim M, Spector AR, Costanzo MR, et al. Phrenic nerve stimulation for the treatment of central sleep apnea: a pooled cohort analysis. J Clin Sleep Med 2019;15:1747–1755.

68. Potratz M, Sohns C, Dumitrescu D, et al. Phrenic nerve stimulation improves physical performance and hypoxemia in heart failure patients with central sleep apnea. J Clin Med 2021. doi: 10.3390/jcm10020202.

69. Javaheri S. Pembrey's dream: the time has come for a long-term trial of nocturnal supplemental nasal oxygen to treat central sleep apnea in congestive heart failure. Chest 2003;123(2):322–325.

70. Hanly PJ, Millar TW, Steljes DG, Baert R, Frais MA, Kryger MH. The effect of oxygen on respiration and sleep in patients with congestive heart failure. Ann Intern Med 1989;111(10):777–782.

71. Andreas S, Clemens C, Sandholzer H, Figulla HR, Kreuzer H. Improvement of exercise capacity with treatment of Cheyne-Stokes respiration in patients with congestive heart failure. J Am Coll Cardiol 1996;27(6):1486–1490.

72. Staniforth AD, Kinnear WJ, Starling R, Hetmanski DJ, Cowley AJ. Effect of oxygen on sleep quality, cognitive function and sympathetic activity in patients with chronic heart failure and Cheyne-Stokes respiration. Eur Heart J 1998;19(6):922–928.

73. Sasayama S, Izumi T, Matsuzaki M, et al. Improvement of quality of life with nocturnal oxygen therapy in heart failure patients with central sleep apnea. Circ J 2009;73(7):1255–1262.

74. Sasayama S, Izumi T, Seino Y, Ueshima K, Asanoi H, Group C-HS. Effects of nocturnal oxygen therapy on outcome measures in patients with chronic heart failure and Cheyne-Stokes respiration. Circ J 2006;70(1):1–7.

75. Toyama T, Seki R, Kasama S, et al. Effectiveness of nocturnal home oxygen therapy to improve exercise capacity, cardiac function and cardiac sympathetic nerve activity in patients with chronic heart failure and central sleep apnea. Circ J 2009;73(2):299–304.

76. Hu K, Li Q, Yang J, Hu S, Chen X. The effect of theophylline on sleep-disordered breathing in patients with stable chronic congestive heart failure. Chin Med J (Engl) 2003;116(11):1711–1716.

77. Javaheri S, Parker TJ, Wexler L, Liming JD, Lindower P, Roselle GA. Effect of theophylline on sleep-disordered breathing in heart failure. N Engl J Med 1996;335(8):562–567.

78. Javaheri S, Sands SA, Edwards BA. Acetazolamide attenuates Hunter-Cheyne-Stokes breathing but augments the hypercapnic ventilatory response in patients with heart failure. Ann Am Thorac Soc 2014;11(1):80–86.

79. Javaheri S. Acetazolamide improves central sleep apnea in heart failure: a double-blind, prospective study. Am J Respir Crit Care Med 2006;173(2):234–237.

80. Yamauchi M, Dostal J, Kimura H, Strohl KP. Effects of buspirone on posthypoxic ventilatory behavior in the C57BL/6J and A/J mouse strains. J Appl Physiol (1985) 2008;105:518–526.

81. Giannoni A, Borrelli C, Mirizzi G, Richerson GB, Emdin M, Passino C. Benefit of buspirone on chemoreflex and central apnoeas in heart failure: a randomized controlled crossover trial. Eur J Heart Fail 2020;23(2):312–320. doi: 10.1002/ejhf.1854. Epub Ahead of Print.

82. Javaheri S, Brown LK, Abraham WT, Khayat R. Apneas of heart failure and phenotype-guided treatments: part one: OSA. Chest 2020;157(2): 394–402.

83. Javaheri S, Brown LK, Khayat RN. Update on apneas of heart failure with reduced ejection fraction: emphasis on the physiology of treatment: part 2: central sleep apnea. Chest 2020;157(6): 1637–1646.

13 Breathing at Altitude

David Patz

INTRODUCTION

The physiologic consequences of high-altitude hypobaric pressure were discovered by balloonists in the eighteenth century, some of whom did not survive. There was some controversy whether the ailments related to altitude were related to hyperventilation and hypocarbia, per Angelo Musso, or hypoxemia, per Paul Bert. Three physiologists (Nathan Zuntz, Joseph Barcroft, and C.G. Douglas – of "the Douglas Bag"), around 1900, studied their own alveolar gases after ascending to 3,350 m (10,990 ft), at the Alta Vista hut in the Canary Islands. Douglas' and Zuntz's personal findings showed hyperventilation, with alveolar partial pressure of carbon dioxide ($PaCO_2$) falling (compared to sea level values) from 41 to 32 and 35 to 27, respectively, and both did not develop mountain sickness. Barcroft, on the other hand, had no drop in his alveolar $PaCO_2$ at altitude and developed severe mountain sickness. The three investigators' findings supported the suggestion of Paul Bert that the mountain sickness was caused by hypoxemia rather than the hypocarbia at altitude. Conversely, this example helps us understand that it is the hyperventilation that relatively improves PO_2, that helps us acclimate to altitude and minimize mountain sickness (1).

Sleep apnea at altitude was first commented on by an English physicist and mountaineer, Tyndall, in 1860 and later Egli-Sinclair, in 1894, noted that at an altitude of 4,400 m (14,436 ft), during sleep, breathing "had the Stokes character", alluding to William Stokes, of Cheyne-Stokes's respiration (2). Angelo Mosso published a recording of this breathing pattern at the Margherita hut at 4,550 m (14,900 ft) in 1898. His brother slept with a bar placed across his chest, with a stylet at the end, marking a rotating drum beside the bed. Every 2 or 3 breaths were followed by a 12-second pause (Figure 13.1) (3).

ACCLIMATIZATION TO ALTITUDE
Ventilatory Acclimatization

Ascending quickly, in a high-altitude hot air balloon, one hyperventilates in response to the hypoxia but has little time for further physiologic adjustments. In a less precipitous ascent, acclimatization describes the additional physiologic changes which provide further improvement in oxygen delivery to the tissues at altitude (4). The most immediate response is the hypoxic ventilatory response (HVR) leading to hyperventilation and thus improvement in PaO_2. The primary site for the oxygen (O_2) chemoreceptors is the carotid body (CB), signaling through the carotid sinus nerve (CSN) to the medullary respiratory centers (5). There is significant individual variation in HVR, as demonstrated by the data above, from the three early physiologists, which may contribute to a person's ability to acclimate. While the three physiologists in 1900 could not measure O_2 or HVR, presumably Barcroft, who failed to hyperventilate at altitude, was more hypoxemic, explaining his development of altitude sickness.

At altitude, within hours, there is a progressive further increase in resting ventilation and the HVR due to CB hypertrophy. While some cells in the human body sicken or die from hypoxemia, unique glomus cells in the CB grow and multiply in hypoxemia (6). This hypertrophy of the CB occurs within hours, continuing to grow, up to several weeks at altitude (7). The carotid hypertrophy leads to hypersensitization to hypoxemia, increased HVR, and is the primary site responsible for the time-dependent increasing ventilation at altitude, resulting in acclimatization. Animal studies have shown that denervation of the CB eliminates acclimatization, i.e. eliminates the progressively increased ventilation in response to hypoxemia. In cat and goat models, where the CB is vascularly isolated, studies evaluating CSN activity (the main neural output of the CB) show a progressive increase in CSN activity from 1 hour to several days after initiating hypoxic exposure to the CB, reflecting the progressive CB hypertrophy. In this same model, with isolated CBs perfused with hypoxic blood, there was a normal acclimatization with a progressive increase in ventilation over time (8).

The renal excretion of bicarbonate is an important part of ventilatory acclimatization. The initial boost in ventilation, due to the HVR, produces a respiratory alkalosis, with the alkalosis braking further increase in ventilation until bicarbonate loss in the urine, promotes a compensatory metabolic acidosis, "un-braking" the alkalosis and thus allowing a further increase in ventilation (4). Within days, arterial blood gases will reveal a hypoxic, compensated respiratory alkalosis.

DOI: 10.1201/9781003000631-16

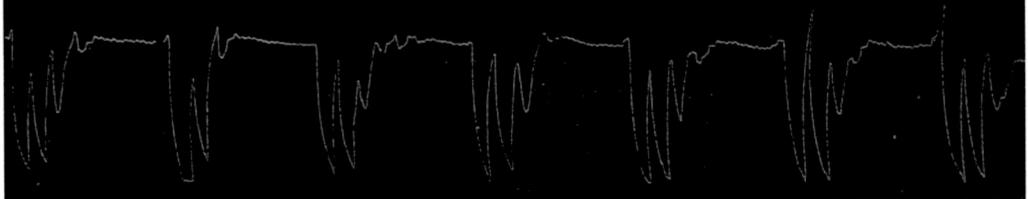

Figure 13.1 Tracing on a rotating smoked drum from a stylette at the end of a bar lying across the chest of Angelo Mosso's brother while asleep at the Margherita Hut on Mt. Rosa, at 4,550 m (14,900 ft) in the 1890s, demonstrating periodic breathing at altitude. The pauses between breaths are about 12 s each. (From Life of Man in the High Alps, A Musso (3).)

Non-Ventilatory Factors Contributing to Acclimatization

Cardiovascular

The immediate cardiovascular response to arrival at altitude is to maintain O_2 delivery to the tissues and to compensate for the hypoxemia by increasing cardiac output. This is achieved by increasing heart rate without a change in stroke volume. Over a couple of weeks at moderate altitudes, as hematocrit increases, increasing blood O_2 content, heart rate returns to near sea level heart rate, though above 4,500 m, many sojourners will remain tachycardic. There is hypoxic pulmonary vasoconstriction (HPV) at altitude, which can affect maximal exercise performance in some climbers/travelers to altitude. Within a couple of weeks at extreme elevations, pulmonary vascular remodeling may begin, with decreased reversibility in response to O_2 (65).

Erythropoiesis

Hypoxemia stimulates the O_2 sensing cells in the kidney to produce erythropoietin within 2 hours of altitude, subsequently increasing red cell mass and hemoglobin (Hgb), improving O_2 content and delivery. However, the increase in blood viscosity at Hgb concentrations above 18 g/dL is curvilinear, and further increases can affect systemic and pulmonary vascular resistance and cardiac output (9).

Hemoglobin's Oxygen Affinity

At altitude, there is an increase in 2, 3, diphosphoglycerate (2,3, DPG), a product of red blood cell metabolism. 2, 3, DPG causes a decrease in Hgb affinity to O_2, which enhances the ability to deliver O_2 to the tissues (10). However, this benefit is debated because decreased affinity may decrease the ability of the blood traveling through the pulmonary capillaries to pick up O_2 in the lung (11). This latter factor is especially relevant at extreme altitudes or with vigorous exercise when there is a diffusion limitation in the lungs. Samaja concluded that at altitudes up to 5,000 m (16,400 ft), the reduced affinity promoted by increased 2, 3, DPG was beneficial, but that above 5,000 m, increased affinity to improve O_2 capture at the pulmonary capillaries is beneficial. Hemoglobin's oxygen affinity is also affected by pH, and, in fact, at the higher altitudes, due to vigorous respiratory alkalosis from hyperventilation, the hemoglobin affinity is increased. A Caucasian, at 6,300 m (20,669 ft), had an increase in DPG/Hgb ratio from 0.80 (sea level) to 1.36. Yet pH was 7.5, causing a net increased Hgb affinity to O_2, and with increased pulmonary O_2 uptake, Oxygen saturation (SaO_2) was comparable to what would be expected 1,300 m (4,260 ft) lower (12). Venous blood gas collected by a scientist/climber on the summit of Everest, when removing supplemental O_2 for 10 minutes, showed a PCO_2 of 7.5 mm Hg and a pH of 7.7–7.8. The marked respiratory alkalosis greatly increased Hgb–O_2 affinity at the extreme elevation, enhancing pulmonary uptake of O_2 (13).

Acute Mountain Sickness, AMS

The main symptoms of insufficient acclimatization are symptoms of acute mountain sickness, of which headache, GI upset, insomnia, and fatigue are the primary symptoms. Without gradual ascent to allow time for acclimatization, mild acute mountain sickness is seen in 10%–25% of people ascending to 2,500 m (8,200 ft). More severe acute mountain sickness is seen in 50%–85% of people ascending abruptly to 4,500–5,500 m (14,760–18,040 ft) (14). Investigators have researched how to predict who may acclimate poorly and develop AMS. Tools including measurement of sea level HVR, improvement in HVR after 1 day at altitude, and pulse oximetry after 30 minutes of simulated hypoxia have been useful (7). One predictor of developing AMS is a prior history of AMS. The speed of ascent is also important. For trekkers and mountaineers, the recommendation is, above 2,000 m (6,560 ft), to go slowly and try not to increase net altitude by more than 600 m (2,000 ft) per day. Abbreviated exposures to altitude, simulated, or real, in the month prior to travel may also reduce the incidence of AMS. Acetazolamide (ACZ) at doses from 125 mg twice per day, up to 250 mg 3 times per day, can be valuable in preventing or treating AMS. For prevention, initiate therapy 1 day prior to travel. ACZ is a carbonic anhydrase inhibitor and accelerates the acclimatization process. By causing renal bicarbonate excretion, it causes metabolic acidosis, increasing ventilation and thus increasing SaO_2 (1.295). The main other therapeutic interventions include descent from altitude, supplemental oxygen, or for extreme symptoms without the option of descent, dexamethasone 4 mg to 8 mg, 3 to 4 times daily, up to 1 week (14).

PERIODIC BREATHING AT ALTITUDE

Periodic breathing/central sleep apnea (CSA) at altitude is very common, and at high enough elevation is seen in almost all mountaineers or inhabitants. It may be seen in some people at altitudes as low as 2,000 m (6,560 ft) (15). In healthy fit subjects living at 1,430 m (4,700 ft), 5 of 16 developed a central apnea index (CAI) of >20/hr sleeping one night in a tent simulating 3,660 m (12,000 ft) (16). During a progressive climb in the Himalayas, 13 of 14 subjects had CSA at 5,050 m (16,570 ft) with an average apnea-hypopnea index (AHI) of 55.7/hr (17). The breathing pattern is not the gradual waxing and waning seen in

Cheyne-Stokes's respirations of CHF, but more similar to the periodic breathing of infancy, where 2–4 breaths are followed by an apnea, etc. (15). The intermittent arousals from sleep can contribute to sleep difficulties, daytime fatigue, and cognitive and attention decline. For mountaineers on Mt. McKinley, 25% of climbers complained of frequent awakenings because of periodic breathing (18).

A brief review of some of the factors which allow central apneas (in general, not specifically at altitude) to repeat and perpetuate a pattern of repetitive apneas is helpful in subsequently understanding how hypoxemia increases this tendency. Skatrud and Dempsey first described the concept of the apneic threshold in 1983. For any given situation and person, this is the PCO_2 value at which central ventilatory drive stops, and apnea occurs in non-rapid eye movement (NREM) sleep (19). For any person, at any elevation, if there is a movement or an arousal during sleep that triggers some hyperpnea, this may drive PCO_2 below this apnea threshold and possibly trigger a chain of repetitive apneas (Figure 13.2). During the apnea, SaO_2 is falling, and PCO_2 is rising. The hypoxemia AND the rising PCO_2 stimulate resumption in breathing, but even after breathing resumes, because of the time delay due to circulation, the CB and central CO_2 chemoreceptors are still seeing further dropping SaO_2 and further increased PCO_2 over the next few seconds. These values trigger deeper breaths, with hyperpnea, again driving PCO_2 down, potentially again below the apnea threshold (point A in Figure 13.2), thus potentially triggering another central apnea. With a second

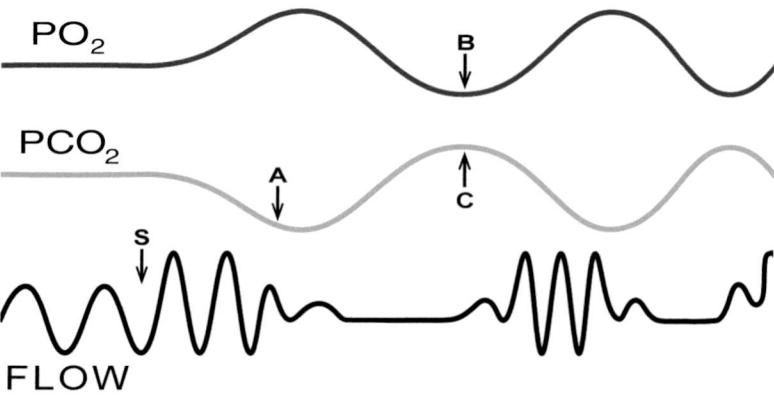

Figure 13.2 Repetitive central apneas: A stimulus (S) causes some deeper breaths, increasing PO_2 and decreasing PCO_2 to and beyond apnea threshold (A). Breathing stops, and PO_2 falls and PCO_2 rise to points (B) and (C), both triggering hyperpnea, dropping PCO_2 below apnea threshold leading to another apnea. Circulatory time delay is not taken into account in this diagram.

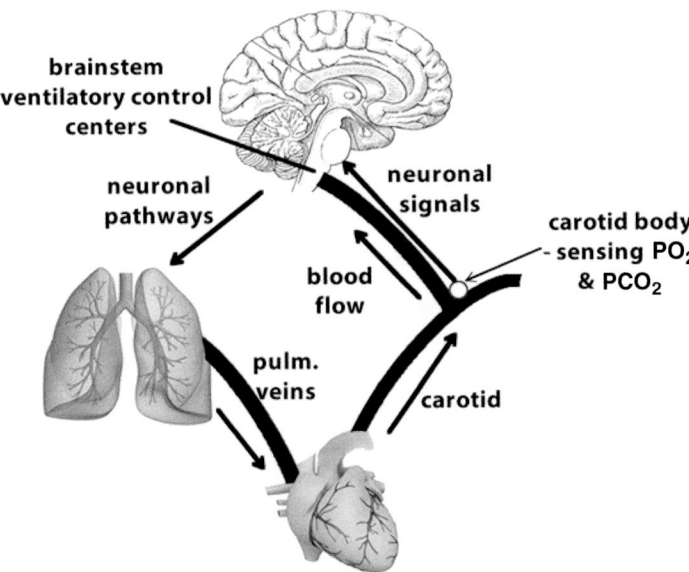

Figure 13.3 Ventilatory feedback loop. The ventilatory feedback loop is responsible for the stability of breathing. The brainstem receives neural signals from the carotid body, and from its own blood flow, regarding PO_2, PCO_2, and pH and sends neuronal signals to respiratory muscles controlling ventilation. This affects gas exchange and PO_2, PCO_2, and pH exiting pulmonary capillaries to the heart. The heart pumps the blood to the body, including to carotid body and brainstem, where chemosignals are interpreted responded to with signals relayed to the respiratory motor center in the brainstem. Any problem along the way, i.e. with cardiac function affecting circulation time or with the brainstem, can affect the smooth operation of this feedback loop system and lead to loop gain instability.

apnea, the pattern repeats and perhaps repeats again and again. At altitude, the main factor destabilizing the feedback loop (Figure 13.3) is hypoxemia. The sequence of events leading to unstable breathing is detailed in the chapter by Morgan and Dempsey (Chapter 2).

In the hypoxic environment, at altitude, following an apnea, SaO_2 (having started at a lower baseline) falls much lower (point B in Figure 13.2) and thus leads to a much stronger ventilatory response than with the same length apnea at sea level. This stronger ventilatory response increases the likelihood of ventilatory overshoot, with the hyperpnea subsequently driving the PCO_2 again below the apnea threshold. Some authors suggest that the magnitude of a person's HVR is related to the severity of his/her CSA at altitude. Men, at sea level, have a greater HVR than women, related to testosterone and men on average have more severe periodic breathing at altitude (20). Almitrine, which increases HVR, increases the severity of CSA at altitude (18). Lahiri described a unique adaptation of some Sherpa, who avoid the problem of CSA at altitude, having a very reduced HVR (21).

An important factor also promoting a pattern of periodic breathing at altitude is that hypoxemia steepens the ventilatory response to PCO_2. The CB responds not only to O_2 but also has some direct chemoreceptor response to CO_2. The CB response to hypercarbia is sluggish in normoxia but brisk in hypoxia, the asphyxia response (5). Daristotle showed, in awake goats, that the CB neural output (and measured resultant ventilation) with combined hypoxia and hypercarbia was much more than the simple addition of the same degree normocarbic hypoxia and normoxic hypercarbia (22). With the immediate CB neuronal response to hypercarbia increased in the hypoxia of altitude, this further increases the chance for ventilatory overshoot following an apnea, blowing pCO_2 again below the apnea threshold, with one apnea triggering the next, etc.

In addition, CB hypoxemia affects the central ventilatory response to CO_2. Blain et al. quantitated the degree that carotid chemoreceptor hypoxia vs. normoxia, vs. hyperoxia, affected the ventilatory response to various levels of central hypercarbia.

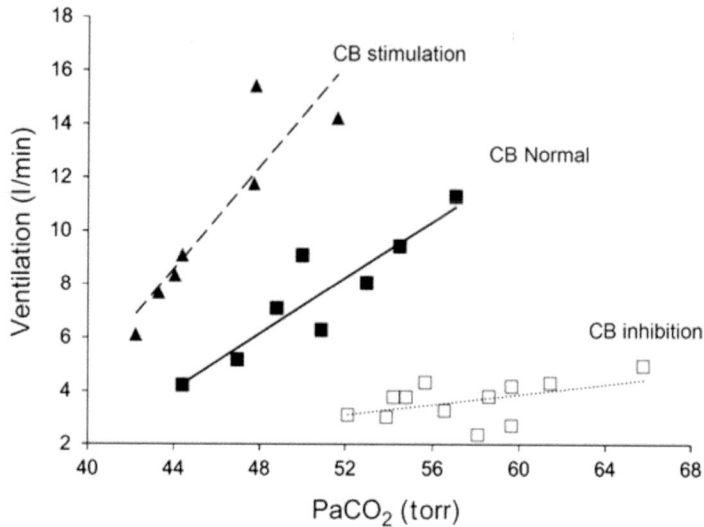

Figure 13.4 In a canine, the carotid chemoreceptor is denervated on one side. The remaining carotid chemoreceptor is vascularly isolated from the systemic and cerebral circulation and perfused extracorporeally. The central chemoreceptor response to CO_2, by itself, is determined by steady-state inhalation of CO_2-enriched air. Note that, when the isolated CB is inhibited (CB Pco_2 = 20 torr and CB Po_2 >500 torr), the central CO_2 response was reduced to about one-fifth of normal, and when the isolated CB was stimulated (CB Po_2 = 40 torr, CB Pco_2 = 40 torr), the central CO_2 response increased an average of twofold. (Borrowed with permission from Dempsey et al. (8), adapted from Blain et al. (23).)

Findings are displayed in Figure 13.4 (23). In carotid chemoreceptor hypoxemia, there is steepening of the central ventilatory response to PCO_2, compared with normoxia. With carotid chemoreceptor hyperoxia inhibiting CB response, there is flattening of the central ventilatory response to PCO_2. This provides the physiologic background displayed with the different slopes on the central CO_2 ventilatory response lines in Figure 13.5 regarding normoxia, hypoxia, and hyperoxia. This dependence of central chemosensitivity on peripheral chemoreceptor input may explain the steepening CO_2 response slope during altitude acclimatization.

The steepened ventilatory response to PCO_2 i.e. increased controller gain, is important in two ways regarding central apnea, at both the top and bottom of this ventilatory response curve. Regarding the top portion of the hypoxia line in Figure 13.5, the hypoxemia increases the response to hypercarbia, thus hypercarbia following the apnea gives an even greater push toward ventilatory overshoot (point C in Figure 13.2). Regarding the bottom portion of the curve, with the steepened ventilatory response, the apneic threshold is even closer to the eupneic PCO_2, i.e. the CO_2 reserve (the difference between eupneic PCO_2 and apneic

threshold PCO_2) has been reduced, so less hyperpnea is required, to trigger the next apnea. The fact that hypoxemia decreases the CO_2 reserve, was demonstrated by Xie et al., studying nine sleeping humans on pressure support ventilation. In the normoxic environment, it required an average of 12.2 seconds of hyperventilation to trigger a central apnea, at an average $P_{ET}CO_2$ of 35.8 torr. In a hypoxic setting, with the same amount of pressure support, it required just 6.3 seconds, and central apnea occurred at a PCO_2 of 38.9 torr (24).

Role of Cerebral Blood Flow Influencing Periodic Breathing at Altitude

Increased cerebral blood flow, as may be triggered by hypercarbia at the end of apnea, helps wash out the CO_2 from the interstitium of the central chemoreceptor nuclei, reducing ventilatory stimulus. This reduces the interstitial hypercarbia at the end of the apnea, reducing the likelihood of ventilatory overshoot (25). Even at sea level, there is normally a drop in cerebral blood flow at sleep onset thought due to reduced cerebral O_2 consumption in sleep stages 1 and 2. Ainslie found that at high altitude, the magnitude of the drop in middle cerebral artery velocity

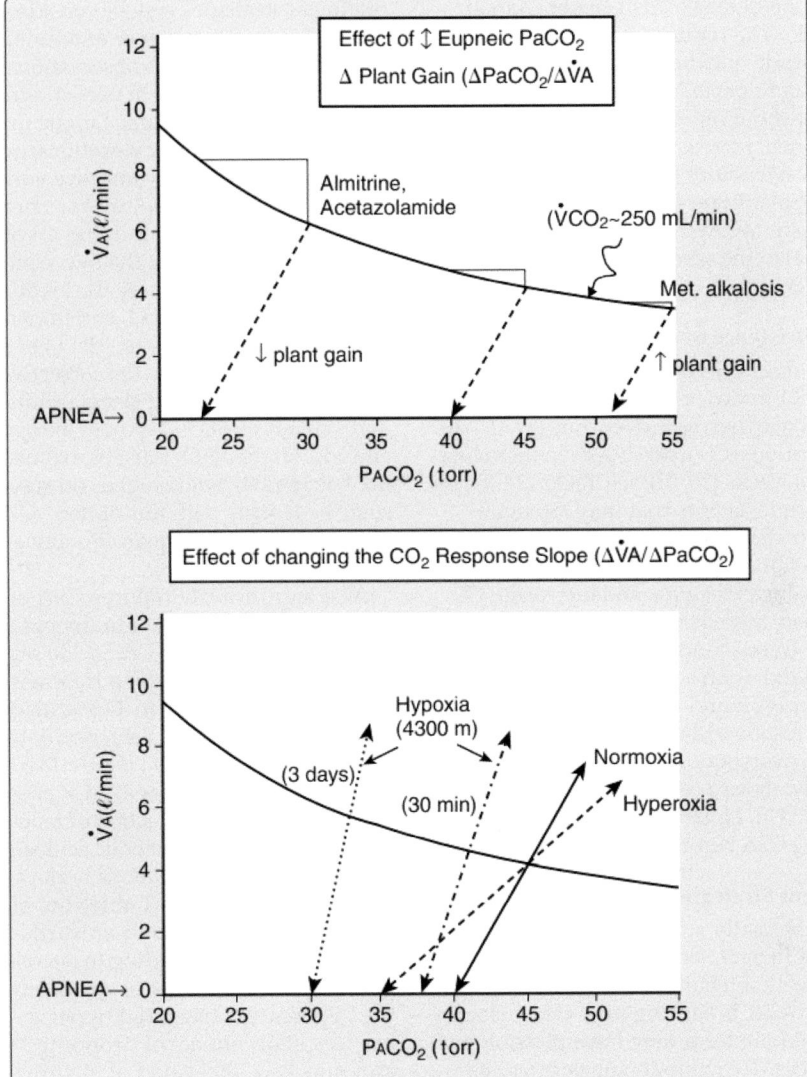

Figure 13.5 At rest, during eupnea, values of PCO_2 and ventilation will lie on the curvilinear isometabolic line, which is determined by the inverse relationship of alveolar ventilation and PCO_2 in the alveolar gas equation. Plant gain represents the power of increased ventilation to reduce PCO_2. The further to the left and upward on the isometabolic curve, the greater the ventilation is, while eupneic, but also, the lower the plant gain is because the isometabolic line is steeper. For example, far to the left, increasing minute ventilation by 2 l/min creates a small drop in PCO_2, while far to the right, where the isometabolic line is flatter, a 2 l/min increase in minute ventilation causes a great drop in PCO_2. Thus, on the right side of this graph, plant gain is greater. The steepness of the ventilatory response to PCO_2 lines, the controller gain, for different settings is determined experimentally. The steeper ventilatory response in hypoxia is determined by studies measuring the ventilatory response to changes in PCO_2 in the hypoxic setting. Xie determined that, in hypoxia, the eupneic ventilation increases, pushing the eupneic point and the whole line to the left. The PCO_2 that reduces the ventilatory drive to zero (in non-REM sleep) is the apnea threshold. In hypoxia, the subject becomes apneic at a PCO_2 quite close to the eupneic PCO_2 (compared to in normoxia), thus the line from eupnea to the X-axis (where ventilation is 0) is steeper, and thus there is reduced CO_2 reserve in hypoxia. Likewise, in hypoxia, the ventilatory response to hypercarbia is greater, steepening the upper portion of this line, as well. Acetazolamide (ACZ) causes an increase in tonic eupneic ventilation, moving eupnea to the left and up on the metabolic response curve. Without changing the slope of the ventilatory response curve, this decreases plant gain and increases CO_2 reserve, both decreasing tendency for central apnea. (With permission from Mohensin et al. (37), adapted from Dempsey et al. (62).)

(MCAv) at sleep onset was greater than at low altitude. The reduced cerebral blood flow at altitude may be an additional factor contributing to periodic breathing, with reduced washout of the CO_2 that has built up post apnea, increasing the likelihood of ventilatory overshoot post apnea. Also, in a series of high-altitude subjects, the magnitude of the drop in MCAv at sleep onset was proportional to the severity of their periodic breathing (26).

Persistence of CSA at Altitude

Over time, does CSA at altitude decrease or persist? At altitudes of 4,300 m (14,100 ft) and below, CSA may decrease over time (27–29). At higher elevations, CSA persists even increases over several weeks (30, 31); see Table 13.1. Over time at altitude, factors that may attenuate CSA include increasing ventilation, which moves the eupneic point to the left in Figure 13.5, decreasing plant gain, and increasing CO_2 reserve. Also, there is improvement in SaO_2. These four trends tend to decrease CSA. On the other hand, with acclimatization, there is increased HVR and HCVR (hypercarbic ventilatory response), both favoring post-apneic ventilatory overshoot and accentuating CSA (15). Possibly, above a certain altitude threshold of about 4,300 m, 14,100 ft, these latter factors accentuating CSA become dominant (Table 13.1).

Treatment Strategies for CSA at Altitude

It is not universally accepted that the oscillations in SaO_2 from CSA (with mean SaO_2 relatively unchanged), are detrimental. But the, periodic breathing may affect sleep quality, and long term may have physiologic consequences. Two human subject studies found that nightly exposure to 9 hours of intermittent hypoxia over 2–4 weeks increased blood pressure and muscle sympathetic nerve activity (32, 33). When sleep quality is impaired by periodic breathing at altitude, several treatment strategies may be considered. One strategy is simply patience and time, given Nussbaumer-Ochsner's observations that while periodic breathing might persist, symptoms of sleeplessness and daytime fatigue may improve with time (31). At lower elevations, even the periodic breathing may improve with time (28).

Oxygen during sleep reverses periodic breathing at altitude, undoing all of the mechanisms by which the hypoxemia at altitude triggered the periodic breathing. Piped in oxygen for bedroom O_2 enrichment to a fraction of inspired oxygen (FiO_2) of 24% has been shown to improve the subjective quality of sleep and measured sleep architecture and acute mountain sickness symptoms at altitude. Higher FiO_2 must be avoided due to fire hazard (34). Some higher ski resorts have some bedrooms with this option, as do some astronomy telescope quarters, above 4,570 m (15,000 ft) in the Andes.

ACZ significantly reduces CSA at altitude. Sutton studied nine mountaineers at 5,360 m (17,590 ft) and found ACZ 250 mg TID decreased percent of sleep time with period breathing from 80.4% to 34.9%, also greatly reduced amplitude of SaO_2 oscillation and increased baseline SaO_2, Figure 13.6 (35). The main effect of oral doses of ACZ is on the renal tubules, leading to reduction of reabsorption of bicarbonate and to metabolic acidosis (36). The acidosis undoes the alkalotic brake and allows for further increased ventilation, moving the person to the left and upward along the isometabolic curve, leading to decreased plant gain (Figure 13.5). Thus, at apnea termination, the hypercarbia triggered hyperventilation has less of an impact of dropping PCO_2 and thus less likelihood of pushing PCO_2 below the apnea threshold to trigger the next apnea. Additionally, with increased baseline ventilation moving the eupneic point upward to the left, even without a change in slope of the ventilatory response line, the eupneic

Table 13.1: Course of Central Sleep Apnea, Over Time, at Altitude (Compared to Upon Arrival): Review of Studies

Altitude	# Subjects	Time at Altitude	Findings	Reference
3,200 m (10,500 ft)	9	6 days	AHI ↓ 16.3 to 13.6	(29)
4,300 m (14,100 ft)	6	1 wk	% TST with PB ↓ 67% to 43%	(27)
4,300 m (14,100 ft)	6	1 wk	AHI ↓ 21.6 to 7.1	(28)
4,559 m (15,000 ft)	16	3 days	AHI ↑ 60.1 to 85.9	(31)
5,050 m (16,570 ft)	5	4 wk	%TST with PB ↑ 52 to 72%	(30)

Abbreviations: AHI apnea-hypopnea index, PB periodic breathing, TST total sleep time, ↓ indicates reduced, ↑ indicates increased.

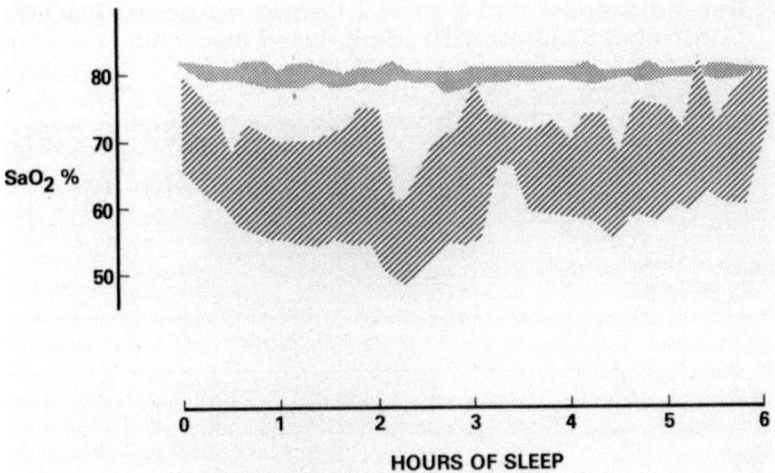

Figure 13.6   Effect of acetazolamide on periodic breathing at altitude. Ranges of SaO_2 peaks and nadirs in one subject during sleep at 5,360 m (17,590 ft), with acetazolamide (upper stippled area) and without it (lower crosshatched area). (With permission from Sutton et al. (35).)

PCO_2 is farther from the apnea threshold (the CO_2 reserve is increased), another factor discouraging repetitive central apnea (37). Swenson has postulated additional carbonic anhydrase inhibitor effects may further ACZ's effect reducing CSA at altitude, including slight CB inhibition blunting both HVR and HCVR to reduce ventilatory overshoot. Also, the release of CO_2 from brainstem vascular endothelial cells may increase ventilation and thus further increase CO_2 reserve and plant gain (38).

Benzodiazepine and non-benzodiazepine receptor agonists have been evaluated for benefit and safety to improve sleep quality at altitude, to help sleep through periodic breathing. The multiple studies in Table 13.2 together suggest that the short-acting benzodiazepine and the non-benzodiazepine receptor agonists, at these doses, can be taken safely and may provide subjective benefit without negatively affecting AHI or mean SaO_2 or next day performance (39–42). Interestingly in Nickol's temazepam study, 14 of 33 subjects felt they slept better with placebo (41). Despite these studies showing a minimal reduction in average SaO_2, individuals may vary, and one must have safety concerns prescribing a hypnotic with respiratory depressant properties to a person traveling to a high-altitude hypoxic environment.

Using a deadspace mask (without positive pressure machinery) has been shown to reduce periodic breathing at altitude. The idea for this stems from Pembrey and Allen's observation in 1905 that breathing a mixture with CO_2 added

to the inspired air stabilized Cheyne-Stokes respiration at low elevation (43). Bersenbrugge found that CO_2 by nasal cannula suppressed the central apnea of hypoxemia/altitude (44). Patz used a deadspace mask, a Quatro CPAP mask with no CPAP machine, but with a cup attached, titrating the size of the cup to provide sufficient dead space to eliminate central apneas. In all 5 of 5 subjects with CAI above 20/hr, at simulated 3,660 m (12,000 ft), the deadspace reduced CAI below 5/hr, or below 10% of baseline CAI, without reduction in average SaO_2 (16). Lovis took 12 subjects to 3,500 m (11,480 ft), where 5 had significant periodic breathing. A 500 cc dead space mask improved AHI from 72.9/hr to 42.5/hr without changing average SaO_2 or altering measures of sleep (45). Likely the mechanism of benefit with dead space (or CO_2 by cannula) is that, with post-apneic deep breathing, one is inhaling CO_2 and thus less able to drop PCO_2 below the apneic threshold to trigger a subsequent apnea. Thus, the rebreather mask, and inhaled CO_2, reduce the impact of hyperventilation on changing PCO_2, they decrease plant gain. This treatment has not had enough corroboration to be recommended as a field strategy (16).

With 18 subjects with CSA at altitude, Orr evaluated adaptive servo ventilation (CPAP-adaptive-servo ventilation, ASV) therapy at 3,800 m (12,470 ft), comparing to oxygen therapy at 2 L/m and to no therapy. The treatment arm had ODI's of 8.3/hr (ASV), 0.5/hr (02), and 15.2/hr (no therapy) (46). While ASV provided significant benefit, it was not nearly

Table 13.2: Benzodiazepine and Non-BDZ Receptor Agonist Placebo-Controlled Studies: Altitude-Related Insomnia

Drug, Dose	Altitude	Subjects	Findings	Reference
Lorazepam 1 mg	4,800m (15,750 ft)	12	Improved sleep structure	(39)
Temazepam 10 mg	5,300 m (17,390 ft)	11	ODI improved 100.8 to 75.0	(40)
			Avg SaO$_2$ 75.7% Plac. 74.7% Tem	
			11 of 11 subjective benefit	
Temazepam 10 mg	5,000 m (16,400 ft)	33	AHI 35.9 pla, 31.1 Tem.	(41)
			Avg SaO$_2$ 78% plac, 76% Tem	
			TST actig. 7.25 hr plac, 7.05 hr Tem	
			17 of 33 subjective benefit	
Zolpidem 10 mg	3,613 m (11,850 ft)	12	ODI plac. 10, Zo. 10, Za. 12	(42)
Zaleplon 10 mg			Avg. SaO$_2$ plac 83%, Zo. 82%, Za. 84%	
			Meds increase %SWS, subjective sleep	
			No increase in TST	

Abbreviations: ODI, oxygen desaturation index, Avg., average, plac, placebo, Tem, temazepam, TST, total sleep time, actig, actigraphy, non-BDZ, non-benzodiazepine, Zo., zolpidem, Za., zaleplon, Meds, medications, SWS, slow wave sleep.

as helpful as nasal O$_2$ if one has the luxury of electricity at altitude.

ADAPTATIONS TO ALTITUDE

Several populations have lived thousands of years at altitude and have developed various adaptations to improve survival in the hypoxic environment. While the HVR is critical for the newcomer traveling to altitude, there is significant metabolic cost maintaining this increased demand on the respiratory muscles even at rest. Tibetan, Sherpa, and Andean native populations all have diminished HVR (8). A way that the Andean native population compensates for the hypoxia, and allows less hyperventilation, is lung growth, and Andean body morphology is altered with a barrel chest to accommodate the increased lung volume. The increased lung volume and thus increased diffusion capacity allows for sufficient oxygenation with reduced HVR (47).

The civilizations that have been at high altitude longer, in Ethiopia, and Asia, have adapted in part by a reduced erythropoietic response to hypoxemia, and thus, at similar altitudes, native Tibetans, Sherpa, and Ethiopians have a lower hemoglobin level than Andeans (who have been at altitude only 15,000 years) (48). Perhaps to help accommodate for the increased blood viscosity, the Andeans have reduced HPV compared to acclimated newcomers at similar altitudes (47).

Another problem at altitude is increased infant and maternal perinatal mortality and increased perinatal problems including pre-eclampsia and reduction in birth weight, all likely reflecting fetal hypoxemia. Andean women, during pregnancy, have increased uterine artery diameter and enhanced placental villous capillarization compared with pregnant European woman at altitude. Due to the improved fetal oxygenation, the Andean women have a relative improvement in birthweights, rates of pre-eclampsia, and mortality compared with Caucasian women living at the same altitude (47).

CHRONIC MOUNTAIN SICKNESS

Chronic mountain sickness (CMS), or "Monge's disease," is an illness seen in 5%–10% of high-altitude residents, characterized by relative hypoventilation with more severe hypoxemia, especially during sleep, development of excessive erythrocytosis (Hgb >19 for women, >21 for men) and the consequences of the increased blood viscosity, in particular, right heart strain. With 140 million people living above 2,500 m (8,200 ft), CMS is not uncommon. It is believed that the civilizations that have been at altitude longer, in Ethiopia, and Asia, have adapted in part by a reduced erythropoietic response to hypoxemia, and thus, at similar altitudes, native Tibetans, Sherpa, and Ethiopians have a lower hemoglobin level than Andeans (who have been at altitude only 15,000 years). Thus the Himalayans and Ethiopians at a given elevation, have a lower incidence of CMS (49). In addition, the Tibetans have very reduced HPV, further protecting them from CMS. Tibetans, in La Hasa, at 3,657 m (12,000 ft), have minimal HPV and normal pulmonary pressures (65). With increasing elevation and with age, the incidence of CMS increases. In the Andes, in La Paz at 3,600 m (11,810 ft), the incidence of CMS is 5.6%. At Cerro de Pasco at 4,340 m (14,240 ft), 15.4% of men 30–39 years old have CMS, and 33% of men at 60 have CMS. Symptoms include breathlessness, palpitations, insomnia, paresthesia, headache, tinnitus. Clubbing, oral cyanosis, hyperemic conjunctivae, dilated varicose veins, and dilated retinal veins are common. Pulmonary hypertension and, in advanced cases, cor pulmonale and congestive heart failure are seen (49).

The cause of CMS is unclear and may be different in different individuals. Is the main cause hypoventilation, from an insufficient ventilatory response to the hypoxemia? (erythrocytosis being secondary to the hypoxemia). Patients with CMS have considerably lower average minute ventilation than the average resident at the same altitude (49). Julian found that young men in La Paz who had suffered some perinatal hypoxemia (with mothers with pre-eclampsia or hypertension of pregnancy) had an odds ratio of 5–6× greater than a control group of developing excessive erythrocytosis, a preclinical form of CMS. This suggested the perinatal exposure to hypoxemia caused an epigenetic change affecting them, possibly their HVR (50). Or is the problem contributing to CMS the excessive erythrocytosis itself? The SENP 1 protein suppresses erythropoiesis. Fibroblasts from CMS patients express less than the normal amount of SENP 1 in response to hypoxemia, suggesting a possible genetic origin to their tendency for excessive erythropoiesis (49). Given the fact that CMS is more common in the obese, Julian evaluated whether sleep apnea might contribute to the development of CMS. In La Paz, in 20 young men (age 18–25), with excessive erythrocytosis, EE (Hgb avg. 19.1), and in 19 control young men, polysomnography (PSG) was performed. The average AHI in the group with EE was 8.6/hr, compared with 2.2/hr in the control group, p <0.05 (52). On the other hand, Richalet did not find an increased AHI in 30 CMS subjects compared to 10 control subjects at Cerro de Pasco, 4,340 m (14,240 ft). AHI in the CMS subjects was 2.2/hr, compared with 3.8/hr in the controls (51).

Treatment for CMS has included phlebotomy, but the benefit is not lasting, and repeated phlebotomies lead to iron deficiency which increases pulmonary hypertension. Descent is most beneficial but separates patients from their families (49). Stimulating respiratory drive has been a strategy for pharmacotherapy. Medroxyprogesterone improved SaO_2 and hematocrit, but with negative effects on libido (66). ACZ 250 mg daily, at 4,300 m, decreased hematocrit from 69% to 64% and improved average SaO_2 from 82% to 84%, and improved some symptoms (51). Oxygen therapy, while effective, has some problems of cost and requirement for electricity.

OBSTRUCTIVE SLEEP APNEA (OSA) AT ALTITUDE

OSA severity worsens in lowlanders traveling to altitude with lower average SaO_2 and SaO_2 nadirs and increased AHI, primarily by the addition of central apneas and central hypopneas. In a study including 34 Swiss lowlander OSA patients, the average AHI (without CPAP) increased from 48/hr at 490 m (1,600 ft), to 80/hr at 1,860 m (6,100 ft), to 90/hr at 2,590 m (8,500 ft). Respectively, avg. SaO_2 decreased from 94% to 90% to 87%. The fraction of apnea and hypopnea events that were central increased with increasing altitude from 1/10 to 1/2 to 2/3, respectively. With OSA untreated, simulated driving performance and blood pressure worsened at altitude (53). ACZ (without CPAP) reduced the central events at altitude without reducing the obstructive events (54). CPAP alone for the traveler to altitude led to CPAP persistent central apneas. Effective therapy in subjects traveling to altitude was achieved by combining CPAP with ACZ therapy (55).

For the trekker with OSA, camping at altitude without electricity available, and unable to take battery packs for the CPAP, advice is to obtain an adjustable mandibular advancement device and work with it at sea level until it has been advanced sufficiently to significantly reduce AHI. Then during travel, use this for the OSA and take ACZ, to also reduce the central events (56). If effective results at sea level cannot be achieved with the dental appliance, the travel plans might need to be reconsidered. There is a report of a single OSA patient trekking on the Annapurna Circuit in Nepal, who developed high altitude pulmonary edema symptoms missing electricity for his CPAP at the huts one night, finally improving, back on his CPAP at the next hut (57).

Residents at altitudes with OSA also have an increased percentage of central respiratory events. Pagel evaluated sleep lab patients of 3 sleep labs at altitudes 1,370–2,440 m (4,500–8,000 ft) and found more central apneas

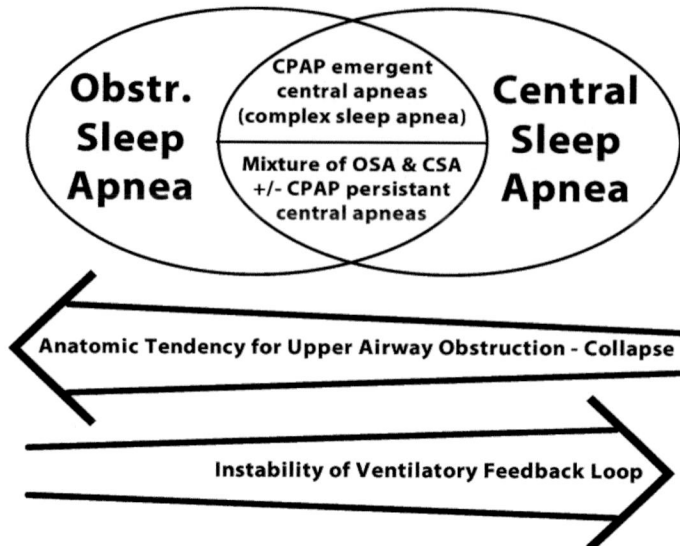

Figure 13.7 Influences on Type of Apnea. The degree of a person's tendency to obstruct and his/her ventilatory instability determine his/her nature of sleep apnea. The hypoxia of altitude contributes to ventilatory instability. (With permission from Patz et al. (63), adapted from Kuzniar et al. (64).)

in their mixture of events than OSA patients at sea level, with the greatest proportion of central events in patients at the highest of these elevations. The higher the altitude in this range, the higher the incidence of unsuccessful CPAP titrations with CPAP persistent central apneas. Hypoxemia is the factor destabilizing the ventilatory feedback loop, causing an increased incidence of central apneas in the diagnostic studies and during the titrations (Figure 13.7). The addition of in line oxygen allowed 95% of Pagel's patients with complex sleep apnea at altitude to achieve optimal titrations (58). Patz studied 11 residents living above 2,440 m (8,000 ft), also noting a "centralization" of their sleep apnea. One subject at home had severe sleep apnea with almost exclusively mixed apneas, yet coming down to a lab at 1,430 m (4,700 ft), he had exclusively obstructive apneas. One subject with exclusively CSA at his home altitude had just upper airway resistance syndrome at sea level with a normal AHI (59). In a comparison cross-sectional population survey, Pham found the sea level residents in Lima, Peru, had an average obstructive AHI of 4.3/hr and a central AHI of 0.6/hr. Residents at altitude, in Puno, at 3,825 m (12,550 ft) had a similar obstructive AHI of 4.6/hr, with a central AHI of 4.4/hr (60). Vargus-Ramirez evaluated patients of Bogota, 2,640 m (8,660 ft), hospitalized for decompensated CHF, and found the percentage of patients in Bogota with primarily CSA or CSR, was greater than in lowlanders with decompensated CHF. Her

subjects had two factors destabilizing their ventilatory feedback loop, both the hypoxemia of altitude and decompensated CHF (61).

Residents in the mountains often need to descend in elevation to be evaluated in an urban sleep lab. However, this descent reduces AHI and affects SaO_2 measures. Patz found that of eight patients living above 2,440 m (8,000 ft), with home AHI 15–50/hr, 3 dropped their AHI below 5/hr descending for PSG evaluation (59). To assess a mountain resident's severity of OSA most accurately, degree of desaturation, absence or presence of central apneas, and absence or presence of CPAP persistent central apneas, polysomnographic assessment should be as close to his/her home elevation as possible (59). If a symptomatic altitude resident has a normal PSG at low elevation, a home sleep test at home altitude should be arranged. If a CPAP titration is done lower than the home elevation, close follow up with data downloads and pulse oximetry on therapy will be needed at the home elevation.

SUMMARY

At altitude, hypoxia immediately triggers CB hypertrophy with new glomus cells, which hypersensitizes the HVR and mediates much of the time-dependent ventilatory acclimatization to high altitude. This minimizes the reduction in PO_2 at altitude. Failure to acclimate, at times from ascending to altitude too rapidly, may lead to acute mountain sickness.

In addition, in hypoxia, the CB increases its response to CO_2. The increased HVR, hypercarbic ventilatory response, and reduced CO_2 reserve in the hypoxia of altitude immediately increase ventilatory loop gain favoring periodic breathing. Insomnia may result, but also hypertension and other consequences of sympathetic activation are potential results of the intermittent hypoxemia of CSA. Supplemental nocturnal oxygen will eliminate periodic breathing. ACZ may help treat both acute mountain sickness and periodic breathing at altitude.

Patients with OSA traveling to altitude or living at altitude may be affected by central apneas and central hypopneas adding into their mixture of respiratory events and may develop complex sleep apnea on CPAP. For complex sleep apnea at altitude, the addition of in line oxygen, or for the traveler, adding ACZ, is helpful.

Some indigenous populations have adapted to altitude with adjustments in HVR, lung volume, erythropoietic response, and uterine-placental circulation. CMS is an unfortunate maladaptation with hypoventilation, hypoxemia, excessive erythrocytosis, and right heart strain.

ACKNOWLEDGMENT

Great thanks are extended to Jerry Dempsey for encouraging and reviewing this chapter.

REFERENCES

1. West JB, Schoene RB, Luks AM, Milledge JS, History. In: High Altitude Medicine and Physiology, 5th edn. Boca Raton, CRC Press, Taylor and Francis Group; 2013: 1–15.

2. West JB, Schoene RB, Luks AM, Milledge JS, Sleep. In: High Altitude Medicine and Physiology, 5th edn. Boca Raton, CRC Press, Taylor and Francis Group; 2013: 202–15.

3. Musso A, Life of Man on the High Alps. London, Unwin; 1898.

4. Ainslie PN, Burgess KR, Respiratory Physiology: Sleep at High Altitudes. In: Kryger MH, Roth T, Dement WC, eds, Principles and Practice of Sleep Medicine, 6th edn. Amsterdam, Elsevier; 2015: 182–92.

5. Dempsey JA, Smith CA, Update on chemoreception: influence on cardiorespiratory regulation and pathophysiology. Clin Chest Med, 2019;40:269–283.

6. Wang ZY, Olson EB, Bjorling DE, et al., Sustained hypoxia-induced proliferation of carotid body type 1 cells in rats. J Appl Physiol, 2008;104(3):803–8.

7. West JB, Schoene RB, Luks AM, Milledge JS, Control of Breathing at High Altitude. In: High Altitude Medicine and Physiology, 5th edn. Boca Raton, CRC Press, Taylor and Francis Group; 2013; 65–81.

8. Dempsey JA, Powell FL, Bisgard GE, et al. Role of chemoreception in cardiorespiratory acclimatization to, and deacclimatization from, hypoxia. J Appl Physiol, 2014;116:858–66.

9. West JB, Shoene RB, Luks AM, Milledge JS, Hematology. In: High Altitude Medicine and Physiology, 5th edn. Boca Raton, CRC Press, Taylor and Francis Group; 2013:121–36.

10. West JB, Shoene RB, Luks AM, Milledge JS, Blood-Gas Transport and Acid-Base Balance. In: High Altitude Medicine and Physiology, 5th edn. Boca Raton, CRC Press, Taylor and Francis Group; 2013:137–49.

11. Dominelli PB, Wiggins CC, Baker SE, et al., Influence of high affinity haemoglobin on the response to normoxic and hypoxic exercise. J Physiol, 2020;598(8):1475–90.

12. Samaja M, Crespi T, Guarzzi M, et al., Oxygen transport in blood at high altitude: the role of the hemoglobin-oxygen affinity and impact of the phenomenon related to hemoglobin allosterism and red cell function. Eur J Appl Physiol, 2003;90:351–9.

13. West JB, Hackett, PH, Maret KH, et al., Pulmonary gas exchange on the summit of Mount Everest. J Appl Physiol Respir Environ Exerc Physiol, 1983;55(3):678–87.

14. Bartsch P, Swenson ER, Acute high-altitude illnesses. N Engl J Med, 2013;368:2294–302.

15. Burgess KR, Ainslie PN, Central Sleep Apnea at High Altitude. In: Roach RC, Hackett PH, Wagner PD, eds, Hypoxia, Advances in Experimental Medicine and Biology. New York, Springer Science + Business; 2016: 275–83.

16. Patz DS, Patz MD, Hackett PH, Dead space mask eliminates central apnea at altitude. High Alt Med Biol, 2013;14(2):168–74.

17. Burgess KR, Johnson PL, Edwards N, Central and obstructive sleep apnoea during ascent to high altitude. Respirology, 2004;9(2):222–9.

18. Hackett PH, Roach RC, Harrison GL, et al., Respiratory stimulants and sleep periodic breathing at high altitude. Am Rev Respir Dis, 1987;135:896–8.

19. Skatrud, JB, Dempsey JA, Interaction of sleep state and chemical stimuli in sustaining rhythmic ventilation. J Appl Physio Respir Environ Exerc Physiol, 1983;553:813–22.

20. Caravita S, Faini A, Lombardi C, et al., Sex and acetazolamide effects on chemoreflex and periodic breathing during sleep at altitude. Chest, 2015;147(1):120–31.

21. Lahiri S, Maret K, Sherpa MG, Dependence of high altitude sleep apnea on ventilatory sensitivity to hypoxia. Resp Physiol, 1983;52:281–301.

22. Daristotle L, Berssenbrugge AD, Bisgard GE. Hypoxic-hypercapnic ventilatory interaction at the carotid body of awake goats. Respir Physiol, 1987;70:63–72.

23. Blain GM, Smith CA, Henderson KS, et al. Peripheral chemoreceptors determine the respiratory sensitivity of central chemoreceptors to CO_2. J Physiol, 2010;588(13):2455–71.

24. Xie A, Skatrud JB, Puleo DS, Dempsey JA. Influence of arterial O_2 on the susceptibility to posthyperventilation apnea during sleep. J Appl Physiol, 2006;100(1):171–7.

25. Xie A, Skatrud JB, Barczi SR, et al. Influence of cerebral blood flow on breathing stability. J Appl Physiol, 2009;106(3):850–6.

26. Ainslie PN, Burgess K, Subedi P, et al. Alterations in cerebral dynamics at high altitude following partial acclimatization in humans: wakefulness and sleep. J Appl Physiol, 2007;102:658–64.

27. Reite M, Jackson D, Cahoon RL, et al. Sleep physiology at high altitude. Electroencephalogr Clin Neurophysiol, 1975;38(5):463–71.

28. White DP, Gleeson K, Pickett CK, et al. Altitude acclimatization: influence on periodic breathing and chemoresponsiveness during sleep. J Appl Physiol, 1987;63(1):401–12.

29. Zielinski J, Koziej M, Mankowski M, et al. The quality of sleep and periodic breathing in healthy subjects at an altitude of 3200m. High Altitude Med Biol, 2000;1(4):331–6.

30. Salvaggio A, Insalaco G, Marrone O, et al. Effects of high-altitude periodic breathing on sleep and arterial oxyhaemoglobin saturation. Eur Respir J, 1998;12:408–13.

31. Nussbaumer-Ochsner Y, Ursprung J, Siebenmann C, et al. Effect of short-term acclimatization to high altitude on sleep and nocturnal breathing. Sleep, 2012;35(3):419–23.

32. Gilmartin GS, Lynch M, Tasmier R, et al. Chronic intermittent hypoxia in humans during 28 nights results in blood pressure elevation and increased muscle sympathetic nerve activity. Am J Physiol Heart Circ Physiol, 2010;299:H925–31.

33. Tamsier R, Pepin JL, Remy J, et al. 14 nights of intermittent hypoxia elevate daytime blood pressure and sympathetic activity in healthy humans. Eur Respir J, 2011;37:119–28.

34. Luks AM, van Melick H, Batarse RR, et al. Room oxygen enrichment improves sleep and subsequent day-time performance at high altitude. Respir Physiol, 1998;113(3):247–58.

35. Sutton JR, Houston CS, Mansell AL, et al. Effect of acetazolamide on hypoxemia during sleep at high altitude. N Engl J Med, 1979;301(24):1329–31.

36. Swenson ER, Leatham KL, Roach RC, et al. Renal carbonic anhydrase inhibition reduces high altitude sleep period breathing. Respir Physiol. 1991;86:333–43.

37. Mohensin V, Javaheri S, Dempsey J., Sleep and Breathing at High Altitude. In: Kryger MH, Roth T, Dement WC, eds, Principles and Practice of Sleep Medicine, 6th edn. Amsterdam, Elsevier; 2015: 1211–21.

38. Swenson ER, Carbonic anhydrase inhibitors and ventilation: a complex interplay of stimulation and suppression. Eur Respir J, 1998;12:1242–7.

39. Goldenberg F, Richalet JP, Jouhandin M, et al. Periodic respiration during sleep at high altitude. Effects of a hypnotic benzodiazepine, loprazolam. Presse Med, 1988;17(10):471–4.

40. Dubowitz G. Effect of temazepam on oxygen saturation and sleep quality at high altitude: randomized placebo controlled crossover trial. BMJ, 1998;316:587–9.

41. Nickol AH, Leverment J, Richards P, et al. Temazepam at high altitude reduces periodic breathing without impairing next-day performance: a randomized cross-over double-blind study. J Sleep Res, 2006;15:445–54.

42. Beaumont M, Batejat D, Pierard C. Zaleplon and zolpidem objectively alleviate sleep disturbances in mountaineers at a 3,613 meter altitude. Sleep, 2007;30(11):1527–33.

43. Pembry MS, Allen RW. Observations upon Cheyne Stokes respiration. Proc Physiol Soc, 1905;21:18–20.

44. Berssenbrugge A, Dempsey J, Iber C, et al. Mechanisms of hypoxia-induced periodic breathing during sleep in humans. J Physiol, 1983;343:507–24.

45. Lovis A, DeRelmatten M, Greiner D, et al. Effect of added dead space on sleep disordered breathing at high altitude. Sleep Med, 2012;13:663–7.

46. Orr JE, Heinrich EC, Djokic M, et al. Adaptive servo ventilation as treatment for central sleep apnea due to high-altitude periodic breathing in nonacclimatized healthy individuals. High Alt Med Biol, 2018;19(2):178–84.

47. Julian CG, Moore LG. Human genetic adaptation to high altitude: evidence from the Andes. Genes, 2009;10(2):150–70.

48. Beall CM. Andean, Tibetan, and Ethiopian patterns of adaptation to high-altitude hypoxia. Integr Comp Biol, 2005;46(1):18–24.

49. Villafuerte FC, Corante N. Chronic mountain sickness: clinical aspects, etiology, management and treatment. High Alt Med Biol, 2016;17(2):61–9.

50. Julian CG, Gonzalez M, Rodriquez A. Perinatal hypoxia increases susceptibility to high-altitude polycythemia and attendant pulmonary vascular dysfunction. Am J Physiol Heart Circ Physiol, 2015;309(4):H565–73.

51. Richalet JP, Rivera M, Bouchet P, et al. Acetazolamide a treatment for chronic mountain sickness. Am J Respir Crit Care Med, 2005;172:1427–33.

52. Julian CG, Vargas E, Gonzales M, et al. Sleep-disordered breathing and oxidative stress in preclinical chronic mountain sickness (excessive erythrocytosis). Respir Physiol Neurobiol, 2013;186:188–96.

53. Nussbaumer-Ochsner Y, Schuepfer N, Ulrich S, et al. Exacerbation of sleep apnoea by frequent central events in patients with the obstructive sleep apnoea syndrome at altitude: a randomized trial. Thorax, 2010;65(5):429–35.

54. Nussbaumer-Oschner Y, Latshang T, Ulrich S, et al. Patients with obstructive sleep apnea syndrome benefit from acetazolamide during an altitude sojourn: a randomized, placebo-controlled, double-blind trial. Chest, 2012;141(1):131–8.

55. Latshang TD, Nussbamumer-Ochsner Y, Henn RM, et al. Effect of acetazolamide and auto-CPAP therapy on breathing disturbances among patients with obstructive sleep apnea syndrome who travel to altitude: a randomized controlled trial. JAMA, 2013;308(22):2390–8.

56. Latshang TD, Bloch KE. How to treat patients with obstructive sleep apnea syndrome during an altitude sojourn. High Alt Med Biol, 2011;12(4):303–7.

57. Ginoar Y, Malhotra A, Schwartz E. High altitude, continuous positive airway pressure and obstructive sleep apnea: subjective observations and objective data. High Alt Med Biol, 2013;14(2):186–9.

58. Pagel JF, Kwiatkowski C, Parnes B. The effects of altitude associated central apnea on the diagnosis and treatment of obstructive sleep apnea: comparative data from three different altitude locations in the mountain west. J Clin Sleep Med, 2011;7(6):610–5.

59. Patz D, Spoon M, Corbin R, et al. The effect of altitude descent on obstructive sleep apnea. Chest, 2006;130(6):1744–50.

60. Pham LV, Meinzen C, Arias RS, et al. Cross-sectional comparison of sleep-disordered breathing in native Peruvian highlanders and lowlanders. High Alt Med Biol, 2017;18(1):11–9.

61. Vargus-Ramirez L, Gonzales-Garcia M, Franco-Reyes C, et al. Severe sleep apnea, Cheyne-Stokes respiration and desaturation in patients with decompensated heart failure at high altitude. Sleep Sci, 2018;11(3):146–51.

62. Dempsey JA, Smith CA, Blain GM, et al. Role of central/peripheral chemoreceptors and their interdependence in the pathophysiology of sleep apnea. Adv Exp Med Biol, 2012;758:343–9.

63. Patz DS, Complex Sleep Apnea (CPAP Emergent Central Apneas), and Apnea Related to Narcotics and to Altitude. In: Pagel JF, Pandi-Perumal SR, eds, Primary Care Sleep Medicine – A Practical Guide, 2nd edn. New York, Springer Verlag; 2014.

64. Kuzniar TJ, Morgenthaler TI. Treatment of complex sleep apnea. Chest. 2012;142(4):1049–57.

65. West JB, Schoene RB, Luks AM, Milledge JS, Cardiovascular System. In: High Altitude Medicine and Physiology, 5th edn. Boca Raton, CRC Press, Taylor and Francis Group; 2013: 101–20.

66. Kryger MH, McCullough RE, Collins D, et al. Treatment of excessive polycythemia of high altitude with respiratory stimulant drugs. Am Rev Respir Dis. 1978;117(3):455–64.

14 Sleep-Disordered Breathing Associated with Chronic Lung Diseases

Bernie Y Sunwoo, Ana Sanchez-Azofra, and Atul Malhotra

SLEEP-DISORDERED BREATHING ASSOCIATED WITH CHRONIC LUNG DISEASES

With almost 1 billion adults having obstructive sleep apnea (OSA) and hundreds of millions affected by chronic lung diseases worldwide, recognizing and understanding the links between sleep and sleep-disordered breathing (SDB) on chronic lung diseases is essential (1, 2). Normal physiologic changes in respiration that occur during sleep can result in profound hypoxemia and hypercapnia in patients with chronic lung disease. In the sleep community, the overlap syndrome (OVS) refers to OSA plus chronic obstructive pulmonary disease (COPD). OVS is associated with a unique pattern of nocturnal oxygen desaturation (NOD) and worse outcomes, but SDB remains underdiagnosed and undertreated in patients with chronic lung disease.

As the prevalence of chronic lung diseases increases, additional research is needed to determine the optimal management of SDB in these patients (3). While we focus on SDB in specific lung diseases, many of the principles likely hold for chronic lung disease in general.

SLEEP IN COPD

COPD is a common disease characterized by persistent respiratory symptoms and airflow obstruction due to airway and/or alveolar abnormalities usually caused by exposure to noxious particles or gases (4). Diagnosis requires demonstration of airflow obstruction by the presence of a post-bronchodilator ratio of forced expiratory volume in one second (FEV_1) to forced vital capacity (FVC), FEV_1/FVC <0.70.

COPD is estimated to affect 10% of adults over age 40, but prevalence data on COPD vary depending on diagnostic criteria and analytical approaches used (5–8). COPD is a leading cause of morbidity and currently the fourth leading cause of death globally (4). Given the situation with air pollution in developing countries, the COPD figures are worsening over time, particularly given that air pollution may already be the commonest cause of COPD, surpassing cigarette smoking.

Patients with COPD often report poor sleep quality, both quantitatively and qualitatively (9–13). Complaints of difficulties falling and staying asleep and fatigue are common. In 146 COPD patients asked to rate the frequency of 89 symptoms and experiences, sleep difficulties ranked third after dyspnea and fatigue (14). In a study questioning sleep in 50 COPD patients, more than twice as many patients with COPD reported regular use of hypnotics compared to controls (13). Overnight polysomnography in COPD patients corroborates complaints of disturbed sleep. Compared to non-COPD, COPD patients have been shown to have reduced sleep efficiency with delayed sleep onset, reduced total sleep time, a lower arousal threshold, increased periods of wakefulness, and changes in sleep architecture with increased N1 and decreased rapid eye movement (REM) sleep (11–13, 15). The poor sleep quality in COPD is likely multi-factorial in etiology including disease-specific symptoms such as cough, hypoxemia, sleep apnea, medications, and comorbidities including depression.

Sleep is associated with stage specific changes in ventilatory control: a decrease in the minute ventilation largely driven by reduced tidal volume, reduced muscle contractility, increased upper airway resistance, and blunted hypoxic and hypercapnic ventilatory responses, resulting in hypoxemia and hypercapnia (16, 17). In healthy individuals, these changes are usually not clinically significant, but in patients with COPD, hypoventilation can result in marked hypoxemia (18–21). NOD is common in COPD and can be severe depending on where the patient lies on the oxyhemoglobin dissociation curve (13, 20). Many COPD patients lie on the steep portion of the oxyhemoglobin dissociation curve, where a minor reduction in partial pressure of oxygen is accompanied by a disproportionately large decrease in oxygen saturation. NOD is particularly evident during REM sleep. In COPD patients, there is often cephalad displacement of the diaphragm with hyperinflation and increasing reliance on accessory muscles of respiration to maintain ventilation. This contribution from the accessory muscles is lost during the skeletal muscle hypotonia that occurs during REM sleep (22). Additionally, ventilation perfusion mismatch and a reduced functional residual capacity, exaggerated in the supine position, can contribute to NOD. In fact, Mulloy et al. compared ventilation and gas exchange in 19 patients with severe stable COPD (mean FEV_1 32% predicted) during sleep and incremental treadmill exercise, and SaO_2 fell twice as much

DOI: 10.1201/9781003000631-17

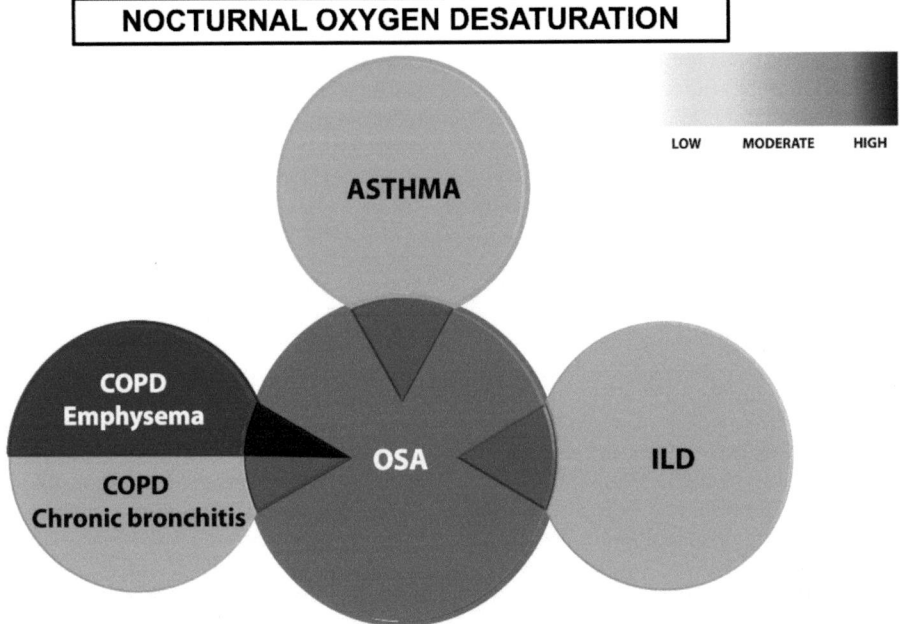

Figure 14.1 Figure depicts the interactions between OSA (obstructive sleep apnea) and ILD (interstitial lung disease) and COPD (chronic obstructive pulmonary disease). Marked desaturations can be seen in Overlap Syndrome (OSA plus COPD).

during sleep as during maximum exercise, 13.1 vs. 6% (p <0.01)(23). NOD may be a factor in the higher nocturnal death rate reported in COPD (24).

In 1985, David Flenley described a unique pattern of sleep hypoxemia in OVS, characterized by more profound hypoxemia, particularly during REM sleep, and a distinctive swinging pattern of nocturnal desaturation even outside REM sleep. He coined the term "overlap syndrome" to the co-existence of OSA and COPD, but in his cardinal 1985 paper, he recognized this unique pattern of nocturnal hypoxemia was likely to occur with OSA and other chronic lung diseases including cystic fibrosis and interstitial lung disease, as depicted in Figure 14.1 (20).

OSA is common and like COPD, prevalence data vary depending on the diagnostic criteria used and population studied. Using the Wisconsin Sleep Cohort Study, an ongoing community-based study established in 1988 and a total apnea-hypopnea index (AHI) ≥15/hr, the prevalence of OSA has been estimated at 13% in men and 6% in women (25). There has been ongoing interest in whether the presence of OSA increases the risk for COPD and vice versa. Epidemiological studies to date that have tried to address this question

have shown mixed results with prevalence estimates ranging from less than 1% to as high as 65% depending on the population studied (26–33). This wide variation in prevalence likely reflects differing definitions used to diagnose both OSA and COPD and study populations (29). Nonetheless, as both OSA and COPD are common, even by chance alone, the OVS is bound to occur commonly. In a systematic review by Shawon et al., the prevalence of OVS in the general and hospital population was estimated at 1%–3.6% (26).

One of the limitations in determining OVS prevalence is the ongoing debate regarding the optimal diagnostic testing and criteria for OSA in chronic lung disease. The diagnosis of OSA relies on calculation of the AHI, and the scoring of hypopneas is dependent on desaturation and/or detection of arousals. However, there has not been consistency in both the use of arousals and the degree of desaturation required to define hypopneas in the sleep community. This issue is of particular relevance in patients with chronic lung disease who sit on the steep portion of the oxyhemoglobin dissociation curve where even a small drop in arterial oxygen tension can result in a major difference in SaO_2. Additionally, COPD patients may be more prone to arousals. Consequently, hypopneas may be scored more readily in patients with chronic lung disease. In contrast, the use of supplemental oxygen eliminates one of the main criteria for scoring hypopneas and the AHI may be under-estimated in patients on supplemental oxygen (3). The presence of carboxyhemoglobin in the blood of severe COPD patients may dampen arousals, potentially also under-estimating the AHI in COPD.

Studies comparing in-laboratory polysomnography to an ambulatory sleep testing pathway have excluded patients with major cardiopulmonary disease and guidelines have not recommended the use of home sleep apnea testing in COPD (34). More recently, some investigators have compared home sleep apnea testing to in-laboratory polysomnography in COPD (35–37). Generalizability of these studies is limited by the use of different portable diagnostics devices and exclusion of patients with severe disease, especially requiring nocturnal oxygen, but portable sleep apnea testing may be an option for diagnosing OSA in milder COPD. There was a tendency for type 3 portable monitors to underestimate the AHI for more severe disease and suggestion of a higher failure rate; thus, additional studies including a range of COPD severities are required (35–37).

OVS has been associated with worse outcomes than OSA or COPD alone (38). Greater sleep-related hypoxemia and hypercapnia have been described with OVS than OSA alone or COPD patients with the same degree of airflow obstruction (39–41). Pulmonary hypertension is more common and more severe in patients with the OVS than OSA or COPD alone (40, 42). When evaluating COPD with hypoxemia, hypercapnia, or pulmonary hypertension out of proportion for their degree of airflow obstruction, polysomnography should be considered. Conversely, in OSA with hypoxemia, hypercapnia, and pulmonary hypertension out of proportion for the severity of OSA, pulmonary function testing should be considered.

OVS is particularly important given its association with poor quality of life and evidence suggesting increased mortality (31, 43, 44). Marin compared 213 patients with OVS to 210 COPD patients without OSA for a median follow up of 9.4 years and found higher mortality (relative risk 1.79, 95% CI 1.21–2.38) and first-time COPD exacerbation (relative risk 1.70, 95% CI 1.21–2.38) leading to hospitalization in those with the OVS (38). In this cohort, patients with untreated OVS had significantly higher number of cardiovascular deaths when compared to COPD alone. Both

COPD and OSA have been associated with similar pathophysiological pathways including hypoxemia, systemic inflammation, oxidative stress, and vascular endothelial dysfunction, factors implicated in the development of cardiovascular disease. Additional mechanistic research is needed regarding SDB, COPD, and cardiovascular disease (45, 46).

Few studies have specifically addressed optimal treatment for OVS, and currently management is directed at the treatment of SDB and COPD individually.

In COPD, smoking cessation is key. Pharmacologic treatment is centered around bronchodilators and anti-inflammatory drugs and can reduce symptoms, reduce the frequency and severity of exacerbations and improve health status and exercise tolerance (4). Long-acting bronchodilators have been shown to improve hypoxemia during sleep in COPD (47, 48). This improvement in sleep hypoxemia, however, has not been consistently associated with improvements in sleep quality, likely reflecting the multi-factorial etiology behind disturbed sleep in COPD.

Long-term administration of oxygen >15 hr/day has been shown to improve survival in patients with COPD and severe daytime resting hypoxemia (49–51). However, randomized controlled trials have failed to demonstrate clinically significant benefits in patients with less severe hypoxemia (51, 52). It remains unknown whether correction of sleep hypoxemia in COPD patients with isolated nocturnal desaturation leads to clinically meaningful outcomes. The International Nocturnal Oxygen study was a multi-center randomized placebo-controlled trial designed to try and address this question, but the study was terminated early and underpowered, limiting any definitive conclusions (53). Supplemental oxygen alone is not recommended as the primary treatment for OSA (54). Supplemental oxygen will improve hypoxemia in OSA, but it does not address the multiple pathophysiological mechanisms driving the hypoxemia and caution must be exercised in targeting oxygen saturation alone in OSA. This issue was highlighted in a randomized controlled trial comparing CPAP to nocturnal supplemental oxygen in 318 OSA patients with cardiovascular or multiple cardiovascular risk factors (55). Despite improvement in oxygenation with supplemental oxygen use, only the CPAP group saw significant reductions in blood pressure at 12 weeks. Only one study, to our knowledge, has investigated nocturnal oxygen in the OVS. Alford et al. studied 20 males with the OVS (mean FEV_1 59% predicted) with polysomnography on two separate nights, with and without nocturnal supplemental oxygen at 4 l/min (56). Supplemental oxygen administration again improved saturation recordings, but it also increased the mean duration of obstructive events by 5.7 seconds and increased end-apneic partial pressure of carbon dioxide by 9.5 mm Hg. Consequently, nocturnal oxygen alone cannot be recommended in the management of OVS.

Continuous positive airway pressure (CPAP) is the mainstay of treatment for OSA. In the same study by Marin et al. showing worse outcomes in patients with OVS compared to COPD alone, CPAP was associated with improved survival and decreased hospitalizations in OVS (38). Similar results were demonstrated by Machado et al., who compared hypoxemic COPD patients with moderate to severe OSA adherent to CPAP treatment to those non-adherent (57). The CPAP adherent group had a 5-year survival estimate of 71% (95% CI 53%–83%) compared to 26% (95% CI 12%–43%) in the CPAP non-adherent group, again supporting the use of CPAP in OVS. Interestingly, this survival benefit of CPAP in the OVS may be particularly true for hypercapnic patients. Jaoude et al. studied 271 patients with OVS, 104 who were hypercapnic at baseline (58). Similar to prior studies, CPAP was associated with reduced mortality, but this reduced mortality was only seen in hypercapnic patients, despite a comparable AHI between the hypercapnic and normocapnic patients. This is of relevance given increasing evidence showing the benefits of nocturnal non-invasive ventilation (NIV) in stable COPD patients is greater in patients with persistent and more severe hypercapnia (59–61). There are currently no major studies on NIV in OVS and it remains unknown whether NIV offers additional benefits over CPAP in OVS, especially in the subset of patients who are hypercapnic. Likely more important than the mode of PAP is adherence to therapy. In an observational cohort, Stanchina et al. showed a clear association between CPAP usage and mortality in patients with OVS (62).

SLEEP IN ASTHMA

Asthma is a heterogeneous disease characterized by chronic airway inflammation (63). Diurnal variation of airflow obstruction in asthma has been well described and symptoms are often worse at night or early morning (64, 65). Complaints of difficulties falling and staying asleep and daytime sleepiness are common in asthma and have been associated with worse quality of life (66–68). Lal et al. used the National Health and Nutritional Examination Survey to examine the association between self-reported sleep problems among 3,204 adults with obstructive lung diseases, 5.2% with asthma alone (69). All obstructive lung diseases were associated with a higher prevalence of sleep problems, defined as any complaints which affect or involve sleep, but there was a stronger association between asthma and sleep problems as compared to COPD and asthma-COPD overlap (69). The authors speculated that the nocturnal burden of asthma contributes to sleep problems, suggesting adults with asthma be aggressively screened for sleep disturbances. Additionally, some of the nocturnal symptoms perceived as asthma may be symptoms of OSA (70–72).

Again, both asthma and OSA are among the most common respiratory disorders making the coexistence of both quite common. A high prevalence of OSA has been reported in asthma patients, ranging from 19% up to 95%, and meta-analyses of 26 studies estimated the prevalence of OSA at 49.5% (95% CI 35.39–62.60) of adults with asthma (69, 70, 73–80). This wide range reflects the heterogeneity of the populations studied and varying diagnostic methods used. A particularly high prevalence of OSA has been described in patients with severe asthma, and using the Wisconsin Sleep Cohort incident, OSA risk was dose-dependent on the duration of asthma (76, 81–84).

It remains unclear whether this association between asthma and OSA represents correlation (i.e. shared risk factors including obesity, rhinitis, and gastroesophageal reflux (GER) chance) or causation (84). A potential bidirectional relationship between asthma and OSA exists, but many confounders challenge attempts to ascertain better the interaction between the two. For example, both OSA and asthma are more common in obese than non-obese individuals. Obese asthmatics have been shown to have more symptoms, more frequent and severe exacerbations, reduced response to asthma medications and decreased quality of life (85). Obesity, however, is also a common risk factor for OSA, and a complex interplay like exists between obesity, asthma, and OSA (86).

Nonetheless, overlap with asthma and OSA has been associated with worse clinical outcomes including worse asthma control and severe asthma exacerbations, worse quality of life, and increased health resource utilization (79, 87–89). Wang compared 77 patients with asthma and varying severities of OSA and found the FEV_1 decline among patients with severe OSA was greater at 72.4 ± 61.7 mL/year as compared to 41.9 ± 45.3 mL/year in those with mild to moderate OSA and 24.3 ± 27.5 mL/year in those without OSA (90). For those patients with severe OSA, the FEV_1 decline was significantly attenuated after CPAP treatment, reinforcing the importance of recognizing OSA in people with asthma.

Given the known benefits of CPAP in OSA, studies have explored the use of CPAP in patients with coexistent asthma and OSA (66, 83, 91–95). In one of the larger studies, Serrano-Pariente examined asthma outcomes in 99 adults with coexisting mild asthma and moderate to severe OSA after 6 months of CPAP treatment. CPAP use was associated with improved asthma control and quality of life (94). Smaller observational clinical studies have shown similar improvements in asthma symptoms and quality of life with CPAP but have failed to show improvements in objective measures of bronchial responsiveness, such as the provocative concentration causing a 20% fall in FEV_1 (PC_{20}) or FEV_1 (91, 93, 95).

Randomized controlled studies are needed to evaluate better the impact of CPAP on asthma OSA overlap, but this issue is further complicated by some interesting studies looking at CPAP in people with asthma without coexisting OSA. By increasing the stretch of the airway during sleep, CPAP has been proposed to suppress airway smooth muscle contractility and improve asthma control (96–99). Small animal and human studies suggest improvement in bronchial hyperreactivity in asthmatics without OSA with CPAP use, but these results have not been reproduced in a larger clinical study (66, 99–102). PC_{20} change was compared in 194 asthma patients randomized to CPAP at levels either less than 1 cm H_2O (sham), 5 cm H_2O, or 10 cm H_2O after 12 weeks (96). While all groups had a significant improvement in PC_{20} at 12 weeks, no significant difference was seen between the active and sham CPAP groups. The study was limited by poor adherence, compromising any firm conclusions.

SLEEP IN INTERSTITIAL LUNG DISEASES

Interstitial lung diseases (ILDs) are a heterogeneous group of diseases characterized by inflammation and fibrosis of lung parenchyma, resulting in a restrictive ventilatory pattern and impaired gas exchange. Of the idiopathic ILDs, idiopathic pulmonary fibrosis (IPF) is the most common. IPF is a chronic, progressive, fibrotic interstitial lung disease of unknown cause associated with important morbidity and mortality (103). In the

United States, the prevalence of IPF has been reported to range from 10 to 60 cases per 100K, although in one study, the prevalence was 494 cases per 100K among adults over 65 years (103).

Less research exists examining sleep and SDB in ILDs than for obstructive lung diseases, but many similarities exist. Like obstructive lung diseases, ILD patients have poor sleep quality and impaired daytime functioning (104–107). This poor sleep quality yields a poor quality of life (104). Similarly, overnight polysomnography in patients with ILD has shown decreased sleep efficiency, worse sleep fragmentation, and altered sleep architecture with reduced REM sleep (105, 106, 108). In a study comparing 11 patients with ILD to 11 age- and sex-matched controls with polysomnography, patients with ILD with awake SaO_2 <90% (in the absence of OSA) had greater disruptions in sleep architecture when compared to those with SaO_2 >90%, suggesting hypoxemia as one mechanism for poor sleep (106).

Like obstructive lung disease, nocturnal desaturation, especially during REM sleep, is common in ILD, although one small study suggested a smaller degree of nocturnal desaturation in ILD compared to COPD (105, 106, 109–113). Sleep hypoxemia has been associated with not only worse sleep quality, daytime impairment, and quality of life but worse disease outcomes in IPF (105, 109, 114, 115). It is predicted by daytime oxygenation and where patients live on the oxyhemoglobin dissociation curve (106, 108, 112, 113). The SaO_2 fall in sleep can again be greater than the SaO_2 fall during exercise, although in a small study of 16 ILD patients, despite similar maximum SaO_2 fall during sleep and maximum exercise, the mean SaO_2 fall during sleep was less than during moderate exercise (111, 113).

While NOD is common in ILD, it is again important to recognize the possibility of co-existing OSA causing desaturations. There is growing evidence to suggest OSA is common in ILD but studies are methodologically limited (31, 107, 111, 116–123). Of 50 patients with IPF followed in one clinic who completed polysomnography, all but six subjects had OSA, 10 (20%) with mild OSA and 34 (68%) with moderate to severe OSA (124). Other cohorts have shown similarly high rates of moderate to severe OSA of between 51% and 72% in patients with incident IPF (125).

The relationship between ILD and OSA remains unclear, but a possible causal interaction has been suggested. Cross-sectional analyses of 1,690 adults in the Multi-Ethnic

Study of Atherosclerosis cohort who underwent both chest CT and polysomnography found an association between moderate to severe OSA and subclinical ILD (117). An obstructive AHI ≥15/hr was associated with a 35% increased odds (95% CI 13%–61%, p = 0.001) of interstitial lung abnormalities on CT, although the association varied by body mass index with the strongest association seen among normal-weight individuals. A greater AHI was also associated with higher serum matrix metalloproteinase-7 and surfactant protein-A levels, again largely in non-obese individuals, suggesting a possible association between OSA and alveolar epithelial injury and extracellular matrix remodeling (117). Oxidative stress and inflammation due to the intermittent hypoxemia seen in OSA may further exacerbate the alveolar epithelial injury. Additionally, the small lung volumes in ILD have been associated with reduced caudal traction in the upper airways, increasing collapsibility, but the exact relationship between ILD and OSA remains to be determined (126). GER is common to both disorders. It has also been implicated in the relationship between ILD and OSA, but in a study of 54 patients with non-connective tissue disease-related fibrosing ILD who underwent screening polysomnography and pH or pH/impedance probe, the AHI did not predict the presence of GER and GER was no more frequent or severe among OSA subjects versus those without OSA (127). Further research is needed to understand better the relationship between ILD and SDB.

OSA in ILD has also been associated with worse clinical outcomes than ILD alone including worse quality of life, disease progression, and even survival (107, 114, 115, 128, 129). In a cohort of 31 newly diagnosed patients with IPF, the lowest SpO_2 and intermittent oxygen desaturation were associated with survival (114). While the AHI itself was not related to survival when the entire study population was examined, after excluding the subgroup of IPF patients assigned to CPAP treatment for OSA, the AHI predicted decreased survival.

Consequently, addressing SDB in ILD is important, yet there are few studies on the optimal treatment of SDB in ILD. The use of supplemental oxygen in patients with ILD is largely extrapolated from studies in COPD. The AmbOx study was a prospective, open-label, crossover randomized trial that looked at the effects of ambulatory oxygen on health-related quality of life in 84 patients with ILD and isolated exertional hypoxemia based on a SaO_2 ≤88% on 6-minute walk

(130). Ambulatory oxygen for 2 weeks was associated with significant improvements in some measures of the King's Brief Interstitial Lung Disease questionnaire. Given data suggesting equivalent to worse desaturations during sleep than during exercise, the findings suggest a possible role for nocturnal oxygen in ILD patients with sleep hypoxemia, but interventional studies are needed. Furthermore, nocturnal oxygen should not be used merely to mask sleep hypoxemia caused by OSA.

To date, there are no randomized controlled trials of CPAP for OSA in ILD to our knowledge, but retrospective data suggest that treating sleep disorders may improve ILD outcomes including sleep and life quality (125, 126, 131–134). CPAP was associated with significant improvement in daily living activities based on the Functional Outcomes in Sleep Questionnaire in a small study of 12 patients with newly diagnosed IPF and moderate to severe OSA (134). The same investigators compared 38 ILD patients with OSA adherent with CPAP to 18 non-adherent with CPAP and again found significant improvements in quality of sleep and quality of life measures after 1 year (131).

CONCLUSION

With one-third of human life spent sleeping, understanding the impact of sleep and SDB on chronic lung diseases and vice versa is essential, especially given the prevalence of these conditions. A comprehensive sleep evaluation should be included in the evaluation of any patient with chronic lung disease. Additional research is needed to delineate the complex relationship between the different phenotypes and severities of SDB and chronic lung disease better.

REFERENCES

1. Benjafield AV, Ayas NT, Eastwood PR, Heinzer R, Ip MSM, Morrell MJ, et al. Estimation of the global prevalence and burden of obstructive sleep apnoea: a literature-based analysis. Lancet Respir Med. 2019;7(8):687–98.

2. World Health Organization. Global Surveillance, Prevention and Control of Chronic Respiratory Diseases: A Comprehensive Approach. World Health Organization; 2007. 1–155 pp.

3. Malhotra A, Schwartz AR, Schneider H, Owens RL, DeYoung P, Han MK, et al. Research priorities in pathophysiology for sleep-disordered breathing in patients with chronic obstructive pulmonary disease. An official American Thoracic Society research statement. Am J Respir Crit Care Med. 2018;197(3):289–99.

4. Singh D, Agusti A, Anzueto A, Barnes PJ, Bourbeau J, Celli BR, et al. Disease. Global Strategy for the Diagnosis, Management, and Prevention of Chronic Obstructive Pulmonary Disease: the GOLD science committee report. 2020 Report. 2020:1–141 PMID: 30846476.

5. Adeloye D, Chua S, Lee C, Basquill C, Papana A, Theodoratou E, et al. Global and regional estimates of COPD prevalence: systematic review and meta-analysis. J Glob Health. 2015;5(2):020415.

6. BOLD. Burden of Obstructive Lung Disease Initiative Webpage, published by Imperial College London. https://www.boldstudy.org/.

7. Halbert RJ, Natoli JL, Gano A, Badamgarav E, Buist AS, Mannino DM. Global burden of COPD: systematic review and meta-analysis. Eur Respir J. 2006;28(3):523–32.

8. GBD 2015 Chronic Respiratory Disease Collaborators. Global, regional, and national deaths, prevalence, disability-adjusted life years, and years lived with disability for chronic obstructive pulmonary disease and asthma, 1990–2015: a systematic analysis for the Global Burden of Disease Study 2015. Lancet Respir Med. 2017;5(9):691–706. doi: 10.1016/S2213-2600(17)30293-X. Epub 2017 Aug 16

9. Agusti A, Hedner J, Marin JM, Barbe F, Cazzola M, Rennard S. Night-time symptoms: a forgotten dimension of COPD. Eur Respir Rev. 2011;20(121):183–94.

10. Hynninen MJ, Pallesen S, Hardie J, Eagan TM, Bjorvatn B, Bakke P, et al. Insomnia symptoms, objectively measured sleep, and disease severity in chronic obstructive pulmonary disease outpatients. Sleep Med. 2013;14(12):1328–33.

11. McSharry DG, Ryan S, Calverley P, Edwards JC, McNicholas WT. Sleep quality in chronic obstructive pulmonary disease. Respirology. 2012;17(7):1119–24.

12. Valipour A, Lavie P, Lothaller H, Mikulic I, Burghuber OC. Sleep profile and symptoms of sleep disorders in patients with stable mild to moderate chronic obstructive pulmonary disease. Sleep Med. 2011;12(4):367–72.

13. Cormick W, Olson LG, Hensley MJ, Saunders NA. Nocturnal hypoxaemia and quality of sleep in patients with chronic obstructive lung disease. Thorax. 1986;41(11):846–54.

14. Kinsman RA, Yaroush RA, Fernandez E, Dirks JF, Schocket M, Fukuhara J. Symptoms and experiences in chronic bronchitis and emphysema. Chest. 1983;83(5):755–61.

15. Yamaguchi Y, Shiota S, Kusunoki Y, Hamaya H, Ishii M, Kodama Y, et al. Polysomnographic features of low arousal threshold in overlap syndrome involving obstructive sleep apnea and chronic obstructive pulmonary disease. Sleep Breath. 2019;23(4):1095–100.

16. Douglas NJ, White DP, Pickett CK, Weil JV, Zwillich CW. Respiration during sleep in normal man. Thorax. 1982;37(11):840–4.

17. Sowho M, Amatoury J, Kirkness JP, Patil SP. Sleep and respiratory physiology in adults. Clin Chest Med. 2014;35(3):469–81.

18. Catterall JR, Douglas NJ, Calverley PM, Shapiro CM, Brezinova V, Brash HM, et al. Transient hypoxemia during sleep in chronic obstructive pulmonary disease is not a sleep apnea syndrome. Am Rev Respir Dis. 1983;128(1):24–9.

19. Douglas NJ, Calverley PM, Leggett RJ, Brash HM, Flenley DC, Brezinova V. Transient hypoxaemia during sleep in chronic bronchitis and emphysema. Lancet. 1979;1(8106):1–4.

20. Flenley DC. Sleep in chronic obstructive lung disease. Clin Chest Med. 1985;6(4):651–61.

21. McNicholas WT, Verbraecken J, Marin JM. Sleep disorders in COPD: the forgotten dimension. Eur Respir Rev. 2013;22(129):365–75.

22. Lu J, Sherman D, Devor M, Saper CB. A putative flip-flop switch for control of REM sleep. Nature. 2006;441(7093):589–94.

23. Mulloy E, McNicholas WT. Ventilation and gas exchange during sleep and exercise in severe COPD. Chest. 1996;109(2):387–94.

24. McNicholas WT, Fitzgerald MX. Nocturnal deaths among patients with chronic bronchitis and emphysema. Br Med J (Clin Res Ed). 1984;289(6449):878.

25. Peppard PE, Young T, Barnet JH, Palta M, Hagen EW, Hla KM. Increased prevalence of sleep-disordered breathing in adults. Am J Epidemiol. 2013;177(9):1006–14.

26. Shawon MS, Perret JL, Senaratna CV, Lodge C, Hamilton GS, Dharmage SC. Current evidence on prevalence and clinical outcomes of co-morbid obstructive sleep apnea and chronic obstructive pulmonary disease: a systematic review. Sleep Med Rev. 2017;32:5868.

27. Bednarek M, Maciejewski J, Wozniak M, Kuca P, Zielinski J. Prevalence, severity and underdiagnosis of COPD in the primary care setting. Thorax. 2008;63(5):402–7.

28. Lopez-Acevedo MN, Torres-Palacios A, Elena Ocasio-Tascon M, Campos-Santiago Z, Rodriguez-Cintron W. Overlap syndrome: an indication for sleep studies?: a pilot study. Sleep Breath. 2009;13(4):409–13.

29. Owens RL, Macrea MM, Teodorescu M. The overlaps of asthma or COPD with OSA: a focused review. Respirology. 2017;22(6):1073–83.

30. Soler X, Gaio E, Powell FL, Ramsdell JW, Loredo JS, Malhotra A, et al. High prevalence of obstructive sleep apnea in patients with moderate to severe chronic obstructive pulmonary disease. Ann Am Thorac Soc. 2015;12(8):1219–25.

31. Zhang XL, Dai HP, Zhang H, Gao B, Zhang L, Han T, et al. Obstructive sleep apnea in patients with fibrotic interstitial lung disease and COPD. J Clin Sleep Med. 2019;15(12):1807–15.

32. Schreiber A, Cemmi F, Ambrosino N, Ceriana P, Lastoria C, Carlucci A. Prevalence and predictors of obstructive sleep apnea in patients with chronic obstructive pulmonary disease undergoing inpatient pulmonary rehabilitation. COPD. 2018;15(3):265–70.

33. Greenberg-Dotan S, Reuveni H, Tal A, Oksenberg A, Cohen A, Shaya FT, et al. Increased prevalence of obstructive lung disease in patients with obstructive sleep apnea. Sleep Breath. 2014;18(1):69–75.

34. Collop NA, Anderson WM, Boehlecke B, Claman D, Goldberg R, Gottlieb DJ, et al. Clinical guidelines for the use of unattended portable monitors in the diagnosis of obstructive sleep apnea in adult patients. Portable Monitoring Task Force of the American Academy of Sleep Medicine. J Clin Sleep Med. 2007;3(7):737–47.

35. Chang Y, Xu L, Han F, Keenan BT, Kneeland-Szanto E, Zhang R, et al. Validation of the Nox-T3 portable monitor for diagnosis of obstructive sleep apnea in patients with chronic obstructive pulmonary disease. J Clin Sleep Med. 2019;15(4):587–96.

36. Jen R, Orr JE, Li Y, DeYoung P, Smales E, Malhotra A, et al. Accuracy of WatchPAT for the diagnosis of obstructive sleep apnea in patients with chronic obstructive pulmonary disease. COPD. 2020;17(1):34–9.

37. Oliveira MG, Nery LE, Santos-Silva R, Sartori DE, Alonso FF, Togeiro SM, et al. Is portable monitoring accurate in the diagnosis of obstructive sleep apnea syndrome in chronic pulmonary obstructive disease? Sleep Med. 2012;13(8):1033–8.

38. Marin JM, Soriano JB, Carrizo SJ, Boldova A, Celli BR. Outcomes in patients with chronic obstructive pulmonary disease and obstructive sleep apnea: the overlap syndrome. Am J Respir Crit Care Med. 2010;182(3):325–31.

39. Weitzenblum E, Chaouat A, Kessler R, Canuet M. Overlap syndrome: obstructive sleep apnea in patients with chronic obstructive pulmonary disease. Proc Am Thorac Soc. 2008;5(2):237–41.

40. Chaouat A, Weitzenblum E, Krieger J, Ifoundza T, Oswald M, Kessler R. Association of chronic obstructive pulmonary disease and sleep apnea syndrome. Am J Respir Crit Care Med. 1995;151(1):82–6.

41. Sanders MH, Newman AB, Haggerty CL, Redline S, Lebowitz M, Samet J, et al. Sleep and sleep-disordered breathing in adults with predominantly mild obstructive airway disease. Am J Respir Crit Care Med. 2003;167(1):7–14.

42. Kessler R, Chaouat A, Schinkewitch P, Faller M, Casel S, Krieger J, et al. The obesity-hypoventilation syndrome revisited: a prospective study of 34 consecutive cases. Chest. 2001;120(2):369–76.

43. Mermigkis C, Kopanakis A, Foldvary-Schaefer N, Golish J, Polychronopoulos V, Schiza S, et al. Health-related quality of life in patients with obstructive sleep apnoea and chronic obstructive pulmonary disease (overlap syndrome). Int J Clin Pract. 2007;61(2):207–11.

44. Zohal MA, Yazdi Z, Kazemifar AM, Mahjoob P, Ziaeeha M. Sleep quality and quality of life in COPD patients with and without suspected obstructive sleep apnea. Sleep Disord. 2014;2014:508372.

45. Kendzerska T, Leung RS, Aaron SD, Ayas N, Sandoz JS, Gershon AS. Cardiovascular outcomes and all-cause mortality in patients with obstructive sleep apnea and chronic obstructive pulmonary disease (overlap syndrome). Ann Am Thorac Soc. 2019;16(1):71–81.

46. McNicholas WT. Chronic obstructive pulmonary disease and obstructive sleep apnea: overlaps in pathophysiology, systemic inflammation, and cardiovascular disease. Am J Respir Crit Care Med. 2009;180(8):692–700.

47. McNicholas WT, Calverley PM, Lee A, Edwards JC, Tiotropium Sleep Study in CI. Long-acting inhaled anticholinergic therapy improves sleeping oxygen saturation in COPD. Eur Respir J. 2004;23(6):825–31.

48. Ryan S, Doherty LS, Rock C, Nolan GM, McNicholas WT. Effects of salmeterol on sleeping oxygen saturation in chronic obstructive pulmonary disease. Respiration. 2010;79(6):475–81.

49. Continuous or nocturnal oxygen therapy in hypoxemic chronic obstructive lung disease: a clinical trial. Nocturnal Oxygen Therapy Trial Group. Ann Intern Med. 1980;93(3):391–8.

50. Long term domiciliary oxygen therapy in chronic hypoxic cor pulmonale complicating chronic bronchitis and emphysema. Report of the Medical Research Council Working Party. Lancet. 1981;1(8222):681–6.

51. Lacasse Y, Tan AM, Maltais F, Krishnan JA. Home oxygen in chronic obstructive pulmonary disease. Am J Respir Crit Care Med. 2018;197(10):1254–64.

52. Long-Term Oxygen Treatment Trial Research G, Albert RK, Au DH, Blackford AL, Casaburi R, Cooper JA, Jr., et al. A randomized trial of long-term oxygen for COPD with moderate desaturation. N Engl J Med. 2016;375(17):1617–27.

53. Lacasse Y, Bernard S, Series F, Nguyen VH, Bourbeau J, Aaron S, et al. Multi-center, randomized, placebo-controlled trial of nocturnal oxygen therapy in chronic obstructive pulmonary disease: a study protocol for the INOX trial. BMC Pulm Med. 2017;17(1):8.

54. Epstein LJ, Kristo D, Strollo PJ, Jr., Friedman N, Malhotra A, Patil SP, et al. Clinical guideline for the evaluation, management and long-term care of obstructive sleep apnea in adults. J Clin Sleep Med. 2009;5(3):263–76.

55. Gottlieb DJ, Punjabi NM, Mehra R, Patel SR, Quan SF, Babineau DC, et al. CPAP versus oxygen in obstructive sleep apnea. N Engl J Med. 2014;370(24):2276–85.

56. Alford NJ, Fletcher EC, Nickeson D. Acute oxygen in patients with sleep apnea and COPD. Chest. 1986;89(1):30–8.

57. Machado MC, Vollmer WM, Togeiro SM, Bilderback AL, Oliveira MV, Leitao FS, et al. CPAP and survival in moderate-to-severe obstructive sleep apnoea syndrome and hypoxaemic COPD. Eur Respir J. 2010;35(1):132–7.

58. Jaoude P, Kufel T, El-Solh AA. Survival benefit of CPAP favors hypercapnic patients with the overlap syndrome. Lung. 2014;192(2):251–8.

59. Duiverman ML. Noninvasive ventilation in stable hypercapnic COPD: what is the evidence? ERJ Open Res. 2018;4(2).

60. Struik FM, Lacasse Y, Goldstein RS, Kerstjens HA, Wijkstra PJ. Nocturnal noninvasive positive pressure ventilation in stable COPD: a systematic review and individual patient data meta-analysis. Respir Med. 2014;108(2):329–37.

61. Murphy PB, Rehal S, Arbane G, Bourke S, Calverley PMA, Crook AM, et al. Effect of home noninvasive ventilation with oxygen therapy vs oxygen therapy alone on hospital readmission or death after an acute COPD exacerbation: a randomized clinical trial. JAMA. 2017;317(21):2177–86.

62. Stanchina ML, Welicky LM, Donat W, Lee D, Corrao W, Malhotra A. Impact of CPAP use and age on mortality in patients with combined COPD and obstructive sleep apnea: the overlap syndrome. J Clin Sleep Med. 2013;9(8):767–72.

63. Bateman ED, Hurd SS, Barnes PJ, Bousquet J, Drazen JM, FitzGerald M, et al. Global strategy for asthma management and prevention: GINA executive summary. Eur Respir J. 2008;31(1):143–78. doi: 10.1183/09031936.00138707

64. Barnes P, FitzGerald G, Brown M, Dollery C. Nocturnal asthma and changes in circulating epinephrine, histamine, and cortisol. N Engl J Med. 1980;303(5):263–7.

65. Soutar CA, Costello J, Ijaduola O, Turner-Warwick M. Nocturnal and morning asthma. Relationship to plasma corticosteroids and response to cortisol infusion. Thorax. 1975;30(4):436–40.

66. Kavanagh J, Jackson DJ, Kent BD. Sleep and asthma. Curr Opin Pulm Med. 2018;24(6):569–73.

67. Janson C, De Backer W, Gislason T, Plaschke P, Bjornsson E, Hetta J, et al. Increased prevalence of sleep disturbances and daytime sleepiness in subjects with bronchial asthma: a population study of young adults in three European countries. Eur Respir J. 1996;9(10):2132–8.

68. Auckley D, Moallem M, Shaman Z, Mustafa M. Findings of a Berlin Questionnaire survey: comparison between patients seen in an asthma clinic versus internal medicine clinic. Sleep Med. 2008;9(5):494–9.

69. Lal C, Kumbhare S, Strange C. Prevalence of self-reported sleep problems amongst adults with obstructive airway disease in the NHANES cohort in the United States. Sleep Breath. 2020 Sep;24(3):985–93.

70. Larsson LG, Lindberg A, Franklin KA, Lundback B. Symptoms related to obstructive sleep apnoea are common in subjects with asthma, chronic bronchitis and rhinitis in a general population. Respir Med. 2001;95(5):423–9.

71. Senaratna CV, Walters EH, Hamilton G, Lowe AJ, Lodge C, Burgess J, et al. Nocturnal symptoms perceived as asthma are associated with obstructive sleep apnoea risk, but not bronchial hyper-reactivity. Respirology. 2019;24(12):1176–82.

72. Sunwoo BY, Owens RL. All that wheezes at night is not asthma. Respirology. 2019;24(12):1127–8.

73. Kong DL, Qin Z, Shen H, Jin HY, Wang W, Wang ZF. Association of obstructive sleep apnea with asthma: a meta-analysis. Sci Rep. 2017;7(1):4088.

74. Shen TC, Lin CL, Wei CC, Chen CH, Tu CY, Hsia TC, et al. Risk of obstructive sleep apnea in adult patients with asthma: a population-based cohort study in Taiwan. PLoS One. 2015;10(6):e0128461.

75. Sweeney J, Patterson CC, Menzies-Gow A, Niven RM, Mansur AH, Bucknall C, et al. Comorbidity in severe asthma requiring systemic corticosteroid therapy: cross-sectional data from the Optimum Patient Care Research Database and the British Thoracic Difficult Asthma Registry. Thorax. 2016;71(4):339–46.

76. Teodorescu M, Barnet JH, Hagen EW, Palta M, Young TB, Peppard PE. Association between asthma and risk of developing obstructive sleep apnea. JAMA. 2015;313(2):156–64.

77. Damianaki A, Vagiakis E, Sigala I, Pataka A, Rovina N, Vlachou A, et al. Tauhe co-existence of obstructive sleep apnea and bronchial asthma: revelation of a new asthma phenotype? J Clin Med. 2019 Sep 16;8(9):1476. doi: 10.3390/jcm8091476

78. Ioachimescu OC, Janocko NJ, Ciavatta MM, Howard M, Warnock MV. Obstructive Lung Disease and Obstructive Sleep Apnea (OLDOSA) cohort study: 10-year assessment. J Clin Sleep Med. 2020;16(2):267–77.

79. Teodorescu M, Broytman O, Curran-Everett D, Sorkness RL, Crisafi G, Bleecker ER, et al. Obstructive sleep apnea risk, asthma burden, and lower airway inflammation in adults in the Severe Asthma Research Program (SARP) II. J Allergy Clin Immunol Pract. 2015;3(4):566–75.e1.

80. Davies SE, Bishopp A, Wharton S, Turner AM, Mansur AH. The association between asthma and obstructive sleep apnea (OSA): A systematic review. J Asthma. 2019;56(2):118–29.

81. Julien JY, Martin JG, Ernst P, Olivenstein R, Hamid Q, Lemiere C, et al. Prevalence of obstructive sleep apnea-hypopnea in severe versus moderate asthma. J Allergy Clin Immunol. 2009;124(2):371–6.

82. Teodorescu M, Consens FB, Bria WF, Coffey MJ, McMorris MS, Weatherwax KJ, et al. Predictors of habitual snoring and obstructive sleep apnea risk in patients with asthma. Chest. 2009;135(5):1125–32.

83. Yigla M, Tov N, Solomonov A, Rubin AH, Harlev D. Difficult-to-control asthma and obstructive sleep apnea. J Asthma. 2003;40(8):865–71.

84. Prasad B, Nyenhuis SM, Imayama I, Siddiqi A, Teodorescu M. Asthma and obstructive sleep apnea overlap: what has the evidence taught us? Am J Respir Crit Care Med. 2020 June 1;201(11):1345–1357

85. Peters U, Dixon AE, Forno E. Obesity and asthma. J Allergy Clin Immunol. 2018;141(4):1169–79.

86. Owens RL, Campana LM, Foster AM, Schomer AM, Israel E, Malhotra A. Nocturnal bilevel positive airway pressure for the treatment of asthma. Respir Physiol Neurobiol. 2020;274:103355.

87. Becerra MB, Becerra BJ, Teodorescu M. Healthcare burden of obstructive sleep apnea and obesity among asthma hospitalizations: results from the U.S.-based Nationwide Inpatient Sample. Respir Med. 2016;117:2306.

88. Kim MY, Jo EJ, Kang SY, Chang YS, Yoon IY, Cho SH, et al. Obstructive sleep apnea is associated with reduced quality of life in adult patients with asthma. Ann Allergy Asthma Immunol. 2013;110(4):253–7, 7 e1.

89. Wang Y, Liu K, Hu K, Yang J, Li Z, Nie M, et al. Impact of obstructive sleep apnea on severe asthma exacerbations. Sleep Med. 2016;26:15.

90. Wang TY, Lo YL, Lin SM, Huang CD, Chung FT, Lin HC, et al. Obstructive sleep apnoea accelerates FEV1 decline in asthmatic patients. BMC Pulm Med. 2017;17(1):55.

91. Ciftci TU, Ciftci B, Guven SF, Kokturk O, Turktas H. Effect of nasal continuous positive airway pressure in uncontrolled nocturnal asthmatic patients with obstructive sleep apnea syndrome. Respir Med. 2005;99(5):529–34.

92. Kauppi P, Bachour P, Maasilta P, Bachour A. Long-term CPAP treatment improves asthma control in patients with asthma and obstructive sleep apnoea. Sleep Breath. 2016;20(4):1217–24.

93. Lafond C, Series F, Lemiere C. Impact of CPAP on asthmatic patients with obstructive sleep apnoea. Eur Respir J. 2007;29(2):307–11.

94. Serrano-Pariente J, Plaza V, Soriano JB, Mayos M, Lopez-Vina A, Picado C, et al. Asthma outcomes improve with continuous positive airway pressure for obstructive sleep apnea. Allergy. 2017;72(5):802–12.

95. Ng SSS, Chan TO, To KW, Chan KKP, Ngai J, Yip WH, et al. Continuous positive airway pressure for obstructive sleep apnoea does not improve asthma control. Respirology. 2018;23(11):1055–62.

96. Holbrook JT, Sugar EA, Brown RH, Drye LT, Irvin CG, Schwartz AR, et al. Effect of continuous positive airway pressure on airway reactivity in asthma. A randomized, sham-controlled clinical trial. Ann Am Thorac Soc. 2016;13(11):1940–50.

97. Irvin CG, Pak J, Martin RJ. Airway-parenchyma uncoupling in nocturnal asthma. Am J Respir Crit Care Med. 2000;161(1):50–6.

98. Skloot G, Permutt S, Togias A. Airway hyperresponsiveness in asthma: a problem of limited smooth muscle relaxation with inspiration. J Clin Invest. 1995;96(5):2393–403.

99. Busk M, Busk N, Puntenney P, Hutchins J, Yu Z, Gunst SJ, et al. Use of continuous positive airway pressure reduces airway reactivity in adults with asthma. Eur Respir J. 2013;41(2):317–22.

100. Xue Z, Yu Y, Gao H, Gunst SJ, Tepper RS. Chronic continuous positive airway pressure (CPAP) reduces airway reactivity in vivo in an allergen-induced rabbit model of asthma. J Appl Physiol (1985). 2011;111(2):353–7.

101. Xue Z, Zhang L, Liu Y, Gunst SJ, Tepper RS. Chronic inflation of ferret lungs with CPAP reduces airway smooth muscle contractility in vivo and in vitro. J Appl Physiol (1985). 2008;104(3):610–5.

102. Xue Z, Zhang L, Ramchandani R, Liu Y, Antony VB, Gunst SJ, et al. Respiratory system responsiveness in rabbits in vivo is reduced by prolonged continuous positive airway pressure. J Appl Physiol (1985). 2005;99(2):677–82.

103. Lederer DJ, Martinez FJ. Idiopathic pulmonary fibrosis. N Engl J Med. 2018;379(8):797–8.

104. Krishnan V, McCormack MC, Mathai SC, Agarwal S, Richardson B, Horton MR, et al. Sleep quality and health-related quality of life in idiopathic pulmonary fibrosis. Chest. 2008;134(4):693–8.

105. Mermigkis C, Stagaki E, Amfilochiou A, Polychronopoulos V, Korkonikitas P, Mermigkis D, et al. Sleep quality and associated daytime consequences in patients with idiopathic pulmonary fibrosis. Med Princ Pract. 2009;18(1):10–5.

106. Perez-Padilla R, West P, Lertzman M, Kryger MH. Breathing during sleep in patients with interstitial lung disease. Am Rev Respir Dis. 1985;132(2):224–9.

107. Bosi M, Milioli G, Parrino L, Fanfulla F, Tomassetti S, Melpignano A, et al. Quality of life in idiopathic pulmonary fibrosis: The impact of sleep disordered breathing. Respir Med. 2019;147:517.

108. McNicholas WT, Coffey M, Fitzgerald MX. Ventilation and gas exchange during sleep in patients with interstitial lung disease. Thorax. 1986;41(10):777–82.

109. Corte TJ, Wort SJ, Talbot S, Macdonald PM, Hansel DM, Polkey M, et al. Elevated nocturnal desaturation index predicts mortality in interstitial lung disease. Sarcoidosis Vasc Diffuse Lung Dis. 2012;29(1):41–50.

110. Hira HS, Sharma RK. Study of oxygen saturation, breathing pattern and arrhythmias in patients of interstitial lung disease during sleep. Indian J Chest Dis Allied Sci. 1997;39(3):157–62.

111. Bye PT, Issa F, Berthon-Jones M, Sullivan CE. Studies of oxygenation during sleep in patients with interstitial lung disease. Am Rev Respir Dis. 1984;129(1):27–32.

112. Clark M, Cooper B, Singh S, Cooper M, Carr A, Hubbard R. A survey of nocturnal hypoxaemia and health related quality of life in patients with cryptogenic fibrosing alveolitis. Thorax. 2001;56(6):482–6.

113. Midgren B, Hansson L, Eriksson L, Airikkala P, Elmqvist D. Oxygen desaturation during sleep and exercise in patients with interstitial lung disease. Thorax. 1987;42(5):353–6.

114. Kolilekas L, Manali E, Vlami KA, Lyberopoulos P, Triantafillidou C, Kagouridis K, et al. Sleep oxygen desaturation predicts survival in idiopathic pulmonary fibrosis. J Clin Sleep Med. 2013;9(6):593–601.

115. Troy LK, Young IH, Lau EMT, Wong KKH, Yee BJ, Torzillo PJ, et al. Nocturnal hypoxaemia is associated with adverse outcomes in interstitial lung disease. Respirology. 2019;24(10):996–1004.

116. Aydogdu M, Ciftci B, Firat Guven S, Ulukavak Ciftci T, Erdogan Y. Assessment of sleep with polysomnography in patients with interstitial lung disease. Tuberk Toraks. 2006;54(3):213–21.

117. Kim JS, Podolanczuk AJ, Borker P, Kawut SM, Raghu G, Kaufman JD, et al. Obstructive sleep apnea and subclinical interstitial lung disease in the Multi-Ethnic Study of Atherosclerosis (MESA). Ann Am Thorac Soc. 2017;14(12):1786–95.

118. Mermigkis C, Chapman J, Golish J, Mermigkis D, Budur K, Kopanakis A, et al. Sleep-related breathing disorders in patients with idiopathic pulmonary fibrosis. Lung. 2007;185(3):173–8.

119. Mermigkis C, Stagaki E, Tryfon S, Schiza S, Amfilochiou A, Polychronopoulos V, et al. How common is sleep-disordered breathing in patients with idiopathic pulmonary fibrosis? Sleep Breath. 2010;14(4):387–90.

120. Pascual N, Jurado B, Rubio JM, Santos F, Lama R, Cosano A. Respiratory disorders and quality of sleep in patients on the waiting list for lung transplantation. Transplant Proc. 2005;37(3):1537–9.

121. Pihtili A, Bingol Z, Kiyan E, Cuhadaroglu C, Issever H, Gulbaran Z. Obstructive sleep apnea is common in patients with interstitial lung disease. Sleep Breath. 2013;17(4):1281–8.

122. Bingol Z, Pihtili A, Gulbaran Z, Kiyan E. Relationship between parenchymal involvement and obstructive sleep apnea in subjects with sarcoidosis. Clin Respir J. 2015;9(1):14–21.

123. Gille T, Didier M, Boubaya M, Moya L, Sutton A, Carton Z, et al. Obstructive sleep apnoea and related comorbidities in incident idiopathic pulmonary fibrosis. Eur Respir J. 2017;49(6).

124. Lancaster LH, Mason WR, Parnell JA, Rice TW, Loyd JE, Milstone AP, et al. Obstructive sleep apnea is common in idiopathic pulmonary fibrosis. Chest. 2009;136(3):772–8.

125. Myall KJ, West A, Kent BD. Sleep and interstitial lung disease. Curr Opin Pulm Med. 2019;25(6):623–8.

126. Mermigkis C, Bouloukaki I, Schiza SE. Sleep as a new target for improving outcomes in idiopathic pulmonary fibrosis. Chest. 2017;152(6):1327–38.

127. Pillai M, Olson AL, Huie TJ, Solomon JJ, Fernandez-Perez ER, Brown KK, et al. Obstructive sleep apnea does not promote esophageal reflux in fibrosing interstitial lung disease. Respir Med. 2012;106(7):1033–9.

128. Bosi M, Milioli G, Fanfulla F, Tomassetti S, Ryu JH, Parrino L, et al. OSA and prolonged oxygen desaturation during sleep are strong predictors of poor outcome in IPF. Lung. 2017;195(5):643–51.

129. Mavroudi M, Papakosta D, Kontakiotis T, Domvri K, Kalamaras G, Zarogoulidou V, et al. Sleep disorders and health-related quality of life in patients with interstitial lung disease. Sleep Breath. 2018;22(2):393–400.

130. Visca D, Mori L, Tsipouri V, Fleming S, Firouzi A, Bonini M, et al. Effect of ambulatory oxygen on quality of life for patients with fibrotic lung disease (AmbOx): a prospective, open-label, mixed-method, crossover randomised controlled trial. Lancet Respir Med. 2018;6(10):759–70.

131. Mermigkis C, Bouloukaki I, Antoniou K, Papadogiannis G, Giannarakis I, Varouchakis G, et al. Obstructive sleep apnea should be treated in patients with idiopathic pulmonary fibrosis. Sleep Breath. 2015;19(1):385–91.

132. Mermigkis C, Bouloukaki I, Antoniou KM, Mermigkis D, Psathakis K, Giannarakis I, et al. CPAP therapy in patients with idiopathic pulmonary fibrosis and obstructive sleep apnea: does it offer a better quality of life and sleep? Sleep Breath. 2013;17(4):1137–43.

133. Mermigkis C, Bouloukaki I, Mermigkis D, Kallergis E, Mavroudi E, Varouchakis G, et al. CRP evolution pattern in CPAP-treated obstructive sleep apnea patients. Does gender play a role? Sleep Breath. 2012;16(3):813–9.

134. Mermigkis C, Mermigkis D, Varouchakis G, Schiza S. CPAP treatment in patients with idiopathic pulmonary fibrosis and obstructive sleep apnea–therapeutic difficulties and dilemmas. Sleep Breath. 2012;16(1):1–3.

15 Obesity Hypoventilation Syndrome

Amanda Piper

The term "Pickwick Syndrome" entered the medical vocabulary in the middle of the last century when the first clinical descriptions of patients presenting with obesity, hypersomnolence, and daytime hypercapnia were published (1, 2). This syndrome is now more commonly referred to as obesity hypoventilation syndrome (OHS). It is defined by the presence of awake hypercapnia ($PaCO_2$ >45 mm Hg) in obese individuals (body mass index [BMI] >30 kg m^{-2}) with sleep-disordered breathing when other disorders such as neuromuscular or lung disease which would better explain the development of hypoventilation have been excluded. Over the past two decades, significant advances in our understanding of the mechanisms, treatment, and outcomes of this disorder have occurred (3, 4).

MECHANISMS

Respiratory abnormalities associated with OHS are related to changes in pulmonary function, sleep-disordered breathing, and altered respiratory control (Figure 15.1). Although obesity is the most obvious feature of OHS, a purely mechanical constraint to breathing is insufficient to explain the emergence of awake hypoventilation that occurs in some obese individuals and not others. Rather, differences in the magnitude of abnormality in each of these three mechanisms and the complex interaction between them likely determine whether or not an individual with obesity is able to compensate adequately for the loads placed on their respiratory system by excess weight. The relative contribution of each of these mechanisms to hypoventilation will also impact on how effective a specific mode of positive airway pressure, the first-line therapy for this condition, is likely to be for a particular individual.

Obesity-Associated Changes in Pulmonary Mechanics

Lung volumes (in particular functional residual capacity and expiratory reserve volume) as well as respiratory system compliance are reduced as a consequence of morbid obesity (5, 6). At the same time, breathing at lower lung volumes promotes small airway closure and increases airway resistance (7), placing a ventilatory load on breathing (8). These alterations in pulmonary mechanics are more marked in OHS compared to those with eucapnic obesity (5, 9), and contribute to the increased work of

breathing seen, which can be two-fold higher in OHS compared to normal controls (10).

While the load on breathing is increased, capacity to cope with this load is reduced, with inspiratory muscle performance impaired in the face of severe obesity or OHS (11–13). This may be related to breathing at low lung volumes or to mechanical overstretching of the diaphragm created by increased abdominal mass. Adopting a supine position for sleep exacerbates the problem by further splinting of the diaphragm, limiting inspiratory excursion (9) or from the development of intrinsic positive end-expiratory pressure (PEEP) (8). Structural changes in the respiratory muscles related to obesity may also occur. In a mouse model of obesity, a chronic high-fat diet altered diaphragm structure with progressive intradiaphragmatic adiposity and fibrosis, resulting in impaired motion *in vivo* and contraction *ex vivo* (14). Although there are no systematic studies of diaphragm morphology in humans with OHS, one study of autopsy findings has reported marked fat infiltration of the respiratory musculature in a patient with OHS (15).

To reduce the high work of breathing, individuals with morbid obesity alter their respiratory pattern to one characterized by a higher breathing frequency and lower tidal volumes (16). This pattern is more marked in those with OHS than in eucapnic obesity (17). Although this may assist in reducing the oxygen cost of breathing while maintaining high overall minute ventilation, such a pattern also increases dead space ventilation and eventually becomes disadvantageous as it worsens gas exchange, favoring a rise in CO_2. The increased basal metabolic rate associated with obesity results in an increased CO_2 production. At the same time, small airway closure arising from reduced lung volumes serves to worsen ventilation-perfusion matching, resulting in more pronounced hypoxemia in OHS compared to eucapnic obesity. These factors all contribute to the increased $PaCO_2$ and reduced PaO_2 characteristic of OHS.

Given the above mechanisms and the observation that OHS prevalence increases as BMI rises (18), it is easy to view OHS simply as a disorder of excess weight, arising from the high mechanical load on the respiratory system producing reduced tidal volumes and

DOI: 10.1201/9781003000631-18

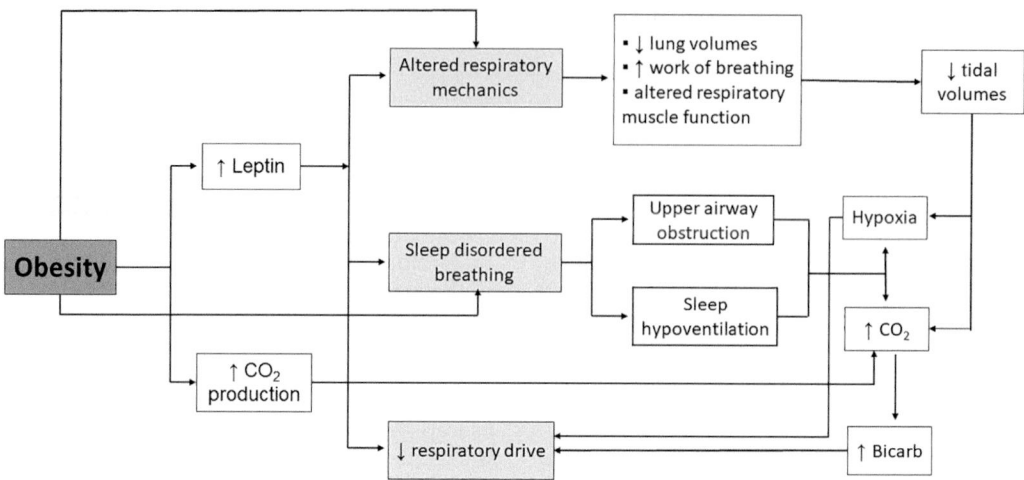

Figure 15.1 Schematic illustrating how the complex interactions between altered respiratory mechanics, respiratory drive, and sleep-disordered breathing could produce hypercapnia in some individuals with obesity.

consequent alveolar hypoventilation in parallel with increased CO_2 production, resulting in hypercapnia during wakefulness and sleep. However, not all morbidly obese individuals develop daytime hypoventilation, even those in the super-obese weight ranges (19), suggesting that other factors must be present for awake hypercapnia to emerge.

Sleep-Disordered Breathing

Hypoventilation during sleep is universal in OHS. In around 10% of individuals, this will be due purely to reduced inspiratory efforts and resultant low tidal volumes, most marked in REM sleep. However, the majority of individuals will demonstrate concomitant upper airway obstruction, with this being severe in nature in around 70% of cases (i.e. apnea-hypopnea index >30/hr) (20). The high prevalence of obstructive sleep apnea (OSA) in this disorder is not surprising.

Excess fat deposition in the pharyngeal tissue in conjunction with reduced lung volumes from central obesity would decrease inspiratory-related caudal traction of the trachea (21), predisposing these individuals to an increased likelihood of upper airway collapse. Even awake, upper airway resistance is higher in OHS individuals both seated and in a supine position compared to eucapnic OSA individuals (22). Nevertheless, the presence of obstructed sleep breathing alone is insufficient to explain the development of daytime hypercapnia, suggesting there must be some impairment in the compensatory response to acute CO_2 loading that occurs in the presence

of upper airway obstruction in OHS since most individuals with OSA maintain eucapnia. Studies measuring breath-by-breath whole body CO_2 balance during sleep have shown that both the duration of the obstructive period relative to the ventilatory recovery period (23) as well as the magnitude of recovery ventilation (24) are key in determining the degree to which CO_2 is eliminated following obstructed breathing. A shortened interapnea duration relative to the apneic period, in concert with a reduced ventilatory response for a given CO_2 load during the interapnea period would reduce the ability of the individual to sufficiently "blow off" the excess CO_2 accumulated during periods of obstructed breathing. This would permit the gradual accumulation of CO_2 overnight (3). In turn, this would trigger a small but elevated rise in serum bicarbonate concentration, which if not eliminated before the next sleep period, would begin to diminish the ventilatory responsiveness to CO_2 (HCVR) (25, 26). Over time, hypoventilation occurring during sleep would spill over into wakefulness as serum bicarbonate rose. This proposal is supported by elevated daytime bicarbonate levels seen in OHS patients (27), including those with early-stage disease without daytime CO_2 retention (28, 29).

In a prospective observational study, Manuel and colleagues (28) showed that a raised bicarbonate, even in the absence of awake hypercapnia, could represent "early OHS." Seventy-one stable obese subjects without significant lung or neuromuscular disease not currently on positive airway pressure therapy were categorized into three groups. Those with normal blood gas and acid-base balance, those with a raised BE (≥2 mmol/L) but normal awake CO_2 or those with awake hypercapnia (>45 mm Hg). All underwent overnight sleep studies and ventilatory response testing. Those individuals with an isolated raised BE generally demonstrated sleep and ventilatory response measurements that fell between the eucapnic obese and conventionally defined OHS groups.

Individuals with OHS also experience a higher hypoxic burden that those with eucapnic OSA, which could also contribute to the development of awake hypercapnia (18, 30). In healthy nonobese individuals, sustained hypoxia delays arousal from sleep in response to external loading (31). This could provide a further mechanism by which periods of abnormal breathing during sleep could be prolonged, thereby further permitting higher levels of CO_2 retention during sleep. It is possible that severe hypoxia could interfere with the synthesis of important neurotransmitters involved in central respiratory drive and chemoresponsiveness (32, 33).

Recent *in vitro* studies by Kikuchi *et al.* (34) have suggested the potential for a positive feedback loop whereby sleep-disordered breathing associated with hypoventilation and hypercapnia could increase adipogenesis and consequently weight gain, in turn further impairing lung mechanics and worsening sleep-disordered breathing and nocturnal gas exchange. These authors took human visceral and subcutaneous preadipocytes and induced them to differentiate into adipocytes under hypocapnic, normocapnic, and hypercapnic conditions, with and without hypoxia. They found that these preadipocytes underwent adipogenesis faster when cultured in high levels of CO_2, independent of extracellular acidosis, oxygen concentration, or whether the exposure to CO_2 was intermittent or sustained. In this way, a vicious spiral of increasing weight worsening nocturnal gas exchange which further promotes weight gain could be set up.

Alterations in Ventilatory Control

In order to compensate for increased respiratory loads, alterations in lung mechanics and increased CO_2 production associated with excess weight (8, 16, 35), an increase in neural drive occurs in the morbidly obese that is 2–3 fold higher than that seen in normal-weight individuals (8). This helps in maintaining eucapnia. Further increases in neural drive are seen when these obese individuals adopt a supine position (8). In OHS, this augmented drive is absent, and hence the ability to maintain eucapnia is lost (36, 37). In contrast to eucapnic OSA, where ventilatory responses to O_2 and CO_2 are normal or augmented (38–40), these responses are diminished in OHS (41–43). A correlation between the percentage of REM sleep spent in hypoventilation and the baseline CO_2 sensitivity has been demonstrated (41). Measuring airway occlusion pressure ($P_{0.1}$) during a modified hypercapnic rebreathing test in 36 subjects with newly diagnosed OHS, Fernandez Alvarez and colleagues (44) found that 23 (63%) exhibited a $P_{0.1}$/ $pEtCO_2$ response that was below that of a reference value obtained from age-adjusted controls. Repeat testing after 6 months of non-invasive ventilation (NIV) demonstrated that in a third of patients (n = 12) suboptimal respiratory responsiveness persisted. Apart from a lower baseline AHI in those with a suboptimal response, no other differences in baseline respiratory characteristics, adherence to NIV or gas exchange response to NIV was seen between the two groups. Similarly, in 15 stable patients with OHS studied by Chouri-Pontarollo and colleagues (41), seven had a low HCVR, while in the remaining eight, the HCVR was in the normal range at baseline. While ventilatory responses were increased by 47% in the group of low responders following NIV, the mean value remained close to the lower limit for normal values with only two of the seven showing a return of HCVR into the normal range. Furthermore, patients with lower responses to CO_2 were the sleepiest and had more significant improvements in objective daytime vigilance following NIV. Whether these differences represent potential different phenotypic traits in OHS or simply reflect the severity of the disorder is not known.

Although a genetic basis for ventilatory responsiveness exists, there is no evidence that this is the cause of the reduced chemoresponsiveness seen in OHS (45, 46), since treatment of sleep-disordered breathing in OHS produces improvement in ventilatory responsiveness to both CO_2 and O_2, albeit limited in some individuals (41, 42). Similarly, it has been known for some time weight loss in OHS reduces daytime $PaCO_2$ and improves chemosensitivity to CO_2 (13, 47). However, the relationship between obesity and sleep-disordered breathing and their relative influence on blunted chemosensitivity has not been fully elucidated.

Leptin as a Link between Mechanisms Associated with Hypoventilation in Obesity

Leptin is a peptide secreted by adipose tissue involved in the regulation of metabolism and satiety. (48) It also acts as a respiratory stimulant, involved in regulating central and peripheral structures that control breathing. Hence, increasing interest has been directed toward leptin as a link between obesity, hypoventilation, reduced lung volumes, and diminished respiratory control in OHS. However, much of the current data regarding leptin and its effects on breathing have come from rodent studies, using either leptin-deficient mice or diet-induced obesity models.

Leptin deficiency in ob/ob mice results in obesity, diminished ventilatory responsiveness to CO_2, and raised levels of CO_2.(49, 50) This respiratory depression is exacerbated with sleep, especially REM sleep. Leptin receptors are also expressed in lung tissue (51), with alterations in the mechanical properties of the lung observed in adult leptin-deficient mice compared with wild-type mice (52). This includes significantly lower lung volumes for a given airway pressure and changes in diaphragm composition, which would favor resistance to fatigue (52). Although human obesity is characterized by resistance to the effects of leptin rather than a deficiency, hyperleptinemia has been implicated in a number of respiratory disorders including reduced lung function, chronic obstructive pulmonary disease, and asthma (53, 54). While associations between leptin levels and lung volumes have not been specifically studied in OHS, the alterations in lung volumes and respiratory system compliance seen in this population (5, 35) are consistent with those reported in the murine model of OHS (52). Leptin replacement in these mice can reverse or at least significantly improve these respiratory abnormalities, in the absence of altering food intake, weight, or CO_2 production (49, 52).

Diet-induced and leptin-deficient obesity also promote sleep-disordered breathing in the mouse model. Using lean and obese wild-type and leptin-deficient mice, Polotsky and colleagues (55) found that both obesity and leptin deficiency were associated with a more collapsible upper airway. Furthermore, compared with the wild-type mice, those with leptin deficiency showed a higher frequency and severity of inspiratory flow limitation (IFL) along with elevations in the nasal pressure threshold at IFL onset, suggesting blunted neuromuscular responses to airway obstruction. Compared to non-REM sleep, marked IFL during REM sleep has also been shown in leptin-deficient mice (56). Leptin replacement reduces this IFL during wakefulness (55) and sleep (56). Hence, it appears that obesity and leptin

deficiency produce defects in upper airway neuromechanical control, with leptin mitigating upper airway mechanical loads by stimulating compensatory neuromuscular responses. The increase in ventilation seen with leptin replacement suggests leptin provides a generalized increase in ventilatory drive to both the upper airway muscles and the diaphragm during sleep (55, 56).

The role of leptin in regulating upper airway neuromuscular control in obese human subjects during sleep has been less well studied. Shapiro and colleagues (57) investigated the relationship between leptin and control of upper airway patency during sleep in 26 morbidly obese subjects (BMI 40–50 kg m^{-2}), 23 of whom were female. They found a significant association between upper airway neuromuscular responses and circulating leptin concentration in these obese women during sleep, independent of measures of adiposity, severity of sleep-disordered breathing, pharyngeal collapsibility, or ventilation.

Although the above findings link leptin with obesity, reduced ventilatory responsiveness to CO_2 and sleep-disordered breathing, in humans, obesity and OSA are associated with increased levels of serum leptin rather than a deficiency (58). High levels of circulating leptin would have a protective effect on ventilation by increasing respiratory drive in response to the high ventilatory loads, thereby allowing eucapnia to be maintained (59). The higher serum leptin levels seen in OHS patients compared to eucapnic obese individuals suggests the stimulatory effects of leptin have become attenuated (59). Makinodan et al. (60) found that despite similar levels of serum leptin, HCVR was significantly lower in hypercapnic OSA patients compared with those who maintained eucapnia. Likewise, in a study of morbidly obese individuals (mean BMI >40 kg m^{-2}), hyperleptinemia was associated with a reduction in respiratory drive and ventilatory responsiveness to CO_2 (61). This suggests the high circulating serum leptin levels in OHS reflects a state of leptin resistance, with reduced permeability of leptin across the blood-brain barrier likely playing a major role (58, 62). In diet-induced obese (DIO) mice, delivery of leptin intranasally to bypass the blood-brain barrier significantly reduced obstructed breathing during sleep acutely, resulting in a reduction in oxygen desaturation events in REM sleep and increasing minute ventilation during flow limited breathing (63). Leptin receptor signaling in the hypothalamic and medullary centers was augmented, indicating successful bypass of the blood-brain barrier. In contrast, administration of intraperitoneal leptin did not alter breathing and had no impact on leptin receptor signaling. How this translates to humans and whether awake breathing could also be improved awaits further studies.

While most studies have investigated the role of leptin in the control of breathing in terms of its influence on central nervous system structures, leptin receptors are also expressed peripherally in the carotid bodies (64). In rodent models, leptin has been shown to act in the carotid body to augment ventilation and the hypoxic ventilatory responses (65, 66). However, high-fat diet-fed rats demonstrate a blunting of the effect of leptin on respiratory responsiveness to hypoxia. Again, given the difference in receptors, cell types, and ventilatory responses between rodents and humans, how these findings pertain to humans remains unclear.

A leptin-dependent mechanism may also underlie improvements in ventilation and sleep-disordered breathing seen following bariatric surgery. Arble et al. (67) performed vertical sleeve gastrectomy in two murine models comprising DIO wild-type mice and obese, leptin-deficient *ob/ob* mice, measuring ventilation and HCVR prior to and 3 weeks following surgery. Improved chemosensitivity and reduced leptin levels were seen in the DIO wild-type mice, independent of body and fat mass. In contrast, no improvement in HCVR was seen in the leptin-deficient *ob/ob* mice despite significant reductions in body mass, fat mass, and improvements in glucose metabolism. However, the HCVR of *ob/ob* mice could be restored to levels similar to wild-type mice with leptin treatment, even before significant loss of body or fat mass. These findings led the authors to speculate that vertical sleeve gastrectomy improved chemosensitivity and ventilatory drive through a leptin-dependent mechanism rather than through weight loss alone.

In humans (57, 68) as well as wild-type mice (69), serum and cerebrospinal fluid (62) leptin levels are significantly higher in females than in males. Polotsky et al. (69) examined the interaction of gender and obesity on ventilatory control during wakefulness and sleep in male and female mice, comparing wild-type normal weight, diet-induced, and leptin-deficient groups. As expected, HCVR was depressed in both male and female leptin-deficient mice, with the female group demonstrating more severe depression than the weight-matched males in all sleep stages. This difference could not be attributed to differences in sex hormones. Furthermore, in normal weight

and obese wild-type groups, HCVR was similar between weight-matched female and male groups. Consequently, it appears that the development of obesity with leptin resistance would place females at a higher risk of experiencing more significant respiratory depression compared to males despite similar serum leptin levels or BMI. In clinical studies, it has been shown that women are more likely to present with isolated REM hypoventilation (70, 71), be more hypoxic and hypercapnic prior to initiating home therapy (72), and have a higher risk of cardiovascular morbidity (73).

SUMMARY

Obesity hypoventilation is characterized by obesity, reduced lung volumes, increased CO_2 production, and sleep-disordered breathing. Unlike obese individuals who can maintain daytime eucapnia, those with OHS fail to respond appropriately to the added ventilatory loads imposed by obesity. In contrast to simple obesity, those with OHS fail to augment neural drive to increase ventilation and demonstrate blunted ventilatory responsiveness to O_2 and CO_2. Work in murine models of leptin-deficiency and diet-induced obesity have shown the importance of leptin in stimulating ventilation in obesity as well as its role in protecting against sleep-disordered breathing. Hyperleptinemia in OHS likely represents a state of leptin resistance where the stimulatory effects of leptin on respiratory control are lost. This resistance to the respiratory effects of leptin in OHS would link the three major mechanisms underlying this disorder, namely obesity, sleep-disordered breathing, and altered respiratory control.

REFERENCES

1. Auchincloss JH, Jr., Cook E, Renzetti AD. Clinical and physiological aspects of a case of obesity, polycythemia and alveolar hypoventilation. J Clin Invest. 1955;34(10):1537–45.

2. Burwell CS, Robin ED, Whaley RD, Bickelmann AG. Extreme obesity associated with alveolar hypoventilation; a Pickwickian syndrome. Am J Med. 1956;21(5):811–8.

3. Berger KI, Goldring RM, Rapoport DM. Obesity hypoventilation syndrome. Semin Respir Crit Care Med. 2009;30:25361.

4. Masa JF, Pepin JL, Borel JC, Mokhlesi B, Murphy PB, Sanchez-Quiroga MA. Obesity hypoventilation syndrome. Eur Respir Rev. 2019;28(151):180097.

5. Naimark A, Cherniack RM. Compliance of the respiratory system and its components in health and obesity. J Appl Physiol. 1960;15:37782.

6. Pelosi P, Croci M, Ravagnan I, Vicardi P, Gattinoni L. Total respiratory system, lung, and chest wall mechanics in sedated-paralyzed postoperative morbidly obese patients. Chest. 1996;109(1):144–51.

7. Zerah F, Harf A, Perlemuter L, Lorino H, Lorino AM, Atlan G. Effects of obesity on respiratory resistance. Chest. 1993;103(5):1470–6.

8. Steier J, Jolley CJ, Seymour J, Roughton M, Polkey MI, Moxham J. Neural respiratory drive in obesity. Thorax. 2009;64(8):719–25.

9. Sharp JT, Henry JP, Sweany SK, Meadows WR, Pietras RJ. The total work of breathing in normal and obese men. J Clin Invest. 1964;43(4):728–39.

10. Lee MY, Lin CC, Shen SY, Chiu CH, Liaw SF. Work of breathing in eucapnic and hypercapnic sleep apnea syndrome. Respiration. 2009;77(2):146–53.

11. Collet F, Mallart A, Bervar JF, Bautin N, Matran R, Pattou F, et al. Physiologic correlates of dyspnea in patients with morbid obesity. Int J Obes. 2006;31(4):700–6.

12. Monneret D, Borel JC, Pepin JL, Tamisier R, Arnol N, Levy P, et al. Pleiotropic role of IGF-I in obesity hypoventilation syndrome. Growth Horm IGF Res. 2010;20(2):127–33.

13. Rochester DF, Enson Y. Current concepts in the pathogenesis of the obesity-hypoventilation syndrome. Mechanical and circulatory factors. Am J Med. 1974;57(3):402–20.

14. Buras ED, Converso-Baran K, Davis CS, Akama T, Hikage F, Michele DE, et al. Fibro-adipogenic remodeling of the diaphragm in obesity-associated respiratory dysfunction. Diabetes. 2019;68(1):45–56.

15. Fadell EJ, Richman AD, Ward WW, Hendon JR. Fatty infiltration of respiratory muscles in the Pickwickian syndrome. N Engl J Med. 1962;266:8613.

16. Chlif M, Keochkerian D, Choquet D, Vaidie A, Ahmaidi S. Effects of obesity on breathing pattern, ventilatory neural drive and mechanics. Respir Physiol Neurobiol. 2009;168(3):198–202.

17. Pankow W, Hijjeh N, Schuttler F, Penzel T, Becker H, Peter J, et al. Influence of noninvasive positive pressure ventilation on inspiratory muscle activity in obese subjects. Eur Respir J. 1997;10(12):2847–52.

18. Kaw R, Hernandez AV, Walker E, Aboussouan L, Mokhlesi B. Determinants of hypercapnia in obese patients with obstructive sleep apnea: a systematic review and metaanalysis of cohort studies. Chest. 2009;136(3):787–96.

19. Sivam S, Yee B, Wong K, Wang D, Grunstein R, Piper A. Obesity hypoventilation syndrome: early detection of nocturnal-only hypercapnia in an obese population. J Clin Sleep Med. 2018;14(9):1477–84.

20. Masa JF, Corral J, Alonso ML, Ordax E, Troncoso MF, Gonzalez M, et al. Efficacy of different treatment alternatives for obesity hypoventilation syndrome. Pickwick Study. Am Respir Crit Care Med. 2015;192(1):86–95.

21. Van de Graaff WB. Thoracic influence on upper airway patency. J Appl Physiol. 1988;65(5):2124–31.

22. Lin CC, Wu KM, Chou CS, Liaw SF. Oral airway resistance during wakefulness in eucapnic and hypercapnic sleep apnea syndrome. Respir Physiol Neurobiol. 2004;139(2):215–24.

23. Ayappa I, Berger KI, Norman RG, Oppenheimer BW, Rapoport DM, Goldring RM. Hypercapnia and ventilatory periodicity in obstructive sleep apnea syndrome. Am J Respir Crit Care Med. 2002;166(8):1112–5.

24. Berger KI, Ayappa I, Sorkin IB, Norman RG, Rapoport DM, Goldring RM. Postevent ventilation as a function of CO(2) load during respiratory events in obstructive sleep apnea. J Appl Physiol. 2002;93(3):917–24.

25. Goldring RM, Turino GM, Heinemann HO. Respiratory-renal adjustments in chronic hypercapnia in man. Extracellular bicarbonate concentration and the regulation of ventilation. Am J Med. 1971;51(6):772–84.

26. Norman RG, Goldring RM, Clain JM, Oppenheimer BW, Charney AN, Rapoport DM, et al. Transition from acute to chronic hypercapnia in patients with periodic breathing: predictions from a computer model. J Appl Physiol. 2006;100(5):1733–41.

27. Mokhlesi B, Tulaimat A, Faibussowitsch I, Wang Y, Evans A. Obesity hypoventilation syndrome: prevalence and predictors in patients with obstructive sleep apnea. Sleep Breath. 2007;11(2):117–24.

28. Manuel ARGM, Mbbs RG, Hart NP, Stradling JRMD. Is a raised bicarbonate, without hypercapnia, part of the physiologic spectrum of obesity-related hypoventilation? Chest. 2015;147(2):362–8.

29. Randerath W, Verbraecken J, Andreas S, Arzt M, Bloch KE, Brack T, et al. Definition, discrimination, diagnosis and treatment of central breathing disturbances during sleep. Eur Respir J. 2017;49(1):1600959.

30. Banerjee D, Yee BJ, Piper AJ, Zwillich CW, Grunstein RR. Obesity hypoventilation syndrome: hypoxemia during continuous positive airway pressure. Chest. 2007;131(6):1678–84.

31. Hlavac MC, Catcheside PG, McDonald R, Eckert DJ, Windler S, McEvoy RD. Hypoxia impairs the arousal response to external resistive loading and airway occlusion during sleep. Sleep. 2006;29(5):624–31.

32. Lee S-D, Nakano H, Farkas GA. Adenosinergic modulation of ventilation in obese Zucker rats. Obes Res. 2005;13(3):545–55.

33. Yang AL, Lo MJ, Ting H, Chen JS, Huang CY, Lee SD. GABA(A) and GABA(B) receptors differentially modulate volume and frequency in ventilatory compensation in obese Zucker rats. J Appl Physiol. 2007;102(1):350–7.

34. Kikuchi R, Tsuji T, Watanabe O, Yamaguchi K, Furukawa K, Nakamura H, et al. Hypercapnia accelerates adipogenesis: a novel role of high CO_2 in exacerbating obesity. Am J Respir Cell Mol Biol. 2017;57(5):570–80.

35. Sampson MG, Grassino AE. Load compensation in obese patients during quiet tidal breathing. J Appl Physiol. 1983;55(4):1269–76.

36. Lopata M, Onal E. Mass loading, sleep apnea, and the pathogenesis of obesity hypoventilation. Am Rev Respir Dis. 1982;126(4):640–5.

37. Sampson MG, Grassino K. Neuromechanical properties in obese patients during carbon dioxide rebreathing. Am J Med. 1983;75(1):81–90.

38. Han F, Chen E, Wei H, He Q, Ding D, Strohl KP. Treatment effects on carbon dioxide retention in patients with obstructive sleep apnea-hypopnea syndrome. Chest. 2001;119(6):1814–9.

39. Verbraecken J, De Backer W, Willemen M, De Cock W, Wittesaele W, Van de H. Chronic CO_2 drive in patients with obstructive sleep apnea and effect of CPAP. Respir Physiol. 1995;101(3):279–87.

40. Wang D, Grunstein R, Teichtahl H. Association between ventilatory response to hypercapnia and obstructive sleep apnea–hypopnea index in asymptomatic subjects. Sleep Breath. 2007;11(2):103–8.

41. Chouri-Pontarollo N, Borel JC, Tamisier R, Wuyam B, Levy P, Pepin JL. Impaired objective daytime vigilance in obesity-hypoventilation syndrome: impact of noninvasive ventilation. Chest. 2007;131(1):148–55.

42. Lin CC. Effect of nasal CPAP on ventilatory drive in normocapnic and hypercapnic patients with obstructive sleep apnoea syndrome. Eur Respir J. 1994;7(11):2005–10.

43. Zwillich CW, Sutton FD, Pierson DJ, Greagh EM, Weil JV. Decreased hypoxic ventilatory drive in the obesity-hypoventilation syndrome. Am J Med. 1975;59(3):343–8.

44. Fernandez Alvarez R, Rubinos Cuadrado G, Ruiz Alvarez I, Hermida Valverde T, Iscar Urrutia M, Vazquez Lopez MJ, et al. Hypercapnia response in patients with obesity-hypoventilation syndrome treated with non-invasive ventilation at home. Arch Bronconeumol. 2018;54(9):455–9.

45. Javaheri S, Colangelo G, Corser B, Zahedpour MR. Familial respiratory chemosensitivity does not predict hypercapnia of patients with sleep apnea-hypopnea syndrome. Am Rev Respir Dis. 1992;145(4 Pt 1):837–40.

46. Jokic R, Zintel T, Sridhar G, Gallagher CG, Fitzpatrick MF. Ventilatory responses to hypercapnia and hypoxia in relatives of patients with the obesity hypoventilation syndrome. Thorax. 2000;55(11):940–5.

47. Sugerman HJ, Fairman RP, Sood RK, Engle K, Wolfe L, Kellum JM. Long-term effects of gastric surgery for treating respiratory insufficiency of obesity. Am J Clin Nutr. 1992;55(2 Suppl):597S–601S.

48. Friedman JM. Leptin and the endocrine control of energy balance. Nat Metab. 2019;1(8):754–64.

49. O'Donnell CP, Schaub CD, Haines AS, Berkowitz DE, Tankersley CG, Schwartz AR, et al. Leptin prevents respiratory depression in obesity. Am J Respir Crit Care Med. 1999;159(5 Pt 1):1477–84.

50. Tankersley C, Kleeberger S, Russ B, Schwartz A, Smith P. Modified control of breathing in genetically obese (ob/ob) mice. J Appl Physiol. 1996;81(2):716–23.

51. Bruno A, Pace E, Chanez P, Gras D, Vachier I, Chiappara G, et al. Leptin and leptin receptor expression in asthma. J Allergy Clin Immunol. 2009;124(2):230–7, 7 e1–e4.

52. Tankersley CG, O'Donnell C, Daood MJ, Watchko JF, Mitzner W, Schwartz A, et al. Leptin attenuates respiratory complications associated with the obese phenotype. J Appl Physiol. 1998;85(6):2261–9.

53. Sin DD, Man SF. Impaired lung function and serum leptin in men and women with normal body weight: a population based study. Thorax. 2003;58(8):695–8.

54. Sood A, Ford ES, Camargo CA, Jr. Association between leptin and asthma in adults. Thorax. 2006;61(4):300–5.

55. Polotsky M, Elsayed-Ahmed AS, Pichard L, Harris CC, Smith PL, Schneider H, et al. Effects of leptin and obesity on the upper airway function. J Appl Physiol. 2012;112(10):1637–43.

56. Pho H, Hernandez AB, Arias RS, Leitner EB, Van Kooten S, Kirkness JP, et al. The effect of leptin replacement on sleep-disordered breathing in the leptin-deficient ob/ob mouse. J Appl Physiol. 2016;120(1):78–86.

57. Shapiro SD, Chin CH, Kirkness JP, McGinley BM, Patil SP, Polotsky VY, et al. Leptin and the control of pharyngeal patency during sleep in severe obesity. J Appl Physiol. 2014;116(10):1334–41.

58. Caro JF, Sinha MK, Kolaczynski JW, Zhang PL, Considine RV. Leptin: the tale of an obesity gene. Diabetes. 1996;45(11):1455–62.

59. Phipps PR, Starritt E, Caterson I, Grunstein RR. Association of serum leptin with hypoventilation in human obesity. Thorax. 2002;57(1):75–6.

60. Makinodan K, Yoshikawa M, Fukuoka A, Tamaki S, Koyama N, Yamauchi M, et al. Effect of serum leptin levels on hypercapnic ventilatory response in obstructive sleep apnea. Respiration. 2008;75(3):257–64.

61. Campo A, Fruhbeck G, Zulueta JJ, Iriarte J, Seijo LM, Alcaide AB, et al. Hyperleptinemia, respiratory drive and hypercapnic response in obese patients. Eur Respir J. 2007;30:22331.

62. Schwartz MW, Peskind E, Raskind M, Boyko EJ, Porte D, Jr. Cerebrospinal fluid leptin levels: relationship to plasma levels and to adiposity in humans. Nat Med. 1996;2(5):589–93.

63. Berger S, Pho H, Fleury-Curado T, Bevans-Fonti S, Younas H, Shin MK, et al. Intranasal leptin relieves sleep disordered breathing in mice with diet induced obesity. Am J Respir Crit Care Med. 2019;199(6):773–83.

64. Porzionato A, Rucinski M, Macchi V, Stecco C, Castagliuolo I, Malendowicz LK, et al. Expression of leptin and leptin receptor isoforms in the rat and human carotid body. Brain Res. 2011;1385:5667.

65. Caballero-Eraso C, Shin MK, Pho H, Kim LJ, Pichard LE, Wu ZJ, et al. Leptin acts in the carotid bodies to increase minute ventilation during wakefulness and sleep and augment the hypoxic ventilatory response. J Physiol. 2019;597(1):151–72.

66. Ribeiro MJ, Sacramento JF, Gallego-Martin T, Olea E, Melo BF, Guarino MP, et al. High fat diet blunts the effects of leptin on ventilation and on carotid body activity. J Physiol. 2018;596(15):3187–99.

67. Arble DM, Schwartz AR, Polotsky VY, Sandoval DA, Seeley RJ. Vertical sleeve gastrectomy improves ventilatory drive through a leptin-dependent mechanism. JCI Insight. 2019;4(1): e124469. doi:10.1172/jci.insight.124469

68. Kennedy A, Gettys TW, Watson P, Wallace P, Ganaway E, Pan Q, et al. The metabolic significance of leptin in humans: gender-based differences in relationship to adiposity, insulin sensitivity, and energy expenditure. J Clin Endocrinol Metab. 1997;82(4):1293–300.

69. Polotsky VY, Wilson JA, Smaldone MC, Haines AS, Hurn PD, Tankersley CG, et al. Female gender exacerbates respiratory depression in leptin-deficient obesity. Am J Respir Crit Care Med. 2001;164(8 Pt 1):1470–5.

70. Masa JF, Corral J, Caballero C, Barrot E, Teran-Santos J, Alonso-Alvarez ML, et al. Non-invasive ventilation in obesity hypoventilation syndrome without severe obstructive sleep apnoea. Thorax. 2016;71(10):899–906.

71. Ojeda Castillejo E, de Lucas Ramos P, Lopez Martin S, Resano Barrios P, Rodriguez Rodriguez P, Moran Caicedo L, et al. Noninvasive mechanical ventilation in patients with obesity hypoventilation syndrome. Long-term outcome and prognostic factors. Arch Bronconeumol. 2015;51(2):61–8.

72. Palm A, Midgren B, Janson C, Lindberg E. Gender differences in patients starting long-term home mechanical ventilation due to obesity hypoventilation syndrome. Respir Med. 2016;110:738.

73. Masa JF, Corral J, Romero A, Caballero C, Teran-Santos J, Alonso-Alvarez ML, et al. Protective cardiovascular effect of sleep apnea severity in obesity hypoventilation syndrome. Chest. 2016;150(1):68–79.

SECTION IV

PATHOPHYSIOLOGY-DIRECTED THERAPIES FOR SLEEP-DISORDERED BREATHING

16 Effect of Positive Airway Pressure on Ventilatory Control and Sleep-Disordered Breathing

James A Rowley

INTRODUCTION

Obstructive sleep apnea-hypopnea syndrome (OSAHS) is a common medical disorder (1, 2) characterized by recurrent episodes of either complete (apnea) or partial (hypopnea) upper airway collapse and obstruction during sleep. These episodes of obstruction are associated with recurrent oxyhemoglobin desaturations and arousals from sleep. OSAHS is associated with significant clinical sequelae including excessive daytime sleepiness, decreased quality of life (3), metabolic and inflammatory abnormalities (4–7), and cardiovascular morbidity and mortality (8–12). Positive airway pressure (PAP) therapy is the mainstay of therapy for moderate to severe OSAHS (13). PAP therapy works primarily by mechanically splinting the upper airway, preventing the soft tissues from collapsing. By this mechanism, PAP effectively eliminates apneas and hypopneas, decreases recurrent arousals, and normalizes oxygen saturation. Evolving evidence suggests that PAP treatment leads to improvement in the sequelae of OSAHS. Specifically, most studies have shown that PAP treatment improves daytime sleepiness and quality of life (13). While studies are mixed on the effect of PAP treatment on blood pressure and hypertension (14–16), a recent meta-analysis did show significant reductions in both systolic and diastolic blood pressure as well as daytime and 24-hour blood pressure (13). In observational studies, patients using PAP therapy were found to have improved survival compared to patients not wearing PAP therapy (9, 17, 18). However, in several large-scale randomized trials investigating the impact of PAP therapy on clinical cardiovascular disease, PAP therapy has not been shown to be effective in preventing heart disease and mortality (19–21).

One of the known sequelae of PAP therapy on patients with OSA is treatment-emergent central sleep apnea (TE-CSA), frequently referred to as "complex sleep apnea." TE-CSA is a form of sleep-disordered breathing in which central breathing events emerge after the resolution of obstructive events on PAP therapy (22). First described in 2005 (23), the prevalence of TE-CSA has since been estimated at 4% to 19% of OSA patients receiving PAP therapy (24–26) and may possibly be higher in patients taking opioids and/or have congestive heart failure (22). Studies have not shown

clear clinical factors that identify patients who develop this syndrome (22, 26) though having severe OSA at baseline may be predictive (25) as may male gender (26) or older age (27). Other risk factors for central sleep apnea, such as congestive heart failure or opioid use, have not been consistently found to be associated with TE-CSA (25, 26). Patients with TE-CSA are more likely to abandon continuous positive airway pressure (CPAP) therapy compared to patients who did not develop TE-CSA (27).

Subsequent studies have shown that many patients with TE-CSA may have resolution of the central events with continued use of CPAP therapy. Javaheri et al. found that 84 of 1,286 patients developed a central apnea index >5/hr while on CPAP therapy (25). Forty-two of these patients had a repeat study and of these, 33 no longer had CSA on the second study. Nine patients with persistent CSA were in general less adherent to PAP therapy (approximate use 1 hr less per night). In a study comparing different modalities of positive pressure treatment for TE-CSA, Morgenthaler et al. found that 64.5% of the patient assigned to CPAP therapy had resolution of the CSA at 90 days (28). Finally, Liu et al. using a large tele-monitoring database looked for the presence of emergent CSA at weeks 1 and 13 of treatment with CPAP (27). At both time points, 3.5% of the patients had CSA with 55% of the patients who had CSA at week 1 showing no CSA at week 13. However, it should be noted that studies have also shown the emergence of TE-CSA after treatment of PAP. For instance, in the Liu study above, 912 (19.7%) patients were identified who had no CSA at week 1 of treatment but had CSA at week 13. Wessel et al. studied a group of 436 patients with OSA treated with CPAP at 3 months follow-up (29). While the majority (74%) of the 54 patients with TE-CSA had resolution at 3 months, they too found that a small minority (7.9%) of the patients without TE-CSA on initial titration had evidence of CSA at 3 months follow-up.

DOES CPAP ALTER VENTILATORY CONTROL ABNORMALITIES IN PATIENTS WITH OSA?

The fact that central sleep apnea can emerge upon PAP treatment in patients with obstructive sleep apnea indicates that central mechanisms of breathing control during sleep

DOI: 10.1201/9781003000631-20

are important in the pathogenesis of OSA. In other words, while OSA is believed to primarily be an upper airway/structural syndrome, in actuality, instability of the ventilatory control system has an important role as well. Evidence for this statement comes from many sources of research. One manifestation is the persistence of periodic breathing and repetitive central apnea following "curative" tracheotomy in patients with OSA (30). Other evidence includes the response to hypercapnia administered in the pseudorandom binary stimulation test (31), and the finding, using proportional-assist ventilation, that the patients with severe OSA have a higher magnitude of chemical control system instability than patients with milder OSA (32). In addition, several lines of evidence suggest a mechanistic interaction between obstructive and central sleep apnea. Multiple studies demonstrate that oscillating ventilatory motor output during periodic breathing is associated with reciprocal changes in upper airway resistance (33, 34); complete upper airway obstruction occurs in individuals with unfavorable upper airway anatomy. Similarly, upper airway narrowing or occlusion occurs during central apnea or hypopnea (35, 36). Finally, there has been significant research showing that patients with OSA have different endotypes, with some showing high airway collapsibility with others showing either high loop gain or arousal threshold (37).

Ventilatory control can be assessed using differing methodologies, many of which are more fully discussed in this book. This section will explore whether there are differences in measurements of ventilatory control and chemoresponsiveness in OSA patients compared to control and whether there are changes in these measurements with the use of CPAP. This section will discuss ventilatory responses to hypoxia and hypercapnia as well as loop gain and its elements, controller, and plant gain.

Ventilatory Responses to Hypercapnia and Hypoxia

It has been postulated that an increased chemoresponsiveness to CO_2 could lead to ventilatory overshoots, leading to reductions in $PaCO_2$ below the level required to stimulate breathing (during sleep, the apneic threshold) and to recruit upper airway dilator muscles. Hence, multiple groups have studied the hypercapnic ventilatory response (HCVR) in subjects with OSA in comparison to control subjects. The majority of these studies have been performed during wakefulness. In one of the earlier studies, Verbraecken et al. found that

in normocapnic OSA subjects, the HCVR was increased compared to control subjects, while in hypercapnic OSA subjects, it was decreased. The subjects in this study were not matched prior to analysis but the groups were similar in age and BMI (38). In contrast, other groups have found no difference in HCVR. In a large cohort study, Sin et al. studied HCVR in 104 subjects with OSA and 115 subjects without OSA and found no difference in HCVR between the two groups (39). Important factors correlating with HCVR were age and daytime PCO_2 in men and BMI in women. In smaller research studies, both Narkiewicz et al. (40) and Foster et al. (41) studied subjects with and without OSA that were matched for both age and BMI. Both groups found no difference in HCVR. It is important to note that both studies included control subjects with obesity as it has also been shown that obesity itself may be associated with increased HCVR in both adults (42) and adolescents (43). Thus, the lack of difference in the Narkiewicz and Foster studies may be related to the control subjects having similar BMI to the OSA subjects. Finally, it should be noted that in one study that specifically studied the ventilatory response to CO_2 during sleep, there was evidence of a blunted ventilatory response to CO_2 in obese adolescents with obesity compared to obese adolescents without OSA (43). Further studies during sleep need to be performed to determine if there is a blunted HCVR during sleep in patients with OSA and whether this is an effect of obesity or OSA.

The effect of CPAP on hypercapnic chemoresponsiveness has been investigated by different groups, with most showing no effect of short-term CPAP on HCVR. Both Verbraecken et al. (38) and Spicuzza et al. (44) studied 15 subjects before and after use of CPAP for 1 month. Neither found any change in HCVR with the use of CPAP. Adherence to CPAP was not reported in either study. Note that Spicuzza et al.'s study did not include control subjects, so unclear if the HCVR was elevated in the OSA subjects. Foster et al. studied the effects of 4 weeks of CPAP on HCVR; average use was about 5 hours per night (41). There was no change in the HCVR with CPAP despite the reasonable adherence during the study. However, it should be noted that in a subsequent study by the Verbracken group, the use of CPAP for 1 year did result in a decrease in HCVR (45).

Hypoxic ventilatory response (HVR) has also been studied. In the aforementioned study by Narkiweicz et al., the group also studied the response to hypoxia in 12 subjects with OSA compared to controls matched for age and BMI (40).

The OSA subjects showed a heightened response to hypoxia compared to controls. In Spicuzza et al.'s study, the response to hypoxia was also studied after 1 month of CPAP use (44). They found that the slope of the HVR was reduced in the group of subjects treated with CPAP for 1 month; the group that received sham CPAP had no change in HVR.

Finally, one group has investigated the effect of CPAP on a brief hypercapnic hypoxic stimulus. In previous work, Younes et al. found that a combination of hypercapnia and hypoxia led to a large increase in ventilatory response in patients with OSA under an experimental condition of brief decreases in CPAP from holding pressure (46). Note that in this study, control subjects were not studied. In a subsequent study, around 12 patients had this dynamic response re-tested after using CPAP for 1 month. The authors found a significant decrease in the magnitude of the response to mixed hypercapnia-hypoxia after CPAP use (47). It should be noted that compliance was noted as "excellent" but hours or days of use were not reported.

The changes in hypoxic sensitivity above is consistent with other data in animals and humans that acute intermittent hypoxia enhances hypoxic sensitivity (48–50). It has been theorized that the acute intermittent hypoxia causes neuroplastic changes leading to increased hypoxic sensitivity (51). Normalization of hypoxia (return to normoxia) in these intermittent hypoxia models leads to return of hypoxic sensitivity to baseline values, confirming that the neuroplasticity is reversible (52, 53). In contrast, intermittent hypoxia is not associated with changes in hypercapnic sensitivity (54).

In summary, the hypercapnic response to hypercapnia has not been consistently found to be different between subjects with and without OSA and the limited data indicates that CPAP may alter HCVR after 1 year but not after a shorter period of time. In contrast, limited data indicates that the response to hypoxia may be more consistently higher in OSA subjects with evidence that CPAP can reduce the response.

Loop Gain

Loop gain is an engineering concept used as a framework to express the overall ventilatory change for a given initial perturbation. This concept and its relationship to OSA pathogenesis is discussed in Chapter 8. In brief, the overall loop gain of the ventilatory system reflects the ratio of the ventilatory response to the disturbance that provoked the response. In general, a loop gain >1 indicates that the ventilatory response is disproportionately larger than the disturbance. Higher loop gain reflects less stable ventilatory control (51). From an engineering standpoint, loop gain is composed of two components, controller gain and plant gain. Controller gain reflects the sensitivity of the chemoreceptors and is generally measured as the slope of the ventilatory response (as measured by minute ventilation) to increasing PCO_2. Plant gain reflects the effectiveness of the lungs to alter blood gases and is measured as a function of the hyperbolic relationship between alveolar ventilation and arterial PCO_2.

Early studies of loop gain indicated that loop gain was higher in patients with more severe OSA (32, 55). However, these early studies did not include control groups of subjects without sleep-disordered breathing. Subsequent studies have included control groups but have come to differing conclusions. For instance, Hudgel et al. compared loop gain between 9 subjects with OSA and 16 subjects without OSA; groups were not matched for gender, age, or BMI. Subjects with OSA were found to have a larger loop gain in this study. Based upon the responses, the authors concluded that the increased loop gain was due to increases in plant gain, not controller gain (31). Using a similar methodology, Deacon-Diaz et al. studied eight males with severe OSA with a control group of seven, height, weight, and age-matched controls and found a higher loop gain in the OSA subjects when measured during the daytime (56). However, despite the increased loop gain, neither controller gain or plant gain were increased in this study.

In contrast, Eckert et al. studied 58 subjects with overall moderate to severe OSA and compared them to 17 patients without OSA; the groups were not matched for age or BMI (37). Overall they found no difference in loop gain during the daytime between the two groups. Finally, Sands et al. compared loop gain between three groups during sleep: overweight subjects with moderate to severe OSA and without OSA and normal-weight subjects without OSA (57). The overweight groups were matched for BMI, age, and sex. This group found no difference in loop gain between the overweight OSA and non-OSA subjects with both groups having a higher loop gain than the normal-weight controls. This study suggests that obesity may be an underlying factor for higher loop gain (presumably through an increased plant gain that has been seen associated with obesity (51, 58)). However, the role of obesity in influencing loop gain is not clear. Bokov et al. compared loop, plant, and controller gain between three groups of women: obese women with and without moderate OSA and lean women without OSA. There was no difference in loop gain between the three groups. While a higher plant gain was found in the obese women with OSA compared to obese women without OSA, there was no difference in plant gain between the obese women without OSA and the lean women.

Differences in methodologies for measuring loop gain may explain the differing findings. Both the Hudgel and Deacon-Diaz groups measured loop gain during wakefulness and using the pseudorandom binary CO_2 stimulation test. In contrast, the Eckert and Sands studies measured loop gain during sleep, using the ventilatory response to drops in CPAP (a methodology that does not allow differentiation of plant and controller gain). It should also be noted that while several studies have shown no difference in loop gain between groups, these studies do show subsets of subjects with higher loop gain that may explain their propensity to have OSA. For instance, in the Eckert study, subjects with a less collapsible airway had overall higher loop gain (37).

Another reason for the difference in results may be the effect of CPAP. In both the Eckert (37) and Sands (57) studies discussed in the previous paragraph, the subjects with OSA had been consistent users of CPAP for >3 months at the time of enrollment in the study. In contrast, in the Deacon-Diaz study (56), the eight males with OSA were all CPAP naïve. Thus, the contrasting results could indicate that there is higher loop gain in OSA patients that is attenuated with the regular use of CPAP. However, the Deacon-Diaz study is the only study that has studied the effect of CPAP on loop gain. In this study, the effects of CPAP were studied after 2 and 6 weeks of use. Adherence was measured during the 6 week interval and showed decline though subjects were still using CPAP about 60% of nights for more than 4 hours at 6 weeks. However, despite the consistent use of CPAP, there was no change in loop gain with CPAP use. Given that the other studies included CPAP use >3 months, however, it is still not totally clear if CPAP use would change loop gain over a longer period of use.

There has been one study that specifically studied the effect of CPAP on controller gain in OSA patients vs. control subjects. Salloum et al. studied 11 pairs of subjects with and without OSA that were matched for gender, age, and BMI (59). In this study, hypocapnia was induced via nasal mechanical ventilation,

allowing measurement of the apneic threshold, CO_2 reserve, and controller gain. The authors found no difference in the apneic threshold but did find a smaller CO_2 reserve in the OSA patients associated with an increase in the controller gain. Seven subjects were restudied after 1 month of use of CPAP; average daily use was 3.8 hours. With CPAP, CO_2 reserve increased and the controller gain decreased.

In summary, studies with different subject recruitment, different methodologies, differing CPAP use for the OSA groups, and control groups that may or may not be matched, do not show a consistent increase in loop gain between subjects with and without moderate-severe OSA. Also, the one study that showed a clear increase in loop gain between subjects with OSA and matched control subjects, there was no decrease in loop gain with CPAP use. However, another group did find an improvement in controller gain with the use of CPAP. Thus, it is not clear if the loop gain is higher at baseline in subjects with OSA and whether CPAP leads to more ventilatory stability over time.

SUMMARY

There are several lines of evidence that while obstructive sleep apnea is primarily related to obstruction of the upper airway, changes in the control of breathing are also important determinants of the propensity for airway collapse during sleep. However, the literature investigating differences in common measures of control of breathing between subjects with and without sleep apnea is sparse, dependent upon small numbers of subjects, and often conflicting. Other reasons for making it difficult to interpret the literature include subject selection, including whether patients are CPAP naïve when studied and not controlling well for the effects of obesity. Methodological differences are also important; these include including different methods to measure control of breathing and whether the study is performed during wakefulness or sleep.

There is a clear need for further research on the effects of CPAP on measures of ventilatory control. These studies will need to (1) better select subjects and control for differences in age, gender, body mass index, and prior CPAP use; (2) study control of breathing primarily during sleep, which is the most relevant sleep state for sleep-disordered breathing; (3) better understand how different methodologies used may or may not be measuring the same parameters so that comparisons between studies are possible.

ACKNOWLEDGMENT

At the time of this publication, Dr Rowley is a member of the board of directors of the American Academy of Sleep Medicine. The views expressed are his own and do not necessarily represent the views of the American Academy of Sleep Medicine.

REFERENCES

1. Young T, Palta M, Dempsey J, Skatrud J, Weber S, Badr S. The occurrence of sleep-disordered breathing among middle-aged adults. N Engl J Med. 1993;328(17):1230–5.

2. Peppard PE, Young T, Barnet JH, Palta M, Hagen EW, Hla KM. Increased prevalence of sleep-disordered breathing in adults. Am J Epidemiol. 2013;177(9):1006–14.

3. Weaver TE, Laizner AM, Evans LK, Maislin G, Chugh DK, Lyon K, et al. An instrument to measure functional status outcomes for disorders of excessive sleepiness. Sleep. 1997;20(10):835–43.

4. Punjabi NM, Shahar E, Redline S, Gottlieb DJ, Givelber R, Resnick HE. Sleep-disordered breathing, glucose intolerance, and insulin resistance: the Sleep Heart Health Study. Am J Epidemiol. 2004;160(6):521–30.

5. McArdle N, Hillman D, Beilin L, Watts G. Metabolic risk factors for vascular disease in obstructive sleep apnea: a matched controlled study. Am J Respir Crit Care Med. 2007;175(2):190–5.

6. Geovanini GR, Wang R, Weng J, Jenny NS, Shea S, Allison M, et al. Association between obstructive sleep apnea and cardiovascular risk factors: variation by age, sex, and race. The multi-ethnic study of atherosclerosis. Ann Am Thorac Soc. 2018;15(8):970–7.

7. Geovanini GR, Wang R, Weng J, Tracy R, Jenny NS, Goldberger AL, et al. Elevations in neutrophils with obstructive sleep apnea: the Multi-Ethnic Study of Atherosclerosis (MESA). Int J Cardiol. 2018;257:318–23.

8. Punjabi NM, Caffo BS, Goodwin JL, Gottlieb DJ, Newman AB, O'Connor GT, et al. Sleep-disordered breathing and mortality: a prospective cohort study. PLoS Med. 2009;6(8):e1000132.

9. Marin JM, Carrizo SJ, Vicente E, Agusti AG. Long-term cardiovascular outcomes in men with obstructive sleep apnoea-hypopnoea with or without treatment with continuous positive airway pressure: an observational study. Lancet. 2005;365(9464):1046–53.

10. Butler MP, Emch JT, Rueschman M, Sands SA, Shea SA, Wellman A, et al. Apnea-hypopnea event duration predicts mortality in men and women in the Sleep Heart Health Study. Am J Respir Crit Care Med. 2019;199(7):903–12.

11. Roca GQ, Redline S, Claggett B, Bello N, Ballantyne CM, Solomon SD, et al. Sex-specific association of sleep apnea severity with subclinical myocardial injury, ventricular hypertrophy, and heart failure risk in a community-dwelling cohort: the atherosclerosis risk in communities—Sleep Heart Health Study. Circulation. 2015;132(14):1329–37.

12. Gottlieb DJ, Yenokyan G, Newman AB, O'Connor GT, Punjabi NM, Quan SF, et al. Prospective study of obstructive sleep apnea and incident coronary heart disease and heart failure: the sleep heart health study. Circulation. 2010;122(4):352–60.

13. Patil SP, Ayappa IA, Caples SM, Kimoff RJ, Patel SR, Harrod CG. Treatment of adult obstructive sleep apnea with positive airway pressure: an American Academy of Sleep Medicine systematic review, meta-analysis, and GRADE assessment. J Clin Sleep Med. 2019;15(2):301–34.

14. Barbe F, Duran-Cantolla J, Capote F, de la Pena M, Chiner E, Masa JF, et al. Long-term effect of continuous positive airway pressure in hypertensive patients with sleep apnea. Am J Respir Crit Care Med. 2010;181(7):718–26.

15. Pedrosa RP, Drager LF, de Paula LKG, Amaro ACS, Bortolotto LA, Lorenzi-Filho G. Effects of OSA treatment on BP in patients with resistant hypertension: a randomized trial. Chest. 2013;144(5):1487–94.

16. Martinez-Garcia MA, Capote F, Campos-Rodriguez F, Lloberes P, Diaz de Atauri MJ, Somoza M, et al. Effect of CPAP on blood pressure in patients with obstructive sleep apnea and resistant hypertension: the HIPARCO randomized clinical trial. JAMA. 2013;310(22):2407–15.

17. Campos-Rodriguez F, Martinez-Garcia MA, de la Cruz-Moron I, Almeida-Gonzalez C, Catalan-Serra P, Montserrat JM. Cardiovascular mortality in women with obstructive sleep apnea with or without continuous positive airway pressure treatment: a cohort study. Ann Intern Med. 2012;156(2):115–22.

18. Campos-Rodriguez F, Pena-Grinan N, Reyes-Nunez N, De la Cruz-Moron I, Perez-Ronchel J, De la Vega-Gallardo F, et al. Mortality in obstructive sleep apnea-hypopnea patients treated with positive airway pressure. Chest. 2005;128(2):624–33.

19. Barbe F, Duran-Cantolla J, Sanchez-de-la-Torre M, Martinez-Alonso M, Carmona C, Barcelo A, et al. Effect of continuous positive airway pressure on the incidence of hypertension and cardiovascular events in nonsleepy patients with obstructive sleep apnea: a randomized controlled trial. JAMA. 2012;307(20):2161–8.

20. Peker Y, Glantz H, Eulenburg C, Wegscheider K, Herlitz J, Thunstrom E. Effect of positive airway pressure on cardiovascular outcomes in coronary artery disease patients with nonsleepy obstructive sleep apnea. The RICCADSA randomized controlled trial. Am J Respir Crit Care Med. 2016;194(5):613–20.

21. McEvoy RD, Antic NA, Heeley E, Luo Y, Ou Q, Zhang X, et al. CPAP for prevention of cardiovascular events in obstructive sleep apnea. N Engl J Med. 2016;375(10):919–31.

22. Khan MT, Franco RA. Complex sleep apnea syndrome. Sleep Disord. 2014;2014:798487.

23. Gilmartin GS, Daly RW, Thomas RJ. Recognition and management of complex sleep-disordered breathing. Curr Opin Pulm Med. 2005;11(6):485–93.

24. Lehman S, Antic NA, Thompson C, Catcheside PG, Mercer J, McEvoy RD. Central sleep apnea on commencement of continuous positive airway pressure in patients with a primary diagnosis of obstructive sleep apnea-hypopnea. J Clin Sleep Med. 2007;3(5):462–6.

25. Javaheri S, Smith J, Chung E. The prevalence and natural history of complex sleep apnea. J Clin Sleep Med. 2009;5:205–11.

26. Morgenthaler TI, Kagramanov V, Hanak V, Decker PA. Complex sleep apnea syndrome: is it a unique clinical syndrome? Sleep. 2006;29(9):1203–9.

27. Liu D, Armitstead J, Benjafield A, Shao S, Malhotra A, Cistulli PA, et al. Trajectories of emergent central sleep apnea during CPAP therapy. Chest. 2017;152(4):751–60.

28. Morgenthaler TI, Kuzniar TJ, Wolfe LF, Willes L, McLain WC, 3rd, Goldberg R. The complex sleep apnea resolution study: a prospective randomized controlled trial of continuous positive airway pressure versus adaptive servoventilation therapy. Sleep. 2014;37(5):927–34.

29. Cassel W, Canisius S, Becker HF, Leistner S, Ploch T, Jerrentrup A, et al. A prospective polysomnographic study on the evolution of complex sleep apnoea. Eur Respir J. 2011;38(2):329–37.

30. Badr MS, Grossman JE, Weber SA. Treatment of refractory sleep apnea with supplemental carbon dioxide. Am J Respir Crit Care Med. 1994;150(2):561–4.

31. Hudgel DW, Gordon EA, Thanakitcharu S, Bruce EN. Instability of ventilatory control in patients with obstructive sleep apnea. Am J Respir Crit Care Med. 1998;158(4):1142–9.

32. Younes M, Ostrowski M, Thompson W, Leslie C, Shewchuk W. Chemical control stability in patients with obstructive sleep apnea. Am J Respir Crit Care Med. 2001;163(5):1181–90.

33. Hudgel DW, Chapman KR, Faulks C, Hendricks C. Changes in inspiratory muscle electrical activity and upper airway resistance during periodic breathing induced by hypoxia during sleep. Am Rev Respir Dis. 1987;135(4):899–906.

34. Badr MS, Kawak A, Skatrud JB, Morrell MJ, Zahn BR, Babcock MA. Effect of induced hypocapnic hypopnea on upper airway patency in humans during NREM sleep. Respir Physiol. 1997;110(1):33–45.

35. Badr MS, Toiber F, Skatrud JB, Dempsey J. Pharyngeal narrowing/occlusion during central sleep apnea. J Appl Physiol. 1995;78(5):1806–15.

36. Sankri-Tarbichi AG, Rowley JA, Badr MS. Expiratory pharyngeal narrowing during central hypocapnic hypopnea. Am J Respir Crit Care Med. 2009;179(4):313–9.

37. Eckert DJ, White DP, Jordan AS, Malhotra A, Wellman A. Defining phenotypic causes of obstructive sleep apnea. Identification of novel therapeutic targets. Am J Respir Crit Care Med. 2013;188(8):996–1004.

38. Verbraecken J, De Backer W, Willemen M, De Cock W, Wittesaele W, Van de H. Chronic CO_2 drive in patients with obstructive sleep apnea and effect of CPAP. Respir Physiol. 1995;101(3):279–87.

39. Sin DD, Jones RL, Man GC. Hypercapnic ventilatory response in patients with and without obstructive sleep apnea: do age, gender, obesity, and daytime PaCO(2) matter? Chest. 2000;117(2):454–9.

40. Narkiewicz K, van de Borne PJ, Pesek CA, Dyken ME, Montano N, Somers VK. Selective potentiation of peripheral chemoreflex sensitivity in obstructive sleep apnea. Circulation. 1999;99(9):1183–9.

41. Foster GE, Brugniaux JV, Pialoux V, Duggan CT, Hanly PJ, Ahmed SB, et al. Cardiovascular and cerebrovascular responses to acute hypoxia following exposure to intermittent hypoxia in healthy humans. J Physiol. 2009;587(Pt 13):3287–99.

42. Narkiewicz K, Kato M, Pesek CA, Somers VK. Human obesity is characterized by a selective potentiation of central chemoreflex sensitivity. Hypertension. 1999;33(5):1153–8.

43. Yuan H, Pinto SJ, Huang J, McDonough JM, Ward MB, Lee YN, et al. Ventilatory responses to hypercapnia during wakefulness and sleep in obese adolescents with and without obstructive sleep apnea syndrome. Sleep. 2012;35(9):1257–67.

44. Spicuzza L, Bernardi L, Balsamo R, Ciancio N, Polosa R, Di Maria G. Effect of treatment with nasal continuous positive airway pressure on ventilatory response to hypoxia and hypercapnia in patients with sleep apnea syndrome. Chest. 2006;130(3):774–9.

45. Verbraecken J, Willemen M, De Cock W, Wittesaele W, Govaert K, Van de HP, et al. Influence of longterm CPAP therapy on CO(2) drive in patients with obstructive sleep apnea. Respir Physiol. 2000;123(1–2):121–30.

46. Younes M, Ostrowski M, Atkar R, Laprairie J, Siemens A, Hanly P. Mechanisms of breathing instability in patients with obstructive sleep apnea. J Appl Physiol. 2007;103(6):1929–41.

47. Loewen A, Ostrowski M, Laprairie J, Atkar R, Gnitecki J, Hanly P, et al. Determinants of ventilatory instability in obstructive sleep apnea (OSA): inherent or acquired? Sleep. 2009; 32:1355–65.

48. Peng YJ, Overholt JL, Kline D, Kumar GK, Prabhakar NR. Induction of sensory long-term facilitation in the carotid body by intermittent hypoxia: implications for recurrent apneas. Proc Natl Acad Sci U S A. 2003;100(17):10073–8.

49. Harris DP, Balasubramaniam A, Badr MS, Mateika JH. Long-term facilitation of ventilation and genioglossus muscle activity is evident in the presence of elevated levels of carbon dioxide in awake humans. Am J Physiol Regul Integr Comp Physiol. 2006;291(4):R1111–R9.

50. Lee DS, Badr MS, Mateika JH. Progressive augmentation and ventilatory long-term facilitation are enhanced in sleep apnoea patients and are mitigated by antioxidant administration. J Physiol. 2009;587(Pt 22):5451–67.

51. Deacon-Diaz N, Malhotra A. Inherent vs. induced loop gain abnormalities in obstructive sleep apnea. Front Neurol. 2018;9:896.

52. Peng YJ, Prabhakar NR. Effect of two paradigms of chronic intermittent hypoxia on carotid body sensory activity. J Appl Physiol (1985). 2004;96(3):1236–42; discussion 196.

53. Pialoux V, Hanly PJ, Foster GE, Brugniaux JV, Beaudin AE, Hartmann SE, et al. Effects of exposure to intermittent hypoxia on oxidative stress and acute hypoxic ventilatory response in humans. Am J Respir Crit Care Med. 2009;180(10):1002–9.

54. Mateika JH, Mendello C, Obeid D, Badr MS. Peripheral chemoreflex responsiveness is increased at elevated levels of carbon dioxide after episodic hypoxia in awake humans. J Appl Physiol. 2004;96(3):1197–205.

55. Wellman A, Jordan AS, Malhotra A, Fogel RB, Katz ES, Schory K, et al. Ventilatory control and airway anatomy in obstructive sleep apnea. Am J Respir Crit Care Med. 2004;170(11):1225–32.

56. Deacon-Diaz NL, Sands SA, McEvoy RD, Catcheside PG. Daytime loop gain is elevated in obstructive sleep apnea but not reduced by CPAP treatment. J Appl Physiol (1985). 2018;125(5):1490–7.

57. Sands SA, Eckert DJ, Jordan AS, Edwards BA, Owens RL, Butler JP, et al. Enhanced upper-airway muscle responsiveness is a distinct feature of overweight/obese individuals without sleep apnea. Am J Respir Crit Care Med. 2014;190(8):930–7.

58. Bokov P, Essalhi M, Delclaux C. Loop gain in severely obese women with obstructive sleep apnoea. Respir Physiol Neurobiol. 2016;221:49–53.

59. Salloum A, Rowley JA, Mateika JH, Chowdhuri S, Omran Q, Badr MS. Increased propensity for central apnea in patients with obstructive sleep apnea: effect of nCPAP. Am J Respir Crit Care Med. 2009;181:189–93.

17 Mild Intermittent Hypoxia and Supplemental Oxygen
Potential Therapeutic Interventions to Treat Breathing Instability

Sreenavya Gandikota and Jason H Mateika

INTRODUCTION TO SLEEP-DISORDERED BREATHING

Obstructive sleep apnea is a disorder associated with persistent collapse or narrowing of the upper airway during sleep. Various risk factors are implicated in the pathogenesis of obstructive sleep apnea, including obesity (1), increased neck circumference (1), and sex (i.e. a greater occurrence in males compared to females) (2). Obstructive sleep apnea has been linked to several detrimental health outcomes including excessive daytime sleepiness, enhanced sympathetic nervous system activity, increased cardiovascular risk, and impaired cognition (1, 3, 4). There are at least four principal phenotypes that contribute to sleep apnea (i) increased collapsibility of the upper airway (obstructive sleep apnea), (ii) a blunted upper airway muscle response to adjustments in the partial pressure of carbon dioxide (obstructive sleep apnea), (iii) a low arousal threshold (central and obstructive sleep apnea), and (iv) instability of the ventilatory control system (i.e. increased loop gain) (central and obstructive sleep apnea) (1, 5, 6) (Figure 17.1).

Upper Airway Collapsibility and Responsiveness

The human upper airway is predominantly composed of muscle and soft tissues and is largely devoid of rigid, bony structures. As a result, the upper airway is susceptible to collapse from various anatomical or physiological perturbations. Individuals with a narrow upper airway, and/or increased tissue pressure around the upper airway due to fat deposits, have a greater likelihood of airway collapse compared to an airway with a larger diameter (7). The pressure at which the upper airway collapses is referred to as the critical closing pressure. A more positive critical closing pressure is associated with increased pharyngeal collapsibility (8).

Individuals with poor upper airway anatomy generally display increased upper airway dilator muscle activity as a compensatory mechanism to maintain upper airway patency during wakefulness (8). Upper airway dilator muscle tone decreases during the transition from wakefulness to sleep as a result of the loss of wakefulness drive (9). Despite this response, dilator muscle activity is greater during

deeper stages of non-rapid eye movement sleep (i.e. slow-wave sleep vs. N2) due to input from the central pattern generator, negative pressure reflex, and short-term potentiation (10, 11). However, patients with sleep apnea experience difficulty reaching deeper sleep levels due to arousals from hypopneas and apneas throughout the night (12). Thus, patients achieving slow-wave sleep may have important implications for mitigating sleep apnea severity.

Arousal Threshold

Arousal from sleep is often associated with the termination of breathing events (i.e. apnea or hypopnea) in patients with obstructive sleep apnea. Arousals play an essential role in the restoration of upper airway patency because they are accompanied by increased upper airway dilator muscle activity (13). Despite this important role, arousal from sleep in response to minor increases in ventilatory drive may occur in patients with a low arousal threshold. A low arousal threshold coupled to a high loop gain (see Loop Gain for details) leads to destabilized breathing and results in the perpetuation of apneic events (14). Thus, treatments to reduce the number of arousals by increasing the arousal threshold could improve sleep quality. Published findings have shown that airflow may be re-established without arousal, if a patient experiences an adequate sleep duration to allow respiratory stimuli (i.e. negative pressure and carbon dioxide) to activate upper airway dilatory muscles (15). Thus, therapies to modify the arousal threshold could play a significant role in mitigating sleep-disordered breathing in patients with an inherent low arousal threshold (14).

Loop Gain

The stability of the ventilatory control system also plays a significant role in the pathophysiology of obstructive sleep apnea. An unstable ventilatory control system results in fluctuations in ventilatory drive, ultimately leading to an unstable upper airway and airway collapse (1, 16, 17). Ventilatory stability is quantified using an engineering concept referred to as loop gain. Loop gain is comprised of controller gain and plant gain and is a measure of the response of the ventilatory control system to one or more inputs (e.g.

DOI: 10.1201/9781003000631-21

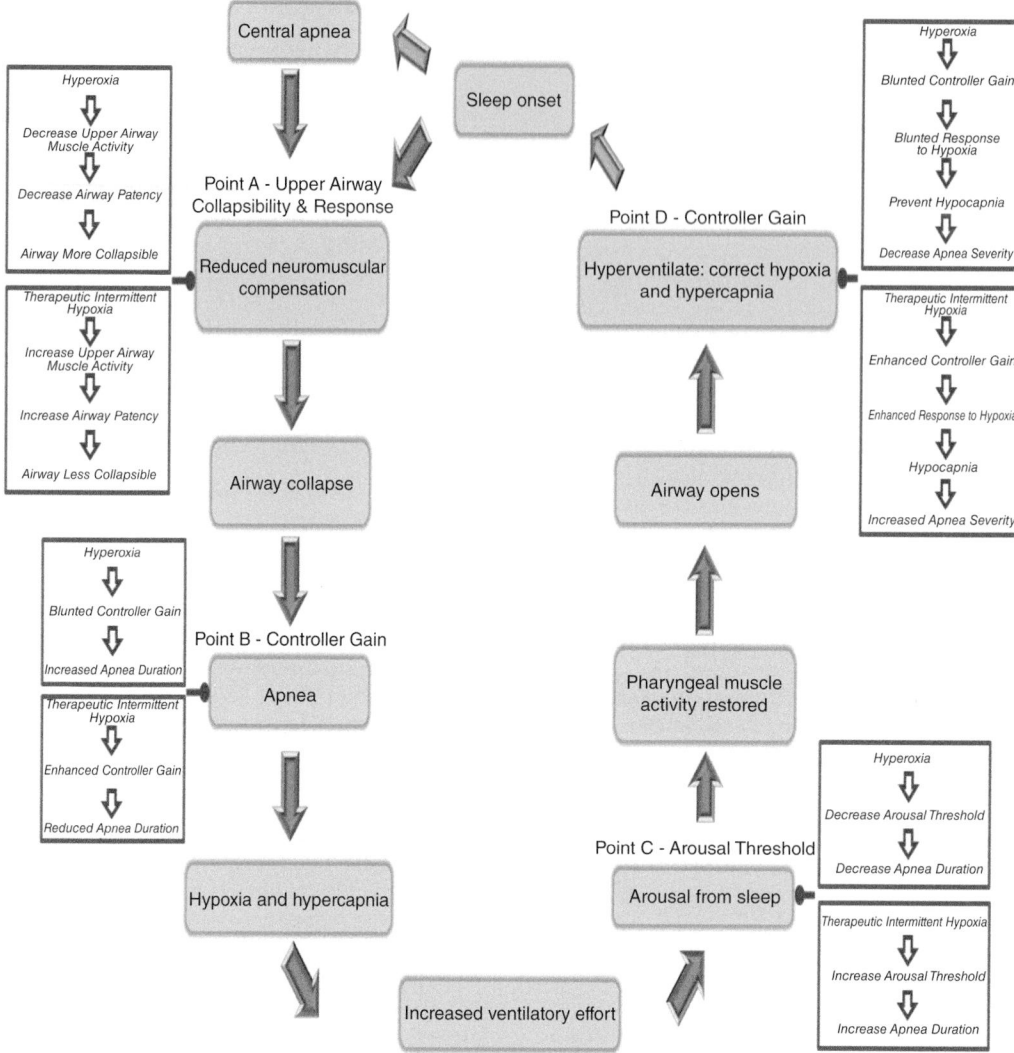

Figure 17.1 Schematic diagram showing the sequence of events leading to the development of a central and/or obstructive apnea, and subsequent events that re-establish patency of the upper airway. In addition, various points along the pathway (see Points A–D) are highlighted. The phenotypic mechanisms that contribute to sleep apnea (i.e. controller/loop gain, arousal threshold, upper airway collapsibility, and responsiveness) are shown at each point. In addition, the impact that therapeutic intermittent hypoxia and supplemental oxygen has on each phenotypic trait and the potential outcome is highlighted at each point (see boxes with blue outline and white fill). For example, administration of supplemental oxygen at point D would blunt controller gain, leading to a blunted ventilatory response hypoxia, thwarting the induction of hypocapnia and the development of an apnea.

hypoxia, hypercapnia) (1, 18). An unstable ventilatory control system is characterized by a loop gain value greater than one. Controller gain is altered by modifications in chemoreflex sensitivity (Figure 17.2) (19). The greater the ventilatory response to a given level of hypoxia or hypercapnia, the greater the controller gain. Measures of plant gain denote the efficiency of

the ventilatory system in the maintenance of homeostatic carbon dioxide levels. Typically, an equilibrium between the arterial partial pressure of carbon dioxide and ventilation is maintained. As the arterial partial pressure of carbon dioxide increases, an accompanying increase in ventilation is initiated by the peripheral and central chemoreceptors.

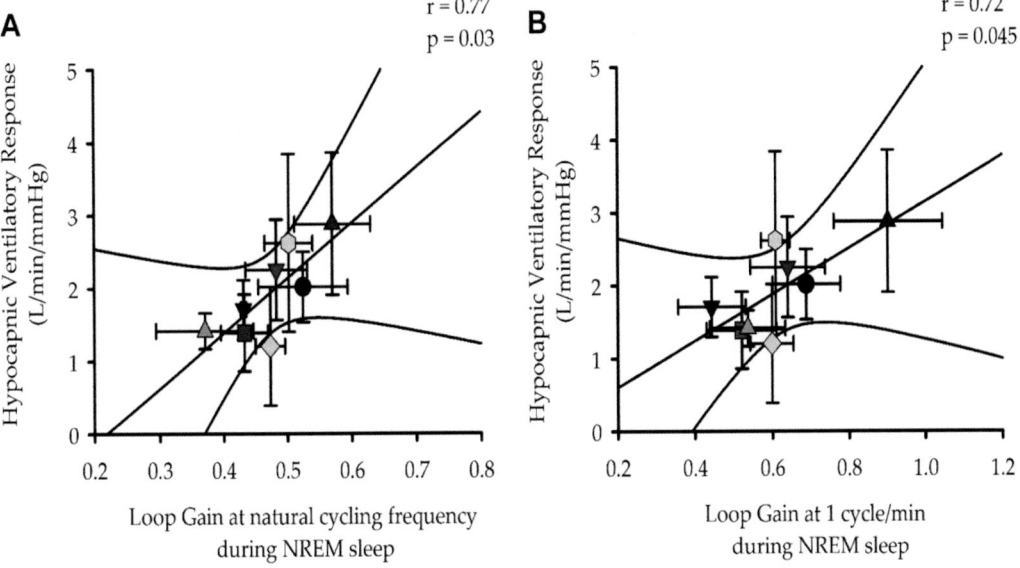

Figure 17.2 Scatterplots showing the relationship between loop gain at the natural cycling frequency and chemoreflex sensitivity (i.e. the hypocapnic ventilatory response) **(A)** and loop gain at 1 cycle/min and chemoreflex sensitivity **(B)** during non-rapid eye movement (NREM) sleep in the evening [10 PM (1)], morning (6 AM), and afternoon (2 PM). Each symbol and corresponding color represent a participant. Each data point represents the mean value ± standard deviation obtained from measures in the evening, morning, and afternoon. Note that in all cases, loop gain was correlated to measures of chemoreflex sensitivity. $n = 8$ participants. A Pearson correlation was used to examine the relationships. (Reprinted from "Variations in loop gain and arousal threshold during NREM sleep are affected by time of day over a 24-hr period in participants with obstructive sleep apnea" by S. Puri et al. J. Appl. Physiol. 129 (4), 800–809, 2020.)

Activation of the receptors returns the arterial partial pressure of carbon dioxide to a homeostatic equilibrium.

However, if the ventilatory response to increases in the partial pressure of carbon dioxide and decreases in oxygen induced by an apnea is inappropriately high, because of an increase in chemoreflex sensitivity, this will lead to a significant reduction in carbon dioxide below homeostatic levels (i.e. hypocapnia) (20) (Figure 17.1). The induction of hypocapnia during sleep will result in a central apneic event that is often coupled to an obstructive event (Figure 17.1). A number of these events will often present in a cyclical manner, because the hypoxia and hypercapnia induced by a given apneic event, coupled with an enhanced chemoreflex sensitivity, initiates hyperventilation and hypocapnia at the termination of the event (Figure 17.1).

While obstructive sleep apnea may be induced by a combination of phenotypic traits, central sleep apnea is frequently caused by an enhanced loop gain. Approximately fifty percent of patients with congestive heart failure experience central sleep apnea (21). Central sleep apnea in these patients is often accompanied by the waxing and waning of breathing known as Cheyne-Stokes respiration (21). An enhanced controller gain that leads to the induction of hypocapnia contributes to Cheyne-Stokes respiration. In addition, Cheyne-Stokes respiration is exacerbated by a delay in blood circulation that accompanies heart failure. Detection of changes in the partial pressure of oxygen and carbon dioxide by the peripheral and central chemoreceptors is typically delayed based on the time required for blood to circulate from the lungs to the location of the chemoreceptors. However, differences in systemic arterial partial pressure measurements of carbon dioxide and the partial pressure of carbon dioxide detected by the chemoreceptors are buffered. In contrast, a delay in circulation time in individuals with congestive heart failure augments the delay in peripheral chemoreceptor stimulation (22). As a result, the partial pressure of carbon dioxide at the site of chemoreceptors lags significantly relative to systemic arterial blood values, which further promotes cyclical breathing (23). Thus, the circulatory delay coupled to an enhanced controller gain contributes to ventilatory instability during sleep. Blunting of chemoreflex sensitivity, and concomitantly loop gain, could mitigate the cyclical breathing events in individuals with obstructive or central sleep apnea.

Based on the identification of the phenotypic traits outlined above, investigators have begun to explore novel therapeutic treatments that target these traits to mitigate the outcomes associated with the complex pathology of central and/or obstructive sleep apnea. This chapter explores the role that therapeutic intermittent hypoxia and hyperoxia have in targeting and mitigating the influence of those phenotypic traits known to exacerbate sleep apnea.

TREATMENT OF OBSTRUCTIVE SLEEP APNEA WITH THERAPEUTIC INTERMITTENT HYPOXIA

Respiratory Plasticity

Intermittent hypoxia is characterized by episodes of hypoxia that are interspersed with periods of normoxia (24) (Figure 17.3). Intermittent hypoxia can be induced experimentally or naturally in response to obstructive sleep apnea (24). Over the past 3–4 decades, exposure to intermittent hypoxia was predominantly linked to detrimental outcomes including hypertension, impaired metabolic and cognitive function (25, 26). The evidence for this viewpoint was initially derived from animal studies that employed protocols in which the dose and length of exposure were severe (25, 26). These findings were significant in the context of sleep apnea, since intermittent hypoxia is a hallmark of sleep-disordered breathing.

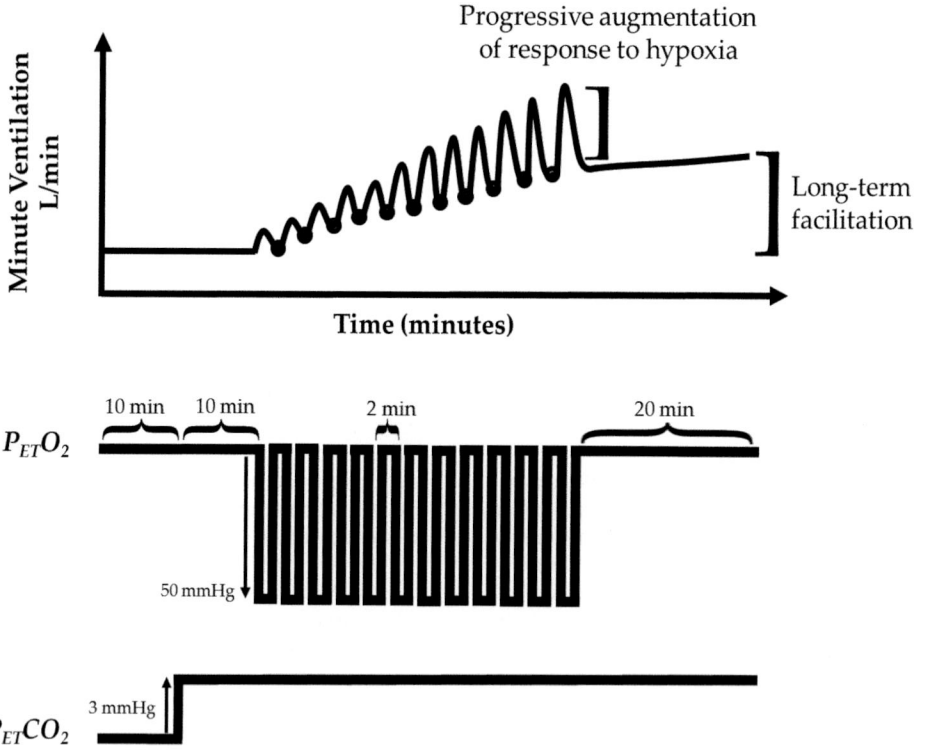

Figure 17.3 A schematic diagram showing two forms of respiratory plasticity (*top*) (i.e. progressive augmentation of the hypoxic ventilatory response and long-term facilitation) initiated during exposure to intermittent hypoxia. In this example, note that the minute ventilation response to hypoxia progressively increased from the initial to the final hypoxic episode. In addition, note that following exposure to intermittent hypoxia, the magnitude of minute ventilation was elevated and sustained above baseline levels. Also note some of the variables that must be considered when determining the appropriate dose of intermittent hypoxia (middle and bottom). These variables include the number of episodes, the duration of episodes, the intensity of hypoxia, and whether or not carbon dioxide levels will be sustained at or above baseline levels.

Within a similar time frame, published results indicated that milder forms of intermittent hypoxia initiated two forms of respiratory plasticity. One form of plasticity was deemed progressive augmentation of the hypoxic ventilatory response (27). Progressive augmentation is characterized by an incremental increase in the ventilatory response to hypoxia that is evident from the initial to the final episode of an intermittent hypoxia protocol (Figure 17.3). This progressive enhancement reflects increases in peripheral chemoreflex sensitivity and consequently is also a reflection of increases in controller and loop gain (see *Introduction* for details regarding controller and loop gain).

The other form of plasticity that was initially identified in animal models was referred to as long-term facilitation (27) (Figure 17.3). Long-term facilitation of ventilation or upper airway muscle activity is characterized by sustained increases in ventilation and upper airway muscle activity that persist long after the intermittent hypoxia stimulus is removed. Both forms of respiratory plasticity are unrelated to modifications in blood gases and are induced by neuromodulators (e.g. serotonin, norepinephrine) that activate a cascade of cellular events (28). The outcome of this activation is the enhancement of synaptic connections between bulbospinal respiratory neurons and motoneurons in the spinal cord (i.e. phrenic and intercostal), or medullary motoneurons that innervate upper airway muscles (29).

Following the discovery of these phenomena in animal models, they were also identified in humans. Progressive augmentation and/or long-term facilitation have been documented in healthy humans (30–36), humans with spinal cord injury (37, 38), and humans with obstructive sleep apnea (39–43). Long-term facilitation of ventilation and upper airway muscle activity only manifests in humans if carbon dioxide levels are maintained at or slightly above baseline levels (32). Moreover, the magnitude of long-term facilitation in humans (i) is similar in males and females (36, 43), (ii) is greater during wakefulness compared to sleep (43), (iii) is greater in individuals with obstructive sleep apnea (40), and (iv) is greater following daily repeated exposure to intermittent hypoxia (39).

The discovery that mild forms of intermittent hypoxia could initiate long-term facilitation of upper airway muscle activity in humans was exciting because activation of the phenomenon could potentially lead to increased airway

patency and the mitigation or elimination of apneic events (17).

Therapeutic Intermittent Hypoxia and Apneic Events

Based on the hypothesis stated above, studies were completed to determine if exposure to mild intermittent hypoxia would mitigate apneic events. In contrast to the hypothesis, findings showed that exposure to mild intermittent hypoxia during wakefulness immediately prior to sleep (44), or during sleep (43), generated an increase in the number of apneic events (43, 44). It was hypothesized that the initiation of progressive augmentation of the hypoxic ventilatory response was responsible for the increase in the number of events (17). The initiation of progressive augmentation resulted in an enhanced ventilatory response to hypoxia following arousal and termination of an apneic event (Figure 17.1). The result of the enhanced response is hypocapnia (see *Introduction* for further details), which induces a central and obstructive event once sleep is re-established (17) (Figure 17.1). Based on prior findings (32), it was proposed that apneic events were not mitigated by the initiation of long-term facilitation of upper airway muscle activity, primarily because oscillating levels of carbon dioxide led to unfavorable conditions (i.e. hypocapnia) for the manifestation of long-term facilitation.

Therapeutic Intermittent Hypoxia and Continuous Positive Airway Pressure

In order for long-term facilitation to effectively mitigate apneic events, carbon dioxide levels must be maintained at or above baseline levels for a given arousal state (i.e. wake vs. sleep) and outcomes (i.e. hypocapnia) linked to progressive augmentation effectively eliminated (26). To test this hypothesis, patients were treated with continuous positive airway pressure to mitigate the influence of progressive augmentation by eliminating apneic events (45). Once the therapeutic pressure was established, patients were treated with mild intermittent hypoxia while carbon dioxide levels were maintained 3 mm Hg above baseline (45). Following exposure to intermittent hypoxia, a 15 minute recovery period ensued (carbon dioxide levels were maintained 3 mm Hg above baseline during this time) followed by step-wise 1–2 cm H_2O decrements in continuous positive airway pressure (45). Measurements of airflow and upper airway resistance were obtained. The results were compared to control experiments in which patients were exposed to room air instead of intermittent hypoxia. Collectively, the findings showed that following exposure to intermittent hypoxia, therapeutic continuous positive airway pressure could be reduced substantially (i.e. 5–7 cm H_2O), while maintaining baseline levels of airflow and upper airway resistance (45). This was not the case when step-wise decreases in continuous positive airway pressure occurred following exposure to a sham protocol (i.e. room air) (45). We believe these findings, coupled to previous results (32), indicate that mild intermittent hypoxia initiated long-term facilitation of upper airway muscle activity leads to improved upper airway patency and reduced airway resistance (Figure 17.1).

Therapeutic Intermittent Hypoxia and Outcome Measures

This finding led to the proposal that mild intermittent hypoxia could be used as an adjunctive therapy with continuous positive airway pressure. We hypothesized that reductions in continuous positive airway pressure after exposure to intermittent hypoxia (45), coupled with findings which showed that sustained (46) and mild intermittent hypoxia (47) increases the arousal threshold (Figure 17.1), could serve to improve adherence with this treatment. Moreover, treatment with intermittent hypoxia, independent of continuous positive airway pressure, has elicited reductions in blood pressure (systolic and diastolic pressure), improved cognitive function (improved memory), and reversed metabolic abnormalities (high cholesterol, high low-density lipoprotein, low high-density lipoprotein, obesity) (25). Thus, we proposed that mild intermittent hypoxia could serve as a multipronged approach to treat co-morbidities linked to sleep apnea, both directly and indirectly by increasing compliance with continuous positive airway pressure (26).

Preliminary findings appear to support the premise. Airway patency improved (i.e. the airway was less collapsible) (48) following treatment with mild intermittent hypoxia (accompanied by carbon dioxide levels sustained slightly above baseline levels) for 5 days per week over a 3-week duration. This response was coupled to an increased adherence to continuous positive airway pressure (i.e. increased number of hours used per night) (48). Ultimately, the treatment resulted in decreases in systolic and diastolic blood pressure (10–15 mm Hg) that far exceeded reductions in blood pressure typically reported in individuals treated with

continuous positive airway pressure for 3 weeks (48). Indeed, in those participants that were only treated with continuous positive airway pressure for 3 weeks (i.e. no intermittent hypoxia), adherence with continuous positive airway pressure was poor and improvement in blood pressure measures was not evident (48).

In summary, evidence to date indicates that treatment with mild intermittent hypoxia in conjunction with continuous positive airway pressure might be an effective therapeutic approach to treat co-morbidities linked to sleep apnea. Moreover, it is possible that mild intermittent hypoxia, independent of continuous positive airway pressure, could be used as a treatment to mitigate apneic events if the detrimental effects of progressive augmentation (i.e. enhanced loop gain) are minimized and the beneficial effects of long-term facilitation are promoted.

Dose and Timing of Therapeutic Intermittent Hypoxia

An important issue that has not been addressed in a systematic fashion is the appropriate dose that is required to initiate the beneficial effects of intermittent hypoxia and prevent the detrimental outcomes linked to severe intermittent hypoxia. In considering the dose, a number of variables must be considered including (i) the number of episodes, (ii) the duration of each episode, (iii) the level of oxygen desaturation, (iv) the profile of oxygen desaturation, (e.g. square wave vs. saw tooth), (v) the number of days of exposure to the intermittent hypoxia protocol, (vi) the maintenance of carbon dioxide levels, and (vii) the timing of exposure (24, 49) (Figure 17.3).

To date, the rationales used to incorporate the parameters that comprise an intermittent hypoxia protocol have been implemented arbitrarily. Considering studies completed to date, the typical design of a mild intermittent hypoxia protocol includes episodes ranging from 8 to 15, an episode duration of 15 seconds – 4 minutes, an oxygen desaturation range from 80% to 90%, an intermittent hypoxia profile that is square wave and carbon dioxide levels that are maintained at or above baseline throughout the protocol (24). The timing of exposure has varied from the early morning (39) to late evening (44) during wakefulness and during the sleep period (43). In regards to timing of exposure, we have shown that long-term facilitation of ventilation is greater in the evening compared to the morning (39) and that the continuous positive airway pressure required to maintain airway patency may be lower in the evening compared to the morning (50). Thus, the magnitude of respiratory plasticity might be modulated by the time of day, which could be an indicator of an endogenous circadian rhythm. If this is the case, the efficaciousness of mild intermittent hypoxia may be dependent in part on the time of day the therapeutic protocol is administered.

HYPEROXIA AS A THERAPEUTIC TREATMENT FOR SLEEP APNEA

Hyperoxia, Loop Gain, and Apnea Severity

Several studies have explored if the administration of supplemental oxygen reduces the severity of sleep apnea in individuals with obstructive sleep apnea and in patients with central sleep apnea coupled to heart failure. The rationales for completing these studies were two-fold. Many studies have shown that an enhanced controller gain, and consequently a high loop gain, combined with a reduced carbon dioxide reserve, are phenotypic traits that initiate and promote sleep apnea (see *Introduction* for further details) (1). Moreover, a few studies have revealed that hyperoxia blunts peripheral chemoreflex sensitivity, decreases the apneic threshold, and increases the carbon dioxide reserve (51, 52) (Figure 17.1).

Published results exploring the efficaciousness of supplemental oxygen as a treatment modality have been equivocal, with results revealing that the apnea/hypopnea index was not improved in a majority of patients (~50% – 66%) treated with hyperoxia over a single night (12). On the other hand, hyperoxia has been shown to reduce the apnea/hypopnea index by 30% or greater in a select group of individuals (53). This latter finding resulted in a hypothesis that patients displaying a high loop gain would be the most responsive to treatment with supplemental oxygen (i.e. display the greatest decrease in loop gain and the apnea/hypopnea index). Taken at face value, the published findings are unclear. Wellman et al. (54) reported that patients with a high loop gain responded to supplemental oxygen, in contrast to patients with a low loop gain. Alternatively, Edwards et al. (55) showed that the response to supplemental oxygen was similar in individuals with loop gain measures ranging from low to high. Edwards et al. (55) explained this discrepancy by suggesting the overall loop gain measures were "somewhat high" in the studied group. However, Xie et al. (52) and Sands et al. (53) reported that loop gain was not a univariate predictor of decreases in apnea frequency following treatment with supplemental oxygen. The overall results indicated that there was no difference in

response to supplemental oxygen in patients with high compared to low loop gain measures.

The inconsistent findings were thought to confirm the developing understanding that the interaction between all the identified phenotypic traits responsible for obstructive sleep must be considered when determining the possible therapeutic efficaciousness of supplemental oxygen. Thus, the arousal threshold, upper airway response to respiratory stimuli, propensity for airway collapsibility, and loop gain must be considered in a multivariate manner when determining the impact of supplemental oxygen on apnea severity (Figure 17.1). This suggestion is supported by the findings of Sands et al. (53), who showed that a higher loop gain increased the likelihood of responding to supplemental oxygen in patients with adequate upper airway patency and compensation.

Supplemental oxygen has also been used to treat Cheyne-Stokes respiration-central sleep apnea patients with congestive heart failure. Supplemental oxygen has been shown to be effective in reducing the severity of sleep apnea by 50% in these patients (56). The reduction in breathing instability and central events may be due in part to increases in central ventilatory motor output (51). This increase could be caused by cerebral vasoconstriction induced by the direct effect of hyperoxia on cerebral vasculature or because of the central arterial hypocapnia induced by the increased motor output (51). Independent of the mechanism, the net effect is reduced carbon dioxide washout, which results in an elevated brain tissue partial pressure of carbon dioxide and ultimately an increased $[H^+]$ in the medulla and enhanced stimulation of the central chemoreceptors.

The reduction in breathing instability and central events could also be the consequence of a blunted controller gain, coupled with the maintenance of carbon dioxide levels, which is important since hypocapnia is the predominant factor in the onset of central sleep apnea. In addition, Franklin et al. (56) showed that treatment with inspired air comprised of 50% oxygen led to a significant increase in carbon dioxide and ultimately a 50% decrease in central apnea events. In contrast, a lower concentration of inspired oxygen only caused a minor decrease in apnea frequency, likely because associated increases in carbon dioxide levels were absent. Nonetheless, it is important to note that carbon dioxide administration is not the ideal treatment of choice for Cheyne-Stokes respiration-central sleep apnea patients with congestive heart failure as the resultant hyperventilation may lead to excessive demand for blood flow.

Hyperoxia, Arousal Threshold, and Apnea Severity

The administration of supplemental oxygen might also modify the arousal threshold independently or concomitantly with loop gain. Given that the administration of sustained and intermittent hypoxia elevates the arousal threshold (i.e. it is more difficult to arouse from sleep), the administration of hyperoxia could lower the threshold (Figure 17.1).

Investigators have proposed that a low arousal threshold leads to repetitive arousals that cause a perpetuating cycle of breathing events, when coupled with a high loop gain that initiates a hyperventilatory response at the termination of each arousal (see *Introduction* for additional discussion) (Figure 17.1). In contrast to this scenario, administration of supplemental oxygen blunts controller gain and this outcome measure has been coupled to an arousal threshold that was unchanged (55, 57) or lowered (53) (Figure 17.1). A blunted controller gain coupled to an unchanging arousal threshold (57) would be associated with increases in apnea duration, since the reduced sensitivity to hypoxia and hypercapnia would extend the time required for the ventilatory drive to reach the arousal threshold. Indeed, Wellman et al. (54) and Xie et al. (52) reported that blunting of loop gain was coupled to increases in apnea duration. When this occurs, one must consider if reductions in apnea frequency are simply the consequence of lengthening of apnea events or are due principally to blunting of chemoreflex sensitivity/controller gain. Wellman et al. (54) reported that the reduction in the apnea/hypopnea index following treatment with supplemental oxygen was greater than expected if a lengthening of apneic events were principally responsible for reductions in apnea frequency.

In contrast, a blunted controller gain coupled to a lowered arousal threshold could lead to an unchanged apnea duration, so that any observed reduction in apnea frequency would be a primary consequence of a blunted controller gain. This suggestion is supported by the findings of Sands et al. (53), who reported a reduction in loop gain and apnea frequency following treatment with supplemental oxygen despite lowering of the arousal threshold.

Hyperoxia, Upper Airway Responsiveness/Collapsibility, and Apnea Severity

In addition to loop gain and the arousal threshold, upper airway collapsibility and responsiveness to chemical stimuli should be considered when exploring the efficaciousness of hyperoxia in treating sleep apnea (Figure 17.1). It is unlikely that hyperoxia can serve as an effective treatment to reduce the apnea/hypopnea index via the reduction of loop gain if upper airway patency is difficult to sustain. Thus, baseline measures of upper airway collapsibility might serve as a predictor in determining the effectiveness of hyperoxia in reducing the severity of sleep-disordered breathing. This suggestion is supported by Sands et al. (53), who reported that a reduced propensity toward collapsibility and greater upper airway muscle compensation was associated with an increased effectiveness of hyperoxia in treating sleep apnea.

Despite this relationship, hyperoxia does not have a beneficial effect on upper airway collapsibility and compensation. A number of studies established that reducing feedback from the peripheral chemoreceptors via the administration of hyperoxia reduces upper airway muscle activity and responsiveness in humans (58) and animals (59, 60) (Figure 17.1). Alternatively, hyperoxia might exacerbate sleep apnea by increasing collapsibility via blunting of upper airway muscle activity and load compensation, although evidence for this suggestion is ambiguous (Figure 17.1). On the one hand, hyperoxia does not seem to alter the immediate response of upper airway muscles to load compensation (61) or measures of airway collapsibility in humans (55). On the other hand, hyperoxia is associated with increases in the apnea/hypopnea index in some individuals (52), and increases in apnea duration in most cases (52, 54). The effect on apnea duration could be due to blunting of loop gain but could also be due to blunting of load compensation. In any event, the value of airway collapsibility and responsiveness in predicating the effectiveness of hyperoxia lies in the understanding that reductions in loop gain will be most effective in reducing the apnea/hypopnea index in the presence of a less collapsible and more responsive airway.

Duration of Therapeutic Hyperoxia

Most studies designed to explore the therapeutic effectiveness of supplemental oxygen in treating obstructive sleep apnea have been completed across a single night of sleep. Fewer studies have explored the effects of supplemental oxygen on apnea severity over a longer time frame. Nonetheless, Wang et al. (62) and Gold et al. (63) reported that treatment with supplemental oxygen for 2 and 1 months, respectively, significantly reduced the oxygen desaturation index and reduced the apnea/hypopnea index, although this latter measure did not reach statistical significance (P = 0.068) in Wang et al.'s (62) investigation. These findings are similar to the results obtained from acute studies. However, in contrast to the acute studies, Wang et al. (62) reported that patients with a higher baseline controller gain during wakefulness had the smallest reduction in breathing events following 2 months of treatment. Thus, caution is required when comparing single night effects with those observed after chronic treatment (e.g. 2 months). Decidedly different effects on the mechanisms that impact apnea frequency might be dependent on the duration of treatment with supplemental oxygen. Likewise, although systematic studies have not been completed, the flow rate and the fractional concentration of oxygen administered will likely have an impact on outcome measures.

Therapeutic Hyperoxia and Outcome Measures

Treatment with supplemental oxygen has been associated with a host of beneficial outcomes including decreased sympathetic nerve activity and elimination of nocturnal oxygen desaturation (64, 65). The elimination or improvement in nocturnal oxygen saturation may occur even though the apnea/hypopnea index remains unchanged when based on parameters that are independent of oxygen saturation (66). Likewise, Turnbull et al. (66) recently showed that nocturnal hyperoxia prevented morning increases in blood pressure that were evident under sham conditions. Although these latter findings are intriguing, they were obtained in patients that received treatment with supplemental oxygen during a 2-week withdrawal period from continuous positive airway pressure (66). In contrast, previous studies did not report reductions in blood pressure even though treatment with supplemental oxygen was as long as 3 months (67, 68). Although other variables could explain this difference (oxygen flow rates, adherence to treatment, severity of obstructive sleep apnea) (69), additional work is required to determine if long-term treatment with supplemental oxygen in treatment naïve patients effectively lowers blood pressure.

While supplemental oxygen may prevent the negative consequences of nocturnal oxygen desaturation, it does not improve daytime sleepiness (66, 69). Moreover, treatment is associated with risks of its own. As mentioned, supplemental oxygen typically increases apnea duration because of blunting of controller gain. Modifications in this mechanism, along with others including a ventilation-perfusion ratio

mismatch, could lead to hypercapnia, which induces increases in sympathetic nervous system activity and blood pressure elevations (70). In addition, treatment with supplemental oxygen could lead to decreases in coronary blood cardiac output, increases in peripheral vascular resistance, and decreases in cardiac output (71, 72). Long-term administration of hyperoxia may also be associated with the production of reactive oxygen species, which in turn can promote cardiac dysfunction (51, 64).

CONCLUSION

Both intermittent hypoxia and supplemental oxygen therapy have a profound impact on ventilatory control and both forms of therapy might serve a useful purpose in treating obstructive sleep apnea. Therapeutic mild intermittent hypoxia administered at an optimal dose (i.e. mild intermittent hypoxia) can target a number of co-morbidities linked to obstructive sleep apnea, both directly and by improving adherence to continuous positive airway pressure because of its influence on upper airway muscle activity and the arousal threshold. The utility of supplemental oxygen in treating obstructive sleep apnea is linked principally to its ability to blunt controller gain.

Given the beneficial effects of both treatments, it is intriguing to consider the outcomes that might occur if the therapies are combined. If long-term facilitation of upper airway muscle activity, initiated by therapeutic intermittent hypoxia, can be induced while preventing the initiation of progressive augmentation of the hypoxic ventilatory response, this combination could effectively mitigate apneic events. This possibility might exist if intermittent hypoxia is coupled with intermittent periods of hyperoxia. The presence of hyperoxia might blunt controller gain with little influence on upper airway muscle function as reported in some studies. This combination could be particularly effective if hypocapnia was prevented. Further investigation is required to explore these possibilities.

AUTHOR CONTRIBUTIONS

Sreenavya Gandikota and Jason H Mateika drafted and edited the manuscript. Both authors have approved the final version of the manuscript.

ACKNOWLEDGMENTS

This work was supported by awards (I01CX000125 and 15SRCS003—JHM) from the Department of Veterans Affairs, Veterans Health Administration, Office of Research and Development, and awards (R56HL142757, R01HL085537) from the National Heart, Lung and Blood Institutes.

REFERENCES

1. Dempsey JA, Veasey SC, Morgan BJ, O'Donnell CP. Pathophysiology of sleep apnea. *Physiological Reviews.* 2010;90(1):47–112.

2. Lozo T, Komnenov D, Badr MS, Mateika JH. Sex differences in sleep disordered breathing in adults. *Respiratory Physiology and Neurobiology.* 2017;245:65–75.

3. McNicholas WT, Bonsignore MR, B26 MCECA. Sleep apnoea as an independent risk factor for cardiovascular disease: current evidence, basic mechanisms and research priorities. *European Respiratory Journal.* 2007;29(1):156–178.

4. Parati G, Lombardi C, Narkiewicz K. Sleep apnea: epidemiology, pathophysiology, and relation to cardiovascular risk. *American Journal of Physiology-Regulatory Integrative and Comparative Physiology.* 2007;293(4):R1671–R1683.

5. Eckert DJ, White DP, Jordan AS, Malhotra A, Wellman A. Defining phenotypic causes of obstructive sleep apnea. Identification of novel therapeutic targets. *American Journal of Respiratory and Critical Care Medicine.* 2013;188(8):996–1004.

6. White DP. Pathogenesis of obstructive and central sleep apnea. *American Journal of Respiratory and Critical Care Medicine.* 2005;172(11):1363–1370.

7. Remmers JE, Degroot WJ, Sauerland EK, Anch AM. Pathogenesis of upper airway occlusion during sleep. *Journal of Applied Physiology.* 1978;44(6):931–938.

8. Mezzanotte WS, Tangel DJ, White DP. Waking genioglossal electromyogram in sleep apnea patients versus normal controls (a neuromuscular compensatory mechanism). *The Journal of Clinical Investigation.* 1992;89(5):1571–1579.

9. Lo YL, Jordan AS, Malhotra A, et al. Influence of wakefulness on pharyngeal airway muscle activity. *Thorax.* 2007;62(9):799–805.

10. Hicks A, Cori JM, Jordan AS, et al. Mechanisms of the deep, slow-wave, sleep-related increase of upper airway muscle tone in healthy humans. *Journal of Applied Physiology.* 2017;122(5):1304–1312.

11. Taranto-Montemurro L, Sands SA, Grace KP, et al. Neural memory of the genioglossus muscle during sleep is stage-dependent in healthy subjects and obstructive sleep apnoea patients. *The Journal of Physiology.* 2018;596(21):5163–5173.

12. Osman AM, Carter SG, Carberry JC, Eckert DJ. Obstructive sleep apnea: current perspectives. *Nature and Science of Sleep.* 2018;10:21–34.

13. Jordan AS, O'Donoghue FJ, Cori JM, Trinder J. Physiology of arousal in obstructive sleep apnea and potential impacts for sedative treatment. *American Journal of Respiratory and Critical Care Medicine.* 2017;196(7):814–821.

14. Eckert DJ, Malhotra A. Pathophysiology of adult obstructive sleep apnea. *Proceedings of the American Thoracic Society.* 2008;5(2):144–153.

15. Jordan AS, Wellman A, Heinzer RC, et al. Mechanisms used to restore ventilation after partial upper airway collapse during sleep in humans. *Thorax.* 2007;62(10):861–867.

16. Hudgel DW, Gordon EA, Thanakitcharu S, Bruce EN. Instability of ventilatory control in patients with obstructive sleep apnea. *American Journal of Respiratory and Critical Care Medicine.* 1998;158(4):1142–1149.

17. Mateika JH, Narwani G. Intermittent hypoxia and respiratory plasticity in humans and other animals: does exposure to intermittent hypoxia promote or mitigate sleep apnoea? *Experimental Physiology.* 2009;94(3):279–296.

18. Naughton MT. Loop gain in apnea gaining control or controlling the gain? *American Journal of Respiratory and Critical Care Medicine.* 2010;181(2):103–105.

19. Puri S, ElChami M, Shaheen D, et al. Variations in loop gain and arousal threshold during NREM sleep are affected by time of day over a 24 hour period in participants with obstructive sleep apnea. *Journal of Applied Physiology.* 2020;129(4):800–809.

20. Orr JE, Malhotra A, Sands SA. Pathogenesis of central and complex sleep apnoea. *Respirology.* 2017;22(1):43–52.

21. Yumino D, Bradley TD. Central sleep apnea and Cheyne-Stokes respiration. *Proceedings of the American Thoracic Society.* 2008;5(2):226–236.

22. Franklin KA, Sandstrom E, Johansson G, Balfors EM. Hemodynamics, cerebral circulation, and oxygen saturation in Cheyne-Stokes respiration. *Journal of Applied Physiology.* 1997;83(4):1184–1191.

23. Pryor WW. Cheyne-Stokes respiration in patients with cardiac enlargement and prolonged circulation time. *Circulation.* 1951;4(2):233–238.

24. Mateika JH, Sandhu KS. Experimental protocols and preparations to study respiratory long term facilitation. *Respiratory Physiology & Neurobiology.* 2011;176(1–2):1–11.

25. Mateika JH, El-Chami M, Shaheen D, Ivers B. Intermittent hypoxia: a low-risk research tool with therapeutic value in humans. *Journal of Applied Physiology.* 2015;118(5):520–532.

26. Mateika JH, Komnenov D. Intermittent hypoxia initiated plasticity in humans: a multipronged therapeutic approach to treat sleep apnea and overlapping co-morbidities. *Experimental Neurology.* 2017;287(Pt 2):113–129.

27. Powell FL, Milsom WK, Mitchell GS. Time domains of the hypoxic ventilatory response. *Respiration Physiology.* 1998;112(2):123–134.

28. Turner S, Streeter KA, Greer J, Mitchell GS, Fuller DD. Pharmacological modulation of hypoxia-induced respiratory neuroplasticity. *Respiratory Physiology & Neurobiology*. 2018;256:4–14.

29. Mitchell GS, Baker TL, Nanda SA, et al. Invited review: intermittent hypoxia and respiratory plasticity. *Journal of Applied Physiology*. 2001;90(6):2466–2475.

30. Chowdhuri S, Pierchala L, Aboubakr SE, Shkoukani M, Badr MS. Long-term facilitation of genioglossus activity is present in normal humans during NREM sleep. *Respiratory Physiology & Neurobiology*. 2008;160(1):65–75.

31. Chowdhuri S, Shanidze I, Pierchala L, Belen D, Mateika JH, Badr MS. Effect of episodic hypoxia on the susceptibility to hypocapnic central apnea during NREM sleep. *Journal of Applied Physiology*. 2010;108(2):369–377.

32. Harris DP, Balasubramaniam A, Badr MS, Mateika JH. Long-term facilitation of ventilation and genioglossus muscle activity is evident in the presence of elevated levels of carbon dioxide in awake humans. *American Journal of Physiology—Regulatory Integrative and Comparative Physiology*. 2006;291(4):R1111–R1119.

33. Mateika JH, Mendello C, Obeid D, Badr MS. Peripheral chemoreflex responsiveness is increased at elevated levels of carbon dioxide after episodic hypoxia in awake humans. *Journal of Applied Physiology*. 2004;96(3):1197–1205.

34. Morelli C, Badr MS, Mateika JH. Ventilatory responses to carbon dioxide at low and high levels of oxygen are elevated after episodic hypoxia in men compared with women. *Journal of Applied Physiology*. 2004;97(5):1673–1680.

35. Pierchala LA, Mohammed AS, Grullon K, Mateika JH, Badr MS. Ventilatory long-term facilitation in non-snoring subjects during NREM sleep. *Respiratory Physiology & Neurobiology*. 2008;160(3):259–266.

36. Wadhwa H, Gradinaru C, Gates GJ, Badr MS, Mateika JH. Impact of intermittent hypoxia on long-term facilitation of minute ventilation and heart rate variability in men and women: do sex differences exist? *Journal of Applied Physiology*. 2008;104(6):1625–1633.

37. Sankari A, Bascom AT, Riehani A, Badr MS. Tetraplegia is associated with enhanced peripheral chemoreflex sensitivity and ventilatory long-term facilitation. *Journal of Applied Physiology*. 2015;119(10):1183–1193.

38. Tester NJ, Fuller DD, Fromm JS, Spiess MR, Behrman AL, Mateika JH. Long-term facilitation of ventilation in humans with chronic spinal cord injury. *American Journal of Respiratory and Critical Care Medicine*. 2014;189(1):57–65.

39. Gerst DG, III, Yokhana SS, Carney LM, et al. The hypoxic ventilatory response and ventilatory long-term facilitation are altered by time of day and repeated daily exposure to intermittent hypoxia. *Journal of Applied Physiology*. 2011;110(1):15–28.

40. Lee DS, Badr MS, Mateika JH. Progressive augmentation and ventilatory long-term facilitation are enhanced in sleep apnoea patients and are mitigated by antioxidant administration. *The Journal of Physiology*. 2009;587(Pt 22):5451–5467.

41. Rowley JA, Deebajah I, Parikh S, Najar A, Saha R, Badr MS. The influence of episodic hypoxia on upper airway collapsibility in subjects with obstructive sleep apnea. *Journal of Applied Physiology*. 2007;103(3):911–916.

42. Shkoukani M, Babcock MA, Badr MS. Effect of episodic hypoxia on upper airway mechanics in humans during NREM sleep. *Journal of Applied Physiology*. 2002;92(6):2565–2570.

43. Syed Z, Lin HS, Mateika JH. The impact of arousal state, sex, and sleep apnea on the magnitude of progressive augmentation and ventilatory long-term facilitation. *Journal of Applied Physiology*. 2013;114(1):52–65.

44. Yokhana SS, Gerst DG, III, Lee DS, Badr MS, Qureshi T, Mateika JH. Impact of repeated daily exposure to intermittent hypoxia and mild sustained hypercapnia on apnea severity. *Journal of Applied Physiology*. 2012;112(3):367–377.

45. El-Chami M, Sudan S, Lin HS, Mateika JH. Exposure to intermittent hypoxia and sustained hypercapnia reduces therapeutic CPAP in participants with obstructive sleep apnea. *Journal of Applied Physiology*. 2017;123(4):993–1002.

46. Edwards BA, Sands SA, Owens RL, et al. Effects of hyperoxia and hypoxia on the physiological traits responsible for obstructive sleep apnoea. *The Journal of Physiology*. 2014;592(20):4523–4535.

47. Alex RM, Panza GS, Hakim H, et al. Exposure to mild intermittent hypoxia increases loop gain and the arousal threshold in participants with obstructive sleep apnoea. *The Journal of Physiology*. 2019;597(14):3697–3711.

48. Panza GS, Puri S, Rimar C, Lin H-S, Mateika J. Mild intermittent hypoxia and its multipronged effect on obstructive sleep apnea. *The FASEB Journal*. 2020;34(S1):1–1.

49. Mateika JH. A reminder that experimentally induced intermittent hypoxia is an incomplete model of obstructive sleep apnea and its outcome measures. *Journal of Applied Physiology*. 2019;127(6):1620–1621.

50. El-Chami M, Shaheen D, Ivers B, et al. Time of day affects the frequency and duration of breathing events and the critical closing pressure during NREM sleep in participants with sleep apnea. *Journal of Applied Physiology*. 2015;119(6):617–626.

51. Chowdhuri S, Sinha P, Pranathiageswaran S, Badr MS. Sustained hyperoxia stabilizes breathing in healthy individuals during NREM sleep. *Journal of Applied Physiology*. 2010;109(5):1378–1383.

52. Xie AL, Teodorescu M, Pegelow DF, et al. Effects of stabilizing or increasing respiratory motor outputs on obstructive sleep apnea. *Journal of Applied Physiology*. 2013;115(1):22–33.

53. Sands SA, Edwards BA, Terrill PI, et al. Identifying obstructive sleep apnoea patients responsive to supplemental oxygen therapy. *European Respiratory Journal*. 2018;52(3):1–21.

54. Wellman A, Malhotra A, Jordan AS, Stevenson KE, Gautam S, White DP. Effect of oxygen in obstructive sleep apnea: role of loop gain. *Respiratory Physiology & Neurobiology*. 2008;162(2):144–151.

55. Edwards BA, Sands SA, Owens RL, et al. Effects of hyperoxia and hypoxia on the physiological traits responsible for obstructive sleep apnoea. *Journal of Physiology-London*. 2014;592(20):4523–4535.

56. Franklin KA, Eriksson P, Sahlin C, Lundgren R. Reversal of central sleep apnea with oxygen. *Chest*. 1997;111(1):163–169.

57. Berry RB, Light RW. Effect of hyperoxia on the arousal response to airway occlusion during sleep in normal subjects. *The American Review of Respiratory Disease*. 1992;146(2):330–334.

58. Hudgel DW, Hendricks C, Dadley A. Alteration in obstructive apnea pattern induced by changes in oxygen- and carbon-dioxide-inspired concentrations. *The American Review of Respiratory Disease*. 1988;138(1):16–19.

59. Aleksandrova NP. Chemoreceptor and vagal influences on genioglossal muscle responses to inspiratory resistive load. *Journal of Physiology and Pharmacology*. 2004;55(Suppl 3):7–14.

60. Gauda EB, Carroll JL, McColley S, Smith PL. Effect of oxygenation on breath-by-breath response of the genioglossus muscle during occlusion. *Journal of Applied Physiology*. 1991;71(4):1231–1236.

61. Wilson PA, Skatrud JB, Dempsey JA. Effects of slow wave sleep on ventilatory compensation to inspiratory elastic loading. *Respiration Physiology*. 1984;55(1):103–120.

62. Wang D, Wong KK, Rowsell L, Don GW, Yee BJ, Grunstein RR. Predicting response to oxygen therapy in obstructive sleep apnoea patients using a 10-minute daytime test. *European Respiratory Journal*. 2018;51(1):1–9.

63. Gold AR, Schwartz AR, Bleecker ER, Smith PL. The effect of chronic nocturnal oxygen administration upon sleep apnea. *American Review of Respiratory Disease*. 1986;134(5):925–929.

64. Sasayama S, Izumi T, Matsuzaki M, et al. Improvement of quality of life with nocturnal oxygen therapy in heart failure patients with central sleep apnea. *Circulation Journal*. 2009;73(7):1255–1262.

65. Javaheri S, Ahmed M, Parker TJ, Brown CR. Effects of nasal O_2 on sleep-related disordered breathing in ambulatory patients with stable heart failure. *Sleep*. 1999;22(8):1101–1106.

66. Turnbull CD, Sen D, Kohler M, Petousi N, Stradling JR. Effect of supplemental oxygen on blood pressure in obstructive sleep apnea (SOX). A randomized continuous positive airway pressure withdrawal trial. *American Journal of Respiratory and Critical Care Medicine*. 2019;199(2):211–219.

67. Gottlieb DJ, Punjabi NM, Mehra R, et al. CPAP versus oxygen in obstructive sleep apnea. *The New England Journal of Medicine*. 2014;370(24):2276–2285.

68. Norman D, Loredo JS, Nelesen RA, et al. Effects of continuous positive airway pressure versus supplemental oxygen on 24-hour ambulatory blood pressure. *Hypertension*. 2006;47(5):840–845.

69. Gottlieb DJ. Supplemental oxygen for obstructive sleep apnea: is there a role after all? *American Journal of Respiratory and Critical Care Medicine*. 2019;199(2):140–141.

70. Owens RL. Supplemental oxygen needs during sleep. Who benefits? *Respiratory Care*. 2013;58(1):32–47.

71. Mak S, Azevedo ER, Liu PP, Newton GE. Effect of hyperoxia on left ventricular function and filling pressures in patients with and without congestive heart failure. *Chest*. 2001;120(2):467–473.

72. Haque WA, Boehmer J, Clemson BS, Leuenberger UA, Silber DH, Sinoway LI. Hemodynamic effects of supplemental oxygen administration in congestive heart failure. *Journal of the American College of Cardiology*. 1996;27(2):353–357.

18 Pharmacological Management of Sleep-Disordered Breathing

Thomas J Altree, Peter G Catcheside, Sutapa Mukherjee, and Danny J Eckert

INTRODUCTION

There is significant inter-individual variability in the pathophysiology of both obstructive sleep apnea (OSA) and central sleep apnea (CSA). Recent advances in knowledge of the mechanisms that contribute to sleep apnea have highlighted several potential treatment targets for pharmacological intervention.

PHARMACOLOGICAL MANAGEMENT OF OSA

There are at least four underlying predisposing traits, or *endotypes*, that contribute to OSA pathophysiology (Figure 18.1) (1). These are sometimes defined based on their clinical manifestations or *phenotypes*. The degree to which each trait contributes to OSA varies markedly between individuals. This interindividual variance of different combinations of traits offers potential targets for pharmacological therapy (Table 18.1). Although current clinical practice of OSA treatment tends not to consider differences in individual endotypic traits, recent advances in non-invasive methods of endotype characterization via signal processing of standard diagnostic polysomnogram data have the potential to facilitate more nuanced OSA treatment decisions based on "precision medicine" principles (2).

Impaired Upper Airway Anatomy

The predominant trait in most people with OSA is an anatomically narrow or collapsible upper airway. This is the target of most existing therapies for OSA (e.g. continuous positive airway pressure (CPAP) devices, dental devices, surgery, and supine avoidance in patients with a strong positional component to OSA). A narrow pharyngeal airway may occur in the setting of intrinsic craniofacial properties, such as retrognathia, or secondarily to obesity. Adipose tissue deposition in the tongue and in the muscles and soft tissues surrounding the upper airway crowds the airway (3) and increases upper airway collapsibility. Central adiposity may also reduce lung volumes, destabilize respiratory control via reduced lung gas stores (4) and increase upper airway collapsibility via caudal traction effects on the airway (5). Thus, any medications that reduce weight may improve upper airway patency.

Several other factors are likely to contribute to upper airway impairment. One potential mechanism is via changes in fluid distribution during sleep. When supine, fluid redistributes throughout the body including tissues surrounding the upper airway. Rostral fluid shifts increase pharyngeal tissue pressure, reduce upper airway cross-sectional area, and increase airway collapsibility (6). Diuretics may therefore reduce OSA severity, especially in patients with volume overload states such as heart failure.

Weight-Reducing Medications

A double-blind multicenter trial of 359 obese participants with at least moderately severe untreated OSA showed that 3 mg of daily liraglutide, a glucagon-like peptide-1 analog that acts as an appetite suppressant, reduces the apnea-hypopnea index (AHI) versus placebo by ~6 events/hr sleep and body weight by ~4% at 32 weeks when used as an adjunct to calorie reduction and exercise (7). The combination of phentermine and topiramate can also reduce body weight with accompanying therapeutic benefits in OSA. Phentermine is a synthetic sympathomimetic amine that suppresses appetite and has less of an effect on blood pressure and heart rate than other stimulants (8). Topiramate is traditionally used as an anticonvulsant. It is a sulfamate-substituted monosaccharide that blocks voltage-sensitive sodium channels, enhances the activity of gamma-aminobutyric acid (GABA) and some types of $GABA_A$ receptors, and reduces activation of the kainite subtype of glutamate receptors (8). Weight loss in obese individuals was a consistent side-effect in early trials of topiramate, and an extended-release (ER) form when used in combination with phentermine results in weight loss in obese patients (9). In a group of 45 obese patients with at least moderately severe untreated OSA, phentermine 15 mg with ER topiramate 92 mg led to greater weight loss (~10%) and reduction in AHI of ~30 events/hr sleep at 28 weeks (10). The reduction in OSA severity correlated with the degree of weight loss. Approximately 50% of participants taking phentermine/topiramate ER experienced dry mouth, and ~25% experienced altered taste sensation. Sibutramine was previously used as a weight loss agent in OSA (11). However, it has since had marketing approval withdrawn in most western countries due to significant safety concerns of elevated rates of nonfatal myocardial infarction and stroke (12). Current American Thoracic Society clinical practice guidelines make a conditional recommendation that anti-obesity

DOI: 10.1201/9781003000631-22

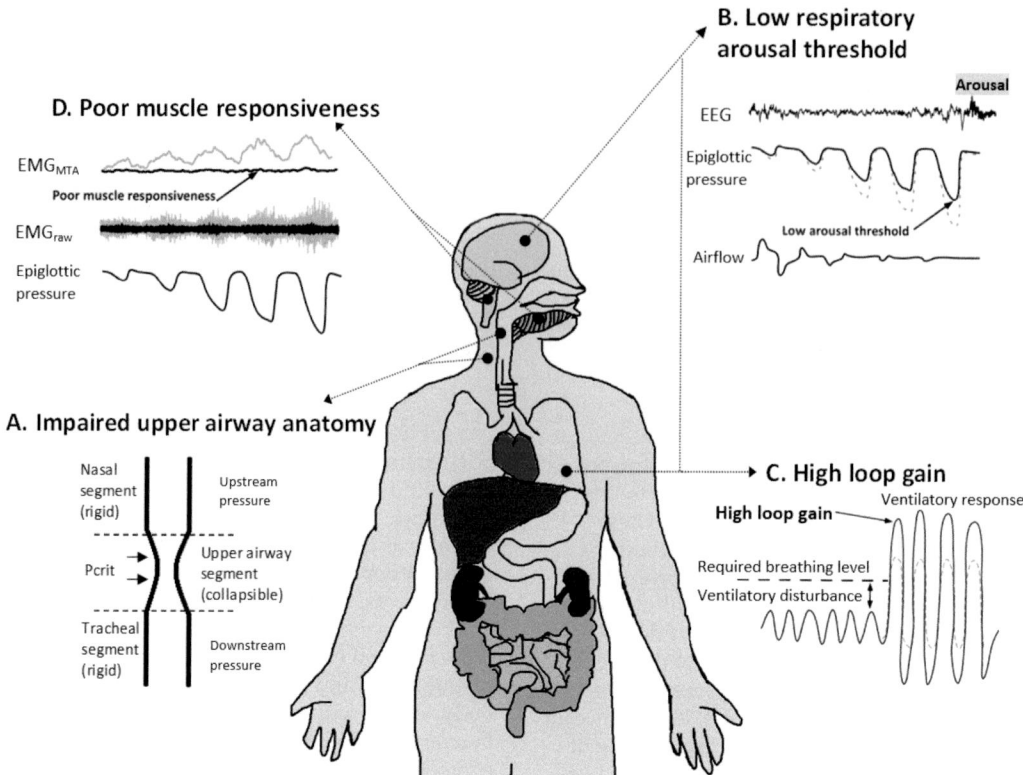

Figure 18.1 Schematic of the four key endotypes understood to contribute to obstructive sleep apnea pathogenesis. A. Impaired upper airway anatomy. Non-anatomical endotypes include: B. Low respiratory arousal threshold (waking up too easily to minor pharyngeal narrowing); C. High loop gain (unstable control of breathing/increased sensitivity to minor changes in CO_2); and D. Poor upper airway muscle responsiveness. Each of these traits offers targets for pharmacological therapy. (Adapted with permission from Carberry et al. Chest, 2018 (108) and Aishah and Eckert, Curr Opin Pulm Med, 2019 (109).)

pharmacotherapy can be considered in patients with OSA with a body mass index >27 kg/m² who have not successfully lost weight with a comprehensive lifestyle weight management program and have no contraindications or active cardiovascular disease (13).

Diuretics

Several studies of diuretics in OSA have shown reductions in AHI via the use of loop and thiazide diuretics, and mineralocorticoid receptor antagonists (14–17). However, overall reductions in AHI have been quite modest. This suggests that rostral fluid shifts are not the main determinant of upper airway collapsibility in most cases.

Upper Airway Dilator Muscles

Upper airway patency relies upon appropriate upper-airway dilator muscle responses to airway narrowing. Many muscles are involved, but two key muscles are genioglossus and tensor palatini. Genioglossus, located at the base of the tongue, is the largest upper airway dilator and is innervated by the hypoglossal nerve. Genioglossus contracts in a phasic pattern, with greater activity during inspiration when negative intraluminal pressures increase the likelihood of upper airway collapse (18). Tensor palatini tends to display a tonic (i.e. constant) level of activation during quiet breathing, and is strongly influenced by the sleep state (19). Tensor palatini activity markedly reduces at sleep onset and then remains relatively constant across sleep stages. Although genioglossus activity also abruptly reduces at sleep onset, subsequent activity can change substantially depending on the level of breathing effort and sleep stage with a progressive reduction from N3 sleep to N2 and REM sleep (19, 20). Impaired upper airway muscle responsiveness likely contributes to OSA pathogenesis in over one-third of patients (1).

Table 18.1: The Endotypic Targets of Medications Used Treat Obstructive and Central Sleep Apnea

Obstructive Sleep Apnea Medications	Endotype	Central Sleep Apnea Medications
Weight loss drugs • Liraglutide • Phentermine + topiramate Diuretics • Loop diuretics • Thiazide diuretics • Mineralocorticoid receptor antagonists	Upper airway anatomy	
Cannabinergic and serotonergic pathways • Dronabinol • Paroxetine • Fluoxetine • Mirtazapine Noradrenergic and muscarinic pathways • Desipramine • Atomoxetine + oxybutynin • Reboxetine	Upper airway dilator muscles	
Carbonic anhydrase inhibitors • Acetazolamide • Zonisamide Supplemental oxygen	Loop gain	Respiratory stimulants • Acetazolamide • Theophylline • Supplemental CO_2 Supplemental oxygen
Sedatives/hypnotics • Zolpidem • Trazodone • Eszopiclone	Arousal threshold	Sedatives/hypnotics • Triazolam • Temazepam • Zopiclone • Zaleplon

Note: A summary of endotypic targets of medications for obstructive and central sleep apnea. Increased loop gain and low arousal thresholds contribute to both obstructive and central sleep apnea pathophysiology. Therefore, there is an overlap in the medications that can be used to target these endotypes. Note: opioid medications have been excluded from this summary as these are covered in more detail in Chapter 19. Other medications that have demonstrated efficacy in very small case series or non-randomized studies have not been included. CO_2: carbon dioxide.

Many neurotransmitters and receptor types are involved in the neural control of upper airway dilator muscle activity. These include excitatory serotonin type 3 (5-HT_3) and inhibitory cannabinoid type 1 (CB_1) receptors in nodose ganglion cells and noradrenergic, serotonergic, and glutamatergic-mediated excitatory inputs to cranial motor pools (21–25). Withdrawal of noradrenergic drive in non-REM (NREM) sleep is a particularly important mediator of genioglossus hypotonia. Muscarinic receptor-mediated inhibition of genioglossus activity plays an additional role in REM sleep (26). These pathways offer potential medication targets to treat OSA. To date, a universally effective pharmacologic therapy for OSA has not been identified, although

agents currently under investigation show considerable promise.

Cannabinergic and Serotonergic Pathways
Dronabinol, a nonselective CB_1 and CB_2 receptor agonist, has been demonstrated to moderately reduce AHI by ~10 events/hr at doses of 2.5 and 10 mg/day (27, 28). Studies assessing enhanced serotonergic transmission with selective serotonin reuptake inhibitors (SSRIs) have shown mixed results. In one study, paroxetine reduced the AHI during NREM sleep but not during REM sleep (29). In a small cohort, fluoxetine reduced AHI during NREM sleep, but with significant inter-individual variability (30). Mirtazapine, a mixed 5-HT_2/5-HT_3 antagonist and α2A

antagonist, showed initial promise in a small randomized, double-blind, placebo-controlled study (31), but two larger subsequent studies failed to demonstrate significant improvements (32). Overall, drugs targeting cannabinergic pathways require further investigation, and drugs targeting serotonergic pathways have not yielded consistent benefits as potential OSA treatments.

Noradrenergic and Muscarinic Pathways

Of all the medications that target upper airway muscles in OSA, those acting on noradrenergic and muscarinic pathways have shown the most promise. Desipramine, a tricyclic antidepressant that inhibits the norepinephrine reuptake receptor in the central nervous system, reduces sleep onset-related reductions in genioglossus activity (33). In a small cohort of OSA patients, desipramine reduced upper airway collapsibility and improved OSA severity in those with impaired upper airway muscle activity (34). Large improvements in OSA severity have been demonstrated with the combination of atomoxetine, a norepinephrine reuptake inhibitor, and oxybutynin, an antimuscarinic agent (35). Reboxetine, as an alternative to atomoxetine, has also shown promise as a therapeutic agent (36). Atomoxetine and reboxetine with oxybutynin are both currently being investigated in randomized, double-blind clinical trials.

Hypnotics

In contrast to the generally accepted view that hypnotics have a detrimental effect on upper airway patency, the non-benzodiazepine hypnotic zolpidem has been shown to increase pharyngeal muscle responsiveness in a detailed physiology study (37). This does not seem to be a class-wide effect, but rather there may be unique receptors through which zolpidem mediates its influence on upper airway muscle control (38). These mechanisms require further study before zolpidem can be recommended for use in a clinical setting to improve upper airway dilator muscle responsiveness, due to the risk of hypnotics worsening hypoxemia in people with high arousal thresholds or severe OSA (39).

Chemogenetics

The use of viral vectors to deliver excitatory designer receptors to hypoglossal motoneurons is a novel concept that is currently under development. These *designer receptors exclusively activated by designer drugs* (DREADDs) are still in the animal model phase of development, but offer major promise for future OSA treatment by using a designer receptor not found elsewhere in the body that would obviate undesirable off-target effects that have plagued other OSA drug treatments to date (40–42).

Arousal Threshold

Respiratory stimuli, such as hypoxia, hypercapnia, and increased resistive loads augment breathing effort and often induce brief arousals or awakenings from sleep (43). The degree of stimulus required to induce an arousal varies from person to person and with sleep depth. Individuals in whom a relatively minor stimulus triggers an arousal are termed to have a low respiratory arousal threshold. A low arousal threshold is a common endotype in patients with OSA, especially in those who are non-obese (1, 44).

Low arousal thresholds contribute to OSA in three main ways. Firstly, arousals prevent the progression from N1 and N2 sleep to N3 (slow-wave) sleep where respiratory control is more stable. Slow-wave sleep is characterized by ventilatory control stability, transiently raised arousal thresholds, increased genioglossus muscle responsiveness, and an overall reduction in frequency of obstructive events (19, 45, 46). Secondly, low arousal thresholds impede upper-airway dilator muscle activation. Arousals may be triggered by the same respiratory stimuli that increase upper airway dilator activity, such as hypoxia, hypercapnia, and more negative airway pressures. Before these stimuli stimulate airway dilator muscles to activate to help re-establish airway patency, they can also trigger arousal before or shortly after airway re-opening, particularly in individuals with low arousal thresholds (47). Thirdly, arousals can precipitate excessive ventilatory responses. Arousals promote rapid airway re-opening and an additional reflex burst in ventilation when the ventilatory drive is already high due to obstruction. The resulting hyperventilation response subsequently promotes low arterial CO_2, sometimes to below the apnea threshold triggering central apneas following chemo-reflex delays and the return to sleep. Relative hypocapnia and consequently low ventilatory and upper airway muscle activity can then precipitate further cyclical obstruction, arousal, and ongoing ventilatory control and sleep instability (48, 49). Medications that raise the arousal threshold may therefore promote more stable ventilatory control and reduce OSA severity in those with low arousal thresholds.

Sedatives and Hypnotics

Sedatives and hypnotics have traditionally been avoided in OSA due to concerns about their effects on pharyngeal muscle relaxation and delayed responses to hypoxia. High hypnotic doses can worsen hypoxemia in people with severe OSA (39). However, in a detailed physiological study of participants with and without OSA that measured arousal thresholds, genioglossus muscle responsiveness, and upper airway collapsibility, zolpidem 10 mg and zopiclone 7.5 mg raised the arousal threshold without worsening muscle responsiveness or upper airway collapsibility as measured by critical closing pressure (37). In the same study, temazepam 10 mg did not alter the arousal threshold or negatively impact upper airway collapsibility. In another detailed study of zopiclone 7.5 mg versus placebo in 12 patients with severe OSA of differing endotypes, zopiclone raised the arousal threshold without reducing genioglossus muscle activity (50). Eszopiclone 3 mg has been shown to increase arousal threshold and reduce OSA severity by ~45% in people with OSA and low arousal thresholds (51). Trazodone has also been shown to increase the arousal threshold in those with a low arousal threshold (52) and reduce OSA severity in unselected patients (53). These small studies suggest a potential role for the use of hypnotics in patients with OSA and low arousal thresholds. However, most hypnotic trials in people with OSA do not systematically alter the AHI (54–58) and as such, further data are required before pharmacologically increasing the arousal threshold can be recommended as a treatment for OSA.

Loop Gain

Ventilation is dependent on sensory feedback and control loops that respond to changes in respiratory stimuli. The overall sensitivity (or *gain*) of a feedback control system is known as loop gain. In terms of ventilatory control, loop gain is the ratio of the magnitude of the ventilatory response to that of the respiratory disturbance that initiated it. Loop gain is a product of both sensory control sensitivity (controller gain) and "plant" gain, which reflects the ability of ventilation to change the sensory stimulus, which for ventilation during sleep is predominantly blood CO_2 levels. The magnitude of an individual's ventilatory response to fluctuations in CO_2 and that of resulting changes in CO_2 varies from person to person and according to a range of dynamically changing factors including ventilation, CO_2 levels, metabolic rate, sleep stage, and lung volume. Individuals with inherently unstable or overly sensitive responses to CO_2 (*high loop gain*) are at increased risk of CSA and OSA (59).

High loop gain can contribute to OSA via two main mechanisms. Firstly, excessive hyperventilation that overcompensates for a relatively small change in CO_2 may cause large negative inspiratory pressures in the pharyngeal airway, beyond the capacity of the upper airway dilator muscles to maintain patency (60). Secondly, breathing patterns in those with high loop gain are characterized by oscillations between hyperventilation or "overshoot" and hypoventilation or "undershoot" instead of stable ventilation and CO_2 at an intermediate stable set-point. During periods of hypocapnia, neural drive to the upper-airway dilator muscles is transiently reduced and a potential mismatch between transmural airway collapsing forces and upper airway muscle dilator activity needed to oppose them can occur, precipitating partial or complete collapse of the pharyngeal airway (1). Medications that reduce loop gain may therefore help to stabilize ventilation and reduce OSA severity.

An important consideration for the clinical use of endotyping to guide precision medicine for SDB is the stability of each trait. While there is some evidence that key traits are quite reproducible in the short term (61, 62), determining immutability versus plasticity for each of the traits requires further investigation. Indeed, components of respiratory control that contribute to loop gain and the arousal threshold have been reported to change following CPAP therapy (63).

Carbonic Anhydrase Inhibitors

Carbonic anhydrase inhibitors reduce bicarbonate reabsorption in the proximal convoluted tubule of the kidney. This induces metabolic acidosis, leading to an increase in ventilation that drives down the blood partial pressure of carbon dioxide ($PaCO_2$), which reduces the alveolar-inspired CO_2 gradient and loop gain (64). In patients with high loop gain, a combination of increased ventilatory drive to upper airway muscles along with reduced $PaCO_2$ and loop gain may be sufficient to achieve stable ventilation in sleep without airway collapse.

The carbonic anhydrase inhibitor acetazolamide at a dose of 500 mg sustained-release twice daily for 1 week reduces loop gain and improves AHI in people with moderate-to-severe OSA without negatively affecting the other key OSA traits (65). Another carbonic anhydrase inhibitor, zonisamide, reduced the AHI by ~30% in a group of 47 patients with moderate-to-severe OSA. Loop gain was not directly measured, but the effect on AHI was heterogeneous, suggesting that zonisamide improved OSA in the subgroup of patients with high loop gain but not in those in whom other endotypes predominate (66).

Supplemental Oxygen

Supplemental oxygen stabilizes ventilatory drive, primarily through reducing peripheral chemosensitivity. In people with high loop gain and OSA, supplemental oxygen administered during sleep between 3 and 5 l/min reduces the AHI and ventilatory instability, although it often does not resolve OSA completely (67). The beneficial effect of oxygen supplementation does not occur in people with OSA who have low loop gain (67). Administration of oxygen does not alter the other key OSA traits (68).

When oxygen is used in conjunction with the hypnotic eszopiclone in patients with OSA, reductions in AHI occur in those with less collapsible upper airways and increased upper airway muscle effectiveness (69). This suggests that benefits occur through a reduction in loop gain and an increase in arousal threshold. These data highlight the benefits of identifying underlying OSA causes or endotypic traits to inform targeted pharmacotherapy for OSA (70).

PHARMACOLOGICAL MANAGEMENT OF CSA

CSA is characterized by cyclical waxing and waning of respiratory drive and consequently ventilation and CO_2 during sleep. This leads to periods of absent ventilation, gas exchange disturbances, and frequent arousals during periods of excessive ventilation. The pathophysiology of CSA and OSA overlap considerably, and both conditions can be present in the same individual. There are many causes of CSA, including the effects of high altitude, narcotics, and several medical conditions including heart failure, stroke, and pulmonary hypertension. While the causes of CSA vary, unstable ventilatory control during sleep is a key underlying feature. Various medications, outlined below, have shown benefit in stabilizing ventilatory drive in CSA.

Steroids

At altitudes high enough to induce alveolar hypoxia, approximately 3,000 m and above, most healthy individuals develop periodic breathing (71–73). Prior to acclimatization, sleep at high altitudes is characterized by lower oxygen saturations, reduced sleep efficiency, higher AHI, and reduced slow-wave sleep (74). At an altitude of 4,559 m, dexamethasone reduces periodic breathing and improves nocturnal oxygen saturations in healthy

mountaineers with a history of susceptibility to high-altitude pulmonary edema (75). In people with chronic obstructive pulmonary disease who live below 800 m, dexamethasone prevents the emergence of CSA when traveling to high altitudes (76). The primary mechanisms for these effects are not clear.

Respiratory Stimulants

Respiratory stimulants such as acetazolamide, theophylline, and carbon dioxide increase ventilation, and can reduce CSA severity arising from high altitude, heart failure, and idiopathic CSA.

Acetazolamide

The metabolic acidosis induced by acetazolamide increases ventilation, causes a leftward shift of the hypercapnic ventilatory response, and lowers the $PaCO_2$ apnea threshold (77, 78). Acetazolamide also reduces plant gain (the change of PCO_2 per unit change in ventilation) (79) and increases the response time of the respiratory circuit to changes in $PaCO_2$ secondary to increased cerebral blood flow (80). These interacting mechanisms reduce unstable breathing in CSA.

A meta-analysis of eight randomized controlled trials assessed the effect of acetazolamide on periodic breathing and AHI in healthy participants and people with OSA from low altitudes ascending above 2,500 m (81). In healthy participants, acetazolamide caused a significant reduction in AHI, periodic breathing, and increased nocturnal oxygen saturation at high altitudes. Acetazolamide was less effective in those with a prior diagnosis of OSA, presumably because acetazolamide would not be expected to improve upper airway muscle activity, anatomical impairment, or alter arousal thresholds. A short-term case series demonstrated beneficial effects of acetazolamide in idiopathic CSA, but there are no randomized controlled trials to support these findings (82).

Acetazolamide is also effective in reducing CSA in patients with heart failure with a reduced ejection fraction. However, the level of evidence available to support its clinical use is low. Acetazolamide reduces central apnea events, nocturnal oxygen desaturations, daytime fatigue and increases perceived sleep quality (83, 84). However, there is heterogeneity in the response with some patients exhibiting large improvements while others respond minimally. In those with minimal AHI improvements, a major contributing factor is acetazolamide-related *increased* CO_2

chemosensitivity, as acetazolamide increased the slope of the hypercapnic ventilatory response in one small but detailed study, with the greatest increases seen in those who achieved smaller reductions in AHI (84). Larger, similarly detailed studies are required to further investigate these complex physiological changes.

Theophylline

The phosphodiesterase inhibitor theophylline improves sleep-disordered breathing (SDB) through several mechanisms. At therapeutic concentrations, theophylline competes with the respiratory depressant adenosine at receptor sites, stimulating central respiratory drive (85). Theophylline also reduces hypoxic ventilatory depression and, in the case of heart failure, reduces circulation time secondary to positive inotropic effects (72, 86).

In healthy men after rapid ascent to high altitude (3,454 m), slow-release theophylline reduced periodic breathing and improved the oxygen desaturation index during sleep compared to placebo, as measured by polysomnography on two consecutive nights (87). Likewise, in a placebo-controlled study of healthy men at 4,559 m, theophylline reduced periodic breathing and the oxygen desaturation index (88). Theophylline also reduced the severity of acute mountain sickness experienced by participants at high altitudes. However, it did not improve mean oxygen saturation during sleep in either study.

In heart failure with a reduced ejection fraction (HFrEF), theophylline reduces periodic breathing. In a double-blind placebo-controlled crossover study of 15 patients with HFrEF, theophylline reduced central apneas by ~20 events/hr sleep versus placebo (89). Overnight oxygen saturation also improved. An important mechanism by which theophylline reduces periodic breathing in HFrEF is through its stimulatory effect on ventilation. In a randomized placebo-controlled study including 22 patients with HFrEF, theophylline reduced awake transcutaneous PCO_2 and increased minute ventilation (90). Despite the potential benefits of theophylline as a treatment for periodic breathing, further studies are required to determine its safety in populations with heart disease, due to its potential arrhythmogenic effects.

Carbon Dioxide

Supplemental CO_2 reduces CSA by maintaining $PaCO_2$ above the CO_2 apnea threshold. In six patients with idiopathic CSA, supplemental CO_2 substantially reduced the AHI when administered continuously or alternating with room air breathing (91). Inhaled CO_2 can also be a beneficial adjunct to positive airway pressure in men with severe refractory mixed SDB (92). In six patients with heart failure and CSA, inhaled CO_2 during sleep administered in 10-minute periods alternating with air inhalation abolished apneas (93). However, these effects have not been studied as a therapeutic intervention for CSA in large numbers. Furthermore, there are safety concerns regarding excessive hypercapnia and potential counter-productive cortical arousal effects of augmented ventilation. Arousals elevate sympathetic nerve activity, potentially contributing to unstable breathing and a poorer prognosis in patients with heart failure and CSA (94–97).

Hypnotics

A limited number of small studies have shown beneficial effects of hypnotic medications on CSA. The proposed mechanism of this effect is to increase the arousal threshold, thereby preventing excessive ventilation that follows an arousal. Triazolam and zolpidem have both been shown to reduce central events and the arousal index and to improve sleep efficiency in idiopathic CSA (98, 99). Other studies have demonstrated improvements in sleep architecture with temazepam, zolpidem, and zaleplon at high altitude, without AHI improvement (100, 101). Larger, randomized studies including detailed measurements of arousal threshold are needed to evaluate the role and mechanisms of hypnotics more thoroughly in CSA treatment.

Oxygen Enrichment

Supplemental oxygen improves CSA in healthy individuals at high altitudes, and in patients with CSA secondary to heart failure or pulmonary hypertension. In Chilean miners who live at low altitude but work and stay at high altitudes for 7 days at a time, oxygen enrichment at 4,200 m to reduce the effective altitude to between 2,700 and 3,300 m (i.e. FiO_2 approximately 24%) markedly reduced the AHI and improved overnight oxygen saturations on a single night (102). Oxygen supplementation modestly reduces AHI in patients with CSA and HFrEF (103, 104) and a subset of patients exhibit much greater reductions (103). The reasons for this heterogeneous response are not well understood, but likely reflect the complex and multifactorial nature of CSA pathogenesis in heart failure, including diversity in oxygen chemosensitivity, arousal threshold, and other factors between patients.

In precapillary pulmonary hypertension, nocturnal supplemental oxygen reduces AHI, although large, high-quality studies have not been performed. In a small cohort of five patients, 2 l/min nocturnal oxygen therapy reduced periodic breathing during sleep (105). In a larger study of 16 participants, nocturnal oxygen therapy moderately reduced AHI and improved daytime exercise capacity (106). The mechanisms underlying oxygen therapy benefits in precapillary pulmonary hypertension-related CSA are unclear, but are likely similar to those in heart failure-related periodic breathing, including prolonged circulation time and hypoxic stimulation of peripheral chemoreceptors (105). Larger studies are needed to determine the significance of and optimal treatments for periodic breathing in pulmonary hypertension (107).

CONCLUSIONS

OSA and CSA are heterogeneous diseases with multiple underlying endotypes and complex and overlapping pathophysiology. The variety of mechanisms that contribute to both diseases provide targets for pharmacological treatment. Some underlying traits, such as impaired muscle responsiveness in OSA, appear to be particularly promising treatment targets for current medications and newer pharmacotherapies that are currently under development. While current evidence supports the use of a wide range of medications as treatment options for OSA and CSA, more detailed studies assessing pathophysiological changes, and larger long-term randomized trials to examine comparative effectiveness and safety are needed to develop more effective future pharmacological therapies.

REFERENCES

1. Eckert DJ, White DP, Jordan AS, Malhotra A, Wellman A. Defining phenotypic causes of obstructive sleep apnea. Identification of novel therapeutic targets. American Journal of Respiratory and Critical Care Medicine 2013;188:996–1004.

2. Sands SA, Edwards BA, Terrill PI, et al. Phenotyping pharyngeal pathophysiology using polysomnography in patients with obstructive sleep apnea. American Journal of Respiratory and Critical Care Medicine 2018;197:1187–97.

3. Kim AM, Keenan BT, Jackson N, et al. Tongue fat and its relationship to obstructive sleep apnea. Sleep 2014;37:1639–48.

4. Sands SA, Edwards BA, Kee K, et al. Loop gain as a means to predict a positive airway pressure

suppression of Cheyne-Stokes respiration in patients with heart failure. American Journal of Respiratory and Critical Care Medicine 2011;184:1067–75.

5. Stadler DL, McEvoy RD, Sprecher KE, et al. Abdominal compression increases upper airway collapsibility during sleep in obese male obstructive sleep apnea patients. Sleep 2009;32:1579–87.

6. White LH, Bradley TD. Role of nocturnal rostral fluid shift in the pathogenesis of obstructive and central sleep apnoea. The Journal of Physiology 2013;591:1179–93.

7. Blackman A, Foster GD, Zammit G, et al. Effect of liraglutide 3.0 mg in individuals with obesity and moderate or severe obstructive sleep apnea: the SCALE sleep apnea randomized clinical trial. Int Journal of Obesity (Lond) 2016;40:1310–9.

8. Garvey WT. Phentermine and topiramate extended-release: a new treatment for obesity and its role in a complications-centric approach to obesity medical management. Expert Opinion on Drug Safety 2013;12:741–56.

9. Garvey WT, Ryan DH, Look M, et al. Two-year sustained weight loss and metabolic benefits with controlled-release phentermine/topiramate in obese and overweight adults (SEQUEL): a randomized, placebo-controlled, phase 3 extension study. The American Journal of Clinical Nutrition 2011;95:297–308.

10. Winslow DH, Bowden CH, DiDonato KP, McCullough PA. A randomized, double-blind, placebo-controlled study of an oral, extended-release formulation of phentermine/topiramate for the treatment of obstructive sleep apnea in obese adults. Sleep 2012;35:1529–39.

11. Yee BJ, Phillips CL, Banerjee D, Caterson I, Hedner JA, Grunstein RR. The effect of sibutramine-assisted weight loss in men with obstructive sleep apnoea. International Journal of Obesity 2007;31:161–8.

12. James WP, Caterson ID, Coutinho W, et al. Effect of sibutramine on cardiovascular outcomes in overweight and obese subjects. New England Journal of Medicine 2010;363:905–17.

13. Hudgel DW, Patel SR, Ahasic AM, et al. The role of weight management in the treatment of adult obstructive sleep apnea. An official American Thoracic Society Clinical Practice Guideline. American Journal of Respiratory and Critical Care Medicine 2018;198:e70–e87.

14. Fiori CZ, Martinez D, Montanari CC, et al. Diuretic or sodium-restricted diet for obstructive sleep apnea-a randomized trial. Sleep 2018;41 (4): zsy016. https://doi.org/10.1093/sleep/zsy016.

15. Bucca CB, Brussino L, Battisti A, et al. Diuretics in obstructive sleep apnea with diastolic heart failure. Chest 2007;132:440–6.

16. Gaddam K, Pimenta E, Thomas SJ, et al. Spironolactone reduces severity of obstructive sleep apnoea in patients

with resistant hypertension: a preliminary report. Journal of Human Hypertension 2010;24:532–7.

17. Kasai T, Bradley TD, Friedman O, Logan AG. Effect of intensified diuretic therapy on overnight rostral fluid shift and obstructive sleep apnoea in patients with uncontrolled hypertension. Journal of Hypertension 2014;32:673–80.

18. Sauerland EK, Harper RM. The human tongue during sleep: electromyographic activity of the genioglossus muscle. Experimental Neurology 1976;51:160–70.

19. Carberry JC, Jordan AS, White DP, Wellman A, Eckert DJ. Upper airway collapsibility (Pcrit) and pharyngeal dilator muscle activity are sleep stage dependent. Sleep 2016;39:511–21.

20. Eckert DJ, Malhotra A, Lo YL, White DP, Jordan AS. The influence of obstructive sleep apnea and gender on genioglossus activity during rapid eye movement sleep. Chest 2009;135:957–64.

21. Carley DW, Radulovacki M. Pharmacology of vagal afferent influences on disordered breathing during sleep. Respiratory Physiology and Neurobiology 2008;164:197–203.

22. Chan E, Steenland HW, Liu H, Horner RL. Endogenous excitatory drive modulating respiratory muscle activity across sleep-wake states. American Journal of Respiratory and Critical Care Medicine 2006;174:1264–73.

23. Fenik VB, Davies RO, Kubin L. REM sleep-like atonia of hypoglossal (XII) motoneurons is caused by loss of noradrenergic and serotonergic inputs. American Journal of Respiratory and Critical Care Medicine 2005;172:1322–30.

24. Sood S, Morrison JL, Liu H, Horner RL. Role of endogenous serotonin in modulating genioglossus muscle activity in awake and sleeping rats. American Journal of Respiratory and Critical Care Medicine 2005;172:1338–47.

25. Burgess C, Lai D, Siegel J, Peever J. An endogenous glutamatergic drive onto somatic motoneurons contributes to the stereotypical pattern of muscle tone across the sleep-wake cycle. Journal of Neuroscience 2008;28:4649–60.

26. Grace KP, Hughes SW, Horner RL. Identification of the mechanism mediating genioglossus muscle suppression in REM sleep. American Journal of Respiratory and Critical Care Medicine 2013;187:311–9.

27. Prasad B, Radulovacki MG, Carley DW. Proof of concept trial of dronabinol in obstructive sleep apnea. Frontiers in Psychiatry 2013;4:1.

28. Carley DW, Prasad B, Reid KJ, et al. Pharmacotherapy of apnea by cannabimimetic enhancement, the PACE clinical trial: effects of dronabinol in obstructive sleep apnea. Sleep 2018;41(1): zsx184. https://doi.org/10.1093/sleep/zsx184.

29. Kraiczi H, Hedner J, Dahlöf P, Ejnell H, Carlson J. Effect of serotonin uptake inhibition on breathing during sleep and daytime symptoms in obstructive sleep apnea. Sleep 1999;22:61–7.

30. Hanzel DA, Proia NG, Hudgel DW. Response of obstructive sleep apnea to fluoxetine and protriptyline. Chest 1991;100:416–21.

31. Carley DW, Olopade C, Ruigt GS, Radulovacki M. Efficacy of mirtazapine in obstructive sleep apnea syndrome. Sleep 2007;30:35–41.

32. Marshall NS, Yee BJ, Desai AV, et al. Two randomized placebo-controlled trials to evaluate the efficacy and tolerability of mirtazapine for the treatment of obstructive sleep apnea. Sleep 2008;31:824–31.

33. Taranto-Montemurro L, Edwards BA, Sands SA, et al. Desipramine increases genioglossus activity and reduces upper airway collapsibility during non-REM sleep in healthy subjects. American Journal of Respiratory and Critical Care Medicine 2016;194:878–85.

34. Taranto-Montemurro L, Sands SA, Edwards BA, et al. Desipramine improves upper airway collapsibility and reduces OSA severity in patients with minimal muscle compensation. European Respiratory Journal 2016;48:1340–50.

35. Taranto-Montemurro L, Messineo L, Sands SA, et al. The combination of atomoxetine and oxybutynin greatly reduces obstructive sleep apnea severity. A randomized, placebo-controlled, double-blind crossover trial. American Journal of Respiratory and Critical Care Medicine 2019;199:1267–76.

36. Lim R, Carberry JC, Wellman A, Grunstein R, Eckert DJ. Reboxetine and hyoscine butylbromide improve upper airway function during nonrapid eye movement and suppress rapid eye movement sleep in healthy individuals. Sleep 2019;42(4): zsy261. https://doi.org/10.1093/sleep/zsy261.

37. Carberry JC, Fisher LP, Grunstein RR, et al. Role of common hypnotics on the phenotypic causes of obstructive sleep apnoea: paradoxical effects of zolpidem. European Respiratory Journal 2017;50:1701344.

38. Che Has AT, Absalom N, van Nieuwenhuijzen PS, Clarkson AN, Ahring PK, Chebib M. Zolpidem is a potent stoichiometry-selective modulator of $\alpha1\beta3$ GABAA receptors: evidence of a novel benzodiazepine site in the $\alpha1$-$\alpha1$ interface. Scientific Reports 2016;6:28674.

39. Berry RB, Kouchi K, Bower J, Prosise G, Light RW. Triazolam in patients with obstructive sleep apnea. American Journal of Respiratory and Critical Care Medicine 1995;151:450–4.

40. Horton GA, Fraigne JJ, Torontali ZA, et al. Activation of the hypoglossal to tongue musculature motor pathway by remote control. Scientific Reports 2017;7:45860.

41. Fleury Curado T, Fishbein K, Pho H, et al. Chemogenetic stimulation of the hypoglossal neurons improves upper airway patency. Scientific Reports 2017;7:44392.

42. Fleury Curado T, Pho H, Freire C, et al. Designer receptors exclusively activated by designer drugs approach to treatment of sleep-disordered breathing. American Journal of Respiratory and Critical Care Medicine 2021;203:102–10.

43. Gleeson K, Zwillich CW, White DP. The influence of increasing ventilatory effort on arousal from sleep. American Review of Respiratory Disease 1990;142:295–300.

44. Gray EL, McKenzie DK, Eckert DJ. Obstructive sleep apnea without obesity is common and difficult to treat: evidence for a distinct pathophysiological phenotype. Journal of Clinical Sleep Medicine 2017;13:81–8.

45. Ratnavadivel R, Chau N, Stadler D, Yeo A, McEvoy RD, Catcheside PG. Marked reduction in obstructive sleep apnea severity in slow wave sleep. Journal of Clinical Sleep Medicine 2009;5:519–24.

46. Jordan AS, White DP, Lo Y-L, et al. Airway dilator muscle activity and lung volume during stable breathing in obstructive sleep apnea. Sleep 2009;32:361–8.

47. Younes M, Ostrowski M, Atkar R, Laprairie J, Siemens A, Hanly P. Mechanisms of breathing instability in patients with obstructive sleep apnea. Journal of Applied Physiology 2007;103:1929–41.

48. Younes M. Role of arousals in the pathogenesis of obstructive sleep apnea. American Journal of Respiratory and Critical Care Medicine 2004;169:623–33.

49. Iber C, Davies SF, Chapman RC, Mahowald MM. A possible mechanism for mixed apnea in obstructive sleep apnea. Chest 1986;89:800–5.

50. Carter SG, Berger MS, Carberry JC, et al. Zopiclone increases the arousal threshold without impairing genioglossus activity in obstructive sleep apnea. Sleep 2016;39:757–66.

51. Eckert DJ, Owens RL, Kehlmann GB, et al. Eszopiclone increases the respiratory arousal threshold and lowers the apnoea/hypopnoea index in obstructive sleep apnoea patients with a low arousal threshold. Clinical Science (Lond) 2011;120:505–14.

52. Eckert DJ, Malhotra A, Wellman A, White DP. Trazodone increases the respiratory arousal threshold in patients with obstructive sleep apnea and a low arousal threshold. Sleep 2014;37:811–9.

53. Smales ET, Edwards BA, Deyoung PN, et al. Trazodone effects on obstructive sleep apnea and non-REM arousal threshold. Annals of the American Thoracic Society 2015;12:758–64.

54. Eckert DJ, Younes MK. Arousal from sleep: implications for obstructive sleep apnea pathogenesis and treatment. Journal of Applied Physiology 2014;116:302–13.

55. Jordan AS, O'Donoghue FJ, Cori JM, Trinder J. Physiology of arousal in obstructive sleep apnea and potential impacts for sedative treatment. American Journal of Respiratory and Critical Care Medicine 2017;196:814–21.

56. Messineo L, Eckert DJ, Lim R, et al. Zolpidem increases sleep efficiency and the respiratory arousal threshold without changing sleep apnoea severity and pharyngeal muscle activity. Journal of Physiology 2020;598:4681–92.

57. Carter SG, Carberry JC, Cho G, et al. Effect of 1 month of zopiclone on obstructive sleep apnoea severity and symptoms: a randomised controlled trial. European Respiratory Journal 2018;52:1800149.

58. Carter SG, Carberry JC, Grunstein RR, Eckert DJ. Randomized trial on the effects of high-dose zopiclone on OSA severity, upper airway physiology, and alertness. Chest 2020;158:374–85.

59. Wellman A, Jordan AS, Malhotra A, et al. Ventilatory control and airway anatomy in obstructive sleep apnea. American Journal of Respiratory and Critical Care Medicine 2004;170:1225–32.

60. Eckert DJ. Phenotypic approaches to obstructive sleep apnoea – new pathways for targeted therapy. Sleep Medicine Reviews 2018;37:45–59.

61. Wellman A, Eckert DJ, Jordan AS, et al. A method for measuring and modeling the physiological traits causing obstructive sleep apnea. Journal of Applied Physiology 2011;110:1627–37.

62. Kirkness JP, Peterson LA, Squier SB, et al. Performance characteristics of upper airway critical collapsing pressure measurements during sleep. Sleep 2011;34:459–67.

63. Loewen A, Ostrowski M, Laprairie J, et al. Determinants of ventilatory instability in obstructive sleep apnea: inherent or acquired? Sleep 2009;32:1355–65.

64. Khoo MC, Kronauer RE, Strohl KP, Slutsky AS. Factors inducing periodic breathing in humans: a general model. Journal of Applied Physiology 1982;53:644–59.

65. Edwards BA, Sands SA, Eckert DJ, et al. Acetazolamide improves loop gain but not the other physiological traits causing obstructive sleep apnea. Journal of Physiology 2012;590:1199–211.

66. Eskandari D, Zou D, Karimi M, Stenlöf K, Grote L, Hedner J. Zonisamide reduces obstructive sleep apnoea: a randomised placebo-controlled study. European Respiratory Journal 2014;44:140–9.

67. Wellman A, Malhotra A, Jordan AS, Stevenson KE, Gautam S, White DP. Effect of oxygen in obstructive sleep apnea: role of loop gain. Respiratory Physiology and Neurobiology 2008;162:144–51.

68. Edwards BA, Sands SA, Owens RL, et al. Effects of hyperoxia and hypoxia on the physiological traits responsible for obstructive sleep apnoea. Journal of Physiology 2014;592:4523–35.

69. Edwards BA, Sands SA, Owens RL, et al. The combination of supplemental oxygen and a hypnotic markedly improves obstructive sleep apnea in patients with a mild to moderate upper airway collapsibility. Sleep 2016;39:1973–83.

70. Messineo L, Magri R, Corda L, Pini L, Taranto-Montemurro L, Tantucci C. Phenotyping-based treatment improves obstructive sleep apnea symptoms and severity: a pilot study. Sleep and Breathing 2017;21:861–8.

71. White DP, Gleeson K, Pickett CK, Rannels AM, Cymerman A, Weil JV. Altitude acclimatization: influence on periodic breathing and chemoresponsiveness during sleep. Journal of Applied Physiology 1987;63:401–12.

72. Eckert DJ, Jordan AS, Merchia P, Malhotra A. Central sleep apnea: pathophysiology and treatment. Chest 2007;131:595–607.

73. West JB, Hackett PH, Maret KH, et al. Pulmonary gas exchange on the summit of Mount Everest. Journal of Applied Physiology: Respiratory, Environmental and Exercise Physiology 1983;55:678–87.

74. Nussbaumer-Ochsner Y, Ursprung J, Siebenmann C, Maggiorini M, Bloch KE. Effect of short-term acclimatization to high altitude on sleep and nocturnal breathing. Sleep 2012;35:419–23.

75. Nussbaumer-Ochsner Y, Schuepfer N, Ursprung J, Siebenmann C, Maggiorini M, Bloch KE. Sleep and breathing in high altitude pulmonary edema susceptible subjects at 4,559 meters. Sleep 2012;35:1413–21.

76. Furian M, Lichtblau M, Aeschbacher SS, et al. Effect of dexamethasone on nocturnal oxygenation in lowlanders with chronic obstructive pulmonary disease traveling to 3100 meters: a randomized clinical trial. JAMA Network Open 2019;2:e190067.

77. White DP, Zwillich CW, Pickett CK, Douglas NJ, Findley LJ, Weil JV. Central sleep apnea: improvement with acetazolamide therapy. Archives of Internal Medicine 1982;142:1816–9.

78. Nakayama H, Smith CA, Rodman JR, Skatrud JB, Dempsey JA. Effect of ventilatory drive on carbon dioxide sensitivity below eupnea during sleep. American Journal of Respiratory and Critical Care Medicine 2002;165:1251–60.

79. Ginter G, Sankari A, Eshraghi M, et al. Effect of acetazolamide on susceptibility to central sleep apnea in chronic spinal cord injury. Journal of Applied Physiology 2020;128:960–6.

80. Fan JL, Burgess KR, Thomas KN, et al. Effects of acetazolamide on cerebrovascular function and breathing stability at 5050 m. Journal of Physiology 2012;590:1213–25.

81. Liu HM, Chiang IJ, Kuo KN, Liou CM, Chen C. The effect of acetazolamide on sleep apnea at high altitude: a systematic review and meta-analysis. Therapeutic Advances in Respiratory Disease 2017;11:20–9.

82. DeBacker WA, Verbraecken J, Willemen M, Wittesaele W, DeCock W, Van deHeyning P. Central apnea index decreases after prolonged treatment with acetazolamide. American Journal of Respiratory and Critical Care Medicine 1995;151:87–91.

83. Javaheri S. Acetazolamide improves central sleep apnea in heart failure: a double-blind, prospective study. American Journal of Respiratory and Critical Care Medicine 2006;173:234–7.

84. Javaheri S, Sands SA, Edwards BA. Acetazolamide attenuates Hunter-Cheyne-Stokes breathing but augments the hypercapnic ventilatory response in patients with heart failure. Annals of the American Thoracic Society 2014;11:80–6.

85. Hudgel DW, Thanakitcharu S. Pharmacologic treatment of sleep-disordered breathing. American Journal of Respiratory and Critical Care Medicine 1998;158:691–9.

86. Lakshminarayan S, Sahn SA, Weil JV. Effect of Aminophylline on ventilatory responses in normal man. American Review of Respiratory Disease 1978;117:33–8.

87. Fischer R, Lang SM, Leitl M, Thiere M, Steiner U, Huber RM. Theophylline and acetazolamide reduce sleep-disordered breathing at high altitude. European Respiratory Journal 2004;23:47–52.

88. Küpper TE, Strohl KP, Hoefer M, Gieseler U, Netzer CM, Netzer NC. Low-dose theophylline reduces symptoms of acute mountain sickness. Journal of Travel Medicine 2008;15:307–14.

89. Javaheri S, Parker TJ, Wexler L, Liming JD, Lindower P, Roselle GA. Effect of theophylline on sleep-disordered breathing in heart failure. New England Journal of Medicine 1996;335:562–7.

90. Andreas S, Reiter H, Lüthje L, et al. Differential effects of theophylline on sympathetic excitation, hemodynamics, and breathing in congestive heart failure. Circulation 2004;110:2157–62.

91. Xie A, Rankin F, Rutherford R, Bradley TD. Effects of inhaled CO_2 and added dead space on idiopathic central sleep apnea. Journal of Applied Physiology 1997;82:918–26.

92. Thomas RJ, Daly RW, Weiss JW. Low-concentration carbon dioxide is an effective adjunct to positive airway pressure in the treatment of refractory mixed central and obstructive sleep-disordered breathing. Sleep 2005;28:69–77.

93. Lorenzi-Filho G, Rankin F, Bies I, Douglas Bradley T. Effects of inhaled carbon dioxide and oxygen on Cheyne-Stokes respiration in patients with heart failure. American Journal of Respiratory and Critical Care Medicine 1999;159:1490–8.

94. Szollosi I, Jones M, Morrell MJ, Helfet K, Coats AJ, Simonds AK. Effect of CO_2 inhalation on central sleep apnea and arousals from sleep. Respiration 2004;71:493–8.

95. Cohn JN, Levine TB, Olivari MT, et al. Plasma norepinephrine as a guide to prognosis in patients with chronic congestive heart failure. New England Journal of Medicine 1984;311:819–23.

96. Leimbach WN, Jr., Wallin BG, Victor RG, Aylward PE, Sundlöf G, Mark AL. Direct evidence from intraneural recordings for increased central sympathetic outflow in patients with heart failure. Circulation 1986;73:913–9.

97. Hanly PJ, Zuberi-Khokhar NS. Increased mortality associated with Cheyne-Stokes respiration in patients with congestive heart failure. American Journal of Respiratory and Critical Care Medicine 1996;153:272–6.

98. Quadri S, Drake C, Hudgel DW. Improvement of idiopathic central sleep apnea with zolpidem. Journal of Clinical Sleep Medicine 2009;5:122–9.

99. Bonnet MH, Dexter JR, Arand DL. The effect of triazolam on arousal and respiration in central sleep apnea patients. Sleep 1990;13:31–41.

100. Beaumont M, Batéjat D, Coste O, et al. Effects of zolpidem and zaleplon on sleep, respiratory patterns and performance at a simulated altitude of 4,000 m. Neuropsychobiology 2004;49:154–62.

101. Nicholson AN, Smith PA, Stone BM, Bradwell AR, Coote JH. Altitude insomnia: studies during an expedition to the Himalayas. Sleep 1988;11:354–61.

102. Moraga FA, Jiménez D, Richalet JP, Vargas M, Osorio J. Periodic breathing and oxygen supplementation in Chilean miners at high altitude (4200m). Respiratory Physiology and Neurobiology 2014;203:109–15.

103. Javaheri S, Ahmed M, Parker TJ, Brown CR. Effects of nasal O_2 on sleep-related disordered breathing in ambulatory patients with stable heart failure. Sleep 1999;22:1101–6.

104. Krachman SL, D'Alonzo GE, Berger TJ, Eisen HJ. Comparison of oxygen therapy with nasal continuous positive airway pressure on Cheyne-Stokes respiration during sleep in congestive heart failure. Chest 1999;116:1550–7.

105. Schulz R, Baseler G, Ghofrani HA, Grimminger F, Olschewski H, Seeger W. Nocturnal periodic breathing in primary pulmonary hypertension. European Respiratory Journal 2002;19:658–63.

106. Ulrich S, Keusch S, Hildenbrand FF, et al. Effect of nocturnal oxygen and acetazolamide on exercise performance in patients with pre-capillary pulmonary hypertension and sleep-disturbed breathing: randomized, double-blind, cross-over trial. European Heart Journal 2015;36:615–23.

107. Randerath W, Verbraecken J, Andreas S, et al. Definition, discrimination, diagnosis and treatment of central breathing disturbances during sleep. European Respiratory Journal 2017;49:1600959.

108. Carberry JC, Amatoury J, Eckert DJ. Personalized management approach for OSA. Chest 2018;153:744–55.

109. Aishah A, Eckert DJ. Phenotypic approach to pharmacotherapy in the management of obstructive sleep apnoea. Current Opinion in Pulmonary Medicine 2019;25:594–601.

19 Neural Mechanisms Regulating Opioid-Induced Respiratory Depression and Therapeutic Strategies to Alleviate the Respiratory Side-Effects of Opioid Drugs

Jean-Philippe Rousseau and Gaspard Montandon

THE OPIOID EPIDEMIC

Opiates were first extracted from the juice obtained from the poppy flower, *Papaver somniferum* (1), and opium poppy was referred to as the "plant of joy" (2). The medicinal analgesic properties of opiates were mentioned in Sumerians archives as far as 6000 BC. The use of opium for medical purposes can also be traced back to the Hippocratic collection around 400 BC. While Hippocrates mostly referred in his texts to the use of opium as a sleep-inducing substance, it is presumed that he knew its analgesic properties as he used it for pain treatment (3). Opiates refer to the natural opioid drugs extracted and/or synthesized from the opium poppy. Morphine, an opioid analgesic widely used in clinical practice, was first isolated in the early 1800s by Wilhelm Sertürner (2). The broader term opioids also includes synthetic drugs such as fentanyl and oxycodone, which are not derived from the opium poppy, but bind to the μ-opioid receptors (MORs) with high affinity (4, 5).

A significant opioid epidemic is currently raging in North America. According to the Centers for Disease Control and Prevention, 67,357 overdose deaths occurred in the United States in 2018, with two out of three opioid-involved overdose deaths involving synthetic opioids. Opioid overdoses can be caused by the misuse of prescribed drugs, such as oxycodone and morphine, or street drugs like heroin and fentanyl (6). While opioid addiction is a major health issue since it often leads to drug abuse, overdose deaths are caused by respiratory depression, asphyxiation, and bradycardia (5). Taken at high dosage or in combination with other centrally depressant drugs (sleep medication or alcohol), opioids substantially depress ventilation by reducing the respiratory rate and tidal volume and can lead to respiratory arrest, hypoxemia, and eventually death if not treated with the opioid antidote naloxone (7). Although the epidemic of opioid overdose is causing severe health and financial burdens on society (8), the pathophysiology underlying the life-threatening respiratory depression due to opioid misuse is still unclear. To better understand the mechanisms of action of opioid drugs on the neural control of breathing, we propose to highlight the recent biomedical and clinical studies investigating these mechanisms.

OPIOID-INDUCED RESPIRATORY DEPRESSION

Opioids are a group of drugs acting on a class of G-protein-coupled opioid receptors in the nervous system. Opioids can bind to μ-, δ-, and κ-opioid receptors (9). The analgesic, addictive and respiratory effects of opioids are mostly mediated by their action on MORs and δ-opioid receptors expressed in the specific cortical, subcortical, brainstem, and spinal cord circuits (5, 10), but also on respiratory muscles (11–13). Opioid drugs decrease respiratory rate (14) and reduce tidal volume (13) (Figure 19.1). These drugs also increase upper airways resistance through vocal cord closure and tracheal constriction (15–17), alter lower airway resistance via a bronchoconstriction, and increase pulmonary vascular resistance, therefore affecting gas exchange (18, 19). They also impair respiratory pump muscle functions induced by thoracic rigidity and inadequate diaphragmatic respiratory timing (20, 21). The sensitivities to oxygen and carbon dioxide are also affected by opioids, as they depress the ability of the respiratory control system to respond to hypoxia and hypercapnia (22–25). With opioid overdose, breathing is shallow and can completely stop leading to severe hypoxia and brain hypoxemia as well as cardiac failure, and eventually organ failure such as brain death (26). Despite years of research investigating opioid drugs and the respiratory system, the neural mechanisms mediating respiratory depression are not well understood.

OPIOID DRUGS ACT ON NEURAL CIRCUITS GENERATING/MODULATING RESPIRATORY RHYTHM AND PATTERN

Respiratory depression by opioid drugs is mediated by activation of MORs in neural circuits generating and/or modulating breathing (27). To better understand the neural mechanisms regulating respiratory depression, a description of the neural circuits mediating and/or modulating respiratory rhythm and pattern generation is critical. A thorough description of these neural circuits and their mechanisms is presented in the chapter of

DOI: 10.1201/9781003000631-23

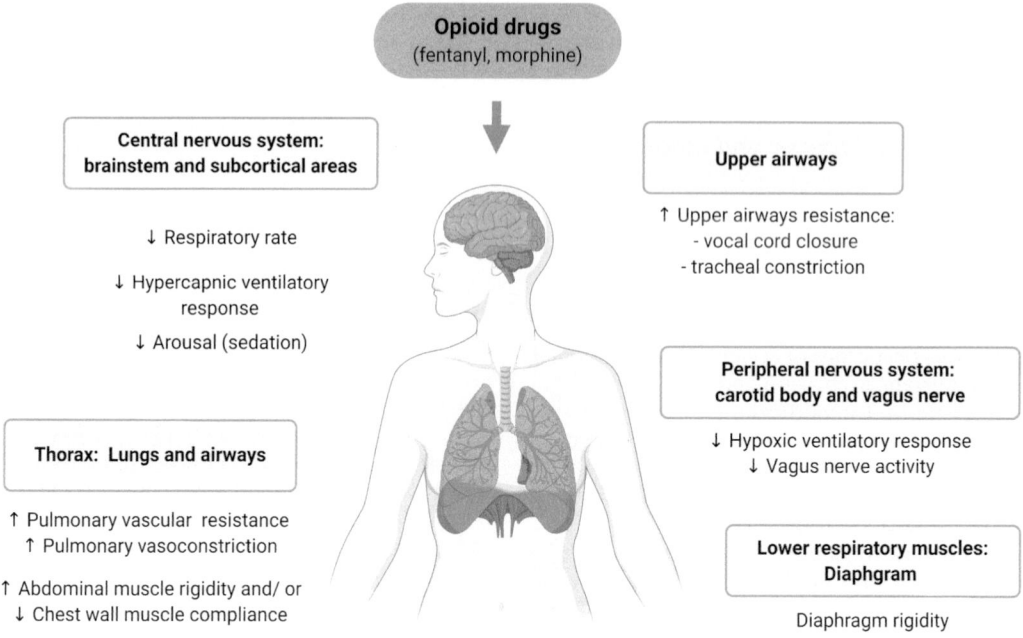

Figure 19.1 Overview of the effects of opioid drugs on the respiratory system including the nervous system, respiratory muscles, and thorax. Opioid drugs such as morphine, fentanyl, heroin, and oxycodone act on μ-opioid receptors and elicit various effects on the respiratory system including parts of the nervous system, respiratory musculature, thorax, and airways. (Illustration created with BioRender.com.)

Del Negro and Wilson in the present book. The current view of these neural circuits highlights three independent circuits which are coordinated to produce respiratory rhythm: the preBötzinger complex (preBötC; inspiration) (28), the post-inspiratory complex (PiCo; post-inspiration) (29), and the lateral parafacial nucleus (pF$_L$; active expiration) (30). While there is substantial work describing the role of the preBötC in regulating respiratory depression by opioid drugs, the roles of PiCo and pF$_L$ are still unclear (Figure 19.2).

The preBötC is a collection of neurons in the medulla critical for respiratory rhythm generation (28, 31). Microperfusion of the MOR agonist DAMGO in the preBötC region (Figure 19.2) of anesthetized rats and rabbits produced a significant depression of respiratory rate, which was reversed by the MOR antagonist naloxone (32–34). Using a transverse slice of the brainstem from rats, local application of DAMGO in the preBötC region also decreased respiratory frequency (35; 36). Using other experimental approaches such as transverse brainstem slices, *en bloc* preparations, and/ or anesthetized/awake animals, it has been demonstrated that activation of MORs in the preBötC directly affects inspiratory activity

(35, 37, 38). Although it is well demonstrated that the preBötC is sensitive to direct activation of its MORs, its role in regulating the respiratory effects of systemic injections of opioid drugs still needs to be demonstrated. Bilateral administration of naloxone to preBötC completely blocked respiratory rate depression by systemic fentanyl in anesthetized rats (38). In rabbits, naloxone microperfused in both preBötC only partially reversed respiratory rate depression by remifentanil (34). Using gene-editing approaches, knockdown of MORs in the preBötC only partially blocked respiratory rate depression by a low dose of morphine in awake mice (39). Low to medium doses (10–20 mg/kg) of injected morphine in intact rats resulted in an attenuated depression of breathing rate (39, 40). However, the complete rescue of breathing was not obtained even at a low dose of opioids and this trend was also absent following medium to high doses of morphine (30–100 mg/kg) or super-saturating dose of fentanyl (150 mg/kg). Similarly, knockdown of MORs in the preBötC reversed respiratory rate depression by morphine in awake mice exposed to hypercapnia (40). Although there is a lack of consistency between these studies, they all demonstrate that the preBötC mediates

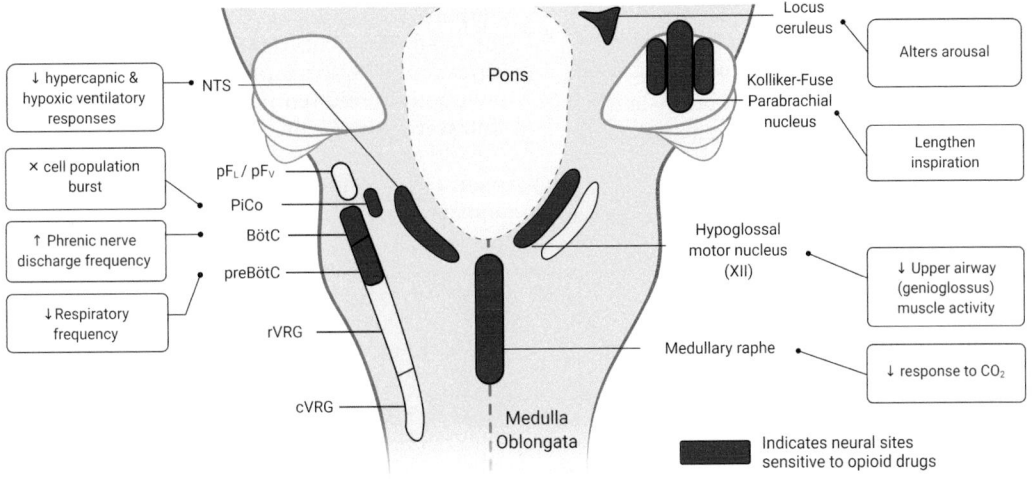

Figure 19.2 Putative neural circuits involved in opioid-induced respiratory depression. Discrete neural sites in the brainstem are sensitive to opioid drugs and mediate respiratory depression. Although the human brain was used as template for this illustration, the roles of these neural sites have been identified in animal studies. NTS, nucleus tractus solitarius; pF_L/pF_V, ventral and lateral parafacial nucleus; PiCo, post-inspiratory complex; BötC, Bötzinger complex; preBötC, preBötzinger complex; rVRG, rostral ventral respiratory group; cVRG, caudal ventral respiratory group. (Illustration created with BioRender.com.)

part of the respiratory rate depression observed with opioid drugs. Such discrepancy may be due to the different animal models used, the presence of volatile anesthetics, the types and dosages of opioid drugs used in these studies, and/or the contribution of arousal states to respiratory depression. Arousal states, i.e. wakefulness, sleep, sedation, are strong modulators of the severity of respiratory depression by opioid drugs (14, 41) and their role is addressed in the next section.

The PiCo is a complex of neurons active during the post-inspiration period. Its role in respiratory depression is not clear, but treatment with DAMGO in horizontal brainstem sections of mice nearly eliminated PiCo cell population burst (Figure 19.2) (29). The role of PiCo in the respiratory rate depression following systemic injection of opioid drugs has not been determined. The lateral part of the parafacial nucleus is active during expiration and is not sensitive to the activation of MORs (42). In the brainstem, other neural circuits also contribute to opioid-induced respiratory depression (Figure 19.2). Neural circuits including the parabrachial nucleus (43), the Kolliker-Fuse nucleus (39, 40), and the ventrolateral medulla (44) are sensitive to opioid drugs. Injection of DAMGO in the Kolliker-Fuse abolished the post-inspiratory phase of the respiratory cycle,

therefore creating lengthened low amplitude inspiration (45). Injection of opioid drugs in the parabrachial and Kolliker-Fuse nucleus slowed breathing in dogs (46, 47). Conditional deletion of MORs in the Kolliker-Fuse dampened the morphine-evoked drop in respiratory rate and inspiratory airflow, but the effect was more moderate than the injection in the preBötC (40). Simultaneous deletion of MORs in both preBötC and parabrachial/KF sites rescued breathing when exposed to opioids and was also resilient to super-saturating doses of opioids that usually slow breathing in control animals (150 mg/kg fentanyl) (40). The Bötzinger Complex, which is critical for the inspiration-expiration phase transition (48), is also sensitive to MOR activation. Injection of the MOR agonist endomorphin-1 in the Bötzinger Complex increased phrenic nerve discharge frequency possibly through a premature termination of expiration (48), which suggests that the Bötzinger Complex may have a limited role in mediating depression of respiratory rate by opioids. In summary, multiple neural circuits can be inhibited by activation of MORs with opioid drugs, but only some mediate respiratory rate depression by systemic opioids. The contribution of these neural circuits depends on the type of opioid drugs, its dosage, the animal model used, and the arousal states.

Factors Modulating the Contributions of Medullary Sites to Respiratory Depression by Opioid Drugs

The relative contributions of brainstem sites to respiratory rate depression may depend on the animal species receiving opioid drugs. Mice (39), rats (38), rabbits (34), and goats (49) present different sensitivities to morphine and fentanyl. Importantly, arousal states strongly modulate the severity of respiratory depression by systemic opioid drugs in rats (38, 41) and humans (14). In states of reduced arousal such as sleep or drowsiness, opioid drugs induced more severe respiratory depression than in wakefulness (41). Conversely, micro-injection of DAMGO into the preBötC of adult awake goats had no effect on respiratory rhythm (49). This state-dependency is reminiscent of the changes observed with obstructive sleep apnea across sleep-wake states, with pronounced upper airway resistance in deep and paradoxical sleep compared to wakefulness. Similarly, concomitant administration of sedatives with opioid drugs may aggravate the severity of respiratory depression and increase the risks of lethal overdose and cardiopulmonary arrest in the hospital setting (50–52). It is unclear whether sedatives aggravate respiratory depression by directly acting on brainstem sites and/or by indirectly reducing arousal. Mechanistic studies are needed to assess the relationship between sedatives and opioid drugs and their synergistic action on the respiratory system. In conclusion, various neural sites in the brainstem are involved in respiratory depression by opioids but differently contribute to its severity depending on the states of arousal, as well as dosage and type of opioid drugs considered, and the concomitant administration of other drugs such as sedatives.

OPIOID DRUGS BLUNT CENTRAL AND PERIPHERAL CHEMORECEPTION

Opioids cause breathing to slow and become irregular, leading to arterial hypercapnia and hypoxia (27). Under normal conditions, changes in partial pressure of oxygen and carbon dioxide in arterial blood and cerebrospinal fluid are sensed by both central and peripheral chemoreceptors but opioids can dampen central and peripheral chemosensitivity and blunt the hypercapnic and hypoxic ventilatory responses (Figure 19.2).

Carbon Dioxide Chemosensitivity

In healthy human subjects, intravenous or subcutaneous injection of morphine showed a depression of both the hypercapnic and hypoxic responses (22–24). A recent study on healthy patients demonstrated a similar effect on the hypercapnic response with the synthetic opioid remifentanil administered intravenously (25). In animal models, systemic opioid drugs blunted the hypercapnic ventilatory response. Morphine injected subcutaneously in rats blunted the ventilatory response to CO_2 (53). Systemic administration of DAMGO also attenuated the ventilatory response to hypercapnia through a reduction of tidal volume (54). Local administration of DAMGO in the caudal medullary raphe region of anesthetized rats significantly inhibited the response to CO_2 via a reduction in tidal volume and respiratory frequency (54). Also, microinjection of DAMGO in the caudomedial nucleus tractus solitarius of conscious and carotid body ablated rats attenuated the hypercapnic response (55). More rostral, the locus coeruleus in the pons (56), and the fastigial nucleus in the cerebellum (57) are also sensitive to opioid drugs and can modulate respiratory depression by opioids. However, although the sensitivity of these neural sites to opioid ligands is well established, their contributions to respiratory depression by systemically applied opioid drugs have not been demonstrated.

Oxygen Chemosensitivity

In patients, intrathecal morphine injection in patients significantly depressed the hypoxic ventilatory response compared to placebo injection. This effect could be due to a central inhibition of neurons located in the brainstem or peripheral sites such as the carotid bodies (58). In conscious rats, intravenous administration of morphine blunted the ventilatory response to hypoxia (10% O_2) as well as the ventilatory response to a combined hypercapnic/hypoxic challenge (59, 60). Microinjection of DAMGO in the caudomedial nucleus tractus solitarius of carotid body ablated rats attenuated their hypoxic response (55). In intact rats, microinjection of DAMGO in the NTS, where afferent nerves of the carotid body terminate, also depressed the hypoxic ventilatory response (55, 61). Overall, these studies support the fact that opioid drugs modulate oxygen chemosensitivity through centrally located neural circuits.

In the periphery, the carotid body is considered the main sensor of O_2. Carotid body cells express MORs, represented by an enkephalin-like immunoreactivity (an endogenous ligand binding to MORs) present in the glomus cells of the carotid body (62). In anesthetized cats, intracardiac injection of morphine depressed carotid sinus nerve activity (63). However, intravenous injection of morphine produced a greater depression of hypercapnic and hypoxic ventilatory responses in bilateral carotid sinus nerve transected rats compared to sham-operated rats (64). These results therefore suggest that carotid bodies may provide stimulation to the respiratory network system when opioid drugs depress respiratory activity and when oxygen blood levels are low.

OPIOID DRUGS IMPAIR RESPIRATORY MUSCLE ACTIVITY

In addition to their effects on respiratory drive and respiratory rhythm generation, opioid drugs affect respiratory motor circuits and muscles directly. In patients, the direct impact of opioid drugs on respiratory muscles may impact upper airway patency and chest inflation (65).

In anesthetized rats, delivery of fentanyl at the hypoglossal motor nucleus (XII) caused a suppression of genioglossus activity and tongue muscle activation (66). Intravenous administration of fentanyl in anesthetized cats decreased vagal (X) motoneuron activity in laryngeal abductors and increased vagal motoneuron activity in laryngeal adductors (67). These combined effects on vagal motoneurons lead to vocal fold closure and pharyngeal obstruction of airflow (67). Lower airways and respiratory pump muscles functions are also directly impaired by opioid drugs. In conscious rats, fentanyl injected intravenously created a mismatch in ventilation-perfusion by either increasing pulmonary vascular resistance or exacerbating the pulmonary vasoconstriction in response to lower arterial blood PO_2 produced by the hypoventilation (13). Subcutaneous administration of the opiate agonist alfentanil in spontaneously breathing adult rats decreased diaphragm inspiratory electromyographic activity and augmented its expiratory activity (68). In conclusion, opioid drugs act directly on motor circuits and respiratory muscles and depress muscle activation.

OPIOID DRUGS AND SLEEP-DISORDERED BREATHING IN PATIENTS

In the postoperative setting, there is a clear association between a history of sleep-disordered breathing in patients and the severity of respiratory depression by opioids (69). Although sleep-disordered breathing, mainly obstructive sleep apneas, is associated with risks of respiratory depression (70), it is

unclear whether opioid drugs directly increase the occurrence of sleep-disordered breathing. A recent systematic review of the literature looked at the impacts of opioid drugs on obstructive sleep apneas and did not find any relationships between opioid drugs and the occurrence of obstructive sleep apnea (71).

Central sleep apnea may, however, be exacerbated by opioid drugs as they directly reduce respiratory sensitivity to CO_2 (72). In fact, a small association has been demonstrated between central sleep apnea and chronic use of methadone, a long-acting MOR agonist (73). A recent case-control study showed that opioid medications substantially increased the occurrence of central sleep apneas (74), suggesting the involvement of opioid drugs in mechanisms mediating apneas. A review of a large cohort of patients also concluded that chronic opioid use increases the central apnea index, with no difference in the obstructive apnea index (75). Opioid dosage seems to be correlated with sleep-disordered breathing incidence as an increase in morphine equivalent dose was associated with higher central apnea index (76). Overall, opioid drugs have multiple effects on sleep and sleep-disordered breathing. Opioids at a morphine equivalent dose of 100 mg/day are associated with increased incidence in central sleep apneas and ataxic breathing, as well as a small increase in sleep-disordered breathing (77). Overall, there is still limited evidence demonstrating the causal role of opioid medications on the occurrence of sleep-disordered breathing, therefore suggesting that additional large-cohort and placebo-controlled studies in patients are needed.

PHARMACOLOGICAL INTERVENTIONS TO ALLEVIATE RESPIRATORY DEPRESSION BY OPIOID DRUGS

The current research investigating the neural mechanisms mediating respiratory depression by opioid drugs may lead to the identification of new therapeutic targets to reverse or prevent respiratory depression by opioid drugs. There are currently three different strategies for novel therapies without the side-effect of respiratory depression (Figure 19.3): (a) Blocking the mechanisms regulating MOR inhibition of the respiratory system, (b) Stimulating breathing to compensate for respiratory depression by opioid drugs, and (c) Designing new opioid ligands with reduced respiratory side-effects.

a. *Blockers of MOR inhibition.* There are currently no therapies to alleviate respiratory depression without reducing

a. Blocking MOR inhibition

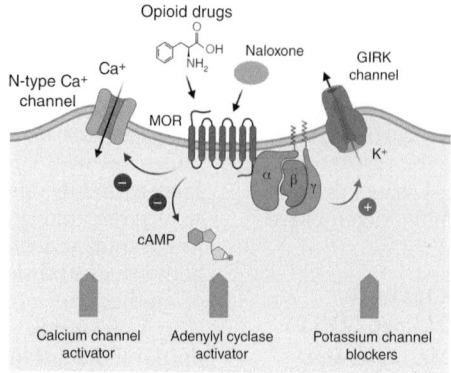

b. Respiratory stimulants

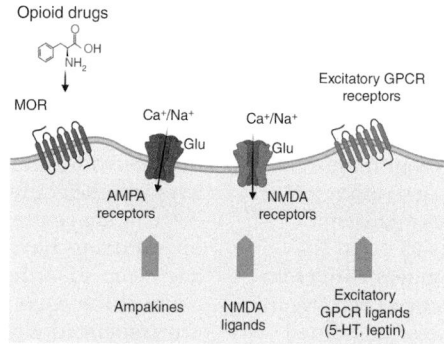

c. Opioid ligands

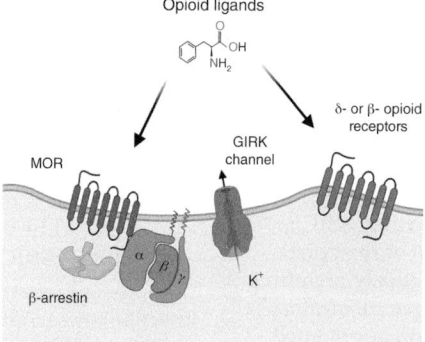

Figure 19.3 Therapeutic strategies to identify safe opioid drugs without respiratory depression by opioid drugs. (a) Blocking or inhibition of the mechanisms of MOR inhibition in the neural circuits regulating respiratory depression. MOR inhibition is mediated by activation of G-protein-inwardly rectifying potassium channels (GIRK) through G-protein signaling, inhibition of N-type calcium channels, and inhibition of the adenylyl cyclase pathway. Drugs targeting these molecular targets have the potential to prevent respiratory depression. (b) Stimulation of excitatory mechanisms in respiratory neural circuits can increase breathing while depressed by opioid drugs. AMPA, NMDA, 5-HT, and leptin receptors may be targeted to alleviate respiratory depression. (c) Novel opioid ligands with reduced respiratory side effects may be used directly as opioid analgesics. MOR, μ-opioid receptors; cAMP, cyclic adenosine monophosphate; K⁺, potassium ion; α, β, and γ G-proteins; GPCR, G-protein-coupled receptors. All receptors represented in this figure are positioned at the post-synapse for clarity. It is not currently known where are located these receptors in respiratory neural circuits. (Illustration created with BioRender.com.)

the analgesic properties of opioids (78). The MOR antagonist naloxone is an effective opioid antidote and it reverses respiratory depression, but it also blocks pain relief (79). In addition, the half-life of naloxone is relatively short compared to the half-lives of synthetic opioid drugs and re-narcotization following naloxone is often observed (79), therefore highlighting the need to find more effective preventive therapies. The withdrawal symptoms associated with naloxone are also substantial and usually discourage chronic opioid users to use naloxone (80). An alternative approach to block or prevent respiratory depression is to directly target the mechanisms mediating MOR inhibition. Ideally, a mechanism not involved in analgesia but mediating respiratory depression would be a potential target. For instance, G-protein–gated inwardly rectifying potassium (GIRK) channels mediate respiratory depression by opioid drugs likely in respiratory circuits including the preBötC (81). GIRK inhibitor tertiapin-Q has shown the ability to attenuate fentanyl-induced respiratory depression, and so did protein kinase A inhibitor, H89 (82). Although the therapeutic potential of GIRK channels may be limited since these channels also mediate opioid analgesia (83), it may lead to the identification of second messengers regulating G-protein coupling and potentially targeted therapies (81). For instance, stimulating adenylyl cyclase with forskolin prevented respiratory rhythm depression in brainstem-spinal cord *in vitro* preparation (84). However, it is unknown whether this strategy would prevent respiratory depression in intact organisms and whether it would also block analgesia.

Outside of the central neural circuits responsible for respiratory generation and modulation, the carotid bodies may provide a protective role against respiratory depression (64). Blockade of peripheral MORs by the peripherally restricted MOR antagonist naloxone methiodide was not sufficient to block respiratory frequency drop with successive morphine systemic administration or stop the initial decrease in tidal volume (12). On the other hand, naloxone methiodide was able to markedly attenuate the decrease in tidal volume following fentanyl systemic injection but once again, the depression in respiratory frequency was unaffected (13). Drugs acting on primary glomus cells in the carotid bodies may be more suitable to stimulate

ventilation (64). Potassium channels are involved in oxygen chemosensitivity in the carotid body and potassium channel blockers are being developed as respiratory stimulants (7). Potassium blockers such as doxapram and GAL021 prevent respiratory depression by opioid drugs in rodent models (85, 86) but has not yet been approved in clinical trials (7).

b. *Respiratory stimulants.* A therapeutic intervention administered concomitantly with opioid drugs and acting directly on brainstem neurons could stimulate breathing and therefore prevent or block respiratory depression. AMPA receptors in the preBötC play a key role in the maintenance of respiratory drive (87). The positive allosteric modulators of AMPA receptors called ampakines stimulate breathing while depressed by opioid, without affecting opioid-induced analgesia (88–90). While one drug has been tested in humans (CX717), a wide variety of ampakine molecules have shown the capacity to antagonize opioid-induced respiratory depression (89–95). Finally, nicotinic acetylcholine receptor agonist A85380 or nicotine itself can reverse opioid-induced respiratory depression following intravenous injection (96). Interestingly, A85380 has a modest effect on opioid-induced analgesia and its receptors $\alpha4\beta2$ are present in the carotid body (96).

Various excitatory G protein-coupled receptors (GPCR) may provide targets to stimulate breathing while it is depressed by opioids. 5-HT receptors agonist can stimulate respiratory activity (97) and bilateral microinjection of 5-HT increased preBötC activity via the 5-HT_{1A} and 5-HT_3 receptors (98). Different agonists for 5-HT_{1A}, 5-HT_4, and 5-HT_{4A} receptors have been shown to increase respiratory activity and counteract opioid-induced respiratory depression (97, 99–102). Dopamine receptors may also be used to stimulate breathing while depressed by opioid drugs. Agonists such as 6-chloro-APB and dihydrexidine can increase neuronal cyclic adenosine monophosphate (cAMP) after administration of opioids and restore breathing (103, 104). Both dopamine receptor agonists have no effect on fentanyl-induced antinociception (7). Other stimulants causing hyperexcitability of respiratory motor neurons by increasing cAMP are phosphodiesterase-4 inhibitors such as caffeine and rolipram (105,

106). The NMDA receptor antagonist esketamine can reverse respiratory depression induced by remifentanil through a stimulatory effect on CO_2 chemosensitivity (25). While antagonizing receptors and blocking channels can prove useful to block respiratory depression, inhibiting the break down of stimulant neurotransmitter can also increase respiratory rate and offer potent results. Acetylcholinesterase, breaking down acetylcholine, was blocked by inhibitors like donepezil or 4-aminopyridine and respiratory depression following morphine administration was reversed (107, 108). The neuropeptide leptin, which activates leptin GPCR receptors, stimulated breathing and prevented morphine-induced sleep-disordered breathing in obese mice (109). In summary, various ligands targeting excitatory GPCRs can stimulate breathing and alleviate respiratory depression in animal models. The fact that these excitatory GPCRs share G-proteins and second messengers with MORs may provide clues on how to stimulate breathing when it is depressed by opioid drugs.

c. *Opioid ligands with reduced side effects.*
Another approach is to develop opioid analgesics impervious to respiratory depression, i.e. drugs that would reduce pain without the side-effect of respiratory depression. Originally, it was suggested that analgesia by opioid drugs was mediated by G-protein signaling, through the activation of G-proteins, GIRK channels, and calcium channels, whereas respiratory depression by opioids would depend on the recruitment of β-arrestin without involving the G-protein pathway (110, 111). According to this idea, biased opioid ligands have been proposed to act mainly through the G-protein pathway with low recruitment of β-arrestin, which would be ideal opioid ligands to promote analgesia without respiratory depression. In 2016, the biased opioid agonist PZM21 was initially thought to have enhanced analgesic effects with a reduced effect on breathing (112) but was later confirmed to cause significant respiratory depression (113). Three biased opioid agonists (TRV130, PZM21, and herkinorin) were tested with patch-clamp electrophysiology and Ca^{2+} imaging and showed lower inhibitory effects than DAMGO (114), which suggests that these opioid ligands are partial

MOR agonists rather than biased opioid ligands. Currently, there is substantial evidence showing that β-arrestin may not be involved in respiratory depression as previously suggested. In fact, in mice with a non-functional G protein-receptor kinase 2, which is not able to recruit β-arrestin, the dose of fentanyl needed to reduce respiratory rate was significantly lower than wild-type mice (115), suggesting that β-arrestin does not mediate respiratory depression by opioid drugs. In fact, the G-protein pathway is equally involved in respiratory depression (81) and analgesia (83), and the role of β-arrestin, albeit intriguing, has been recently challenged by several groups (116). Although there has been considerable interest related to biased ligands over the last decades, it is becoming clear that biased ligands may have selective effects on respiratory depression and analgesia because they are partial agonists for opioid receptors (117). For instance, cebranopadol is a partial opioid agonist with analgesic properties but minimal respiratory side effects (118). Although initially promising, the idea of biased ligands with potent analgesic properties but reduced respiratory side-effect did not hold its promise. While it is likely that some biased opioid ligands activate G protein signaling over β-arrestin recruitment (119), respiratory depression equally involves G-protein signaling, which limits the use of biased ligands as safe opioid analgesics.

CONCLUSION

Even though the North American opioid epidemic is staggering, opioids are still widely prescribed due to their potent analgesic properties. Importantly, opioid drugs are highly addictive and when misused can lead to overdose. Regardless of their origins, opioid drugs, such as fentanyl, heroin, or oxycodone, induce respiratory depression by acting on MORs and can lead to respiratory arrest if not treated. The neural circuits regulating breathing present a relatively high expression of MORs, which make them highly sensitive to opioid drugs. Multiple neural circuits are involved in respiratory depression by opioid drugs, and their activation and role depend on the types of drug used, the sedative properties of the opioid drugs, and the combination with other respiratory depressant drugs, such as sedatives (51, 120). A clear understanding of the mechanisms of action of opioid drugs on respiratory circuits is critical to develop potent analgesics without the lethal side-effect of respiratory depression or to identify new antidotes for overdose.

REFERENCES

1. Radke JB, Owen KP, Sutter ME, Ford JB, Albertson TE (2014) The effects of opioids on the lung. Clin Rev Allergy Immunol 46:54–64.

2. Brook K, Bennett J, Desai SP (2017) The chemical history of morphine: an 8000-year journey, from resin to de-novo synthesis. J Anesth Hist 3:50–55.

3. Astyrakaki E, Papaioannou A, Askitopoulou H (2010) References to anesthesia, pain, and analgesia in the Hippocratic Collection. Anesth Analg 110:188–194.

4. Gutstein HB (2001) Opioid analgesics. In: Goodman and Gilman's the Pharmacological Basis for Therapeutics (Hardman JG, Limbird LE, Gilman AG, eds), pp. 569–618. New York: McGraw-Hill.

5. Montandon G, Slutsky AS (2019) Solving the opioid crisis: respiratory depression by opioids as critical end point. Chest 156:653–658.

6. Schiller EY, Goyal A, Mechanic OJ (2020) Opioid Overdose. Treasure Island: StatPearls.

7. Dahan A, van der Schrier R, Smith T, Aarts L, van Velzen M, Niesters M (2018) Averting opioid-induced respiratory depression without affecting analgesia. Anesthesiology 128:1027–1037.

8. Florence CS, Zhou C, Luo F, Xu L (2016) The economic burden of prescription opioid overdose, abuse, and dependence in the United States, 2013. Med Care 54:901–906.

9. Basbaum AI, Fields HL (1978) Endogenous pain control mechanisms: review and hypothesis. Ann Neurol 4:451–462.

10. Heinricher MM, Tavares I, Leith JL, Lumb BM (2009) Descending control of nociception: Specificity, recruitment and plasticity. Brain Res Rev 60:214–225.

11. Zebraski SE, Kochenash SM, Raffa RB (2000) Lung opioid receptors: pharmacology and possible target for nebulized morphine in dyspnea. Life Sci 66:2221–2231.

12. Henderson F, May WJ, Gruber RB, Young AP, Palmer LA, Gaston B, Lewis SJ (2013) Low-dose morphine elicits ventilatory excitant and depressant responses in conscious rats: Role of peripheral mu-opioid receptors. Open J Mol Integr Physiol 3:111–124.

13. Henderson F, May WJ, Gruber RB, Discala JF, Puskovic V, Young AP, Baby SM, Lewis SJ (2014) Role of central and peripheral opiate receptors in the effects of fentanyl on analgesia, ventilation and arterial blood-gas chemistry in conscious rats. Respir Physiol Neurobiol 191:95–105.

14. Montandon G, Cushing SL, Campbell F, Propst EJ, Horner RL, Narang I (2016a) Distinct cortical signatures associated with sedation and respiratory rate depression by morphine in a pediatric population. Anesthesiology 125:889–903.

15. Yasuda I, Hirano T, Yusa T, Satoh M (1978) Tracheal constriction by morphine and by fentanyl in man. Anesthesiology 49:117–119.

16. Ruiz Neto PP, Auler Junior JO (1992) Respiratory mechanical properties during fentanyl and alfentanil anaesthesia. Can J Anaesth 39:458–465.

17. Bennett JA, Abrams JT, Van Riper DF, Horrow JC (1997) Difficult or impossible ventilation after sufentanil-induced anesthesia is caused primarily by vocal cord closure. Anesthesiology 87:1070–1074.

18. Popio KA, Jackson DH, Ross AM, Schreiner BF, Yu PN (1978) Hemodynamic and respiratory effects of morphine and butorphanol. Clin Pharmacol Ther 23:281–287.

19. Mitaka C, Sakanishi N, Tsunoda Y, Mishima Y (1985) Comparison of hemodynamic effects of morphine, butorphanol, buprenorphine and pentazocine on ICU patients. Bull Tokyo Med Dent Univ 32:31–39.

20. Neidhart P, Burgener MC, Schwieger I, Suter PM (1989) Chest wall rigidity during fentanyl- and midazolam-fentanyl induction: ventilatory and haemodynamic effects. Acta Anaesthesiol Scand 33:1–5.

21. Costa R, Navalesi P, Cammarota G, Longhini F, Spinazzola G, Cipriani F, Ferrone G, Festa O, Antonelli M, Conti G (2017) Remifentanil effects on respiratory drive and timing during pressure support ventilation and neurally adjusted ventilatory assist. Respir Physiol Neurobiol 244:10–16.

22. Weil JV, McCullough RE, Kline JS, Sodal IE (1975) Diminished ventilatory response to hypoxia and hypercapnia after morphine in normal man. N Engl J Med 292:1103–1106.

23. Dahan A, Sarton E, Teppema L, Olievier C (1998) Sex-related differences in the influence of morphine on ventilatory control in humans. Anesthesiology 88:903–913.

24. Sarton E, Teppema L, Dahan A (1999) Sex differences in morphine-induced ventilatory depression reside within the peripheral chemoreflex loop. Anesthesiology 90:1329–1338.

25. Jonkman K, van Rijnsoever E, Olofsen E, Aarts L, Sarton E, van Velzen M, Niesters M, Dahan A (2018) Esketamine counters opioid-induced respiratory depression. Br J Anaesth 120:1117–1127.

26. Grigorakos L, Sakagianni K, Tsigou E, Apostolakos G, Nikolopoulos G, Veldekis D (2010) Outcome of acute heroin overdose requiring intensive care unit admission. J Opioid Manag 6:227–231.

27. Pattinson KT (2008) Opioids and the control of respiration. Br J Anaesth 100:747–758.

28. Smith JC, Ellenberger HH, Ballanyi K, Richter DW, Feldman JL (1991) Pre-Botzinger complex: a brainstem region that may generate respiratory rhythm in mammals. Science 254:726–729.

29. Anderson TM, Garcia AJ, 3rd, Baertsch NA, Pollak J, Bloom JC, Wei AD, Rai KG, Ramirez JM (2016) A novel excitatory network for the control of breathing. Nature 536:76–80.

30. Huckstepp RT, Cardoza KP, Henderson LE, Feldman JL (2015) Role of parafacial nuclei in control of breathing in adult rats. J Neurosci 35:1052–1067.

31. Gray PA, Janczewski WA, Mellen N, McCrimmon DR, Feldman JL (2001) Normal breathing requires preBotzinger complex neurokinin-1 receptor-expressing neurons. Nat Neurosci 4:927–930.

32. Montandon G, Qin W, Liu H, Ren J, Greer JJ, Horner RL (2011a) PreBötzinger complex neurokinin-1 receptor-expressing neurons mediate opioid-induced respiratory depression. J Neurosci 31:1292–1301.

33. Montandon G, Horner R (2014) CrossTalk proposal: The preBotzinger complex is essential for the respiratory depression following systemic administration of opioid analgesics. J Physiol 592:1159–1162.

34. Stucke AG, Miller JR, Prkic I, Zuperku EJ, Hopp FA, Stuth EA (2015) Opioid-induced respiratory depression is only partially mediated by the preBotzinger complex in young and adult rabbits in vivo. Anesthesiology 122:1288–1298.

35. Gray PA, Rekling JC, Bocchiaro CM, Feldman JL (1999) Modulation of respiratory frequency by peptidergic input to rhythmogenic neurons in the preBotzinger complex. Science 286:1566–1568.

36. Stucke AG, Zuperku EJ, Sanchez A, Tonkovic-Capin M, Tonkovic-Capin V, Mustapic S, Stuth EA (2008) Opioid receptors on bulbospinal respiratory neurons are not activated during neuronal depression by clinically relevant opioid concentrations. J Neurophysiol 100:2878–2888.

37. Mellen NM, Janczewski WA, Bocchiaro CM, Feldman JL (2003) Opioid-induced quantal slowing reveals dual networks for respiratory rhythm generation. Neuron 37:821–826.

38. Montandon G, Qin W, Liu H, Ren J, Greer JJ, Horner RL (2011b) PreBotzinger complex neurokinin-1 receptor-expressing neurons mediate opioid-induced respiratory depression. J Neurosci 31:1292–1301.

39. Varga AG, Reid BT, Kieffer BL, Levitt ES (2020) Differential impact of two critical respiratory centres in opioid-induced respiratory depression in awake mice. J Physiol 598:189–205.

40. Bachmutsky I, Wei XP, Kish E, Yackle K (2020) Opioids depress breathing through two small brainstem sites. Elife 9.

41. Montandon G, Horner RL (2019) Electrocortical changes associated with sedation and respiratory depression by the analgesic fentanyl. Sci Rep 9:14122.

42. Janczewski WA, Feldman JL (2006) Distinct rhythm generators for inspiration and expiration in the juvenile rat. J Physiol 570:407–420.

43. Miller JR, Zuperku EJ, Stuth EAE, Banerjee A, Hopp FA, Stucke AG (2017) A subregion of the parabrachial nucleus partially mediates respiratory rate depression from intravenous remifentanil in young and adult rabbits. Anesthesiology 127:502–514.

44. Phillips RS, Cleary DR, Nalwalk JW, Arttamangkul S, Hough LB, Heinricher MM (2012) Pain-facilitating medullary neurons contribute to opioid-induced respiratory depression. J Neurophysiol 108:2393–2404.

45. Levitt ES, Abdala AP, Paton JFR, Bissonnette JM, Williams JT (2015) μ opioid receptor activation hyperpolarizes respiratory-controlling Kölliker-Fuse neurons and suppresses post-inspiratory drive. The Journal of Physiology 593:4453–4469.

46. Mustapic S, Radocaj T, Sanchez A, Dogas Z, Stucke AG, Hopp FA, Stuth EA, Zuperku EJ (2010) Clinically relevant infusion rates of μ-opioid agonist remifentanil cause bradypnea in decerebrate dogs but not via direct effects in the pre-Botzinger complex region. J Neurophysiol 103:409–418.

47. Prkic I, Mustapic S, Radocaj T, Stucke AG, Stuth EA, Hopp FA, Dean C, Zuperku EJ (2012) Pontine mu-opioid receptors mediate bradypnea caused by intravenous remifentanil infusions at clinically relevant concentrations in dogs. J Neurophysiol 108:2430–2441.

48. Lonergan T, Goodchild AK, Christie MJ, Pilowsky PM (2003) Mu opioid receptors in rat ventral medulla: effects of endomorphin-1 on phrenic nerve activity. Respir Physiol Neurobiol 138:165–178.

49. Krause KL, Neumueller SE, Marshall BD, Kiner T, Bonis JM, Pan LG, Qian B, Forster HV (2009) Micro-opioid receptor agonist injections into the presumed pre-Botzinger complex and the surrounding region of awake goats do not alter eupneic breathing. J Appl Physiol 107:1591–1599.

50. Turner BJ, Liang Y (2015) Drug overdose in a retrospective cohort with non-cancer pain treated with opioids, antidepressants, and/or sedative-hypnotics: interactions with mental health disorders. J Gen Intern Med 30:1081–1096.

51. Overdyk FJ, Dowling O, Marino J, Qiu J, Chien HL, Erslon M, Morrison N, Harrison N, Dahan A, Gan TJ (2016) Association of opioids and sedatives with increased risk of in-hospital cardiopulmonary arrest from an administrative database. PLoS One 11:e0150214.

52. Izrailtyan I, Qiu J, Overdyk FJ, Erslon M, Gan TJ (2018) Risk factors for cardiopulmonary and respiratory arrest in medical and surgical hospital patients on opioid analgesics and sedatives. PLoS One 13:e0194553.

53. Emery MJ, Groves CC, Kruse TN, Shi C, Terman GW (2016) Ventilation and the response to hypercapnia after morphine in opioid-naive and opioid-tolerant rats. Anesthesiology 124:945–957.

54. Zhang Z, Xu F, Zhang C, Liang X (2007) Activation of opioid mu receptors in caudal medullary raphe region inhibits the ventilatory response to

hypercapnia in anesthetized rats. Anesthesiology 107:288–297.

55. Zhuang J, Gao X, Gao F, Xu F (2017) Mu-opioid receptors in the caudomedial NTS are critical for respiratory responses to stimulation of bronchopulmonary C-fibers and carotid body in conscious rats. Respir Physiol Neurobiol 235:71–78.

56. Oyamada Y, Ballantyne D, Muckenhoff K, Scheid P (1998) Respiration-modulated membrane potential and chemosensitivity of locus coeruleus neurones in the in vitro brainstem-spinal cord of the neonatal rat. J Physiol 513 (Pt 2):381–398.

57. Martino PF, Davis S, Opansky C, Krause K, Bonis JM, Pan LG, Qian B, Forster HV (2007) The cerebellar fastigial nucleus contributes to CO_2-H+ ventilatory sensitivity in awake goats. Respir Physiol Neurobiol 157:242–251.

58. Bailey PL, Lu JK, Pace NL, Orr JA, White JL, Hamber EA, Slawson MH, Crouch DJ, Rollins DE (2000) Effects of intrathecal morphine on the ventilatory response to hypoxia. N Engl J Med 343:1228–1234.

59. May WJ, Gruber RB, Discala JF, Puskovic V, Henderson F, Palmer LA, Lewis SJ (2013a) Morphine has latent deleterious effects on the ventilatory responses to a hypoxic challenge. Open J Mol Integr Physiol 3:166–180.

60. May WJ, Henderson F, Gruber RB, Discala JF, Young AP, Bates JN, Palmer LA, Lewis SJ (2013b) Morphine has latent deleterious effects on the ventilatory responses to a hypoxic-hypercapnic challenge. Open J Mol Integr Physiol 3:134–145.

61. Guyenet PG, Stornetta RL, Bayliss DA (2010) Central respiratory chemoreception. J Comp Neurol 518:3883–3906.

62. Hansen JT, Brokaw J, Christie D, Karasek M (1982) Localization of enkephalin-like immunoreactivity in the cat carotid and aortic body chemoreceptors. Anat Rec 203:405–410.

63. McQueen DS, Ribeiro JA (1980) Inhibitory actions of methionine-enkephalin and morphine on the cat carotid chemoreceptors. Br J Pharmacol 71:297–305.

64. Baby SM, Gruber RB, Young AP, MacFarlane PM, Teppema LJ, Lewis SJ (2018) Bilateral carotid sinus nerve transection exacerbates morphine-induced respiratory depression. Eur J Pharmacol 834:17–29.

65. Webster LR, Karan S (2020) The physiology and maintenance of respiration: a narrative review. Pain Ther 9:467–486.

66. Hajiha M, DuBord M-A, Liu H, Horner RL (2009) Opioid receptor mechanisms at the hypoglossal motor pool and effects on tongue muscle activity in vivo. The Journal of Physiology 587:2677–2692.

67. Lalley PM (2003) Mu-opioid receptor agonist effects on medullary respiratory neurons in the cat: evidence for involvement in certain types of ventilatory

disturbances. Am J Physiol Regul Integr Comp Physiol 285:R1287–1304.

68. Campbell C, Weinger MB, Quinn M (1995) Alterations in diaphragm EMG activity during opiate-induced respiratory depression. Respir Physiol 100:107–117.

69. Nagappa MW, TN, Montandon G, Sprung J, Chung F. (2017) Opioids, respiratory depression and sleep-disordered breathing. Best Pract Res Clin Anaesthesiol 31(4):469-485.

70. Selvanathan J, Peng PWH, Wong J, Ryan CM, Chung F (2020) Sleep-disordered breathing in patients on opioids for chronic pain. Reg Anesth Pain Med 45:826–830.

71. Ahmad A AR, Meteb M, Ryan CM, Leung RS, Montandon G, Luks V, Kendzerska T (2021) The relationship between opioid use and obstructive sleep apnea: A systematic review and meta-analysis. Sleep Medicine Reviews 58:101441.

72. Teichtahl H, Wang D, Cunnington D, Quinnell T, Tran H, Kronborg I, Drummer OH (2005) Ventilatory responses to hypoxia and hypercapnia in stable methadone maintenance treatment patients. Chest 128:1339–1347.

73. Wang D, Teichtahl H, Drummer O, Goodman C, Cherry G, Cunnington D, Kronborg I (2005) Central sleep apnea in stable methadone maintenance treatment patients. Chest 128:1348–1356.

74. Gavidia R, Emenike A, Meng A, Jansen EC, Hershner S, Goldstein C, Fetterolf J, Dunietz GL (2021) The influence of opioids and non-opioid central nervous system active medications on central sleep apnea: a case-control study. J Clin Sleep Med 17:55-60.

75. Walker JM, Farney RJ, Rhondeau SM, Boyle KM, Valentine K, Cloward TV, Shilling KC (2007) Chronic opioid use is a risk factor for the development of central sleep apnea and ataxic breathing. J Clin Sleep Med 3:455–461.

76. Jungquist CR, Flannery M, Perlis ML, Grace JT (2012) Relationship of chronic pain and opioid use with respiratory disturbance during sleep. Pain Manag Nurs 13:70–79.

77. Cutrufello NJ, Ianus VN, Rowley JA (2020) Opioids and sleep. Curr Opin Pulm Med 26:634–641.

78. van der Schier R, Roozekrans M, van Velzen M, Dahan A, Niesters M (2014) Opioid-induced respiratory depression: reversal by non-opioid drugs. F1000Prime Rep 6:79.

79. Dahan A, Aarts L, Smith TW (2010) Incidence, reversal, and prevention of opioid-induced respiratory depression. Anesthesiology 112:226–238.

80. Dydyk AM, Jain NK, Gupta M (2020) Opioid Use Disorder. Treasure Island: StatPearls.

81. Montandon G, Ren J, Victoria NC, Liu H, Wickman K, Greer JJ, Horner RL (2016b) G-protein-gated inwardly

rectifying potassium channels modulate respiratory depression by opioids. Anesthesiology 124:641–650.

82. Liang X, Yong Z, Su R (2018) Inhibition of protein kinase A and GIRK channel reverses fentanyl-induced respiratory depression. Neurosci Lett 677:14–18.

83. Marker CL, Stoffel M, Wickman K (2004) Spinal G-protein-gated K+ channels formed by GIRK1 and GIRK2 subunits modulate thermal nociception and contribute to morphine analgesia. J Neurosci 24:2806–2812.

84. Ballanyi K, Lalley PM, Hoch B, Richter DW (1997) cAMP-dependent reversal of opioid- and prostaglandin-mediated depression of the isolated respiratory network in newborn rats. J Physiol 504 (Pt 1):127–134.

85. Golder FJ, Dax S, Baby SM, Gruber R, Hoshi T, Ideo C, Kennedy A, Peng S, Puskovic V, Ritchie D, Woodward R, Wardle RL, Van Scott MR, Mannion JC, MacIntyre DE (2015) Identification and characterization of GAL-021 as a novel breathing control modulator. Anesthesiology 123:1093–1104.

86. Haji A, Kimura S, Ohi Y (2016) Reversal of morphine-induced respiratory depression by doxapram in anesthetized rats. Eur J Pharmacol 780:209–215.

87. Shao XM, Ge Q, Feldman JL (2003) Modulation of AMPA receptors by cAMP-dependent protein kinase in preBötzinger complex inspiratory neurons regulates respiratory rhythm in the rat. J Physiol 547:543–553.

88. Ren J, Poon BY, Tang Y, Funk GD, Greer JJ (2006) Ampakines alleviate respiratory depression in rats. Am J Respir Crit Care Med 174:1384–1391.

89. Greer JJ, Ren J (2009) Ampakine therapy to counter fentanyl-induced respiratory depression. Respir Physiol Neurobiol 168:153–157.

90. Ren J, Ding X, Funk GD, Greer JJ (2009) Ampakine CX717 protects against fentanyl-induced respiratory depression and lethal apnea in rats. Anesthesiology 110:1364–1370.

91. Oertel BG, Felden L, Tran PV, Bradshaw MH, Angst MS, Schmidt H, Johnson S, Greer JJ, Geisslinger G, Varney MA, Lotsch J (2010) Selective antagonism of opioid-induced ventilatory depression by an ampakine molecule in humans without loss of opioid analgesia. Clin Pharmacol Ther 87:204–211.

92. Cavalla D, Chianelli F, Korsak A, Hosford PS, Gourine AV, Marina N (2015) Tianeptine prevents respiratory depression without affecting analgesic effect of opiates in conscious rats. Eur J Pharmacol 761:268–272.

93. Haw AJ, Meyer LC, Greer JJ, Fuller A (2016) Ampakine CX1942 attenuates opioid-induced respiratory depression and corrects the hypoxaemic effects of etorphine in immobilized goats (Capra hircus). Vet Anaesth Analg 43:528–538.

94. Dai W, Xiao D, Gao X, Zhou XB, Fang TY, Yong Z, Su RB (2017) A brain-targeted ampakine compound protects against opioid-induced respiratory depression. Eur J Pharmacol 809:122–129.

95. Dai W, Gao X, Xiao D, Li YL, Zhou XB, Yong Z, Su RB (2019) The impact and mechanism of a novel allosteric AMPA receptor modulator LCX001 on protection against respiratory depression in rodents. Front Pharmacol 10:105.

96. Ren J, Ding X, Greer JJ (2019) Activating α4β2 nicotinic acetylcholine receptors alleviates fentanyl-induced respiratory depression in rats. Anesthesiology 130:1017–1031.

97. Manzke T, Guenther U, Ponimaskin EG, Haller M, Dutschmann M, Schwarzacher S, Richter DW (2003) 5-HT4(a) receptors avert opioid-induced breathing depression without loss of analgesia. Science 301:226–229.

98. Iovino L, Mutolo D, Cinelli E, Contini M, Pantaleo T, Bongianni F (2019) Breathing stimulation mediated by 5-HT1A and 5-HT3 receptors within the preBötzinger complex of the adult rabbit. Brain Res 1704:26–39.

99. Sahibzada N, Ferreira M, Wasserman AM, Taveira-DaSilva AM, Gillis RA (2000) Reversal of morphine-induced apnea in the anesthetized rat by drugs that activate 5-hydroxytryptamine(1A) receptors. J Pharmacol Exp Ther 292:704–713.

100. Meyer LC, Fuller A, Mitchell D (2006) Zacopride and 8-OH-DPAT reverse opioid-induced respiratory depression and hypoxia but not catatonic immobilization in goats. Am J Physiol Regul Integr Comp Physiol 290:R405–413.

101. Guenther U, Theuerkauf NU, Huse D, Boettcher MF, Wensing G, Putensen C, Hoeft A (2012) Selective 5-HT(1A)-R-agonist repinotan prevents remifentanil-induced ventilatory depression and prolongs antinociception. Anesthesiology 116:56–64.

102. Ren J, Ding X, Greer JJ (2015) 5-HT1A receptor agonist Befiradol reduces fentanyl-induced respiratory depression, analgesia, and sedation in rats. Anesthesiology 122:424–434.

103. Lalley PM (2004) Dopamine1 receptor agonists reverse opioid respiratory network depression, increase CO_2 reactivity. Respir Physiol Neurobiol 139:247–262.

104. Lalley PM (2005) D1-dopamine receptor agonists prevent and reverse opiate depression of breathing but not antinociception in the cat. Am J Physiol Regul Integr Comp Physiol 289:R45–R51.

105. Kasaba T, Takeshita M, Takasaki M (1997) The effects of caffeine on the respiratory depression by morphine. Masui 46:1570–1574.

106. Kimura S, Ohi Y, Haji A (2015) Blockade of phosphodiesterase 4 reverses morphine-induced ventilatory disturbance without loss of analgesia. Life Sci 127:32–38.

107. Elmalem E, Chorev M, Weinstock M (1991) Antagonism of morphine-induced respiratory depression by novel anticholinesterase agents. Neuropharmacology 30:1059–1064.

108. Tsujita M, Sakuraba S, Kuribayashi J, Hosokawa Y, Hatori E, Okada Y, Kashiwagi M, Takeda J, Kuwana S (2007) Antagonism of morphine-induced central respiratory depression by donepezil in the anesthetized rabbit. Biol Res 40:339–346.

109. Freire C, Pho H, Kim LJ, Wang X, Dyavanapalli J, Streeter SR, Fleury-Curado T, Sennes LU, Mendelowitz D, Polotsky VY (2020) Intranasal leptin prevents opioid-induced sleep-disordered breathing in obese mice. Am J Respir Cell Mol Biol 63:502–509.

110. Bohn LM, Lefkowitz RJ, Gainetdinov RR, Peppel K, Caron MG, Lin FT (1999) Enhanced morphine analgesia in mice lacking beta-arrestin 2. Science 286:2495–2498.

111. Raehal KM, Walker JK, Bohn LM (2005) Morphine side effects in beta-arrestin 2 knockout mice. The Journal of pharmacology and experimental therapeutics 314:1195–1201.

112. Manglik A, Lin H, Aryal DK, McCorvy JD, Dengler D, Corder G, Levit A, Kling RC, Bernat V, Hubner H, Huang XP, Sassano MF, Giguere PM, Lober S, Da D, Scherrer G, Kobilka BK, Gmeiner P, Roth BL, Shoichet BK (2016) Structure-based discovery of opioid analgesics with reduced side effects. Nature 537:185–190.

113. Hill R, Disney A, Conibear A, Sutcliffe K, Dewey W, Husbands S, Bailey C, Kelly E, Henderson G (2018) The novel mu-opioid receptor agonist PZM21 depresses respiration and induces tolerance to antinociception. Br J Pharmacol 175:2653–2661.

114. Yudin Y, Rohacs T (2019) The G-protein-biased agents PZM21 and TRV130 are partial agonists of mu-opioid receptor-mediated signalling to ion channels. Br J Pharmacol 176:3110–3125.

115. Kliewer A, Schmiedel F, Sianati S, Bailey A, Bateman JT, Levitt ES, Williams JT, Christie MJ, Schulz S (2019) Phosphorylation-deficient G-protein-biased mu-opioid receptors improve analgesia and diminish tolerance but worsen opioid side effects. Nat Commun 10:367.

116. Kliewer A, Gillis A, Hill R, Schmidel F, Bailey C, Kelly E, Henderson G, Christie MJ, Schulz S (2020) Morphine-induced respiratory depression is independent of beta-arrestin 2 signalling. Br J Pharmacol.

117. Gunther T, Dasgupta P, Mann A, Miess E, Kliewer A, Fritzwanker S, Steinborn R, Schulz S (2018) Targeting multiple opioid receptors—improved analgesics with reduced side effects? Br J Pharmacol 175:2857–2868.

118. Calo G, Lambert DG (2018) Nociceptin/orphanin FQ receptor ligands and translational challenges: focus on cebranopadol as an innovative analgesic. Br J Anaesth 121:1105–1114.

119. Manglik A (2020) Molecular basis of opioid action: from structures to new leads. Biol Psychiatry 87:6–14.

120. Gupta K, Prasad A, Nagappa M, Wong J, Abrahamyan L, Chung FF (2018) Risk factors for opioid-induced respiratory depression and failure to rescue: a review. Curr Opin Anaesthesiol 31:110–119.

20 Pharmacologic Intervention Studies to Mitigate Breathing Instability – Animal Studies

Carla Freire, Lenise J Kim, and Vsevolod Y Polotsky

INTRODUCTION

Sleep is the vulnerable state for breathing disorders due to diminished cortical output to respiratory control centers in the brainstem and respiratory pump muscles (1). Sleep-disordered breathing (SDB) includes a spectrum of conditions including obstructive sleep apnea (OSA), alveolar hypoventilation, and central sleep apnea.

OSA, the most common type of SDB, is characterized by recurrent upper airway obstruction, which results in intermittent hypoxemia, transthoracic pressure swings, and sleep fragmentation (2). This obstruction is a consequence of unfavorable pharyngeal anatomy in combination with impaired neuromuscular control of the upper airway. Overly robust peripheral chemoreflex and low arousal threshold contribute to the development and progression of the disease (3). Intermittent hypoxia is a key factor in the pathophysiology of SDB. An imbalance between peripheral chemosensitivity and the compensatory ventilatory response results in breathing instability, which plays a key role in the generation of obstructive and central sleep apneas (4). Increased peripheral chemosensitivity leads to central apneas observed at high altitudes and in patients with Cheyne-Stokes respiration (5).

Another type of SDB is alveolar hypoventilation due to inadequate ventilation during sleep leading to carbon dioxide (CO_2) retention. The primary causes of alveolar hypoventilation are blunted response to CO_2 and impaired respiratory pump muscle function (6). Suppressed CO_2 chemosensitivity is most commonly observed in obesity hypoventilation syndrome (OHS) (7) and opioid-induced respiratory depression (8). Respiratory muscle weakness is observed in diseases of respiratory motoneurons such as spinal cord injury (SCI), amyotrophic lateral sclerosis (ALS), and muscular dystrophies of multiple etiologies (9).

In this chapter, we will summarize animal studies dedicated to drug development in different types of SDB.

OSA

Animal Models

Several animal models that mimic anatomical and neuromuscular predisposition to SDB have been described (10). First thoroughly investigated and well-described models of spontaneous OSA are English bulldogs (11), in which anatomy predisposes to SDB and the Yucatan minipigs that develop obesity-related sleep apnea (12). These models have been used for pre-clinical drug studies and a trial of trazodone, a drug with complex serotoninergic and adrenergic effects, in the English bulldog was the earliest attempt to develop pharmacotherapy for OSA (13). However, the utility of these models is limited due to low throughput and genetic variability. Other studies utilized tools such as mechanical upper airway obstruction, muscle lesions or paralyses, injections of solidified substances into the upper airway and flexion of the neck in dogs, cats, and rodents (14–20). These models were fundamental for the understanding of SDB pathophysiology and its consequences, but they do not allow to elucidate structural and functional features of the upper airway in OSA and, therefore, cannot be used for drug development.

Rodents are widely used in translational research because of the availability of genetically engineered models, well-described anatomy and physiology, and low cost. The utility of rodent models in the past was limited by the inability to detect upper airway obstruction. Investigators relied on detection of post-sigh and non-post sigh respiratory pauses (21, 22). Later on, researchers demonstrated that neuromuscular control of the upper airway in rodents and humans is remarkably similar (10), despite unique anatomic evolutionary features in humans, such as an unattached hyoid bone and elongated pharynx predisposing to the development of OSA. Obese rodents exhibit anatomical features of OSA such as fat deposits and narrowing of the pharynx in Zucker rats (23, 24) and New Zealand obese (NZO) mice (25). Increased number of apneas and hypopneas during the resting light phase (26), marked inspiratory flow limitation and obesity hypoventilation with CO_2 retention were described in leptin-deficient *ob/ob* mice (Figure 20.1), diet-induced obese (DIO) C57BL/6J mice (Figure 20.2) and NZO mice (27–29). These models develop a pattern of mild sleep apnea characterized by flow limitation and hypopneas, mostly during REM sleep, as well as hypoventilation throughout sleep-wake states (29, 30).

DOI: 10.1201/9781003000631-24

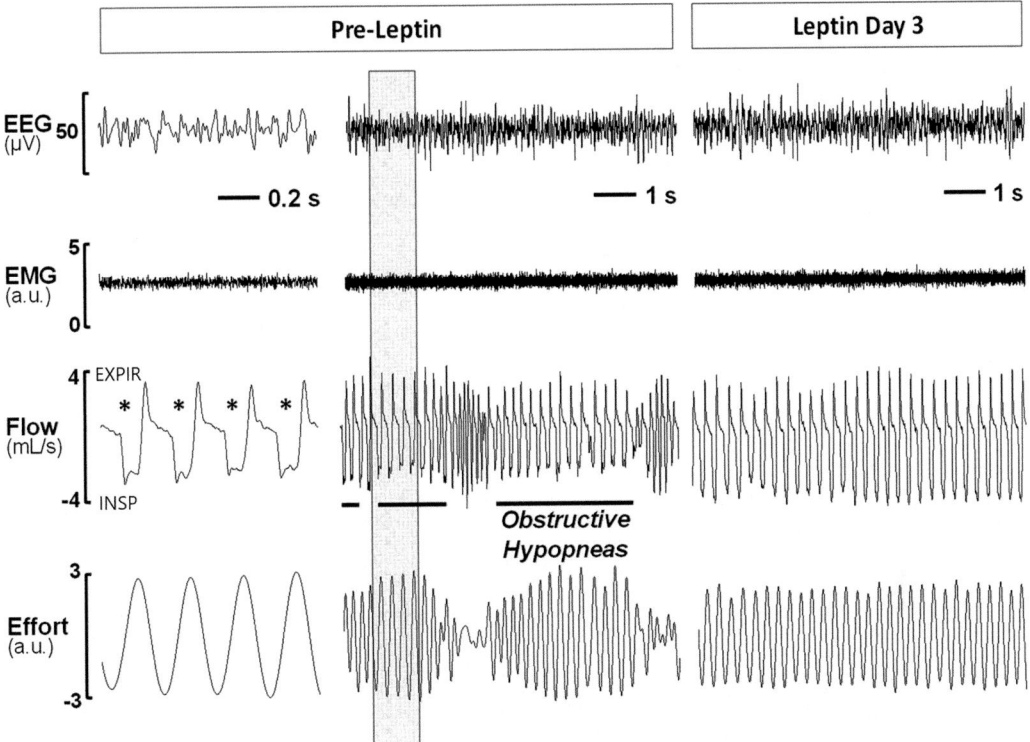

Figure 20.1 Representative tracing of ventilation in leptin-deficient *ob/ob* mice during REM sleep. *Left*, inspiratory flow limitation (IFL, see *) and obstructive hypopneas (underlined) are observed in *ob/ob* mice. *Right*, systemic leptin administration for 3 days abolished the respiratory events. Effort represents respiratory movements recorded from a sensor bladder placed on the bottom of the plethysmography chamber. The shaded area is decompressed on the left panel. (From Pho et al. (28). a.u.: arbitrary units.)

Interventions to Improve Neuromuscular Control

Sleep, especially REM sleep, is characterized by the withdrawal of excitatory drive to the motoneurons that innervate the respiratory muscles (31). Research efforts have been directed at the neuromuscular control of the tongue and genioglossus (GG) muscle, the main pharyngeal dilator (32). The hypoglossal motoneurons innervate most of the muscle fibers in the tongue (33) and evidence suggests that the co-activation of protruder and retractor muscles may be more efficient in stabilizing the pharynx than activation of GG alone (34, 35). Recent advances in hypoglossal electrical stimulation therapy in humans are derived from pivotal animal experiments and illustrate the role of the GG muscle activity modulation in the therapeutic arsenal for OSA (36).

Kubin *et al.* were the first to demonstrate the possibility of pharmacological modulation of hypoglossal activity. Pontine injections of carbachol, a cholinergic receptor agonist, induced pharmacological REM sleep with characteristic atonia and these effects were reversed with the injection of atropine, a muscarinic cholinergic antagonist. Investigators hypothesized that the reduced activity of hypoglossal motoneurons during REM sleep was due to decreased release of excitatory neurotransmitters. Medullary serotoninergic and pontine noradrenergic neuronal populations were potential mediators of this effect because they have reduced activity during sleep and have projections to the XII nucleus (31). The role of serotonin was confirmed by *in vivo* and *in vitro* studies that showed excitatory effects of serotonin (5-hydroxytryptamine [5-HT]) receptor agonists on the hypoglossal motoneurons with increased GG activity (37–39). The decrease in GG activity with serotonin receptor antagonists suggested an endogenous excitatory serotoninergic drive to the hypoglossal motoneurons. Specifically, 5-HT$_2$

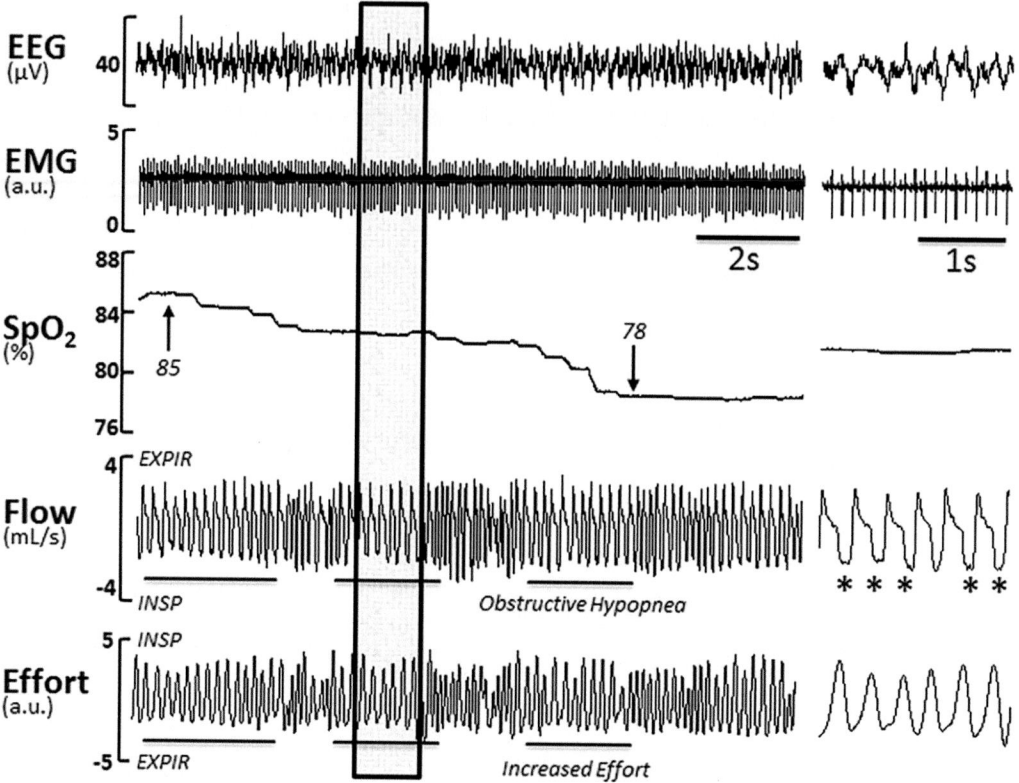

Figure 20.2 Representative tracing of ventilation of diet-induced obese (DIO) mice during REM sleep. Inspiratory flow limitation (IFL, see *) with increases in respiratory effort, obstructive hypopneas, and oxygen desaturations (see the arrows) are prevalent in DIO mice during REM sleep. Effort represents respiratory movements recorded from a sensor bladder placed on the bottom of the plethysmography chamber. The shaded area is decompressed on the right panel. (From Fleury Curado et al. (29). a.u.: arbitrary units.)

receptor subtypes are excitatory and found abundantly in the XII nucleus. Peripherally, serotoninergic stimulation at the nodose ganglion, especially of 5-HT$_3$ subtypes, inhibits respiration and induces central apneas (40). Most studies were performed in vagotomized and anesthetized animals and presented off-target effects such as elevated blood pressure. However, studies during natural sleep were less promising for the role of 5-HT in OSA drug development. Horner and his group showed that, in unanesthetized animals, endogenous 5-HT contributes little to GG muscle tone during sleep (41–43). The magnitude of 5-HT effect on the tonic drive of the upper airway appears to be stronger in cats and dogs than in rats (13, 44, 45). Of note, serotonin contributes to the activity of the GG in naturally awake rats, and the effects of 5-HT are modulated by the circadian cycle. However, the minimal effects of serotoninergic agents on OSA in humans prompted researchers to look for other

neurotransmitters involved in the tonic drive of pharyngeal muscles during sleep (46–48).

Chan et al. showed that infusion of phenylephrine, an α1 receptor agonist, into the hypoglossal nucleus of rats increased GG activity during NREM sleep and wakefulness, whereas α1 antagonist terazosin decreased GG activity. In contrast, the effect of α1 stimulation during REM sleep was minimal (49). However, another study showed that pontine injection of yohimbine, an α2 antagonist, reversed the depression of the hypoglossal motor activity during pharmacologically induced REM sleep (50).

Although the withdrawal of noradrenergic input seems to be an important mechanism for the decrease of pharyngeal muscle activity, administration of noradrenergic agents in animal and human studies did not improve motor activity during REM sleep (49, 51). A more complex network with contribution from the withdrawal of glutamatergic drive and tonic inhibitory drive by GABA and glycine may play a role on the suppression of respiratory motor activity during REM sleep (52). Grace et al., demonstrated that both muscarinic receptor antagonism or blockade of G-protein-coupled inwardly rectifying potassium (GIRK) channels caused GG reactivation during REM sleep and that cholinergic-GIRK channels can be activated by muscarinic inhibition (53).

In order to facilitate future studies, Horner et al. identified 1,492 potential drug targets in the hypoglossal nucleus and its afferents by identifying genes that differentiate these regions from the rest of the brain in an existing database. They listed the genes capable of increasing hypoglossal motor output, highlighting drugs specific to G-protein coupled receptors and ion channel modulators, especially the inward-rectifying potassium 2.4 (Kir2.4) channel, as well as other potential drug targets (54). Based on this mapping, Horner's group tested new targets such as thyrotropin releasing hormone (TRH) and its analog taltirelin. Both agents increased GG activity in anesthetized and in unanesthetized rats across sleep/wake states (55).

Dronabinol, a cannabinoid receptor agonist, reduced the number of apneas and augmented GG activity in rat model of central apneas induced by serotonin. This effect was abolished by cannabinoid receptor blockers (21). However, dronabinol also has effects on sleep architecture and reduces REM sleep. Cannabinoids' effects have been attributed to vagal inhibition, which led to improvement in upper airway muscle activation and breathing stability (56). Cannabinoids are now commonly utilized in a variety of sleep disorders, and further studies to assess the relevance and safety in patients with OSA are necessary.

Polotsky's laboratory has extensively studied leptin's potential as a respiratory stimulant and candidate for SDB pharmacotherapy. Leptin is an adipocyte-secreted hormone which increases metabolic rate and suppresses food intake by acting in hypothalamic centers (57). Initial experiments under anesthesia showed that leptin decreased collapsibility of the upper airway (58). The Johns Hopkins investigators developed a novel approach to analyze breathing throughout sleep-wake states in mice with continuous measurements of airflow (27). They used this model extensively to examine the effects of leptin on SDB. These studies showed mitigation of upper airway obstruction both in leptin deficient (ob/ob) mice (Figure 20.1) and DIO mice (28, 59). However, potential future use of leptin is limited by two major problems. First, obese individuals are leptin resistant and have a high prevalence of OSA despite high levels of circulating leptin. Second, high plasma levels of leptin have been implicated in cardiovascular complications such as hypertension (60). Nevertheless, future therapeutic use of leptin is possible, as we will discuss in the next section of our chapter.

Another potential hormonal treatment is oxytocin. Oxytocin is a neuropeptide capable of modulating the parasympathetic nervous system. Recent research in animal models has shown that activation of oxytocin neurons in the paraventricular nucleus prevented hypertension that occurs in response to intermittent hypoxia/hypercapnia in rats (61). Thus, oxytocin has the potential of regulating the autonomic dysfunction and cardiorespiratory events characteristic of OSA (62).

Preclinical studies, especially in freely behaving animals during natural sleep, are fundamental for the development of pharmacotherapies for OSA. A promising clinical trial in humans utilized a combination of atomoxetine and oxybutynin, a noradrenergic agonist and a muscarinic blocker, respectively (63). This approach was based on animal evidence of the role of noradrenergic and muscarinic modulation on GG activity and is discussed in a separate chapter.

One of the main limitations for pharmacotherapy in OSA is that the targets are not unique, and multiple side effects are possible. In an attempt to selectively activate hypoglossal motoneurons, researchers used genetically engineered G-protein coupled receptors. The designer receptors exclusively activated by designer drugs (DREADDs) are human cholinergic receptors modified to respond exclusively to a specific ligand. Stereotactic injection of DREADDs into the hypoglossal nucleus followed by systemic administration of DREADD-ligand led to increase in tongue muscle EMG and dilation of the pharynx (64, 65). These findings elegantly demonstrate the role of the hypoglossal nucleus to maintain upper airway patency. The injection of retrograde DREADDs directly to the GG muscle was effective for increasing GG muscle activity and improving pharyngeal patency and breathing during sleep in a mouse model of SDB (66). The latter approach has a higher translational potential because stereotactic brain injections are avoided. Chemogenetics are also important tools to understand the mechanisms of SDB. Recent work with inhibitory DREADDs showed

Table 20.1: Summary of Potential Therapeutic Targets for OSA Pharmacotherapy Originated from Pre-Clinical Studies

OSA Trait	Agents
Neuromuscular response	Serotonergic modulation (37–39)
	α1-adrenergic drugs (49)
	Yohimbine (50)
	Muscarinic blockade (53)
	Leptin (28, 59)
	Cannabinoids (56)
	Thyrotropin-releasing hormone (55)
	DREADDs activation of XII neurons (64, 65)
Chemoreflex and breathing stability	Leptin (68, 69)
	Cystathionine-lyase blockade (70)
	H_2S synthesis blockade (70) P2X2/3 receptors blockade (71)
	Sedative-hypnotics (72, 73)
	Optogenetic inhibition of PBel[CGRP] (74)

that catecholaminergic A1/C1 neurons in the medulla have an excitatory effect on the GG muscle, introducing a new potential therapeutic target for SDB (67). Table 20.1 summarizes potential agents for OSA therapy.

Future studies should pursue the identification of unique targets in the XII nucleus and areas of the brain modulating hypoglossal motoneuron activity. Investigators can deploy novel technology including single cell PCR and RNAseq followed by the pharmacological database analysis and drug trials. Similar strategy can be deployed for modulation of chemoreflex and breathing stability.

INTERVENTIONS TARGETING AROUSAL THRESHOLD

Airway occlusion and elevation of CO_2 stimuli can generate arousals with subsequent sleep fragmentation and respiratory instability. The external lateral parabrachial nucleus (PBel) in the pons integrates the chemosensory and mechanical stimuli that mediate arousals (75–77). The selective inhibition of calcitonin gene-related peptide (CGRP) neurons in the PBel prevented arousal during hypercapnia (74). Serotonin also seems to have a role in modulating arousal from hypercapnia. Deletion of serotoninergic neurons in the brainstem prevents arousal. This effect is attributed to the dorsal raphe serotonin neurons (DR[Sert]) that selectively project to the PBel. Deletion of optogenetic inhibition of the DR[Sert] increases arousal latency (78). Thus, serotonergic modulation may increase the arousal threshold and contribute to OSA treatment.

Animal studies have also shown that medications such as zolpidem, lorazepam and pentobarbital increase GG muscle activity during sleep when administered systemically to rodents. This effect is attributed to an increase in arousal threshold that allows a longer and more stable ventilatory response (72, 73). Sedative hypnotic medications have been prescribed with caution in apneic patients due to the potential depression of neuromuscular activity that could exacerbate OSA. One of the challenges for translation of this research is identifying individuals with low arousal threshold where the benefits would outweigh the depression in neuromuscular activity.

INTERVENTIONS IN THE PERIPHERAL CHEMOREFLEX FOR THE TREATMENT OF SDB

Intermittent hypoxia is the main factor in the pathology of sleep apnea (2). Fluctuations in arterial O_2 levels evoke cardiorespiratory responses in order to restore normal arterial blood gases (79–84). The carotid bodies (CB) are major oxygen peripheral sensors localized at the common carotid artery bifurcation (83, 85). Neuron-like O_2-sensitive glomus (type I) cells and glia-like type II cells compose the CB glomerular structure (84). The CB mainly governs the peripheral hypoxic chemoreflex, playing an important role in the control of breathing (79, 80, 82–85). Even modest drops in arterial O_2 levels can be detected by the CB, causing acute hyperventilation (79, 80, 82–84). The hypoxic ventilatory response (HVR) is initiated peripherally by the activation of CB and depolarization of type I cells. Afferent chemosensory input is transmitted through the carotid sinus nerve (CSN), a branch of the glossopharyngeal nerve, to the nucleus of the solitary tract (NTS) and then to the brainstem respiratory network and respiratory motoneurons (83, 84, 86). The activation of this neural circuit leads to hyperventilation and sympatho-excitation in response to hypoxia and hypercapnia (79, 80, 82–85).

Impaired respiratory response to hypoxia leads to breathing instability and is one of the pathophysiological traits of SDB (70, 87–91). Loop gain is an engineering concept that defines the magnitude of ventilation in response to a disturbance, such as an obstruction in the upper airway in OSA patients (92, 93). Loop gain is regulated by both a controller gain and a plant gain (94). The peripheral chemosensitivity to arterial blood gases composes the controller gain, while the ventilatory response to alter the gas exchange refers to the plant gain (93, 94). An exacerbated respiratory response to the upper airway obstructions (high loop gain) is observed in 36% of OSA patients with anatomy predisposition to upper airway collapse (92). The over-exuberant hypoxic response causes breathing instability and augments upper airway obstruction by inducing negative inspiratory pressure swings and attenuating the activity of hypoglossal motoneurons (3, 92, 95–97). Augmented responses to hypoxia and hypercapnia are involved in the emergence and progression of Cheyne-Stokes respiration, a subtype of central apnea predominantly observed in patients with heart failure (98, 99). Central apnea is also uniformly present during hypoxic exposure of high altitudes (100). The modulation of CB chemosensitivity has been proposed as a potential therapeutic approach for SDB. Different molecular pathways in CB have been identified as promising targets for drug development (101).

Potential Pharmacological Targets in CB
Hypoxia-Inducible Factors (HIF)
Intermittent hypoxia induces functional plasticity in the CB (102). The overactivation of CB induced by intermittent hypoxia is related to the production of reactive oxygen species (ROS) (103–106). Transcriptional responses to oxidative stress induced by intermittent hypoxia in CB appear to be regulated by the balance between HIF-1α and HIF-2α signaling (104–106). HIF-1α and HIF-2α are transcriptional factors involved in the expression of pro-oxidant (i.e. NADPH oxidase 2) and antioxidant enzymes (Sod2), respectively (103–105, 107). Intermittent hypoxia increases the levels of HIF-1α and reduces HIF-2α in the CB (103–105). HIF-1α-deficient mice (HIF-1α$^{+/-}$) are resistant to the CB overactivation induced

by intermittent hypoxia, showing reduced HVR (108). On the other hand, the genetic ablation of HIF-2α in mice (HIF-2α$^{+/-}$ mice) reduced the expression of Sod2, augmented HVR, and caused ventilatory instability during sleep, leading to increased post-sigh apneas (109) SDB was abolished in these mice by the administration of the antioxidant MnTMPyP (manganese (III) tetrakis (1-methyl-4-pyridyl) porphyrin pentachloride) (109). Thus, molecular manipulations of HIF-1α and HIF-2α signaling in the CB are promising pharmacological targets for SDB.

Purinergic Receptors
Purinergic system mainly governs the excitatory post-synaptic responses of peripheral chemoreflex through the activation of P2X2/3 receptors in glomus cells and petrosal chemosensitive terminals (110–113). Acute hypoxia modulates the P2X2 receptor in vitro and the P2X-receptor antagonist, suramin, suppresses depolarization induced by hypoxia in petrosal neurons (113). P2X2 deficiency in mice resulted in attenuated HVR and reduced CSN activity during hypoxic stimulus. Double knockout for the P2X2 and P2X3 receptors results in more marked attenuation of these responses (111). Hence, the pharmacological blockade of P2X2/3 receptors in CB may normalize hypoxic chemoreflex and treat SDB. Indeed, administration of P2X3 antagonist AF-454 blunted HVR and decreased the number of apneas in newborn rats (71).

Gasotransmitters: the balance between the gasotransmitters carbon monoxide (CO) and hydrogen sulfide (H$_2$S) appears to be involved in the regulation of CB chemoreflex (106, 114). CO and H$_2$S are generated by the enzymes hemeoxygenase-2 (HO-2) and cystathionine-γ-lyase (CSE), respectively (114, 115). While CO and HO-2 levels are associated with CB inhibition, H$_2$S and CSE increase CB hypoxic response (114, 115). CSE-deficient mice (CSE$^{-/-}$) show reduced CB chemosensory activity and impaired HVR (114). On the other hand, HO-2-null mice (HO-2$^{-/-}$) have irregular breathing with a high frequency of central and obstructive apneas, and hypopneas during NREM and REM sleep (70). The pharmacological blockade of CSE with ʟ-propargylglycine (ʟ-PAG) treated the SDB of HO-2-null mice (70). Thus, interventions in the CB that promote the downregulation of CSE and/or upregulation of HO-2, which balance the levels of H$_2$S and CO, are promising pharmacotherapies for SDB.

Leptin: the long isoform of leptin receptor (LEPR^b) is largely expressed in the CB glomus cells (68, 116) and leptin binding stimulates CB chemoreflex (68, 69). Our group has shown that subcutaneous infusion of leptin augmented CSN activity and increased HVR in lean C57BL/6J mice, which was abolished by the CSN denervation (68). Augmented ventilatory response to hypoxia was also observed in LEPR[b]-deficient *db/db* mice transfected with LEPR[b] in the CB (68) and in obese Zucker rats with leptin infusion (117). LEPR[b] replacement in the CB of *db/db* mice increased ventilation during NREM and REM sleep, which may prevent hypoventilation during sleep (68). However, leptin could also overactivate CB chemoreflex, exacerbating the respiratory response to hypoxia, leading to breathing instability and SDB (101). Different pathways may be involved in the leptin-induced augmented ventilation, including activation of O_2-sensitive channels TRPM7 (118), TASK-1 and -3 (117, 119), TRPC (120–122), BK_{Ca} (123, 124), and K_{ATP} (125). However, the specific role of these channels in the leptin downstream regulation of hypoxic chemoreflex still needs to be determined.

ALVEOLAR HYPOVENTILATION SYNDROMES

Interventions Targeting Control of Breathing

Obesity increases the risk of OSA and predisposes to OHS when the depressed hypercapnic ventilatory response leads to daytime hypercapnia and hypoventilation during sleep. Respiratory stimulants such as medroxyprogesterone and acetazolamide were proposed but had limited efficacy (7). Leptin deficient *ob/ob* mice and DIO mice develop characteristics of OSA and OHS (28, 57, 58, 126–128). *ob/ob* mice have hypercapnia and reduced hypercapnic ventilatory responses that are resolved with leptin replacement (126–129).

DIO mice and obese humans have elevated peripheral plasma levels of leptin and are resistant to its effects (59, 130–133). Higher levels of leptin have also been demonstrated in subjects with OSA when compared to weight-matched controls with a reduction in leptin levels after CPAP treatment (134, 135). Emergent evidence suggests that resistance to the respiratory effects of leptin in obesity is caused by limited leptin transport through the blood-brain barrier (BBB). Intranasal administration of leptin in DIO mice bypassed the BBB and improved SDB by increasing ventilation and decreasing the number of oxygen desaturations during NREM and REM sleep (59). In a separate study in obese mice, intranasal leptin was also effective in relieving inspiratory flow limitation and ventilatory depression induced

by morphine during sleep (136). Agents such as serotonin agonists (137) and ampakines (138) (modulators of glutamate receptor activity) are also potential tools to protect against opioid-induced respiratory depression. Approaches to mitigate opioid-induced respiratory depression are discussed in a separate chapter.

Interventions Targeting Motoneurons

Mutations in the gene encoding the acid α-glucosidase (GAA) enzyme cause progressive respiratory failure and tongue motor dysfunction in Pompe disease due to deposits of glycogen in the muscular system. Evidence suggests that Pompe disease also leads to the accumulation of glycogen in the central nervous system even with the replacement of the enzyme (139). Pre-clinical studies demonstrated that adeno-associated virus (AAV) delivery of alpha-glucosidase gene can effectively restore cardiac and respiratory function in the Pompe mouse model (140, 141). These studies were the foundation for the development of clinical trials to improve respiratory function in patients via direct injection of the AAV mediated gene therapy to the diaphragm (142).

Genetic approach is also being pursued in other neuromuscular diseases such as ALS. Using AAV to deliver microRNA against human SOD1 in neonatal superoxide dismutase (SOD1) mutant mice showed effective silencing of the mutant gene with increased survival, preserved motor function, and reduced neuroinflammation (143). A variety of neuroprotective and anti-inflammatory drugs have been tested in SOD1 mice with unsuccessful translational results in studies in humans (144).

Repetitive acute intermittent hypoxia (AIH) is linked to respiratory plasticity, serotonin release, and brain-derived neurotrophic factor synthesis. Chronic AIH improved respiratory and non-respiratory motor function in rats with cervical spine injury (CSI) (145). Similar approach has also been tested in an ALS model with the improvement of phrenic plasticity (146). However, prolonged exposure to hypoxia may have detrimental effects such as cognitive dysfunction and increased sympathetic activation. Animal studies are fundamental to study different AIH protocols that effectively induce plasticity with minimal side effects (147).

CONCLUSION

Currently, there is no pharmacotherapy for SDB. The complex pathophysiology with different functional circuits for upper airway motor control during NREM and REM sleep and diversity of phenotypes in OSA pose a challenge for the pharmaceutical development in SDB. Animal models have limitations such as the lack of a model of severe OSA, a variety of methodologies with different results depending on the model (induced vs. natural sleep or anesthetized animals), or parameters evaluated (apneas, flow limitation, GG muscle activation). Nevertheless, animal studies are indispensable in identifying potential drug targets and evaluating the effects of drug candidates on different types of SDB and phenotypic traits predisposing to OSA.

REFERENCES

1. Smith JC, Abdala APL, Borgmann A, et al. 2013 Brainstem respiratory networks: building blocks and microcircuits. Trends Neurosci **36**:152–162.

2. Dempsey JA, Veasey SC, Morgan BJ, et al. 2010 Pathophysiology of sleep apnea. Physiol Rev **90**:47–112.

3. Eckert DJ 2018 Phenotypic approaches to obstructive sleep apnoea – New pathways for targeted therapy. Sleep Med Rev **37**:45–59.

4. White DP 2005 Pathogenesis of obstructive and central sleep apnea. Am J Respir Crit Care Med **172**:1363–1370.

5. Orr JE, Malhotra A, Sands SA 2017 Pathogenesis of central and complex sleep apnoea: Central apnoea mechanisms. Respirology **22**:43–52.

6. Martin TJ, Sanders MH 1995 Chronic alveolar hypoventilation: a review for the clinician. Sleep **18**:617–634.

7. Mokhlesi B 2010 Obesity hypoventilation syndrome: a state-of-the-art review. Respir Care **55**:1347–1362.

8. Chowdhuri S, Javaheri S 2017 Sleep disordered breathing caused by chronic opioid use. Sleep Med Clin **12**:573–586.

9. Bourke SC, Gibson GJ 2002 Sleep and breathing in neuromuscular disease. Eur Respir J **19**:1194–1201.

10. Kim LJ, Freire C, Fleury Curado T, et al. 2019 The role of animal models in developing pharmacotherapy for obstructive sleep apnea. J Clin Med **8**:2049.

11. Hendricks JC, Kline LR, Kovalski RJ, et al. 1987 The English bulldog: a natural model of sleep-disordered breathing. J Appl Physiol **63**:1344–1350.

12. Lonergan RP, Ware JC, Atkinson RL, et al. 1998 Sleep apnea in obese miniature pigs. J Appl Physiol **84**:531–536.

13. Veasey SC, Fenik P, Panckeri K, et al. 1999 The effects of trazodone with L-tryptophan on sleep-disordered breathing in the English bulldog. Am J Respir Crit Care Med **160**:1659–1667.

14. Farré R, Nácher M, Serrano-Mollar A, et al. 2007 Rat model of chronic recurrent airway obstructions to study the sleep apnea syndrome. Sleep **30**:930–933.

15. Neuzeret PC, Gormand F, Reix P, et al. 2011 A new animal model of obstructive sleep apnea responding to continuous positive airway pressure. Sleep **34**:541–8.

16. Crossland RF, Durgan DJ, Lloyd EE, et al. 2013 A new rodent model for obstructive sleep apnea: effects on ATP-mediated dilations in cerebral arteries. Am J Physiol Regul Integr Comp Physiol **305**:R334–R342.

17. Lee M-C, Lee CH, Hong S-L, et al. 2013 Establishment of a rabbit model of obstructive sleep apnea by paralyzing the genioglossus. JAMA Otolaryngol Neck Surg **139**:834.

18. Lu H-y., Dong F, Liu C-y, et al. 2015 An animal model of obstructive sleep apnoea-hypopnea syndrome corrected by mandibular advancement device. Eur J Orthod **37**:284–289.

19. Lee M-C, Rhee C-S, Joe S, et al. 2016 A single primary site obstruction may lead to sleep-disordered breathing in multiple sites: an animal model. Ann Otol Rhinol Laryngol **125**:277–283.

20. Kimoff RJ, Makino H, Horner RL, et al. 1994 Canine model of obstructive sleep apnea: model description and preliminary application. J Appl Physiol **76**:1810–1817.

21. Calik MW, Radulovacki M, Carley DW 2014 Intranodose ganglion injections of dronabinol attenuate serotonin-induced apnea in Sprague-Dawley rat. Respir Physiol Neurobiol **190**:20–24.

22. Yamauchi M, Hasan O, Dostal J, et al. 2008 Post-sigh breathing behavior and spontaneous pauses in the C57BL/6J (B6) mouse. Respir Physiol Neurobiol **162**:117–125.

23. Brennick MJ, Delikatny J, Pack AI, et al. 2014 Tongue fat infiltration in obese versus lean Zucker rats. Sleep **37**:1095–1102.

24. Brennick MJ, Pickup S, Cater JR, et al. 2006 Phasic respiratory pharyngeal mechanics by magnetic resonance imaging in lean and obese Zucker rats. Am J Respir Crit Care Med **173**:1031–1037.

25. Brennick MJ, Pack AI, Ko K, et al. 2009 Altered upper airway and soft tissue structures in the New Zealand obese mouse. Am J Respir Crit Care Med **179**:158–169.

26. Baum DM, Morales Rodriguez B, Attali V, et al. 2018 New Zealand obese mice as a translational model of obesity-related obstructive sleep apnea syndrome. Am J Respir Crit Care Med **198**:1336–1339.

27. Hernandez AB, Kirkness JP, Smith PL, et al. 2012 Novel whole body plethysmography system for the continuous characterization of sleep and breathing in a mouse. J Appl Physiol Bethesda Md 1985 **112**:671–680.

28. Pho H, Hernandez AB, Arias RS, et al. 2016 The effect of leptin replacement on sleep-disordered breathing in the leptin-deficient *ob/ob* mouse. J Appl Physiol Bethesda Md 1985 **120**:78–86.

29. Fleury Curado T, Pho H, Berger S, et al. 2018 Sleep-disordered breathing in C57BL/6J mice with diet-induced obesity. Sleep **41** (8):zsy089.

30. Davis EM, O'Donnell CP 2013 Rodent models of sleep apnea. Respir Physiol Neurobiol **188**:355–361.

31. Kubin L, Davies RO, Pack AI 1998 Control of upper airway motoneurons during REM sleep. News Physiol Sci **13**:91–97.

32. Remmers JE, deGroot WJ, Sauerland EK, et al. 1978 Pathogenesis of upper airway occlusion during sleep. J Appl Physiol **44**:931–938.

33. Zaidi FN, Meadows P, Jacobowitz O, et al. 2013 Tongue anatomy and physiology, the scientific basis for a novel targeted neurostimulation system designed for the treatment of obstructive sleep apnea. Neuromodulation **16**:376–386; discussion 386.

34. Fuller D, Mateika JH, Fregosi RF 1998 Co-activation of tongue protrudor and retractor muscles during chemoreceptor stimulation in the rat. J Physiol **507 (Pt 1)**:265–276.

35. Fuller DD, Williams JS, Janssen PL, et al. 1999 Effect of co-activation of tongue protrudor and retractor muscles on tongue movements and pharyngeal airflow mechanics in the rat. J Physiol **519 (Pt 2)**:601–613.

36. Schwartz AR, Bennett ML, Smith PL, et al. 2001 Therapeutic electrical stimulation of the hypoglossal nerve in obstructive sleep apnea. Arch Otolaryngol Head Neck Surg **127**:1216–1223.

37. Sood S, Liu X, Liu H, et al. 2003 5-HT at hypoglossal motor nucleus and respiratory control of genioglossus muscle in anesthetized rats. Respir Physiol Neurobiol **138**:205–221.

38. Fenik VB, Davies RO, Kubin L 2005 REM sleep-like atonia of hypoglossal (XII) motoneurons is caused by loss of noradrenergic and serotonergic inputs. Am J Respir Crit Care Med **172**:1322–1330.

39. Veasey SC 2003 Serotonin agonists and antagonists in obstructive sleep apnea: therapeutic potential. Am J Respir Med Drugs Devices Interv **2**:21–29.

40. Veasey SC 2001 Pharmacotherapies for obstructive sleep apnea: how close are we? Curr Opin Pulm Med **7**:399–403.

41. Sood S, Liu X, Liu H, et al. 2007 Genioglossus muscle activity and serotonergic modulation of hypoglossal motor output in obese Zucker rats. J Appl Physiol Bethesda Md 1985 **102**:2240–2250.

42. Sood S, Morrison JL, Liu H, et al. 2005 Role of endogenous serotonin in modulating genioglossus muscle activity in awake and sleeping rats. Am J Respir Crit Care Med **172**:1338–1347.

43. Sood S, Raddatz E, Liu X, et al. 2006 Inhibition of serotonergic medullary raphe obscurus neurons suppresses genioglossus and diaphragm activities in anesthetized but not conscious rats. J Appl Physiol **100**:1807–1821.

44. Jelev A, Sood S, Liu H, et al. 2001 Microdialysis perfusion of 5-HT into hypoglossal motor nucleus differentially modulates genioglossus activity across natural sleep-wake states in rats. J Physiol **532**:467–481.

45. Kubin L 2014 Sleep-wake control of the upper airway by noradrenergic neurons, with and without intermittent hypoxia. Prog Brain Res **209**:255–274.

46. Berry RB, Yamaura EM, Gill K, et al. 1999 Acute effects of paroxetine on genioglossus activity in obstructive sleep apnea. Sleep **22**:1087–1092.

47. Kraiczi H, Hedner J, Dahlof P, et al. 1999 Effect of serotonin uptake inhibition on breathing during sleep and daytime symptoms in obstructive sleep apnea. Sleep **22**:61–67.

48. Marshall NS, Yee BJ, Desai AV, et al. 2008 Two randomized placebo-controlled trials to evaluate the efficacy and tolerability of mirtazapine for the treatment of obstructive sleep apnea. Sleep **31**:824–831.

49. Chan E, Steenland HW, Liu H, et al. 2006 Endogenous excitatory drive modulating respiratory muscle activity across sleep-wake states. Am J Respir Crit Care Med **174**:1264–1273.

50. Song G, Poon C-S 2017 α2-Adrenergic blockade rescues hypoglossal motor defense against obstructive sleep apnea. JCI Insight **2**:e91456.

51. Taranto-Montemurro L, Sands SA, Edwards BA, et al. 2016 Desipramine improves upper airway collapsibility and reduces OSA severity in patients with minimal muscle compensation. Eur Respir J **48**:1340–1350.

52. Horner RL 2009 Emerging principles and neural substrates underlying tonic sleep-state-dependent influences on respiratory motor activity. Philos Trans R Soc B Biol Sci **364**:2553–2564.

53. Grace KP, Hughes SW, Horner RL 2013 Identification of the mechanism mediating genioglossus muscle suppression in REM sleep. Am J Respir Crit Care Med **187**:311–319.

54. Horner RL, Grace KP, Wellman A 2017 A resource of potential drug targets and strategic decision-making for obstructive sleep apnoea pharmacotherapy. Respirology **22**:861–873.

55. Liu W-Y, Liu H, Aggarwal J, et al. 2020 Differential activating effects of thyrotropin-releasing hormone and its analog taltirelin on motor output to the tongue musculature in vivo. Sleep **43** (9):zsaa053.

56. Suraev AS, Marshall NS, Vandrey R, et al. 2020 Cannabinoid therapies in the management of sleep disorders: A systematic review of preclinical and clinical studies. Sleep Med Rev **53**:101339.

57. Friedman J 2016 The long road to leptin. J Clin Invest **126**:4727–4734.

58. Polotsky M, Elsayed-Ahmed AS, Pichard L, et al. 2012 Effects of leptin and obesity on the upper airway function. J Appl Physiol **112**:1637–1643.

59. Berger S, Pho H, Fleury-Curado T, et al. 2019 Intranasal leptin relieves sleep-disordered breathing in mice with diet-induced obesity. Am J Respir Crit Care Med **199**:773–783.

60. Bravo PE, Morse S, Borne DM, et al. 2006 Leptin and hypertension in obesity. Vasc Health Risk Manag **2**:163–169.

61. Jameson H, Bateman R, Byrne P, et al. 2016 Oxytocin neuron activation prevents hypertension that occurs with chronic intermittent hypoxia/hypercapnia in rats. Am J Physiol Heart Circ Physiol **310**:H1549–H1557.

62. Jain V, Kimbro S, Kowalik G, et al. 2020 Intranasal oxytocin increases respiratory rate and reduces obstructive event duration and oxygen desaturation in obstructive sleep apnea patients: a randomized double blinded placebo controlled study. Sleep Med **74**:242–247.

63. Taranto-Montemurro L, Messineo L, Sands SA, et al. 2018 The combination of atomoxetine and oxybutynin greatly reduces obstructive sleep apnea severity: a randomized, placebo-controlled, double-blind crossover trial. Am J Respir Crit Care Med. https://doi.org/10.1164/rccm.201808-1493OC.

64. Horton GA, Fraigne JJ, Torontali ZA, et al. 2017 Activation of the hypoglossal to tongue musculature motor pathway by remote control. Sci Rep **7**:45860.

65. Curado TF, Fishbein K, Pho H, et al. 2017 Chemogenetic stimulation of the hypoglossal neurons improves upper airway patency. Sci Rep **7**:44392.

66. Fleury Curado T, Pho H, Freire C, et al. 2020 DREADD approach to treatment of sleep disordered breathing. Am J Respir Crit Care Med. https://doi.org/10.1164/rccm.202002-0321OC.

67. Rukhadze I, Carballo NJ, Bandaru SS, et al. 2017 Catecholaminergic A1/C1 neurons contribute to the maintenance of upper airway muscle tone but may not participate in NREM sleep-related depression of these muscles. Respir Physiol Neurobiol **244**:41–50.

68. Caballero-Eraso C, Shin M-K, Pho H, et al. 2019 Leptin acts in the carotid bodies to increase minute ventilation during wakefulness and sleep and augment the hypoxic ventilatory response. J Physiol **597**:151–172.

69. Ribeiro MJ, Sacramento JF, Gallego-Martin T, et al. 2018 High fat diet blunts the effects of leptin on ventilation and on carotid body activity. J Physiol **596**:3187–3199.

70. Peng Y-J, Zhang X, Gridina A, et al. 2017 Complementary roles of gasotransmitters CO and H$_2$S in sleep apnea. Proc Natl Acad Sci **114**:1413–1418.

71. Katayama PL, Abdala AP, Charles I, et al. 2020 P2X3 receptor antagonism reduces the occurrence of apnoeas in newborn rats. Respir Physiol Neurobiol **277**:103438.

72. Younes M, Park E, Horner RL 2007 Pentobarbital sedation increases genioglossus respiratory activity in sleeping rats. Sleep **30**:478–488.

73. Park E, Younes M, Liu H, et al. 2008 Systemic vs. central administration of common hypnotics reveals opposing effects on genioglossus muscle activity in rats. Sleep **31**:355–365.

74. Kaur S, Wang JL, Ferrari L, et al. 2017 A genetically defined circuit for arousal from sleep during hypercapnia. Neuron **96**:1153–1167.e5.

75. Kaur S, Pedersen NP, Yokota S, et al. 2013 Glutamatergic signaling from the parabrachial nucleus plays a critical role in hypercapnic arousal. J Neurosci Off J Soc Neurosci **33**:7627–7640.

76. Yokota S, Kaur S, VanderHorst VG, et al. 2015 Respiratory-related outputs of glutamatergic, hypercapnia-responsive parabrachial neurons in mice. J Comp Neurol **523**:907–920.

77. Kaur S, Saper CB 2019 Neural circuitry underlying waking up to hypercapnia. Front Neurosci **13**:401.

78. Kaur S, De Luca R, Khanday MA, et al. 2020 Role of serotonergic dorsal raphe neurons in hypercapnia-induced arousals. Nat Commun **11**:2769.

79. Gonzalez-Martín MC, Vega-Agapito MV, Conde SV, et al. 2011 Carotid body function and ventilatory responses in intermittent hypoxia. Evidence for anomalous brainstem integration of arterial chemoreceptor input. J Cell Physiol **226**:1961–1969.

80. Silva AQ, Schreihofer AM 2011 Altered sympathetic reflexes and vascular reactivity in rats after exposure to chronic intermittent hypoxia. J Physiol **589**:1463–1476.

81. Prabhakar NR, Kumar GK, Peng Y-J 2012 Sympatho-adrenal activation by chronic intermittent hypoxia. J Appl Physiol Bethesda Md 1985 **113**:1304–1310.

82. Nurse CA, Piskuric NA 2013 Signal processing at mammalian carotid body chemoreceptors. Semin Cell Dev Biol **24**:22–30.

83. Prabhakar NR 2013 Sensing hypoxia: physiology, genetics and epigenetics. J Physiol **591**:2245–2257.

84. Ortega-Sáenz P, López-Barneo J 2020 Physiology of the carotid body: from molecules to disease. Annu Rev Physiol **82**:127–149.

85. Lindsey BG, Nuding SC, Segers LS, et al. 2018 Carotid bodies and the integrated cardiorespiratory response to hypoxia. Physiol Bethesda Md **33**:281–297.

86. Eldridge FL 1974 Central neural respiratory stimulatory effect of active respiration. J Appl Physiol **37**:723–735.

87. Bellville JW, Whipp BJ, Kaufman RD, et al. 1979 Central and peripheral chemoreflex loop gain in normal and carotid body-resected subjects. J Appl Physiol **46**:843–853.

88. Nemati S, Edwards BA, Sands SA, et al. 2011 Model-based characterization of ventilatory stability using spontaneous breathing. J Appl Physiol Bethesda Md 1985 **111**:55–67.

89. Edwards BA, Sands SA, Berger PJ 2013 Postnatal maturation of breathing stability and loop gain: the role of carotid chemoreceptor development. Respir Physiol Neurobiol 185:144–155.

90. Peng Y-J, Zhang X, Nanduri J, et al. 2018 Therapeutic targeting of the carotid body for treating sleep apnea in a pre-clinical mouse model. Adv Exp Med Biol 1071:109–114.

91. Pham LV, Schwartz AR, Polotsky VY 2018 Integrating loop gain into the understanding of obstructive sleep apnoea mechanisms. J Physiol 596:3819–3820.

92. Eckert DJ, White DP, Jordan AS, et al. 2013 Defining phenotypic causes of obstructive sleep apnea. Identification of novel therapeutic targets. Am J Respir Crit Care Med 188:996–1004.

93. Deacon-Diaz N, Malhotra A 2018 Inherent vs. induced loop gain abnormalities in obstructive sleep apnea. Front Neurol 9:896.

94. Khoo MC 2000 Determinants of ventilatory instability and variability. Respir Physiol 122:167–182.

95. Wellman A, Edwards BA, Sands SA, et al. 2013 A simplified method for determining phenotypic traits in patients with obstructive sleep apnea. J Appl Physiol Bethesda Md 1985 114:911–922.

96. Eckert DJ, Malhotra A, Jordan AS 2009 Mechanisms of apnea. Prog Cardiovasc Dis 51:313–323.

97. Younes M 2008 Role of respiratory control mechanisms in the pathogenesis of obstructive sleep disorders. J Appl Physiol Bethesda Md 1985 105:1389–1405.

98. Ahmed M, Serrette C, Kryger MH, et al. 1994 Ventilatory instability in patients with congestive heart failure and nocturnal Cheyne-Stokes breathing. Sleep 17:527–534.

99. Yumino D, Bradley TD 2008 Central sleep apnea and Cheyne-Stokes respiration. Proc Am Thorac Soc 5:226–236.

100. Burgess KR, Ainslie PN 2016 Central sleep apnea at high altitude. Adv Exp Med Biol 903:275–283.

101. Kim LJ, Polotsky VY 2020 Carotid body and metabolic syndrome: mechanisms and potential therapeutic targets. Int J Mol Sci 21 (14), 5117.

102. Peng Y-J, Overholt JL, Kline D, et al. 2003 Induction of sensory long-term facilitation in the carotid body by intermittent hypoxia: implications for recurrent apneas. Proc Natl Acad Sci U S A 100:10073–10078.

103. Prabhakar NR, Semenza GL 2016 Regulation of carotid body oxygen sensing by hypoxia-inducible factors. Pflugers Arch 468:71–75.

104. Semenza GL, Prabhakar NR 2015 Neural regulation of hypoxia-inducible factors and redox state drives the pathogenesis of hypertension in a rodent model of sleep apnea. J Appl Physiol Bethesda Md 1985 119:1152–1156.

105. Semenza GL, Prabhakar NR 2018 The role of hypoxia-inducible factors in carotid body (patho) physiology. J Physiol 596:2977–2983.

106. Prabhakar NR, Peng Y-J, Yuan G, et al. 2018 Reactive oxygen radicals and gaseous transmitters in carotid body activation by intermittent hypoxia. Cell Tissue Res 372:427–431.

107. Nanduri J, Wang N, Yuan G, et al. 2009 Intermittent hypoxia degrades HIF-2alpha via calpains resulting in oxidative stress: implications for recurrent apnea-induced morbidities. Proc Natl Acad Sci U S A 106:1199–1204.

108. Peng Y-J, Yuan G, Ramakrishnan D, et al. 2006 Heterozygous HIF-1α deficiency impairs carotid body-mediated systemic responses and reactive oxygen species generation in mice exposed to intermittent hypoxia. J Physiol 577:705–716.

109. Peng Y-J, Nanduri J, Khan SA, et al. 2011 Hypoxia-inducible factor 2α (HIF-2α) heterozygous-null mice exhibit exaggerated carotid body sensitivity to hypoxia, breathing instability, and hypertension. Proc Natl Acad Sci U S A 108:3065–3070.

110. Zhang M, Zhong H, Vollmer C, et al. 2000 Co-release of ATP and ACh mediates hypoxic signalling at rat carotid body chemoreceptors. J Physiol 525 (Pt 1):143–158.

111. Rong W, Gourine AV, Cockayne DA, et al. 2003 Pivotal role of nucleotide P2X2 receptor subunit of the ATP-gated ion channel mediating ventilatory responses to hypoxia. J Neurosci 23:11315–11321.

112. Moraes DJA, da Silva MP, Spiller PF, et al. 2018 Purinergic plasticity within petrosal neurons in hypertension. Am J Physiol Regul Integr Comp Physiol 315:R963–R971.

113. Prasad M, Fearon IM, Zhang M, et al. 2001 Expression of P2X2 and P2X3 receptor subunits in rat carotid body afferent neurones: role in chemosensory signalling. J Physiol 537:667–677.

114. Peng Y-J, Nanduri J, Raghuraman G, et al. 2010 H₂S mediates O₂ sensing in the carotid body. Proc Natl Acad Sci U S A 107:10719–10724.

115. Prabhakar NR, Dinerman JL, Agani FH, et al. 1995 Carbon monoxide: a role in carotid body chemoreception. Proc Natl Acad Sci U S A 92:1994–1997.

116. Porzionato A, Rucinski M, Macchi V, et al. 2011 Expression of leptin and leptin receptor isoforms in the rat and human carotid body. Brain Res 1385:56–67.

117. Yuan F, Wang H, Feng J, et al. 2018 Leptin signaling in the carotid body regulates a hypoxic ventilatory response through altering TASK channel expression. Front Physiol 9:249.

118. Shin M-K, Eraso CC, Mu Y-P, et al. 2019 Leptin induces hypertension acting on transient receptor potential melastatin 7 channel in the carotid body. Circ Res 125:989–1002.

119. Wei Z, Hao Y, Yu H, et al. 2020 Disordered leptin signaling in the retrotrapezoid nucleus is associated with the impaired hypercapnic ventilatory response in obesity. Life Sci **257**:117994.

120. Qiu J, Fang Y, Rønnekleiv OK, et al. 2010 Leptin excites proopiomelanocortin neurons via activation of TRPC channels. J Neurosci Off J Soc Neurosci **30**:1560–1565.

121. Qiu J, Fang Y, Bosch MA, et al. 2011 Guinea pig kisspeptin neurons are depolarized by leptin via activation of TRPC channels. Endocrinology **152**:1503–1514.

122. Dhar M, Wayman GA, Zhu M, et al. 2014 Leptin-induced spine formation requires TrpC channels and the CaM kinase cascade in the hippocampus. J Neurosci Off J Soc Neurosci **34**:10022–10033.

123. Shanley LJ, Irving AJ, Rae MG, et al. 2002 Leptin inhibits rat hippocampal neurons via activation of large conductance calcium-activated K+ channels. Nat Neurosci **5**:299–300.

124. Shanley LJ, O'Malley D, Irving AJ, et al. 2002 Leptin inhibits epileptiform-like activity in rat hippocampal neurones via PI 3-kinase-driven activation of BK channels. J Physiol **545**:933–944.

125. Harvey J, McKay NG, Walker KS, et al. 2000 Essential role of phosphoinositide 3-kinase in leptin-induced K(ATP) channel activation in the rat CRI-G1 insulinoma cell line. J Biol Chem **275**:4660–4669.

126. O'donnell CP, Schaub CD, Haines AS, et al. 1999 Leptin prevents respiratory depression in obesity. Am J Respir Crit Care Med **159**:1477–1484.

127. Breslow MJ, Min-Lee K, Brown DR, et al. 1999 Effect of leptin deficiency on metabolic rate in ob/ob mice. Am J Physiol **276**:E443–449.

128. Yao Q, Shin MK, Jun JC, et al. 2013 Effect of chronic intermittent hypoxia on triglyceride uptake in different tissues. J Lipid Res **54**:1058–1065.

129. Pho H, Hernandez AB, Arias RS, et al. 2016 The effect of leptin replacement on sleep-disordered breathing in the leptin-deficient *ob/ob* mouse. J Appl Physiol **120**:78–86.

130. Maffei M, Halaas J, Ravussin E, et al. 1995 Leptin levels in human and rodent: measurement of plasma leptin and ob RNA in obese and weight-reduced subjects. Nat Med **1**:1155–1161.

131. Considine RV, Sinha MK, Heiman ML, et al. 1996 Serum immunoreactive-leptin concentrations in normal-weight and obese humans. N Engl J Med **334**:292–295.

132. Scarpace PJ, Zhang Y 2009 Leptin resistance: a predisposing factor for diet-induced obesity. Am J Physiol Regul Integr Comp Physiol **296**:R493–500.

133. Wauman J, Tavernier J 2011 Leptin receptor signaling: pathways to leptin resistance. Front Biosci Landmark Ed **16**:2771–2793.

134. Ip MS, Lam KS, Ho C, et al. 2000 Serum leptin and vascular risk factors in obstructive sleep apnea [see comments]. Chest **118**:580–586.

135. Chin K, Shimizu K, Nakamura T, et al. 1999 Changes in intra-abdominal visceral fat and serum leptin levels in patients with obstructive sleep apnea syndrome following nasal continuous positive airway pressure therapy. Circulation **100**:706–712.

136. Freire C, Pho H, Kim LJ, et al. 2020 Intranasal leptin prevents opioid induced sleep disordered breathing in obese mice. Am J Respir Cell Mol Biol. https://doi.org/10.1165/rcmb.2020-0117OC.

137. Manzke T, Guenther U, Ponimaskin EG, et al. 2003 5-HT4(a) receptors avert opioid-induced breathing depression without loss of analgesia. Science **301**:226–229.

138. Greer JJ, Ren J 2009 Ampakine therapy to counter fentanyl-induced respiratory depression. Respir Physiol Neurobiol **168**:153–157.

139. Byrne BJ, Falk DJ, Pacak CA, et al. 2011 Pompe disease gene therapy. Hum Mol Genet **20**:R61–R68.

140. Doyle BM, Turner SMF, Sunshine MD, et al. 2019 AAV gene therapy utilizing glycosylation-independent lysosomal targeting tagged GAA in the hypoglossal motor system of Pompe mice. Mol Ther Methods Clin Dev **15**:194–203.

141. Mah CS, Falk DJ, Germain SA, et al. 2010 Gel-mediated delivery of AAV1 vectors corrects ventilatory function in Pompe mice with established disease. Mol Ther **18**:502–510.

142. Salabarria SM, Nair J, Clement N, et al. 2020 Advancements in AAV-mediated gene therapy for Pompe disease. J Neuromuscul Dis **7**:15–31.

143. Keeler AM, Zieger M, Semple C, et al. 2020 Intralingual and intrapleural AAV gene therapy prolongs survival in a SOD1 ALS mouse model. Mol Ther Methods Clin Dev **17**:246–257.

144. Browne EC, Abbott BM 2016 Recent progress towards an effective treatment of amyotrophic lateral sclerosis using the SOD1 mouse model in a preclinical setting. Eur J Med Chem **121**:918–925.

145. Fuller DD, Mitchell GS 2017 Respiratory neuroplasticity – Overview, significance and future directions. Exp Neurol **287**:144–152.

146. Nichols NL, Gowing G, Satriotomo I, et al. 2013 Intermittent hypoxia and stem cell implants preserve breathing capacity in a rodent model of amyotrophic lateral sclerosis. Am J Respir Crit Care Med **187**:535–542.

147. Navarrete-Opazo A, Mitchell GS 2014 Therapeutic potential of intermittent hypoxia: a matter of dose. Am J Physiol Regul Integr Comp Physiol **307**:R1181–R1197.

Index

Note: Locators in *italics* represent figures and **bold** indicate tables in the text.

A

Abdominal premotor neurons, 6; *see also* Premotor neurons (first order)
Acetazolamide (ACZ), 64–65, 149, 163, 170, 174, *175*, 226–227
Acetylcholine (ACh) neurons, *87*, 88
Acute mountain sickness (AMS), 169–170
ACZ, *see* Acetazolamide
Adults, SDB in
  apneic threshold, 111
  arousals, 113–114
  brainstem, 108–109
  chemoreceptors, 109
    central, 109
    peripheral, 109
  chemosensitivity, 109, 111
  circulatory delay, 111
  CO$_2$ reserve, 111
  cortical activity, 109
  loop gain, 111–112
  lungs and chest wall, 113
  OSA or CSA, 108, *110*
  upper airway, 112–113
  ventilatory control system, 108
  wake-sleep and sleep stage transitions, 114–115
Aging
  from animal studies, 64
  and chemoreceptor reactivity, 58–62
    cerebrovascular responsiveness, 62
    chemoresponsiveness during sleep, 58–61
    in plasticity, 61–62
    wake chemoresponsivess, 58, **59–60**
  longitudinal studies, 65, **66**
  pathophysiology of SDB, 58–64
  potential therapy for SDB, 64–66
    acetazolamide, 64–65
    supplemental oxygen, 64, *65*
  upper airway mechanics and function, 62–63, *63*
  ventilatory responses to hypoxia and hypercapnia, 58, **59–60**
Airway resistance, 3, 6, 28, 62, 63, 80, 101, 178, 182, 193–194, 203, 213–214, 233, 236
Alpha-amino-3-hydroxy-5-methyl-4-isoxazolepropionic acid (AMPA), 47–48, *238*, 239
Altitude
  acclimatization to
    acute mountain sickness, 169–170
    cardiovascular, 169
    erythropoiesis, 169
    hemoglobin's oxygen affinity, 169
    non-ventilatory factors, 169
    ventilatory, 168
  adaptations to, 176
  CBF, role of, 172, 174
  chronic mountain sickness, 176–179
  CSA at
    persistence of, 174, **174**
    treatment strategies for, 174–176
  OSA at, 177–178, *178*
  periodic breathing at, *169*, 170–172
  sleep apnea at, 168
Alveolar ventilation (VA), 28, *30*, 70–71, 73–76, 133, 149, *173*, 204
AMPA, *see* Alpha-amino-3-hydroxy-5-methyl-4-isoxazolepropionic acid
Ampakines stimulate breathing, 239
AMS, *see* Acute mountain sickness
Animal studies
  alveolar hypoventilation syndromes
    interventions targeting control of breathing, 252
    interventions targeting motoneurons, 252
  B6 animal model, 150
  C57BL/6J mice, 246, 252
  of DIO mice, 196–197, 247–249, *248*, 252
  HO-2-null mice, 251
  interventions targeting arousal threshold, 250
  LEPR[b]-deficient *db/db* mice, 252
  leptin deficient *ob/ob* mice, 196–197, 246, *247*, 249, 252
  NZO mice, 246
  OSA
    interventions to improve neuromuscular control, 247–250, **250**
    in leptin-deficient, 246, *247*
  in peripheral chemoreflex for treatment of SDB
    hypoxia-inducible factors (HIF), 251
    potential pharmacological targets in CB, 251
    purinergic receptors, 251–252
  SOD1 mice, 252
  Zucker rats, 246, 252
Apnea; *see also* Breathing
  alveolar gas equation, *30*
  and hypocapnia, 28
  and isocapnia, 32
  of prematurity, 98
  of prematurity in newborns, 12
  in rats, mechanical ventilation, 11
  during SDB, 31
  termination of, 28
  transient hyperventilation, 26, 28
  ventilation, 108
Apnea begets apnea, 147
Apnea hypopnea index (AHI), 58, 61, 64–65, 118–128, 150, 170, 175–178, 183–184, 195, 222–223, 225–228
  central, 108, 163, 178
  obstructive, 108, 178, 187
Apneic threshold, 28–29, *30*, 60–61, 101, 111, 115, 140, 146, 148, 154–155, 163, 170, 172, 175, 205, 215
Arousals
  arousal threshold, 114
  EEG activity, 113
  harmful effects, 114

in OSA, 114
in SDB, 101, 113–114
as survival mechanism, 114
threshold, 224–225
Asphyxia, 24, 28, 32, 147, 171, 233
Asthma
  CPAP in, 186
  dyspnea in, 31
  life-threatening episodes, 102
  prevalence of OSA, 185
  SDB in, 185–186
  sleep-related desaturation, 101
Autoresuscitation, 2

B

"Balance of forces model," 80, *81*
Benzodiazepine receptor, 159, 175, **176**
Body mass index (BMI), 63, 118, *122*, 123, 125, 127, 159,
    193, 196, 197, 203–205
BötC, *see* Bötzinger complex
Bötzinger complex (BötC), 5
  augmenting expiratory activity (dubbed E-Aug), 14
  decrementing expiratory activity (dubbed E-Dec), 14
  in early expiration (E1), *10*
  rostral VRC, 42, 44
Brainstem
  for breathing, 2
  chemosensors, 2
  DMNX, 3
  interneurons in, 6–15
  noeud vital (vital node), 2
  pF, *see* Parafacial nucleus
  phrenic premotor neurons, 6
  preBötC, *see* Pre-Bötzinger complex
  preBötC in humans, *8*
Breathing
  ataxic, 11
  CNS effects, 2, 33
  deficits, 8
  eupneic, 3
  fetal breathing movements, 42
  initial variability, 98
  inspiratory, 7, 11
  muscles, 3–5, 6
  opioid effects, 8, 11
  regions of brainstem, 2
  and study of sleep, *see* Obstructive sleep apnea
      syndrome
  upper cervical injuries, 2
  vestibulocochlear cranial nerve (CN VIII), 2
Breuer-Hering (B-H) deflation and inflation, 14, 98
Bronchopulmonary dysplasia (BPD), 98–99, 101
Bronchopulmonary reflexes
  C-fiber receptors, 49–50
  rapidly adapting receptors, 49
  slowly adapting stretch receptors, 48–49
Buspirone, 149–150, 163

C

Cardiac resynchronization therapy (CRT), 161
Cardiorespiratory control, 25, *25*, 31, 35

Carotid body (CB)
  dopamine beta-hydroxylase, 24
  eucapnic hypoxic responses, 32
  glomus cell, 24
  hyperadditive effect of, 25, *26*
  hypoxia to denervated animals, 25, *27*
  neural pathways, 24
  NTS neurons, 24
  peripheral arterial chemoreceptors, 52, *52*
  plasticity reversible, 31–32
  sensory input on central CO_2 sensitivity, 25, *26*
  signal transduction, 24
  tyrosine hydroxylase, 24
Caudal ventral respiratory group (cVRG), 5, 6, 42, *45*,
    235
CB, *see* Carotid body
CBF, *see* Cerebral flow regulation
Central congenital hypoventilation syndrome
    (CCHS), 102
Central nervous system (CNS)
  adenosine, 163
  central chemoreceptors, 109
  control breathing, 2
  effects in breathing, 2, 33
  hypoxia, 25, *27*
  leptin receptors, 197
  norepinephrine reuptake receptor, 224
  respiratory regions of, 2, 6, *10*
Central pattern generator (CPG), *25*, 42, 47
Central sleep apnea (CSA), 108
  at altitude, 174–176
  cerebrovascular reactivity and, 140–142
  CO_2 reserve
    effect of pharmacologic agents, 149–150
    effect of sex hormones, 148–149
    PAP therapy and supplemental oxygen, 150
  in HF, *see* Heart failure
  hypercapnic, 108
  mechanical ventilation model, 147–148
  non-hypercapnic, 108
  nonperiodic phenomena
    asphyxia, 147
    increased left atrial pressure, 147
    narrowing or occlusion of pharyngeal airway,
        147
    negative pressure, 147
    opioid-related CSA, 147
    rhythmic breathing, 147
    sighs, 147
    ventilatory instability, 147
  during NREM sleep, 146–148
    experimental induction of central apnea,
        147–148
    initiation of central apnea, 146
    loop gain, 146–147
    perpetuation of central apnea, 146–148
  pharmacological management of, *see*
        Pharmacological management
  plasticity of apneic threshold, 148–150
  propensity of apneic threshold, 148, *148*
  repetitive central apneas, 170, *170*
Cerebral flow (CBF) regulation
  acute CBF reduction, 138–140

ventilatory control system
central chemoreceptor tissue PCO$_2$ (PbtCO$_2$), 133, *134*
cerebral circulation and regulation, 134, *135*
cerebrovascular reactivity (CVR), 134
PaCO$_2$ and vCO$_2$, 133
Cerebrovascular reactivity (CVR)
for CBF, 134
and central sleep apnea, 140–142
Cerebrovascular responsiveness (CVR), 62, *63*, 64, 133, 140
Cervical spinal cord, 2, 6, 7, 146
C-fiber receptors, 49–50
Chemogenetics, 224, 249
Chemoreception
CB, *see* Carotid body
human and rodent, cardiorespiratory chemosensitivity in, 32–35
pathogenesis of SDB, *see* Sleep-disordered breathing
peripheral/central chemoreceptors, 24–28
plasticity in carotid chemoreflex function, 29–32
ventilatory and MSNA, 33, *33*, 34, *34*
Chemoreceptors, 109
central, 109
peripheral, 109
Chemoresponsiveness
with aging
"loop gain," 60
during NREM sleep, 61
during sleep, 58–61
wake, 58, **59–60**
in sleep, 29
Chemosensitivity
carbon dioxide chemosensitivity, 236
central CO$_2$ chemosensitivity, 26
hypoxic ventilatory chemosensitivity, 25, *26*, 52–53
oxygen chemosensitivity, 236–237
SDB in adults, 109, 111
testing in mammals, *see* Mammals
ventilatory *vs.* neurocirculatory, 33–35
Cheyne-Stokes breathing (CSB), 112, 115
Cheyne-Stokes respiration (CSR), 60, 64, 146, 149, 178, 211
CHF, *see* Chronic heart failure
Children
with chronic pulmonary disease, 101–102
pathophysiology of OSAS, *see* Obstructive sleep apnea syndrome
sleep-disordered breathing, 98–102
Chronic heart failure (CHF), 29, *30*, 31–32, 60, 61, 178
Chronic intermittent hypoxia (CIH), 87–88
Chronic lung diseases, 98, 101, 182–187
Chronic mountain sickness (CMS), 176–179
Chronic obstructive pulmonary disease (COPD), 31
ambulatory sleep testing pathway, 184
CB hypersensitivity, 29, 31–32
CPAP, 185
FRC, 113
home sleep apnea testing, 184
long-term administration of oxygen, 184
nocturnal oxygen desaturation, 182, *183*
nocturnal supplemental oxygen, 184–185
non-invasive ventilation (NIV), 185

and OSA, 183
SDB in, 182–185
smoking cessation, 184
in ventilatory control, 182
Circulatory delay, 111, 112, 212
Clonidine, 149
CMS, *see* Chronic mountain sickness
CNS, *see* Central nervous system
Compact NA (NAc), 4, *5*, 6
Complex sleep apnea, 178–179, 202
Congenital central hypoventilation syndrome (CCHS), 12, 44, 102
Continuous positive airway pressure (CPAP) therapy, 118
in asthma, 186
in COPD, 185
in HF, 160
OSAHS, 127
PAP therapy, 202–205
therapeutic intermittent hypoxia, 213–214
COPD, *see* Chronic obstructive pulmonary disease
CO$_2$ reserve, 111, 146
in CSA
effect of pharmacologic agents, 149–150
effect of sex hormones, 148–149
PAP therapy and supplemental oxygen, 150
in CSA, pharmacologic agents
acetazolamide, 149
buspirone, 149–150
clonidine, 149
zolpidem, 149
SDB in adults, 111
CPAP therapy, *see* Continuous positive airway pressure therapy
CPG, *see* Central pattern generator
Cranial nerves (CNs)
accessory CN XI, 6
IX, X, XI, and XII, 3–4, 6, 13–15
vestibulocochlear cranial nerve (CN VIII), 2
Critical closing pressure (Pcrit), *see* Pcrit values
CVRG, *see* Caudal ventral respiratory group

D

Dbx1 (developing brain homeobox 1), 7, 11
De Lorry, Antoine Charles, 2
dogs, experiments on, 2
medulla, locus of vital functions, 2
Designer receptors exclusively activated by designer drugs (DREADDs), 223, 249
Diet-induced obese (DIO) mice, 196–197, 247–249, *248*, 252
DIO, *see* Diet-induced obese mice
Diuretics, 160, 221–222
DMNX, *see* Dorsal motor nucleus of the vagus
Dopamine beta-hydroxylase (DBH), 24
Dorsal motor nucleus of the vagus (DMNX), 3–4, *4*
Dorsal respiratory group (DRG), 14, 42, 44, 49
Down syndrome, 122
DREADDs, *see* Designer receptors exclusively activated by designer drugs
DRG, *see* Dorsal respiratory group
Dronabinol, 223, 249

E

Early expiration (E1), *10*
Ehlers–Danlos syndrome, 122
Electromyogram (EMG), 28, 81–82, *84*, 85, 87–89, 155, *156*, 249
Embryonic parafacial (e-pF), 13
Endothelial nitric oxide synthase (eNOS), 136, *137*
End-stage kidney disease, 31
E-pF, *see* Embryonic parafacial
Erythropoiesis, 169, 177
Exercise
    adjustment of respiratory control system
        arterial PCO$_2$ and minute ventilation, 71, *71*, *72*, *72*, *74*
        breathing regulation, 71
        magnitude of, 70
    control of breathing
        alveolar ventilation and pulmonary gas exchange rate, *72*, 73–76
        blood gas homeostasis, 72
        increase in metabolic rate and a motor activity, 71–72
        increase in ventilation, 73–74, *74*
        peripheral and central, *75*, 75–76
        total obstruction of blood flow, 73, *74*
Extended ventrolateral preoptic nucleus (eVLPO), 88
External NA (NAe), 4

F

Facial (VII) cranial motor nucleus, 12
Flourens, Marie-Jean-Pierre, 2
    breathing center, 2
    experiments on breathing in rabbits, 2, *3*
    medulla as *noeud vital* (vital node), 2
Functional residual capacity (FRC), 49, 53, 98–99, 113–114

G

Galen, 2
Genioglossus (GG) muscle; *see also* Upper airway control during sleep
    reflex increase, 83–85
    sleep-wake patterns of upper airway muscle activity, 81
        effects of REM sleep, 82
        EMG activity of, 81
        in experimental animals, 83, *84*
        at sleep onset and during non-REM sleep, 81–82
        studies of single motor units, 82–83
    of tongue during sleep states in rats, 83, *84*, 89
Glossopharyngeal (IX) nerves, 3
G-protein-coupled inwardly rectifying potassium (GIRK) channels, 249
G-protein-coupled receptors, 46, *46*
Guideline-directed medical therapy (GDMT), 161

H

Heart failure (HF)
    acute and chronic consequences, 154
    adverse cardiac consequences, 155

    CSA in
        acetazolamide, 163
        buspirone (80, 81), 163
        cardiac transplantation, 161
        hospitalization and mortality, 156, 158–159
        low flow nocturnal oxygen therapy, 162–163
        mechanisms of, 154–155
        medications, 163
        in non-REM sleep, 154
        PO$_2$ and PCO$_2$, 154–155
        positive airway pressure devices, 161
        reason for unnoticed, undiagnosed, and under treated patients, 159
        theophylline, 163
        transvenous phrenic nerve stimulation, 161–162, *162*
    HCSB, 154
    OSA in
        CPAP and oral appliance therapy, 160
        exercise, 160
        hospitalization and mortality, 155–156
        mechanisms of, 155–156
        prevalence of, *161*
    phenotypic treatment, 163
    with preserved ejection fraction (HFpEF), 154, *160*
    recommendations, 159
    with reduced ejection fraction (HFrEF), 154, *160*
    treatment of, 159–163
Henneman's size principle, 3
Hering-Breuer (H-B) reflex, *see* Slowly adapting stretch receptors
HF, *see* Heart failure
Human preBötC, 7, *8*
Hunter-Cheyne-Stokes Breathing (HCSB), 154
5-hydroxytryptamine (5HT), 85–86, *86*
Hypercapnia, 12, *26*, 28, 32, 52, 58, 61–62, 100–102, 108–109, 111, 134, *135*, 142, 154, 163, 184, 194–195, 224, 233, 250–251
Hypercapnic ventilatory response (HCVR), 58, **59–60**, 203–204
Hyperoxia
    acute, 29
    CNS, 26, *27*, 33
    isolated CB, *26*, *27*
    isooxic levels of, 32
    nocturnal, 29
    therapeutic, *see* Therapeutic hyperoxia
    transient, 31, *33*
Hyperoxic hypercapnic ventilatory response (HCVR), 140–141
Hyperpneas, 70–71, 73, 109, 111–114, 146, 150, 155, 159, 170–172
Hypertension
    drug-resistant, 31
    human, 29, 31–32
    pulmonary, 102, 177, 184, 226–228
Hypnotics, 182, 224–225, 227
Hypocapnia, *26*, 28–29, 60–62, 71, 109, 113–114, 146–147, *147*, 211, 213, 215, 225
Hypoglossal premotor neurons, 6; *see also* Premotor neurons (first order)
Hypopneas, 29, 64, 80, 101, 108, 111–114, 150, 177, 179, 183, 202, 246–248

Hypoxemia
    at altitude, 171
    carotid chemoreceptor, 172, *172*
    mountain sickness, 168
    in preterm born infants, 99
Hypoxia
    acute, 31, 34
    at altitude, 171–172, *173*
    ATP in, 24
    to awake CB-denervated animals, 25, *27*
    CNS, 25, 26, 27, 33
    eucapnic, 32, *33*, 34, *34*
    with heart failure, 111
    intermittent, 29
    isooxic levels of, 32
    norepinephrine IN, 24
    sympathetic responses, 35
    therapeutic intermittent, *see* Therapeutic
        intermittent hypoxia
    ventilatory responses, 33–35, *34*, 58, **59–60**,
        203–204
Hypoxic pulmonary vasoconstriction (HPV), 169,
    176–177
Hypoxic ventilatory response (HVR), 168, 171, 174,
    176, 178–179, 203, 204, 251–252

I

Idiopathic pulmonary fibrosis (IPF), 186–187
I-γ (gamma) neurons, 15
IH, *see* Intermittent hypoxia
ILD, *see* Interstitial lung diseases
Inhibitory preBötC neurons, 11
Inotropic receptors, *see* Ligand-gated ion channels
Inspiratory flow limitation (IFL), 196, *247*, *248*
Intermediate reticular formation (IRt), 4, *5*, 6
Intermittent hypoxia (IH)
    acute, 61, 204, 252
    chronic, 29, 64, 87, 127
    mild, *see* Mild intermittent hypoxia and
        supplemental oxygen
    therapeutic, *see* Therapeutic intermittent hypoxia
Internal carotid arteries (ICA), 139
International Classification of Sleep Disorders, Third
    Edition (ICSD-3), 108
Interstitial lung diseases (ILD)
    IPF, 186
    nocturnal desaturation, 186
    and OSA, 186–187
    SDB in, 186–187
Isocapnia, 32, 58

J

Juxtacapillary receptors, 49

K

King's Brief Interstitial Lung Disease questionnaire,
    187
Kölliker-Fuse nucleus (KFN), 13–14, 44
Krebs cycle, 70

L

Larynx
    laryngeal chemoreflex (LCR), 50–51, *51*
    responses to saline stimulus, 50, *50*
    vagally mediated mechano- and chemoreceptors,
        49, 50–51
Late expiration (E2), 10
Lateral parafacial (pF$_L$), 4, *5*, 6, *9*, *10*, 12–14
Legallois, Julien-Jean-César, 2
    autoresuscitation, 2
    vestibulocochlear cranial nerve (CN VIII), 2
Leptin
    deficient *ob/ob* mice, 196–197, 246, *247*, 249, 252
    OHS, 195–197
    receptors, 197
Ligand-gated ion channels, 46, *46*
Long-term facilitation, 61–62, 213
Loop gain, 111–112, 115, 119, 120, 146–147, 204–205,
    209–212, *211*, 225–226
Loose NA (NAl), 4
Lorazepam, 250
Loss of wakefulness, 28–29
Lumsden, T.
    experiments on breathing in cats, 2, *3*
Lungs; *see also* Respiration
    and airways, 15
    functional residual capacity, 113
    gas exchange, 70
    loop gain, 204
    mechanoreceptors, 99
    volume of, 113

M

Mammals, 32–35; *see also* Animal studies
    chemoreceptor sensitivity, 34
    chemosensitivity testing, 32–33
        chemoreceptor CO_2 response, 32
        eupneic arterial PCO_2, 32
        iso-oxic levels, CO_2 at, 32
        ventilatory response to hypoxia, 33
    ventilatory *vs.* neurocirculatory chemosensitivity,
        33–35
Medulla
    level of preBötC, 7, *7*
    premotor neurons, 6
    respiratory center, 2, 14
    vestibulocochlear cranial nerve, *3*
Melanin-concentrating hormone (MCH), 88
Metabotropic receptors, *see* G-protein-coupled
    receptors
Middle cerebral artery velocity (MCAv), 139, *142*
Mild intermittent hypoxia and supplemental oxygen
    chemoreflex sensitivity, 210, *211*
    sleep-disordered breathing, *210*
        arousal threshold, 209
        loop gain, 209–212, *211*
        upper airway collapsibility and
            responsiveness, 209
    therapeutic hyperoxia
        arousal threshold and apnea severity, 216
        duration of, 216–217

loop gain and apnea severity, 215
and outcome measures, 217
upper airway responsiveness/collapsibility
and apnea severity, 216
treatment of OSA with therapeutic intermittent
hypoxia
and apneic events, 213
and continuous positive airway pressure,
213–214
dose and timing, 214–215
and outcome measures, 214
respiratory plasticity, 212, 212–213
Minute ventilation (VE), 71, 71, 73–74, 74
Monge's disease, see Chronic mountain sickness
μ-opioid receptors (μORs), 8, 223
Motor neurons, 3
cardiovagal preganglionic, 4
esophagomotor neurons, 4
inspiratory, 11
NAc, 4
pharyngeal and laryngeal, 4
phrenic, 3, 14, 15
scalene, 6
somatic, 4
VII motor neurons, 12
XII motor neurons, 6
MSNA, see Muscle sympathetic nerve activity
Muscle sympathetic nerve activity (MSNA), 33, 33,
34, 34
Myelomeningocele, 102–103

N

NA, see Nucleus ambiguus
NAc, see Compact NA
NAe, see External NA
NAsc, see Semi-compact (NAsc)
National Heart, Lung, and Blood Institute (NHLBI), 162
Neonate-child
mapping respiratory network, 42, 44, 45
dorsal respiratory group, 44
pontine respiratory group, 44
postinspiratory complex, 44
retrotrapezoid nucleus, 44
ventral respiratory column, 42, 44
neuroanatomy of central respiratory network,
42–44
phases of respiration, 42, 43
triple-oscillator hypothesis, 42, 44
neuromodulators, 48
neurotransmitters, 46, 46–48, 47
peripheral inputs, 48–51, 53
bronchopulmonary reflexes, 48–50
peripheral arterial chemoreceptors, 52, 52–53, 53
proprioceptors, 51
vagally mediated mechano- and
chemoreceptors in larynx, 50, 50–51, 51
SDB in, 98–100
apnea of prematurity, 98–99
bronchopulmonary dysplasia (BPD), 99
hypoxemia, 99
OSAS, 99–100
periodic breathing (PB), 98

Neurokinin-1 receptors (NK1Rs), 7, 8, 11, 48
Neuromodulators
acetylcholine, 48
adenosine, 48
adenosine triphosphate (ATP), 48
GABAergic and glutamatergic neurotransmission,
48
neurokinin, 48
serotonin, 48
substance P, 48
Neurotransmitters
GABA and glycine, 46–47, 47
glutamate, 46–48
G-protein-coupled receptors, 46, 46
ligand-gated ion channels, 46, 46
New Zealand obese (NZO) mice, 246
N-methyl-D-aspartate (NMDA), 47
Nocturnal hyperoxia, 29
Nocturnal oxygen (NOX), 162
Nocturnal oxygen desaturation (NOD), 182, 183
Nocturnal supplemental oxygen, 184–185
Noeud vital (vital node), see Medulla
Non-benzodiazepine receptor, 175, **176**
Non-invasive ventilation (NIV), 185
Non-rapid eye movement (NREM) sleep
AHI during, 223
chemoresponsiveness, 61, 119
cortical control of breathing, 109
CSA during, 146–148
fiberoptic nasopharyngoscopy, 63
periodic breathing, 62
SDB in, 28–29
sleep apnea in, 29
wakefulness to, 114–115
Norepinephrine (NE), 85–86, 86
Normoxia, 147, 171–172, 204, 212
NREM, see Non-rapid eye movement sleep
NTS, see Nucleus of solitary tract
Nucleus ambiguus (NA), 3, 8, 13
compact, 4
external, 4
loose, 4
semi-compact, 4, 4
Nucleus of solitary tract (NTS)
carotid body, 24
dorsal respiratory group, 14
glossopharyngeal inputs and neurons, 15
rapidly adapting receptor, 14–15
slowly adapting pulmonary stretch receptor, 14
vagal inputs and neurons, 15

O

Obesity hypoventilation syndrome (OHS)
alterations in ventilatory control, 195
changes in pulmonary mechanics, 193–194
leptin, 195–197
mechanisms, 193–197
respiratory control, 193, 194
sleep-disordered breathing, 194–195
Obstructive sleep apnea (OSA); see also Apnea
at altitude, see Altitude
in HF, see Heart failure

moderate OSA, 126
morphine in, 29
pharmacological management of, *see*
    Pharmacological management
regulatory mechanisms, 80
TE-CSA, 202
Obstructive sleep apnea hypopnea syndrome (OSAHS)
  age and ageism
    by AHI, 126
    anatomy pathway (Pcrit), 127
    CPAP therapy, 127
    gain pathway, 128
    moderate OSA, 126–127
    muscle recruitment pathway, 127–128
    sleep-wake pathway, 127
    stressors and genetic predisposition, 126, *126*
    survivor effect, 126
  causality and risk, 118–120, *119*
  clinical sequelae, 202
  gender and transgender
    external factors, 124, *124*
    higher BMI, 125
    insomnia symptoms, 122
    menopause, 122–124
    muscle recruitment, 124–125
    sleep architecture, 124
  genetic set points, 120–122, *122*, **123**
  interactions among set points, 128
  "loop gain," 119–120, *120*
  PAP therapy, *see* Positive airway pressure therapy
  recurrent apneas, 120, *121*
  related syndromes and interventions
    hormone manipulation, 125
    polycystic ovarian syndrome, 125
    transgender examples, 125–126
  and sleep, 119–120
Obstructive sleep apnea syndrome (OSAS)
  balance of upper airway anatomy and muscle
    tone, 100
  central congenital hypoventilation syndrome, 102
  myelomeningocele, 102–103
  Prader Willi Syndrome, 103
  in preterm born infants, 99–100
  SDB in children with chronic pulmonary disease,
    101–102
  trisomy 21, 103
  ventilatory responses during sleep, 100–101
OHS, *see* Obesity hypoventilation syndrome
Opioid drugs
  addiction, 233
  effects on preBötCneurons, 10
  induced respiratory depression, 12, 233, *234*
    blunt central and peripheral chemoreception,
      236
    carbon dioxide chemosensitivity, 236
    DAMGO, 236
    factors modulating contributions of medullary
      sites, 236–237
    impair respiratory muscle activity, 237
    oxygen chemosensitivity, 236–237
  on neural circuits, *235*
    modulating respiratory rhythm and pattern
      generation, 233–234
      MOR activation, 235
      preBötzinger complex, 234–235
      role of PiCo, 235
  opioid epidemic, 233
  for pain management, 10
  Papaver somniferum, 233
  pharmacological interventions
    blockers of MOR inhibition, 237, *238*, 239
    opioid ligands with reduced side effects, 240
    respiratory stimulants, 239–240
  and SDB in patients, 237
OSAHS, *see* Obstructive sleep apnea hypopnea
    syndrome
OSAS, *see* Obstructive sleep apnea syndrome
Overlap syndrome (OVS), 182, 183
OVS, *see* Overlap syndrome
Oxytocin, 249

P

PaCO$_2$, *see* Partial pressure of arterial CO$_2$
PaO$_2$, *see* Partial pressure of arterial oxygen
Parabrachial nucleus, 13–14
Parafacial nucleus (pF), 6, *9*, 12–15
  BötC, *see* Bötzinger complex
  Kölliker-fuse and parabrachial nucleus, 13–14
  lateral parafacial, 12
  NTS, *see* Nucleus of solitary tract
  pFV or RTN, 12–13
Paraventricular nucleus (PVN), 24, *25*
Partial pressure of arterial CO$_2$ (PaCO$_2$), 28–30, 35, 58,
    61–62, 70–71, 108–109, 111–112, 114, 133–141,
    146–147, 193, 195, 203, 225, 227
Partial pressure of arterial oxygen (PaO$_2$), 58, 64, 70,
    73, 108, 109, 133–134, 168, 193
PB, *see* Periodic breathing
Pcrit values, 63–64, 80, 113, 119–120, 127
  passive, 63–64, 80, 113, 119–120, 127
Periodic breathing (PB), 98, 112, 147
  at altitude, *see* Altitude
  neonate-child, 98
  NREM sleep, 62
Peripheral arterial chemoreceptors
  carotid body, 52, *52*
  hypoxic chemosensitivity, 52–53
Peripheral/central chemoreceptors
  cardiorespiratory control, 25, *25*
  central CO$_2$ chemosensitivity, 26
  CNS hypoxia, 25, *27*
  hypoxic ventilatory chemosensitivity, 25, *26*
  and interconnections, 25, *25*
  perfused CB and humans with CB denervation,
    25, *26*
  regulating ventilation and sympathetic nerve
    activity, 24
  respiratory-sympathetic coupling, 28
PF, *see* Parafacial nucleus
PF$_L$, *see* Lateral parafacial
PFV, *see* Ventral parafacial
Pharmacological management
  of CSA
    acetazolamide, 226–227
    carbon dioxide, 227

endotypic targets of medications, **223**
hypnotics, 227
oxygen enrichment, 227–228
respiratory stimulants, 226–227
steroids, 226
theophylline, 227
to mitigate breathing instability, *see* Animal
studies
of OSA
arousal threshold, 224–225
cannabinergic and serotonergic pathways,
223–224
carbonic anhydrase inhibitors, 225–226
chemogenetics, 224
diuretics, 222
endotypic targets of medications, **223**
hypnotics, 224
impaired upper airway anatomy, 221–222
loop gain, 225–226
noradrenergic and muscarinic pathways, 224
predisposing traits or endotypes, 221, *222*
sedatives and hypnotics, 224–225
supplemental oxygen, 226
upper airway dilator muscles, 222–224
weight-reducing medications, 221–222
Pharynx, 80, 83, 246–247, 249
Phox2b, *9*, 11–12, *25*, 102
Phrenic premotor neurons, 6; *see also* Premotor
neurons (first order)
Henneman's size principle, 3
phrenic nerve, C3–C5, 3
Pickwick Syndrome, *see* Obesity hypoventilation
syndrome
Pierre Robin Prader-Willi syndrome, 122
Plasticity in carotid chemoreflex function
CB plasticity, 31–32
of end-stage kidney disease, 31
in experimental animals, 32
exposure of rats to chronic IH, 29
in human hypertension, 29, 31
in humans with CHF, 31
in patients with COPD, 31
plasticity-induced chemoreflex hypersensitivity,
31
Polycystic ovarian syndrome (PCOS), 125
Pompe disease, 122
Pons; *see also* Brainstem
arrays of microelectrodes, 14
CN IX and CN X, 13
opioids, effects of, 10
rapidly adapting receptors, 15
trigeminal motor nucleus, 6
Pontine respiratory group (PRG), 44
Positive airway pressure (PAP) therapy
on blood pressure and hypertension, 202
CPAP therapy
loop gain, 204–205
in patients with OSA, 202–205
ventilatory responses to hypercapnia and
hypoxia, 203–204
severe OSAHS, 202
TE-CSA, 202
Posterior cerebral artery (PCA), 139

Post-inspiration, *see* Early expiration (E1)
Postinspiratory complex (PiCo), 14, 44, 234
Prader Willi Syndrome (PWS), 103
Pre-Bötzinger complex (PBC); *see also* Bötzinger
complex
cellular composition of, 6, *7*
functional and anatomic definition of, 7–8, 10–11
genetic definition of, 11
human preBötC, 7, *8*
induced respiratory depression, 234
inhibitory preBötC neurons, 11
in perspective, 11–12
pF, RTN nuclei, 6, *9*
respiratory regions of CNS, 6, *10*
rostral VRC, 42, 44
Preinspiratory neurons, 12
Premotor neurons (first order); *see also* Motor neurons
of medulla and cervical spinal cord, 6
abdominal premotor neurons, 6
hypoglossal premotor neurons, 6, 11
phrenic premotor neurons, 6, 11
in rVRG, *10*
Proprioceptors, 51
Pump neurons, 15

R

Rapidly adapting receptors (RARs), 49–50, 98–99
REM sleep
in COPD patients, 182–183
DIO mice, 248
MCH cells, 88
with muscle twitches, 87
phasic, 28
upper airway muscle activity, 82, *86*
Renal failure, 29, 31
Renin-angiotensin system, 29
Renshaw cells, 3
Respiration
neural network anatomy
external NA, 4
historical background and discovery, 2
motor neuron pools, 3–6
noeud vital (vital node), 2
premotor neurons (first order), 6
respiratory center, 2–3, *3*
respiratory nuclei in transverse sections, 3, *4*, *5*
rhythm-generating nuclei and higher order
interneurons, 6–15
phases of, 42, *43*
expiration, 42, *43*
inspiration, 42, *43*
post inspiration, 42, *43*
Respiratory center, 139
historical overview and discovery of, 2–3
in rabbits, 2, *3*
ventral medulla, *3*
Restless Legs syndrome, 122
Retrotrapezoid nuclei (RTN), *4*, 6, *9*, 11–15, 24–25, *25*,
28, 44, 139
RETT syndrome, 47, 54, 150
Rostral ventral respiratory group (rVRG), *5*, 6–7, *10*,
11, 42, *45*, 235

Rostral ventrolateral medulla (RVLM) neurons, 24, 25, 28–29
RTN, *see* Retrotrapezoid nuclei
RVRG, *see* Rostral ventral respiratory group

S

Scalene motor neurons, 6
SDB, *see* Sleep-disordered breathing
Selective serotonin reuptake inhibitors (SSRIs), 223
Semi-compact (NAsc), 4, 6
Sleep apnea; *see also* Apnea
    at altitude, 168
    CB plasticity, 29, 32
    chronic IH, 29
    in NREM sleep, 29
    PB nuclei, 14
    raising blood pressure, 31, *34*
Sleep-disordered breathing (SDB); *see also* Apnea; Breathing
    in adults, *see* Adults, SDB in
    alveolar gas equation, 29, *30*
    and arousals, 101
    associated with chronic lung diseases, 182
    in asthma, 185–186
    chemoresponsiveness and ventilatory instability, 29
    in children, *see* Children
    in chronic pulmonary disease, 101–102
    in COPD, 182–185
    due to HF, *see* Heart failure
    in interstitial lung diseases, 186–187
    loss of vigilance, 28
    loss of wakefulness, 28–29
    lowering chemosensitivity/controller gain, 29, *30*
    in neonates and children born preterm, 98–100
    in NREM sleep, 28
    in OHS, *see* Obesity hypoventilation syndrome
    in older adults, *see* Aging
    and OSAS, *see* Obstructive sleep apnea syndrome
    PAP therapy in, *see* Positive airway pressure therapy
    pathogenesis of, 28–29
    reduced PaCO$_2$/augmented tidal volume/increased resistive loads, 28
    sleep-induced suppression of wakefulness, 28
    structures and processes, 108, *109*
    transient ventilatory overshoots, 28
Sleep Heart Health Study, 118
Slowly adapting stretch receptors (SARs), 48–50
Smoking cessation, 182, 184
Somatic motor neurons, 4
Somatostatin (SST), 7, 8, 11
Starling resistor model, 80
Steroids, 226
Substance P, 86, *87*
Sudden infant death syndrome (SIDS), 12, 44, 48, 51, 54
Supplemental oxygen, 32, 53, 64–65, 98, 150, 170, 184–185, 209–217, 226, 227–228

T

Temazepam, 225, 227
Tertiapin-Q, 88–89, 239

Theophylline, 163, 226–227
Therapeutic hyperoxia
    arousal threshold and apnea severity, 216
    duration of, 216–217
    loop gain and apnea severity, 215
    and outcome measures, 217
    upper airway responsiveness/collapsibility and apnea severity, 216
Therapeutic intermittent hypoxia
    and apneic events, 213
    and continuous positive airway pressure, 213–214
    dose and timing, 214–215
    and outcome measures, 214
    respiratory plasticity, *212*, 212–213
Thyrotropin-releasing hormone (TRH), 86, *87*, 249
"Tracheal tug," 113
Transient ventilatory overshoots, 28, *30*
Transvenous phrenic nerve stimulation (TPNS), 161–162, *162*
Triazolam, 227
Triple-oscillator hypothesis, 42, *44*
Trisomy 21 (T21), 103
XII motor neurons, 6
Tyrosine hydroxylase (TH), *9*, 24

U

Upper airway control during sleep
    biomechanical environment
        "balance of forces model," 80, *81*
        Pcrit values, 80–81, 113
        Starling resistor model, 80
        ventilation during sleep, 113–115
        vulnerable to collapse and its models, 80–81, 112–113
    circadian effects, 89
    negative pressure mechanoreceptors
        awake and asleep, 84–85
        reflex control, 83–85
    neurochemistry of central state-dependent pathways
        active sleep-dependent effects, 88–89
        exposure to CIH, 87–88
        NE and 5HT, 85–86, *86*
        orexins, 85, 86, *87*
        potassium ion (K+) channels, 87
        substance P and TRH, 86, *87*
        wakefulness stimulus for breathing, 85–88
    sleep-wake patterns, *see* Genioglossus muscle

V

Vagal-mediated reflexes, 98
Vagus (X) nerves, 3
Ventilatory control system, 108
    and CBF regulation
        central chemoreceptor tissue PCO$_2$ (PbtCO$_2$), 133, *134*
        cerebral circulation and regulation, 134, *135*
        cerebrovascular reactivity (CVR), 134
        PaCO$_2$ and vCO$_2$, 133

cerebrovascular influences on chemoreceptors
acute CBF reduction, 138–140
cerebrovascular and ventilatory responses, *138*, 138–139, *141*
driving stimuli: [H+], 134–135
hypercapnic vasodilator response, 135
reactivity assessment per se, 140
regional CVR heterogeneity, 139
stimuli sensing and mechanisms of action, 135, 138
vascular CO_2 reactivity, 135–138
cerebrovascular reactivity and central sleep apnea, 140–142
chemoreflex stimulation, 24
CNS hypoxia, 26, 29, 31
control of, 2
DBH+ glomus cells, 24
mechanical, 11
in OHS, 195
Ventilatory instability in sleep, 29
Ventral parafacial (pFV), 12–13
Ventral respiratory column (VRC), 42, 44
caudal VRC, 42
rostral VRC, 42

Bötzinger complex, 42, 44
caudal ventral respiratory group (cVRGroup), 42
pre-Bötzinger complex (PBC), 42, 44
rostral ventral respiratory group (rVRGroup), 42
Vestibulocochlear cranial nerve (CN VIII), 2

W

Wakefulness
loss of, 28–29
in SDB, 28–29, 114–115
sleep-induced suppression of, 28
stimulus for breathing, 85–88
"wakefulness drive," 109
Weight-reducing medications, 221–222
Wisconsin Sleep Cohort, 118

Z

Zaleplon, 227
Zolpidem, 149, 224–225, 227
Zucker rats, 246, 252